Durgin & Hanan's

PHARMACY PRACTICE FOR TECHNICIANS

Fifth Edition

JANE M. DURGIN, CIJ, RPh, EdD
ZACHARY I. HANAN, RPh, MS, FASHP, FASCP

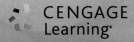

CENGAGE Learning

Australia • Brazil • Japan • Korea • Mexico • Singapore • Spain • United Kingdom • United States

CENGAGE Learning

Durgin & Hanan's Pharmacy Practice for Technicians, Fifth Edition

Jane M. Durgin and Zachary I. Hanan

Vice President, Careers & Computing: Dawn Gerrain

Publisher: Stephan Helba

Acquisitions Editor: Jadin Kavanaugh

Director, Development-Career and Computing: Marah Bellegarde

Product Development Manager: Juliet Steiner

Associate Product Manager: Meghan Orvis

Editorial Assistant: Nicole Manikas

Brand Manager: Wendy Mapstone

Market Development Manager: Erica Glisson

Senior Production Director: Wendy Troeger

Production Manager: Andrew Crouth

Senior Content Project Manager: Kenneth McGrath

Senior Art Director: Jack Pendleton

Media Editor: Deborah Bordeaux

Cover Image: www.Shutterstock.com/OliOpi

Library of Congress Control Number: 2013947956

ISBN-13: 978-1-133-13276-9

Cengage Learning
5 Maxwell Drive
Clifton Park, NY 12065-2919
USA

Cengage Learning is a leading provider of customized learning solutions with office locations around the globe, including Singapore, the United Kingdom, Australia, Mexico, Brazil, and Japan. Locate your local office at: **international.cengage.com/region**

Cengage Learning products are represented in Canada by Nelson Education, Ltd.

To learn more about Delmar, visit **www.cengage.com/delmar**

Purchase any of our products at your local college store or at our preferred online store **www.cengagebrain.com**

Notice to the Reader

Publisher does not warrant or guarantee any of the products described herein or perform any independent analysis in connection with any of the product information contained herein. Publisher does not assume, and expressly disclaims, any obligation to obtain and include information other than that provided to it by the manufacturer. The reader is expressly warned to consider and adopt all safety precautions that might be indicated by the activities described herein and to avoid all potential hazards. By following the instructions contained herein, the reader willingly assumes all risks in connection with such instructions. The publisher makes no representations or warranties of any kind, including but not limited to, the warranties of fitness for particular purpose or merchantability, nor are any such representations implied with respect to the material set forth herein, and the publisher takes no responsibility with respect to such material. The publisher shall not be liable for any special, consequential, or exemplary damages resulting, in whole or part, from the readers' use of, or reliance upon, this material.

Printed in the United States of America
1 2 3 4 5 6 7 17 16 15 14 13

Contents

Preface

In an effort to meet the needs of pharmacy technicians in their various training programs and in their respective careers, this textbook provides the technician with an understanding of the pharmacy profession and its involvement in the many specialty areas of practice in health care. It also provides meaningful basic and educational chapters on the profession of pharmacy and pharmacy technology.

Why We Wrote This Text

More than 40 years ago, we developed an in-house technician training program in our hospital pharmacy for our pharmacy technicians that we subsequently published in textbook form in the early 1970s. We have continued to revise the textbook over the years to include relevant topics for the technician to be able to support optimal pharmacy practice models with pharmacists providing cost-effective use of medications and drug therapy management practices. In the coming years it is projected that technicians will continue to be assigned all distributive functions that do not require clinical judgment, that technicians will be registered and licensed with state boards of pharmacy, and that all technicians will require certification by the Pharmacy Technician Certification Board.

Organization of the Fifth Edition

This textbook is organized into five sections with the respective chapters written by recognized practitioners and academicians with the experience and background to comprehensively cover the topics in each of their respective chapters. The five sections of the textbook are as follows :

Part I: Overview of Health Care
Part II: The Profession of Pharmacy
Part III: Professional Aspects of Pharmacy Technology
Part IV: Clinical Aspects of Pharmacy Technology
Part V: Administrative Aspects of Pharmacy Technology

Features

This fifth edition has been completely revised, with new chapters on topics for the technician relating to career opportunities in mail-order pharmacy and nuclear pharmacy practices, and a chapter on the communication skills that are important for the technician to master.

New to This Edition

Chapter 1

- Added discussion of the contributions of Gerhard Domagk, Karl Scheele, and Hildegard of Bingen to pharmacy
- Added discussion of contributions from various Native American tribes

Chapter 2

- Added discussion of various types and categories of hospitals and services provided by hospitals
- Expanded discussion of the role of the pharmacy technician in hospital settings

Chapter 3

- Updated data and statistics throughout
- Moderate updating to content throughout to incorporate newer ideas, concepts, and technologies applicable to home health care and home infusion therapy

Chapter 4

- Updated data and statistics throughout
- An added section on the role of the technician in an in-house pharmacy in a nursing home that provides an overview of the numerous drug distribution activities of the technician in that environment

Chapter 5

- Updated data and statistics throughout
- Added discussion of central fill operations and telepharmacy

Chapter 6

- New chapter on mail-order pharmacy practice
- Provides an overview of the specialty area of mail-order pharmacy practice with emphasis on the integral role of the pharmacy technician

Chapter 7

- New chapter on nuclear pharmacy practice
- Provides an overview of the specialty area of nuclear pharmacy practice with emphasis on the integral role of the pharmacy technician

Chapter 8

- Extensive expansion of the regulatory standards in this chapter from the perspective of the author, who is a pharmacist with the credentials as an attorney in the pharmaceutical industry

Chapter 9

- New title of *Medication Management: The Foundation of Pharmaceutical Care*

- The American Society of Health-System Pharmacists (ASHP) and the ASHP Research and Education Foundation is supporting the Hospital and Health-System Pharmacy Practice Model Initiative (PPMI). The goal of this initiative is to advance meaningfully the health and well-being of patients by developing and disseminating a futuristic practice model that upholds the most effective use of pharmacists as direct patient care providers. The objectives of the PPMI have been added and are now outlined in this chapter.

Chapter 10

- Now includes examples of competing medical virtues in six ethical dilemmas in pharmacy practice and outlines ethical principles (bioethical decision making) that are helpful in resolving an ethical dilemma

Chapter 11

- New title of *Organizations in Pharmacy*
- Includes an extensive table of selected pharmacy and pharmacy technician organizations and their web site addresses
- Provides descriptions of pharmacy technician organizations along with other national associations in pharmacy representing special segments of the profession

Chapter 12

- Added discussions on e-prescribing and computerized prescriber order entry
- Added ISMP list of error-prone abbreviations, symbols, and dose designations

Chapter 13

- Minor revisions and updating

Chapter 14

- Updating and expansion of some discussions throughout
- Added examples
- Added discussion of orally dissolving tablets

Chapter 15

- Added calculation of days supply and amount to dispense, based on weight and height

Chapter 16

- Updating provided where appropriate related to equipment

Chapter 17

- Updating of terminology and procedures where appropriate

Chapter 19

- Includes discussion of the concept of evidence-based medicine
- Updated resource lists

Chapter 20

- This chapter has been completely revised. It outlines the major activities in the drug distribution process, the roles of the pharmacist, and the current and possible future roles of the pharmacy technician in the drug distribution process and the role of the technician in computerization and automation processes.

Chapter 21

- Added discussion of respiratory hygiene and cough etiquette
- Expanded discussion of the history of herbal products
- Updated statistical information and resources related to the use of herbal products
- Added discussion on the use of international medicines in the United States

Chapter 27

- An extensive review of the drug procurement process for institutional pharmacies, including the roles of group purchasing organizations and prime vendors, the current dilemma with manufacturer's back orders, and review of the technician's roles in supplying medications to areas of the hospital and storing and controlling medications

Chapter 28

- A completely revised chapter outlining the impact of a formulary in pharmacy practice in relation to managed care organizations, technologies that will improve formulary compliance, and the processes for addition of drugs and for regular revision of the formulary

Chapter 29

- Added discussion of the Health Information Technology for Economic and Clinical Health (HITECH) Act

Chapter 30

- A 2006 Institute of Medicine report focused increased attention on medical medication errors. This chapter is written by individuals from the Institute for Safe Medication Practices and presents the most current information on system breakdowns that result in medication errors, commonly used drugs that result in error-related deaths, preventive measures and system enhancements, and the checks and balances needed to provide the maximum degree of safety as pharmacists and technicians prepare, dispense, and control medications in both community and institutional pharmacy settings.

Chapter 31

- New chapter covering communication skills: verbal, written, and cultural considerations
- Provides an overview on the importance of developing communication skills that can be used to provide excellent customer service and interview for jobs successfully

Chapter 32

- A completely revised chapter that provides an overview of prescription drug plans, rising drug costs, and types of prescription drugs plans that cover drugs dispensed in the community pharmacy setting
- Provides a description of the methodologies used for prescription drug payments in the community pharmacy, long-term care facilities, home care pharmacies, and institutional or hospital pharmacies

Chapter 33

- Provides an overview of ASHP accreditation program for pharmacy technicians and their promulgation of the need for standardized training of the pharmacy technician: completion of an ASHP-accredited pharmacy technician training program, successful passing of the Pharmacy Technician Certification Board national exam, and registration

Chapter 34

- Added discussion on the Joint Commission of Pharmacy Practitioners (JCPP) Future Vision of Pharmacy Practice
- Updated content relevant to new Pharmacy Technician Certification Exam guidelines and the 2012 Job Analysis Study
- Added discussion of the C.R.E.S.T. Initiative

Ancillary Package

The complete supplement package for the fifth edition of *Pharmacy Practice for Technicians* was developed to achieve two goals:

1. To assist students in learning and applying the information presented in the book.
2. To assist instructors in planning and implementing their courses in the most efficient manner and providing exceptional resources to enhance their students' experience.

Instructor Companion Website

ISBN 13: 978-1-133-13277-6

Spend less time planning and more time teaching with Cengage Learning's Instructor Resources to Accompany *Pharmacy Practice for Technicians, Fifth Edition.* This content can be accessed through your Instructor SSO account.

To set up your account:

- Go to www.cengagebrain.com/login.
- Choose **Create a New Faculty Account.**
- Select your **Institution.**
- Complete your personal **Account Information.**
- Accept the **License Agreement.**
- Choose **Register.**
- Your account will be pending until validated. You will receive an e-mail notification when the validation process is complete.
- If you are unable to find your institution, complete an **Account Request Form.**

Once your account is set up or if you already have an account:

- Go to www.cengagebrain.com/login.
- Enter your e-mail address and password and select **Sign In.**
- Search for your book by author, title, or ISBN.
- Select the book and click **Continue.**
- You will receive a list of available resources for the title you selected.
- Choose the resources you would like and click **Add to My Bookshelf.**

Components available on the Instructor Companion site include the following:

Instructor's Manual

An electronic *Instructor's Manual* provides instructors with invaluable tools for preparing for class lectures and examinations. Following the text chapter by chapter, the *Instructor's Manual* reiterates three essential components of comprehension: knowledge, attitude, and skills. Additional learning activities and evaluation methods are provided. Answers to the text's end-of-chapter Test Your Knowledge sections are also included. The *Instructor's Manual* provides a synthesized recap of each chapter's main points and goals.

Computerized Test Bank

An electronic test bank makes and generates tests and quizzes in an instant. With a variety of question types, including short answer, multiple choice, and true or false, creating challenging exams will be no barrier in your classroom. This test bank includes a rich bank of questions that tests students on retention and application of what they have learned in the course. Answers are provided for all questions so instructors can focus on teaching, not grading.

Instructor PowerPoint Slides

A comprehensive offering of instructor support slides created in Microsoft® PowerPoint outlines concepts and objectives to assist instructors with lectures.

CourseMate to Accompany *Pharmacy Practice for Technicians, Fifth Edition*

Visit www.cengagebrain.com to access the following resources:

- Printed access code: ISBN 13: 978-1-1331-3-2813
- Instant access code: ISBN: 978-1-1331-3-2820

CourseMate complements your textbook with several robust and noteworthy components:

- An interactive e-book, with highlighting, note-taking, and search capabilities
- Interactive and engaging learning tools including flash cards, quizzes, videos, games, PowerPoint presentations, and much more!
- Engagement Tracker, a first-of-its-kind tool that monitors student participation and retention in the course.

Reviewers

Reviewers of the Fifth Edition

April B. Cortwright, AABA, CPhT, RPhT
Associate Director of Education
Sanford-Brown Institute
Tampa, Florida

Michelle Nunlee, PharmD
Pharmacist, Walgreens
Instructor/Consultant
Adult and Continuing Education
Delaware State University
Dover, Delaware

Kelly Prater, CPhT
Director, Pharmacy Technician Program
Vatterott College
Joplin, Missouri

Diana Rangaves, PharmD, RPh
Director, Pharmacy Technician Program
Santa Rosa Junior College
Santa Rosa, California

Douglas Scibner, BA, CPhT
Director, Pharmacy Technician Program
Central New Mexico Community College
Albuquerque, New Mexico

Idris Bond Smith, MS, BSN
Adjunct Faculty
Ivy Tech Community College
Richmond, Indiana

Karen Snipe, CPhT, MEd
Coordinator, Pharmacy Technician Program
Trident Technical College
Charleston, South Carolina

Lorraine C. Zentz, CPhT, PhD
Instructor
Mesa, Colorado

Reviewers of the Fourth Edition

Glenn D. Appelt, PhD, RPht
Columbia Southern University
Orange Beach, Alabama

Donald Becker
San Jacinto College
Houston, Texas

David P. Elder, RPh
Skagit Valley College
Mt. Vernon, Washington

Michael Ellis
Trinity College
Fairfield, California

Michelle C. McCranie, CPhT, AAS
Ogeechee Technical College
Statesboro, Georgia

Jim Mizner, RPh, MBA
Pharmacy Technician Training Program Coordinator
Applied Career Training
Rosslyn, Virginia

Diana Rangraves, PharmD, RPh
Santa Rosa Junior College
Santa Rosa, California

Traci Tonhofer
Davis Applied Technology College
Kaysville, Utah

Reviewers of Second and Third Editions

Renee Ahrens, PharmD, MBA
Shenandoah University
Winchester, Virginia

Cheri Boggs, BA, CPhT
El Paso Community College
La Mesa, New Mexico

Carolyn Bunker, RPh
Salt Lake City Community College
Salt Lake City, Utah

Sharon Burton-Young, RN
POLY Tech Adult Education
Woodside, Delaware

Jane Doucette, RPh
Salt Lake City Community College
Salt Lake City, Utah

Emery C. Fellows, Jr., CPhT
Pima Medical Institute
Denver, Colorado

Elizabeth Johnson
Houston Community College System
Southeast College
Houston, Texas

Percy M. Johnson
Bidwell Training
Pittsburgh, Pennsylvania

Carol Miller, EdD, CPhT
Miami-Dade Community College
Miami, Florida

Kathy Moscou, BS Pharmacy
North Seattle Community College
Seattle, Washington

Larry Nesmith, BS Ed
Academy of Health Sciences, AMEDD Center & School
Pharmacy Branch, Fort Sam Houston, U.S. Army
San Antonio, Texas

Glen E. Rolfson, RPh
Salt Lake Community College
Salt Lake City, Utah

Peter E. Vondereau, RPh
Cuyahoga Community College
Highland Falls Village, Ohio

Tova R. Wiegand-Green
Ivy Tech State College
Fort Wayne, Indiana

Acknowledgments

We wish to acknowledge and thank our professional colleagues, personal friends, peers, and associates from academia, institutional and community practice, and state and national organizations, who have dedicated their expertise and taken the time to make a personal commitment to participate, and without whom this publication would not have been possible.

Each of our authors has enhanced the content of the fifth edition of our textbook. Their knowledge and experience are evident in their contributions to their respective chapters. Their support of the education and training of pharmacy technicians is very much appreciated.

We would like to thank the team at Cengage Learning and the many other individuals who we worked with for all their contributions to the numerous details required for the publication of the fifth edition.

Lastly, but very importantly, we would like to thank our families, our peers, and our friends for their support and encouragement during the process of the planning, development, composing, and editing of the contents of our fifth edition.

Jane M. Durgin, CIJ, RPh, EdD
Zachary I. Hanan, RPh, MS, FASHP, FASCP

Contributors

Jane Marie Durgin, CIJ, RPh, EdD
Formerly Professor of Pharmacy
St. John's University
College of Pharmacy and Health Sciences
Jamaica, New York
Chapter 1: *A History of Pharmacy*

Douglas E. Miller, PharmD
Senior Director, Hospital & Health System Pharmacy Services
Viscante, Inc.
O'Fallon, Missouri

Principal
Douglas E. Miller, LLC
Pharmacy Consultants
O'Fallon, Missouri
Chapter 2: *Organizational Structure and Function of the Hospital and the Pharmacy Department*

Barbara Limburg Mancini, PharmD, BCNSP
Director of Pharmacy
Walgreens Specialty Infusion Pharmacy
Lombard, Illinois
Chapter 3: *Home Health Care*

Richard J. Lohne, MBA, FACHE, LNHA
Administrator
Nyack Manor
Valley Cottage, New York
Chapter 4: *Long-Term Care*

Jonathan Shataal, RPh, MS
Director of Pharmacy
Parkshore Healthcare LLC
d/b/a Four Seasons Nursing and Rehabilitation
Brooklyn, New York
Chapter 4: *Long-Term Care*

Maria Marzella Mantione, PharmD, CGP
Associate Clinical Professor
Department of Clinical Pharmacy Practice
College of Pharmacy and Health Sciences
St. John's University
Jamaica, New York
Member, NYS Board of Pharmacy
Chapter 5: *Community Pharmacy Practice*

Carmela Avena-Woods, PharmD, CGP
Assistant Clinical Professor
Department of Clinical Pharmacy Practice
College of Pharmacy and Health Sciences
St. John's University
Jamaica, New York
Chapter 5: *Community Pharmacy Practice*

Sam Medure, RPh
Senior Manager, Mail and Specialty Pharmacy
WellCare Health Plans, Inc.
Tampa, Florida
Chapter 6: *Mail-Order Pharmacy Practice*

Dan Palmquist, RPh, AU
Zone Operations Director
Cardinal Health Nuclear Products
Nuclear Pharmacy Services
Chester, New Hampshire
Chapter 7: *Nuclear Pharmacy Practice*

Richard P. Medeiros, PharmD
Pharmacy Manager/Radiation Safety Officer
Cardinal Health Nuclear Products
Hermon, Maine
Chapter 7: *Nuclear Pharmacy Practice*

James Ruger, RPh, PhD, Esq.
Chief FDA/Regulatory Counsel
Quest Diagnostics Legal Department
Madison, New Jersey
Chapter 8: *Regulatory Standards in Pharmacy Practice*

Norberto Alberto, RPh, MS, HScD
Director of Pharmacy Services
New York Presbyterian–Lower Manhattan
New York, New York

Adjunct Professor
Arnold and Marie Schwartz College of Pharmacy and Allied Health Sciences
Brooklyn, New York
Chapter 9: *Medication Management: The Foundation of Pharmaceutical Care*

Shu Jing, RPh, PharmD
Clinical Pharmacist
New York Downtown Hospital
New York, New York
Chapter 9: *Medication Management: The Foundation of Pharmaceutical Care*

William N. Kelly, PharmD, FISPE
Professor of Pharmacotherapeutics and Clinical Research
College of Pharmacy
University of South Florida
Tampa, Florida
Chapter 9: *Medication Management: The Foundation of Pharmaceutical Care*

Martha L. Mackey, JD
Assistant Professor of Pharmacy Administration
St. John's University College of Pharmacy and Health Sciences
Jamaica, New York
Chapter 10: *Ethical Considerations for the Pharmacy Technician*

William N. Kelly, PharmD, FISPE
Professor of Pharmacotherapeutics and Clinical Research
College of Pharmacy
University of South Florida
Tampa, Florida
Chapter 10: *Ethical Considerations for the Pharmacy Technician*

Debra Feinberg, RPh, JD
Executive Director
New York State Council of Hospital Pharmacists
Albany, New York
Chapter 11: *Organizations in Pharmacy*

Robert A. Hamilton, PharmD, MPH
Associate Dean for the Vermont Campus
Albany College of Pharmacy and Health Sciences
Colchester, Vermont
Chapter 12: *The Prescription*

M. Elyse Wheeler, PhD, MT (ASCP)
Chair, Department of Health Sciences
Albany College of Pharmacy and Health Sciences
Albany, New York
Chapter 13: *Medical Terminology and Abbreviations*

Danielle R. Janiak
Former Pharm D Candidate
Albany College of Pharmacy and Health Sciences
Albany, New York
Chapter 13: *Medical Terminology and Abbreviations*

P. L. Madan, PhD
Professor of Pharmaceutics and Industrial Pharmacy
St. John's University
College of Pharmacy and Health Sciences
Jamaica, New York
Chapter 14: *Pharmaceutical Dosage Forms*

Melinda Reed, RPh, MBA
Formerly Instructor, Department of Pharmaceutical Sciences
Albany College of Pharmacy and Health Sciences
Albany, New York
Chapter 15: *Pharmaceutical Calculations*

Lee Anna Obos, RPh
Instructor, Department of Pharmaceutical Sciences
Albany College of Pharmacy and Health Sciences
Albany, New York
Chapter 15: *Pharmaceutical Calculations*

Steve Laddy, RPh, MS, CEO
MasterPharm Compounding Pharmacy
Richmond Hill, New York
Chapter 16: *Extemporaneous Compounding*

Thomas Mastanduono, RPh
Vice President
MasterPharm Compounding Pharmacy
Richmond Hill, New York
Chapter 16: *Extemporaneous Compounding*

Lin Leung, PharmD
Supervising Pharmacist
MasterPharm Compounding Pharmacy
Richmond Hill, New York
Chapter 16: *Extemporaneous Compounding*

Laura Thoma, PharmD
Associate Professor
Pharmaceutics/Pharmacy
Director, Parenteral Medication Laboratory
University of Tennessee
Memphis, Tennessee
Chapter 17: *Sterile Preparation Compounding*

Karen T. Wong, RPh, MBA
Formerly Manager of Major Pharma Companies, Supervising Pharmacist and Clinical Pharmacist in Institutional Pharmacy Practice and Compliance Officer in Compounding Pharmacy Practice
Flushing, New York
Chapter 17: *Sterile Preparation Compounding*

Sabra Boughton, RN, ANP-C, PhD
Director of Patient Education
Co-Chair Nursing Diversity
Stony Brook University Medical Center
Smoking Cessation Counselor
Stony Brook, New York
Chapter 18: *Administration of Medications*

Laura Gianni Augusto, PharmD
Associate Clinical Professor
Department of Clinical Pharmacy Practice
College of Pharmacy and Health Sciences
St. John's University
Jamaica, New York
Chapter 19: *Drug Information*

Gary C. Collins, RPh, MS
Formerly Managing Director, Consulting Services
Pharmacy Healthcare Solutions, Ltd.
An Amerisource Bergen Company
Dallas, Texas
Chapter 20: *Drug Distribution Systems*

Catherine Shannon, FNP-C, CIC
Director, Infection Prevention and Control & Employee Health Services
St. Catherine of Siena Medical Center
Smithtown, New York
Chapter 21: *Infection Control and Prevention in the Pharmacy*

Robert S. Kidd, MS, PharmD, PhD
Professor and Chair
Department of Biopharmaceutical Sciences
Bernard J. Dunn School of Pharmacy
Shenandoah University
Winchester, Virginia
Chapter 22: *Introduction to Biopharmaceutics*

Regina F. Peacock, PhD
Associate Professor
Department of Biopharmaceutical Sciences
Bernard J. Dunn School of Pharmacy
Shenandoah University
Winchester, Virginia
Chapter 22: *Introduction to Biopharmaceutics*

Robert S. Kidd, MS, PharmD, PhD
Professor and Chair
Department of Biopharmaceutical Sciences
Bernard J. Dunn School of Pharmacy
Shenandoah University
Winchester, Virginia
Chapter 23: *The Actions and Uses of Drugs*

L. Michael Marcum, PharmD
Co-Manager
Kroger Pharmacy
Morehead, Kentucky
Chapter 23: *The Actions and Uses of Drugs*

Nicole M. Maisch, PharmD
Associate Clinical Professor
Department of Clinical Pharmacy Practice
College of Pharmacy and Health Sciences
St. John's University
Jamaica, New York

Director, Drug Information Service
Long Island Jewish Medical Center
New Hyde Park, New York
Chapter 24: *Nonprescription Medications*

Dudley G. Moon, PhD
Professor of Biological Sciences
Director, Health and Human Sciences Program
Albany College of Pharmacy and Health Sciences
Albany, New York
Chapter 25: *Natural Products*

Elaine Liu, PhD Candidate
Department of Pathology and Laboratory Medicine
University of Pennsylvania
Philadelphia, Pennsylvania
Chapter 25: *Natural Products*

Zachary I. Hanan, RPh, MS, FASHP
President
ZIH Pharmacy Associates, Inc.
Oakdale, New York
Formerly Director of Pharmaceutical Services
Mercy Medical Center
Rockville Centre, New York
Chapter 26: *The Policy and Procedure Manual*

Gary C. Collins, RPh, MS
Formerly Managing Director, Consulting Services
Pharmacy Healthcare Solutions, Ltd.
An Amerisource Bergen Company
Dallas, Texas
Chapter 27: *Pharmaceutical Supply Chain*

Mark N. Brueckl, RPh, MBA
Assistant Director, Pharmacy Affairs
Academy of Managed Care Pharmacy
Alexandria, Virginia
Chapter 28: *The Pharmacy Formulary System*

Edmund Hayes, RPh, MS, PharmD
Assistant Director of Pharmacy
Stony Brook University Hospital
State University of New York at Stony Brook
Stony Brook, New York

Affiliate Assistant Clinical Professor
College of Pharmacy and Health Sciences
St. John's University
Jamaica, New York
Chapter 29: *Computer Applications in Drug Use Control*

Matthew Grissinger, RPh, FISMP, FASCP
Director, Error Reporting Programs
Institute for Safe Medication Practices
Horsham, Pennsylvania
Chapter 30: *Preventing and Managing Medication Errors: The Technician's Role*

Susan Proulx, PharmD
President
Med-ERRS, A Subsidiary of ISMP
Horsham, Pennsylvania
Chapter 30: *Preventing and Managing Medication Errors: The Technician's Role*

Michael DeCoske, PharmD, BCPS
Associate Chief Pharmacy Officer, Ambulatory Services
Duke University Hospital
Durham, North Carolina
Chapter 31: *Communication Skills*

Angela C. Dominelli, BS, MBA, PhD
Dean, School of Pharmacy and Pharmaceutical Sciences
Associate Vice President for Institutional Effectiveness
Associate Professor of Pharmacy Administration
Albany College of Pharmacy and Health Sciences
Albany, New York 12208
Chapter 32: *Reimbursement for Pharmacy Services*

Lisa S. Lifshin, RPh
Manager, Program Services
Coordinator, Technician Training Programs
Accreditation Services Division
American Society of Health-System Pharmacists
Bethesda, Maryland
Chapter 33: *Accreditation of Technician Training Programs*

Melissa Murer Corrigan, RPh
Formerly Chief Executive Officer
Pharmacy Technician Certification Board
Washington, D.C.
Chapter 34: *Pharmacy Technician Certification*

Megan E. Coder, PharmD
Formerly Director of Professional Affairs
Pharmacy Technician Certification Board
Washington, D.C.
Chapter 34: *Pharmacy Technician Certification*

Introduction

Pharmacy Technicians: Essential Members of the Health Care Team in Securing the Public Health for Patients

So much has happened in the advancement and advocacy for the role of the pharmacy technician since the publication of the fourth edition of *Pharmacy Practice for Technicians*. We have now gone beyond one decade into the twenty-first century. All of the major pharmacy organizations are advocating elevation of the role of the pharmacy technician. For example, one of the major priorities on the advocacy agenda of the American Society of Health-System Pharmacists (ASHP) is for all pharmacy technicians to have completed standardized ASHP-accredited education and training; obtain and maintain Pharmacy Technician Certification Board (PTCB) national certification, and registration. A specific task force known as the Pharmacy Technician Initiative (PTI) has been relegated within ASHP to partner with individual state affiliates to work with their specific boards of pharmacy to make the aforementioned agenda happen. As of 2013, 26 states have signed up and have committed to work on this endeavor. Although this will not happen overnight, more states have started to require completion of an ASHP-accredited program prior to registration and passing of the PTCB since the last publication of this very useful educational tool.

More than 200 pharmacy technician training programs are now ASHP accredited, including some of the major chains' programs. The larger pharmacy chains are now recognizing the value of diverse, standardized training for their employees and the greater span of functions that they can now provide. ASHP-accredited programs are located in 40 states across the country. Let's make it 50 by the time the next edition of *Pharmacy Practice for Technicians* is published. The roles of the pharmacist and pharmacy technician are rapidly changing.

The Pharmacy Practice Model Initiative (PPMI), an endeavor supported by ASHP and the ASHP Research and Education Foundation, was created in 2008. Key thought leaders in pharmacy practice convened for a summit in November 2010 and were engaged to think outside of the box to develop ways in which pharmacists could be more involved in making a bigger impact in the improvement of patient care. A main part of the initiative supports pharmacy technicians as integral members of the health care team and—with education and training—they can fulfill more unique roles than ever before. Pharmacy technicians are key in managing the new innovations in pharmacy technology and informatics that are designed to enhance the safety of the medication distribution process.

The fifth edition of *Pharmacy Practice for Technicians* is an important reference in advancing the education of the pharmacy technician, who need to be ready and able to meet the future medication safety needs of patients. Hand in hand, the time is now for the pharmacy technician to assume a more active role as an essential member of the health care team in supporting the pharmacist in securing the public health of patients. The iron is hot for pharmacy technicians to complete ASHP-accredited pharmacy technician training programs, become PTCB certified, and registered or licensed in their state of employment. All of these criteria will enforce the credibility of the pharmacy technician on this very important team.

Lisa S. Lifshin, RPh
American Society of Health-System Pharmacists
Bethesda, Maryland

PART

I

Overview of Health Care

Chapter 1: A History of Pharmacy

Chapter 2: Organizational Structure and Function of the Hospital and Pharmacy Department

Chapter 3: Home Health Care

Chapter 4: Long-Term Care

Chapter 5: Community Pharmacy Practice

Chapter 6: Mail-Order Pharmacy Practice

Chapter 7: Nuclear Pharmacy Practice

CHAPTER

1

A History of Pharmacy

Competencies

Upon completion of this chapter, the reader should be able to:

1. Describe the Greek and/or Roman influence on present-day health care.
2. Cite the names of pharmacists and/or researchers in the following countries who have contributed to the therapeutic progress of pharmacy in their respective countries: England, France, Germany, Sweden, Canada, and the United States.
3. Describe how research and development of insulin, digoxin, penicillin, and the polio vaccine contributed to the health and well-being of Americans.
4. Trace the development of drugs in the United States from colonial days to the present.
5. Describe how the history of pharmacy has contributed to increasing knowledge and enhancing an appreciation of the profession of pharmacy.

Key Terms

Abbess Hildegard
alkaloid
allopathy
almshouse
antianginal
antiarrhythmic
antidote
antihypertensive
asylum
beta blocker
bile
biologicals
carminative
deinstitutionalization
dispensatory
galenical
herb
Hippocrates
homeopathy
homeostasis
hospice
immunity
immunomodulator
Maimonides
malaria
monastery
Native American
pandemic
pharmacognosy
pharmacotherapy
phlegm
psychiatric
sanatorium
Theophrastus
vasodilator

Introduction

Welcome to the world of pharmacy, an honorable profession that has been in existence for more than 5,000 years. This chapter discusses the many drugs used in the old worlds of Mesopotamia (present Persian Gulf area), China, India, Arabia, and Egypt because many of the drugs mentioned have influenced Eastern medicine for thousands of years. Native Americans have used herbal remedies for thousands of years although their first written records began only with their contact with Europeans. A few selections from particular tribes and the remedies they used are cited as examples later in this chapter.

The Western influence on pharmacy, also known as *materia medica*, was cradled in Greece and Rome, as well as many European countries including Germany, Italy, Switzerland, and Belgium. Many of the drugs brought over from Europe were used by the early colonists in North America.

The history of the field of pharmacology can be pictured as a spiral—it continually evolves and adapts while maintaining and tapping into the roots of previous drug knowledge. Although traditional medical research today emphasizes bioengineered drugs and immunomodulators (drugs that activate the immune system for patients with AIDS or depress the immune system for human organ recipients), the field of natural remedies has also grown and developed into a billion-dollar business. Almost every pharmacy, whether independent or part of a chain, now contains shelves of herbal, mineral, and nutritional supplements. Still lacking, however, is a system of checks and balances for purity, potency, dosage, and contraindications for these natural remedies. Currently, Germany leads in setting standards for natural remedies. In the world of global communications and international scientific exchange, much of the work done in Germany may soon be shared throughout the world of pharmacy.

Greek Influence

Hippocrates a Greek physician; considered the "father of medicine"

Some of the earliest examples of healing centers can be found in Greece. A temple dedicated to Asclepius, the mythical god of medicine, on the island of Cos is one such example. It was here that gods were implored, physicians practiced medicine, and apprentices learned the art of healing. Around 400 B.C. **Hippocrates**, considered to be the "father of medicine," practiced medicine and pharmacy in ancient Greece in such temples (**Figure 1-1**). Patients who came to these temples were diagnosed, treated, and cared for until they were able to return home. Treatments included herbal remedies, mineral baths, exercise, fresh sea air, and sunshine. Archaeologists have found admission records and other medical records inscribed in the columns of these temples.

Hippocrates (ca. 460–377 B.C.)

homeostasis a tendency toward stability in the internal body environment; a state of equilibrium

For thousands of years, the writings of Hippocrates occupied a place in medicine corresponding to that of the Bible in the literature and ethics of Western people. Through the use of rational concepts based on objective knowledge, he liberated medicine from the mystic and the demonic.

The concept of **homeostasis**—the attainment and retainment of equilibrium in the body through the appropriate use of drugs and diet—was the traditional

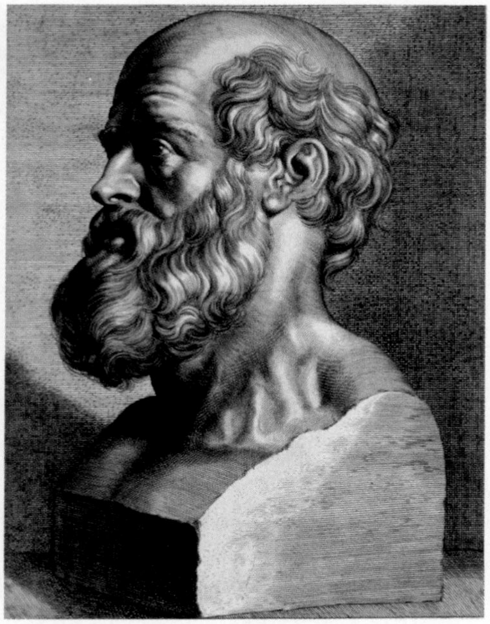
Courtesy of the National Library of Medicine.

FIGURE 1-1 Hippocrates, the father of medicine.

phlegm a viscous mucus secreted orally

bile a fluid secreted by the liver

allopathy a method of treating a disease by administering an agent that has the opposite characteristics of the disease (e.g., antipyretics to reduce fever)

homeopathy a method of treating or preventing disease by administering very dilute substances that cause the same effect as the symptom (e.g., giving a minute quantity of a fever-producing substance to reinforce the body's defense system)

benchmark of his numerous practices and writings. Hippocrates theorized that disease resulted from a disturbance of a body fluid (e.g., blood), **phlegm** (viscous mucus secreted orally), and yellow and black **bile** (fluid secreted by the liver), and was thus treated by restoring equilibrium. He believed that health was preserved by caring for the internal environment (e.g., diet, sleep, exercise) and properly reacting to the external environment (e.g., rain, excess sun, climate changes) to enhance the physical harmony of the body.

More than 200 herbal remedies and a dozen minerals are recommended in the Hippocratic writings. The juice of the poppy, which today we recognize as opium, was among the 200 drugs mentioned. These drugs were available as pills, troches, gargles, eyewashes, ointments, and inhalants. In these writings, the word for *drug*—pharmakon—was defined as a purifying remedy; later it was described as a healing remedy. Many of these drug forms are still used today and will be covered in Chapter 25.

Allopathy, a concept employed by the Greeks and in common medical practice in the Western world, treats symptoms and diseases with drugs that restore health by causing the opposite effect. For example, the common cold, seen as cold and damp, was treated with mustard, which is hot and dry. Modern-day examples of drugs used in this manner are antacids, antibiotics, and antidiarrheals. This is in contrast to an infrequently used therapy known as **homeopathy**, which treats health problems with very dilute substances that cause the same effect as the symptom (e.g., a person with a fever is treated with minute doses of a fever-producing agent to reinforce the body's defense system).

Theophrastus a Greek philosopher and botanist who classified plants by pharmaceutical actions

pharmacognosy the study of therapeutic agents derived from natural sources (e.g., plants)

Theophrastus (ca. 370–287 B.C.)

Theophrastus was a Greek philosopher and botanist who lived circa 300 B.C. Botany, the study of plants, is closely related to **pharmacognosy**, the science that deals with the medicinal ingredients in living plants. Theophrastus classified

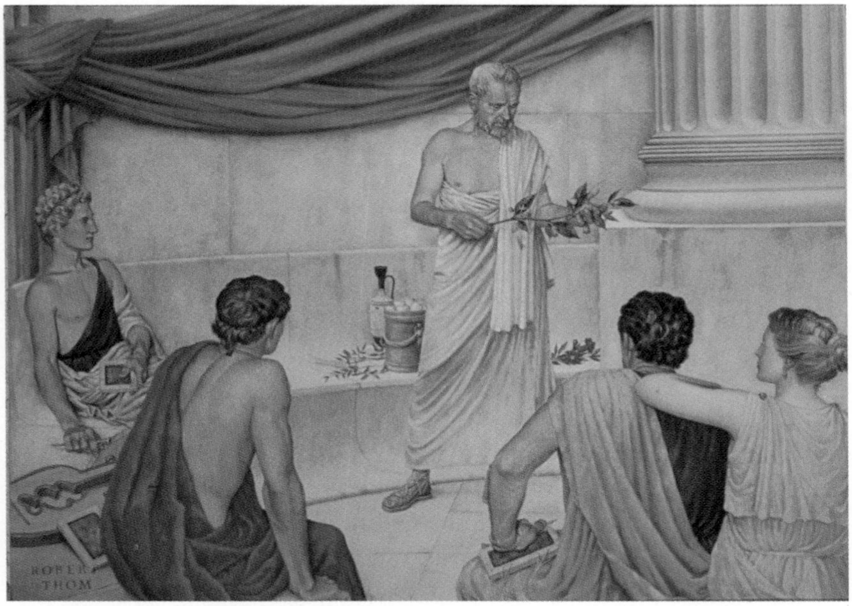

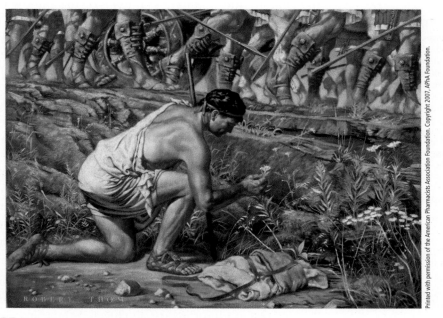

FIGURE 1-2 Theophrastus, the father of botany.

plants by their leaves, roots, seeds, and stems (**Figure 1-2**). His accurate pharmaceutical and pharmacologic observations related to the classification and action of medicinal plants won him the title of "father of botany."

Pedanius Dioscorides (A.D. 100)

The noted botanist and pharmacist Dioscorides was the major authority on drugs for 16 centuries (**Figure 1-3**). He added to the work of Hippocrates the

FIGURE 1-3 Dioscorides, noted botanist and pharmacist.

knowledge he gained while accompanying the Roman armies on their conquests. A major focus of his studies and writings was the use and biological effects of early remedies. For this reason, perhaps he should be called the "father of pharmacology."

Dioscorides' Herbal

The information in Dioscorides' herbal, known in Latin as *De Materia Medica*, contained information on more than 600 plants and 90 minerals. Knowledge was collected by Dioscorides from his extensive travels in Africa, Gaul, Persia, Armenia, and Egypt. The remedies of these countries were incorporated into the herbal, which gave plant/mineral descriptions, instructions for growing and preservation, dosage, medicinal uses, and side effects. Considered the most important pharmaceutical guide of antiquity, 35 translations and commentaries had been issued by the year 1540.

Roman Influence

In early Rome (A.D. 200–500), hospitals were often endowed by wealthy citizens who frequently cared for the sick as volunteers. Fabiola, a wealthy Roman woman, donated her palace for the care of the sick and injured and personally cared for their needs. With the fall of the Roman Empire, major changes occurred. The care of the sick became a civil responsibility, and prostitutes and prisoners were assigned health care tasks.

Claudius Galen (A.D. 130–200)

Until 1950, pharmacy students took a course entitled "Galenical Pharmacy." Galen, a Greek-born physician, practiced and taught both pharmacy and medicine in Rome (**Figure 1-4**). His principles, derived from Hippocrates' theory for the

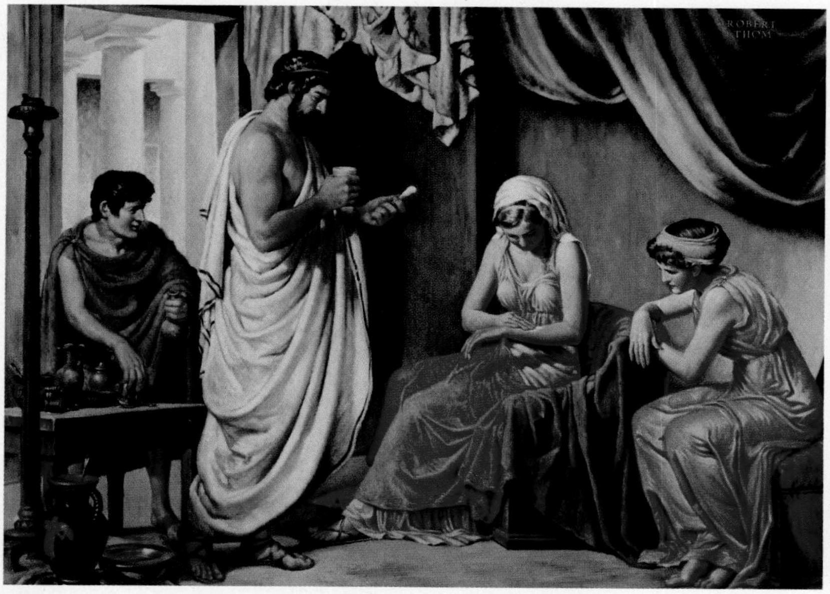

FIGURE 1-4 Galen, a physician, created a scientific system of treating disease with medicine.

pharmacotherapy the treatment of disease with medications

galenical a standard preparation containing one or several organic ingredients (e.g., elixirs, tinctures)

biologicals medicinal preparations made from living organisms or their products; include serums, vaccines, antigens, and antitoxins

preparation and compounding of medicines, were followed in the Western world for 1,500 years. Galen organized the **pharmacotherapy** (treatment of disease with medications) of humoral pathology into a scientific system.

Galen compiled and added to drug information available in Rome in the most famous of his writings, *On the Art of Healing*. This work describes the properties and mixtures of simple remedies and compounded drugs. The treatments describe such **galenicals** (a standard preparation containing one or more natural organic substances) as elixirs, tinctures, fluid extracts, syrups, and ointments (see Chapter 14). Galenicals have recently lost popularity due to the present use of synthetic chemicals, antibiotics, and **biologicals**.

Jewish Influence

Maimonides Rabbi Moses ben Maimon, a Spanish-born Hebrew physician, pharmacist, and rabbi (1135–1204); physician to Sultan Saladin; author of a health book, *Book of Counsels*, and a handbook on poisons

The Jewish influence on health care is demonstrated in biblical records of the Old Testament, as well as by the teachings and works of the famous rabbi and physician Moses **Maimonides** (**Figure 1-5**). The Prayer of Maimonides for many years served as the pledge of service made by pharmacists as they completed school and began professional practice.

Biblical Records (1200 B.C.)

The Old Testament Book of Sirach (38:4–8) states:

> *The Lord created medicines from the earth and a sensible man will not despise them. Was not water made sweet with a tree in order that His power might be known? And he gave skill to men that He might be glorified in His marvelous works. By them He heals and takes away pain; the pharmacist makes of them a compound. His works will never be finished; and from Him health is upon the face of the earth.*

carminative a medicine that relieves stomach/intestinal gas

Genesis, the first book of the Bible, mentions myrrh, a remedy used throughout history as an appetite stimulant, **carminative** (a medicine that relieves intestinal gas), and skin protectant with healing properties. Olibanum (frankincense)

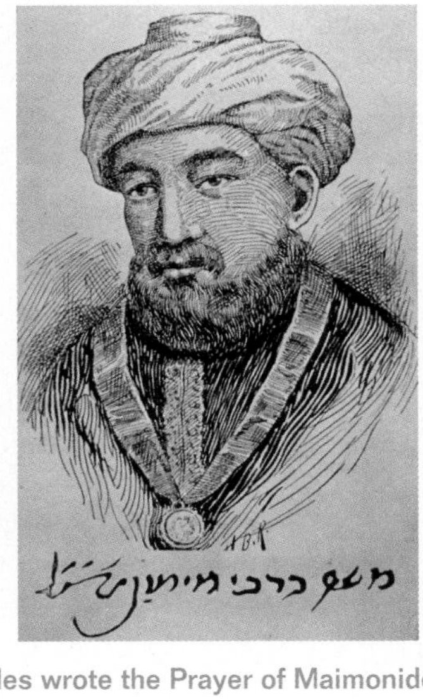

Courtesy of the National Library of Medicine.

FIGURE 1-5 Moses Maimonides wrote the Prayer of Maimonides, a pledge of service for pharmacists.

is a gum resin mentioned in the books of Exodus, Ezra, Jeremiah, Ezekiel, and the Song of Solomon. The Old Testament of the Bible includes the pharmacist's role, professional norms, and many drug examples.

Ancient Hebrews (1200 B.C.)

Several drugs mentioned in the Old Testament are still in use today. Garlic (Numbers 11:5), with a history of thousands of years, is currently being investigated as a means to reduce blood pressure, lower cholesterol, and possibly inhibit the growth of cancer cells. Aloe, mentioned in the New Testament (John 19:39) but available much earlier, is an official ingredient in the compound benzoin tincture. Acacia (Exodus 26:15), used earlier for building purposes, is now commonly used as an emulsifying agent. Other items still in use include coriander, myrrh, almond, and anise. Presently, they are mainly used as foods or flavors.

Moses ben Maimon (Maimonides) (A.D. 1135–1204)

For many decades, pharmacy students were presented with a scroll at graduation containing the Prayer of Maimonides, a Spanish rabbi and scientist. Included are the phrases "May I be filled with love for my art. Preserve my strength that I may be able to preserve the strength of (others). May there never rise in me the notion that I know enough." Although Maimonides is best known for this document, he also published a glossary of drug terms and a manual of poisons.

Christian Influence

The spread of Christianity brought the teachings of Jesus to the care of the sick and infirm. At the Council of Nicaea in the fourth century A.D., bishops were required to provide a shelter for the care of the sick in each diocese. The Basilius, built by St. Basil the Great in the fourth century, has influenced hospital design to this day. Bishop Landry founded the Hotel Dieu in Paris in A.D. 660. This hospital still cares for the sick from its location on the Seine River in Paris.

Cosmas and Damian (d. A.D. 303)

While the early Greeks had their mythical gods and goddesses of healing (e.g., Asclepius, Hygeia, and Panacea), the early Christians venerated those saints who significantly contributed to healings. Cosmas was a physician; Damian, his twin brother, practiced pharmacy (**Figure 1-6**). They were among many who were martyred for their Christian beliefs during Diocletian's persecutions (A.D. 303–313). Over the years, they have been honored as the patron saints of medicine and pharmacy.

monastery a dwelling place for individuals under religious vows who live in ascetic simplicity

The early Christian **monasteries** (dwellings for persons under religious vows) included an infirmary in their structural design. These infirmaries served the sick monks and people in the neighborhood who required special care. During periodic plagues, the monks cared for those who had deadly and frightening diseases. Monasteries also contributed to health service by growing, preserving, and preparing herbal medicines and retaining and printing drug information available at the time. These early manuscripts were the medical textbooks of the day.

Monastic Manuscripts (A.D. 500–1200)

The impact of the political, intellectual, religious, social, and cultural upheavals of the Middle Ages gave rise to medieval monasteries as centers of learning

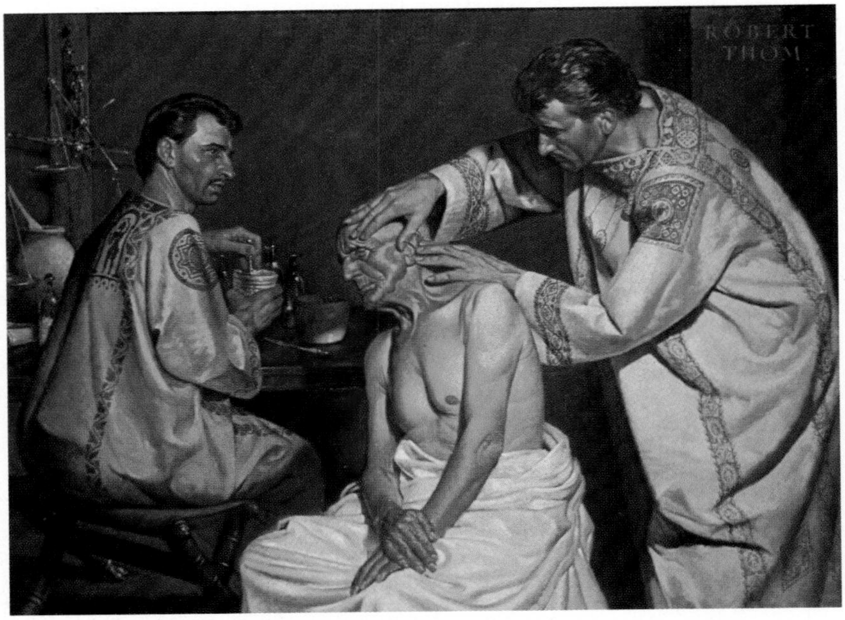

FIGURE 1-6 Damian and Cosmas, the patron saints of medicine and pharmacy, respectively.

Abbess Hildegard writer of *Causae et Curae*.

and science, including medical/pharmaceutical knowledge. Manuscripts from throughout the world were translated or copied in the famous monastic *scriptoria* (libraries). Among the most famous treaties are *De Viribus Herbarum* ("Herbs Used by People"), composed in a French abbey by Abbott Odo, and *Causae et Curae*, written by the **Abbess Hildegard** in a monastery in Bingen, Germany. Both manuscripts were completed during the eleventh to twelfth centuries. In addition to compiling existing knowledge, the monks added to that knowledge by studying the effects of the numerous plants grown in the monastery gardens (**Figure 1-7**).

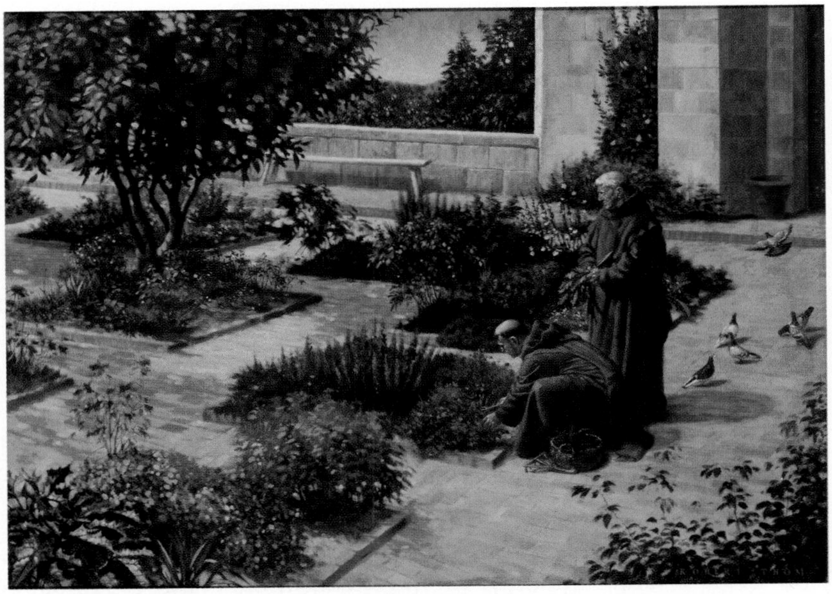

FIGURE 1-7 Herbal remedies and medicines were grown in the gardens at monasteries.

Christian Renaissance Period (A.D. 1300–1550)

At the beginning of the Renaissance, several encouraging events occurred. In 1586, St. Camillus de Lellis founded a religious order, Clerics Regular Servants of the Sick, at the Hospital of St. James in Rome. Through his efforts, the deplorable, filthy conditions in hospitals and miserable treatment by civil servants were scrutinized. St. Camillus took his new community of men and centered their activities in the Hospital of the Holy Spirit, which had been founded in A.D. 717 and was one of the largest hospitals in Europe. The brothers provided personal care for the patients, with special attention to diet. Hospital of the Holy Spirit soon became a major site for the education of lay physicians, with nearly 100 physicians in attendance. The hospital still contains an impressive library of medical literature. Thus, hospitals were beginning to emerge from the Dark Ages. After St. Camillus founded his religious order, Pope Sixtus V authorized the red cross as a special insignia designating the special service provided by the order in the care of patients, many with diseases. To this day, a fourth vow of service, which originated at the time of pestilence, is made by members of this order who wear the red cross on the breast of their habit. The red cross was soon seen on battlefields and ultimately became the insignia of the famous relief organization, the International Red Cross (recently renamed the International Red Cross and Red Crescent Movement).

Eastern Influence

The earliest recordings for the use of healing remedies go back in time to 3000 B.C. These early findings include inscriptions on clay tablets found in Mesopotamia and the *Pen T'sao*, found in China written on bamboo slats, which covered more than 10,000 remedies. Eastern pharmacy and medicine have influenced the health sciences and care and treatment of disease for more than 5,000 years.

Clay Tablets of Mesopotamia (3000–2500 B.C.)

Among thousands of clay tablets unearthed in the present Iraq and Persian Gulf region, more than 800 tablets contained *materia medica* information. These first pharmaceutical texts contained more than 500 remedies from plant, mineral, and other sources. The Code of Hammurabi was also discovered; it contains a section on ethical standards for health practitioners.

Pen T'sao (3000 B.C.)

The Chinese document *Pen T'sao*, freely translated as "the botanical basis of pharmacy," describes more than 1,000 plants and 11,000 prescriptions handed down by oral tradition from Shen-Nung, considered the father of Chinese pharmaceutics. The early Chinese texts were inscribed on bamboo slats. They indicated the name of the drug, the dosage, and the symptoms it was used to treat. About 500 B.C., Lao-tsu, a Taoist philosopher, composed an herbal compendium called *Tao te Ching* ("The Way").

China (500 B.C.)

Drugs used in early China included ephedra, cassia, rhubarb, camphor, and ginseng. "Yin" drugs were cold and wet, and "yang" drugs were warm and dry. "Red" drugs treated heart conditions, and "yellow" drugs were used to treat liver problems.

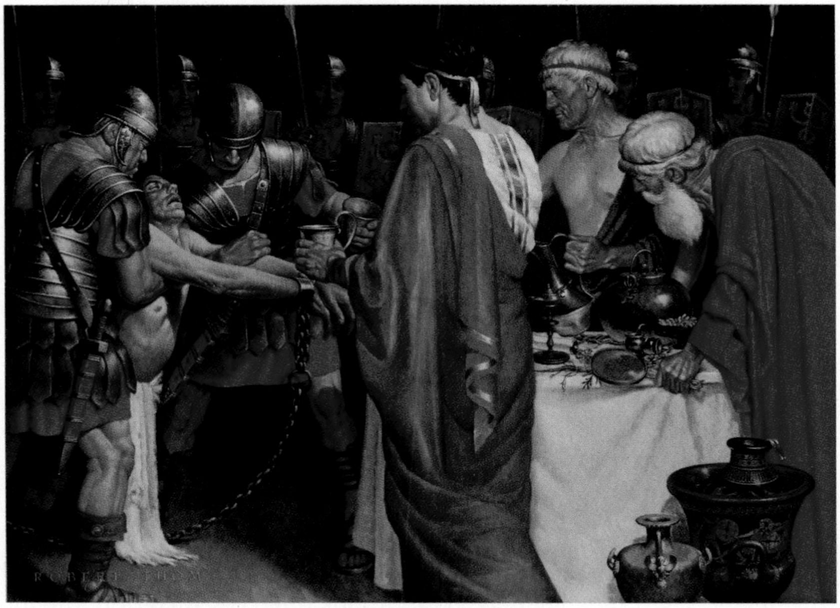
Printed with permission of the American Pharmacists Association Foundation. Copyright 2007, APhA Foundation.

FIGURE 1-8 Mithradates studied prevention of poisoning and possible antidotes.

Mithradates VI (d. 63 B.C.)

Early in history, the adverse or poisonous effects of drugs were a matter of concern. Mithradates might be called the "father of toxicology" for his investigation and writings related to the prevention and counteraction of the poisonous effects of drugs through the use of appropriate **antidotes** (a remedy for counteracting a poison) (**Figure 1-8**).

antidote a remedy for counteracting a poison

Arabia and Persia (A.D. 700–800)

psychiatric relating to the medical treatment of mental disorders

In Arab countries, attitudes were humane and compassionate. Asylums for **psychiatric** patients (those with mental illnesses) were built that provided gardens, fountains, pleasant music, and a healthy setting where drugs, baths, and good nutrition were given to the patients.

New dosage forms were introduced as syrups and jams that contained active ingredients such as aloe, senna, nutmeg, clover, camphor, and musk. The *Minhaj* ("Handbook for the Apothecary Shop") stated that a pharmacist "ought to have deep religious convictions, consideration for others, especially the poor and needy, a sense of responsibility and be careful and God-fearing."

Avicenna (Ibn Sina) (A.D. 980–1037)

Avicenna, also known as Ibn Sina, is called the "Persian Galen" (**Figure 1-9**). His Arabic writings unified pharmaceutical and medical knowledge known at the time. His teachings were accepted in the West until the seventeenth century and to this day remain influential in the East.

India (1000 B.C.)

Charaka, sometimes spelled **Caraka**, born c. 300 B.C. was one of the principal contributors to the ancient art and science of Ayurveda, a system of medicine and lifestyle developed in Ancient India. He is referred to as the Father of Medicine.

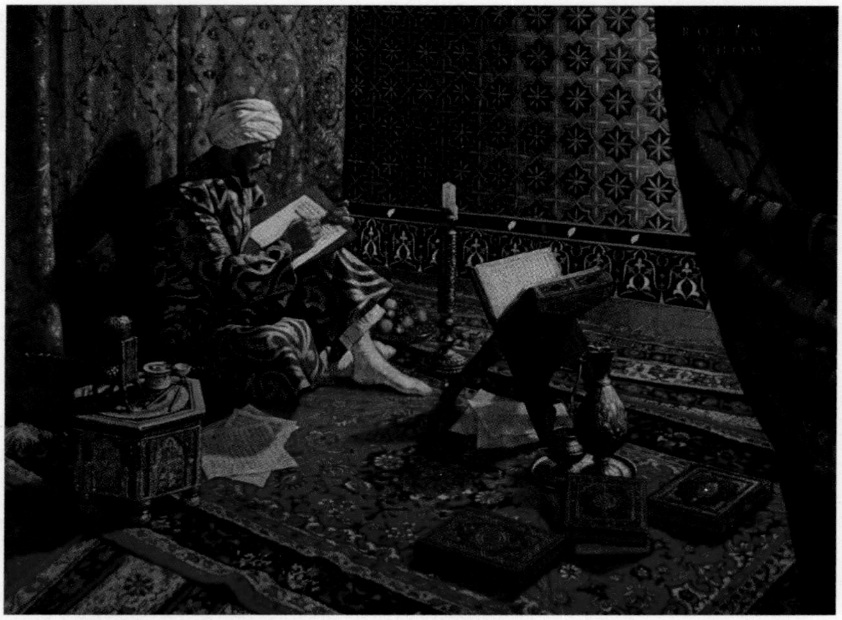

FIGURE 1-9 Avicenna, the "Persian Galen."

More than 2,000 drugs are mentioned in Charaka's writings, including cinnamon, cardamom, ginger, pepper, aconite, and licorice. These condiments and spices are in use today. Mercury was used in numerous preparations and is used today as an external antiseptic in Mercurochrome and Merthiolate.

Egyptian Influence

Ebers Papyrus (1500 B.C.)

The parchment (papyrus) scroll found in Egypt by George Ebers (1837–1898) is one of 11 medical scrolls that preserve the knowledge of early Egyptian medicine. More than 700 drugs are mentioned, with formulas for more than 800 remedies. According to these scrolls, the pharmacist selected the drugs, prepared them in a magically correct way, and then said a prescribed benediction over them. The use of mortars and pestles, hand mills, sieves, and weighing scales is mentioned in the papyrus.

The Great Al-Mansur Hospital (A.D. 1285)

The Great Al-Mansur Hospital in Cairo, Egypt, is an example of the Arabs' interest in and dedication to health care. The hospital had special wards for particular diseases, outpatient clinics, convalescent areas, diet kitchens, and a large medical library. Both men and women were trained to provide care for the sick.

Military Influence

Wars accelerate the need for health care. Military medicine throughout history has provided the stimulus for improvement in infection control, surgical interventions, and trauma management. The Crusaders brought personal and financial support to the hospitals in the areas of conquest between A.D. 1096 and 1291. The Crusaders built hospitals in the Holy Lands. During this period, the Hospitallers of the Order of St. John of God were established to staff the hospitals and care for the wounded on the battlefield. This order continues to maintain health facilities throughout the world.

Hospitals began to take shape in what is now the United States in approximately the same way. It is known that military hospitals functioned during the Revolutionary War in New York (Manhattan), Pennsylvania (Lititz), Massachusetts, and other areas of battle. For the most part, these were temporary field hospitals.

A historic example of a hospital formulary was compiled in Pennsylvania during the Revolutionary War. Known as the "Lititz Pharmacopoeia," it was used in preparing medications for the military hospital located in that town.

During the Civil War in the United States, Louisa May Alcott served as a volunteer and observed the wanton conditions of poor sanitation, the depressing environment, and patient and staff misery at the Union Hospital in Georgetown, Virginia. She describes these conditions in detail in her published book, *Hospital Sketches*. This book influenced President Abraham Lincoln to establish the U.S. Sanitary Commission, which had as its goal a single desire and resolute determination to secure for the men who had enlisted in the war the care that was the duty of the nation to give them. Lincoln also requested the Sisters of Charity to care for the wounded on the battlefields in the Civil War.

During the ensuing decades, rapid changes took place. The wars of the twentieth century brought significant changes to hospitals and health care delivery systems. World War I brought about the need to care for patients suffering from major trauma, burns, poison gas, and infections of all kinds. Hospital design reflected these needs in dealing with the masses of the injured, maimed, and sick. Ships designed as floating hospitals (begun during the Civil War) were in great demand to handle large numbers of casualties away from the immediate battlefield. They were also used to transport the sick under treatment to land-based institutions.

World War II saw major advances in trauma surgery, the introduction of systemic sulfonamides, penicillin, and the wide use of blood and plasma for transfusion. Very large hospitals were built to provide needed services to the large number of injured soldiers. The Cadet Nurse Corps was developed in the early 1940s to answer the need for large numbers of professionally trained people to nurse those who had been injured. Because of the kinds of injuries, new forms of treatment for war injuries were developed. The professions of occupational therapist and physical therapist came into being. Emotional problems resulting from the war gave new impetus for hospital facilities to deal with war-related psychiatric problems.

One vivid reminder of the Korean conflict was the television series *M*A*S*H*. The weekly series brought us the experience of war through the eyes and emotions of a mobile army surgical hospital staff. It was the proximity of these mobile operating rooms and support resources that resulted in saving hundreds, if not thousands, of lives.

Influences of Western Europe (A.D. 500–1200)

herb a leafy plant used as a healing remedy or flavoring agent.

Medieval physicians prescribed approximately 1,000 natural substances, most of plant origin. **Herbs** (leafy plants used as medicinal or flavoring agents) were the main source of medication. *Materia medica* was derived from the Greeks, Romans, and Arabs. The monasteries in England, Germany, and France preserved this information and added to it the medicinal herbs grown in the monastery gardens. Early explorers of American shores brought back to Europe native remedies such as quinine, found in the bark of South American trees.

During the Middle Ages, medical advancement came close to a standstill. A church edict in 1163 forbade clerics from performing any surgery that caused a loss of blood. At this time, monks were the primary health care practitioners, so surgical procedures were eliminated. Between 1347 and 1350, the Black Plague killed almost one-third of the inhabitants of Europe. Although most people were cared for and/or died in their own homes, many either died on the street or were brought to overcrowded hospitals. Hotel Dieu, one of the finest hospitals in Europe at the time, was reported to dismiss up to 500 bodies a day for burial during the height of the plague.

Throughout the centuries, people with mental health problems were often secluded from society in confined custodial care. The poor conditions of care are reflected in the memory of Bethlehem Hospital in London, called Bedlam. (The word continues in the English language to convey the idea of confusion and disorder.) Modern health care requires concern for those who have mental disorders. In France, mental hospitals were built in Metz; in Sweden, in the town of Uppsala; and in Italy, in Bergamo and Florence, in which patients were treated in a humane way. The town of Gheel in Belgium provided outstanding care to patients with psychiatric problems. The focus of the town's employment and activities was on the care of psychiatric patients who resided in the homes of the townspeople. It was in this town that St. Dymphna, the patron saint for mental disorders, was murdered by her deranged father (the king of Ireland), who pursued his daughter in a rage after she had fled his abuse. To this very day, the town of Gheel is given over to the care of those with mental illness with support from the Belgian government.

Swiss Influence

Paracelsus (1493–1541) was born Philippus Aureolus Theophrastus Bombast von Hohenheim. This Swiss alchemist changed his name to indicate his superiority over the great herbalist, Celsus. A product of the Renaissance, Paracelsus revolutionized pharmacy from a botanical science to the beginnings of a chemical orientation in the profession. He replaced the four body fluids identified by Hippocrates (blood, phlegm, yellow bile, and black bile) with three chemical constituents of the body. Paracelsus was the prime mover in bringing pharmacy from a botanical to a chemical science. Sulfur, mercury, and salt were the materials of the body, and drugs were used to overcome excess acid or alkalinity in the body. Alcohols, spirits, acids, and oils were used, as well as mercurials and other minerals.

Carl Scheele (1742–1786) was a Swedish pharmacist who made numerous chemical discoveries in the laboratory of his pharmacy shop. Among his discoveries were arsenic (1771), chlorine (1774), glycerin (1783), and numerous organic acids.

The first *International Pharmacopoeia* was published in Geneva, Switzerland, in 1951 under the auspices of the World Health Organization.

German Influence

Hildegard of Bingen (1098–1179) had a name for the healing force of all remedies: *veriditis*, which literally means "greenness," "growing energy," the "principle of sexuality and life." Her manuscript *Causae et Curae* is based on natural remedies. For example, she wrote that vermouth in deer fat could be used as an anointment; when massaged into an arthritic pain, it would bring relief.

For the first time in the history of Western Europe, pharmacy was declared an independent profession separate from medicine through the official Edict of 1231. Emperor Frederick II of Germany was the author of this edict, known as the Magna

Carta of Pharmacy. By it, pharmacies were subject to government inspections; the pharmacist was obliged, under oath, to prepare drugs as prescribed in a reliable and uniform method. This edict influenced the practice of pharmacy across all of Western Europe.

Currently, more than 400 physicians and health providers in Germany are experimenting with some 2,000 suggested remedies and health suggestions, many of which have been found effective.

Pharmacopeias

dispensatory a treatise on the quality and composition of medicine

Books that contain official drug standards have been known through the ages as recipe books, formularies, **dispensatories**, and pharmacopeias. The distinction of having the first legal pharmacopeia goes to the city of Nuremberg, Germany, where the municipal authorities in 1546 made it the official book of drug standards for that city. This book, known as *Dispensatorium Pharmacopolarum*, also became official in Augsburg, Cologne, Florence, and Rome.

Friedrich Serturner (1783–1841), a pharmacist, won international recognition when he prepared salts of morphine (1804), a drug of universal acclaim in the control of intractable (not easily managed) pain.

Johann Buchner (1783–1852), a pharmacist and professor of pharmacy in Munich, discovered salicin in willow bark and nicotine in tobacco. These discoveries paved the groundwork for aspirin (acetylsalicylic acid) and nicotinic acid. The latter was synthesized from nicotine in 1867 and is used today as niacin, a member of the vitamin B complex.

Rudolph Brandes (1795–1842) isolated hyoscyamine (1819) and, with fellow pharmacist Philipp Geiger (1785–1836), collaborated in research to discover atropine (1835). Atropine, used to this day, is a prototype for antispasmodic drugs.

Although Emil von Behring (1854–1917) was a physician and not a pharmacist, his contribution to pharmacy was a landmark one. His work with antitoxins to combat the effects of diphtheria, and later tetanus, initiated serum therapy. Diphtheria antitoxin (1892) created a whole new category of pharmaceuticals.

The concept of chemotherapy was introduced by Paul Ehrlich (1854–1915), a German physician and a pioneer in cellular pathology (**Figure 1-10**). Ehrlich researched 606 chemical combinations until he found an arsenical that would be effective in combating the contemporary **pandemic** (a disease affecting a global population): syphilis. Arsphenamine was patented in 1907 and achieved fame as

pandemic a global epidemic disease

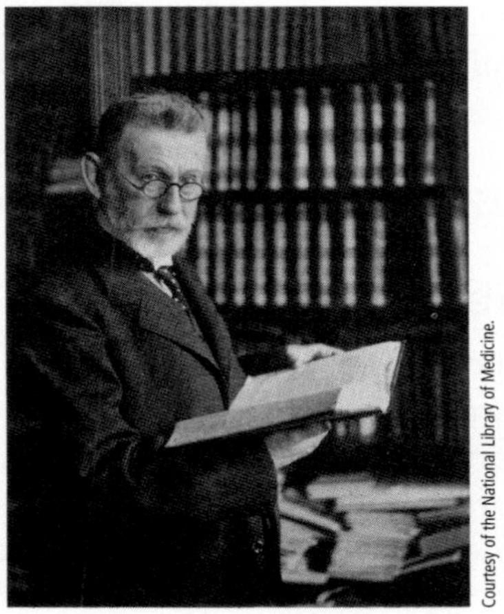
Courtesy of the National Library of Medicine.

FIGURE 1-10 Paul Ehrlich.

the "magic bullet" against syphilis. Specific remedies, many of a chemical nature, were targeted at specific microbial and specific human cells. An intensive warfare against infection had begun.

Gerhard Domagk (1895–1964), a German scientist, discovered a sulfa drug, prontosil, to be effective against hemolytic streptococci. The use of this drug became widespread as its effectiveness against a wide range of microorganisms became evident.

British Influence

During the eighteenth century, many hospitals were built in England to provide treatment for the poor. The Bristol Royal Hospital claims to be the first voluntary hospital in the provinces. One of the most famous hospitals, Guy's Hospital in London, was built in 1740 and provided free care through a ticket admission system.

William Withering (1741–1799), a clinician and a botanist in England, investigated the active ingredient in a folk remedy used to cure dropsy (an accumulation of fluids due to heart impairment). He called attention to digitalis (1741) as the active **alkaloid** (a nitrogenous basic substance found in plants or in synthetic substances with structures similar to plant structures) in the foxglove plant. Digoxin, a form of digitalis, is widely used today as a cardiotonic drug.

alkaloid a nitrogenous basic substance found in plants or in synthetic substances with structures similar to plant structures (e.g., atropine, caffeine, morphine)

Edward Jenner (1749–1823), an English physician, vaccinated against smallpox with the cowpox vaccine (1789) (**Figure 1-11**). This discovery in turn led to the eradication of smallpox in the twentieth century.

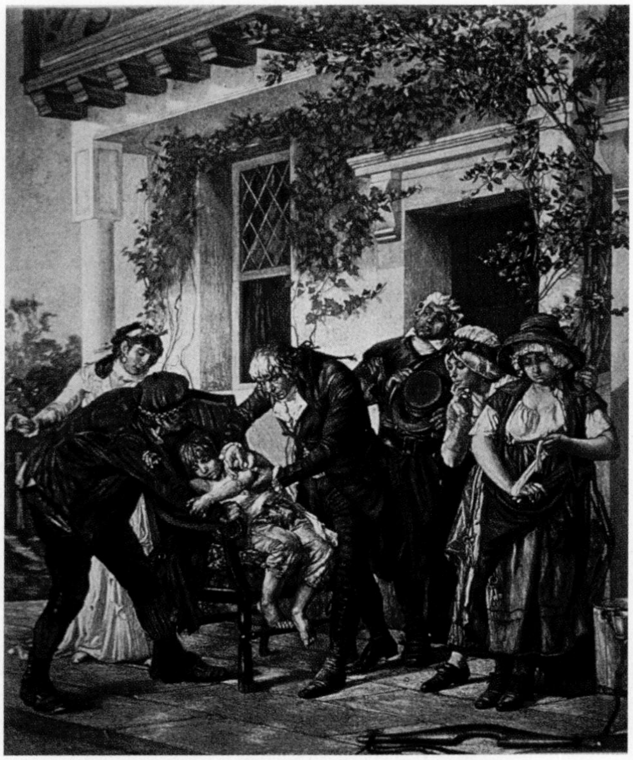

Courtesy of the National Library of Medicine.

FIGURE 1-11 Edward Jenner discovered the vaccine for smallpox.

Ten years later, a new class of anti-infective drugs became available in limited quantities. Early on when penicillin, the first antibiotic to be used in therapy, became available, there was only enough to treat 100 patients. It was first observed as an inhibitor of microbial growth by Alexander Fleming at St. Mary's Hospital in London in 1928. Later, Howard Florey (1898–1968) and his coworkers succeeded in first isolating and then making available large quantities of this lifesaving antibiotic to treat gram-positive infections.

French Influence

Bernard Courtois (1777–1838) discovered iodine (1811) in marine algae. In 1826, the year he graduated from pharmacy school in Montpellier, Antoine Balard (1802–1876) discovered bromine in sea water. He later became a faculty member at the same school.

Joseph Caventou (1795–1877), a pharmacist, collaborated with Pierre Pelletier (1788–1842) in the discovery of quinine (1820), which has become a worldwide treatment for **malaria** (an infectious fever-producing disease, transmitted by infected mosquitoes). He made other discoveries as well, including the identification of caffeine (1821).

malaria an infectious fever-producing disease, transmitted by infected mosquitoes

Pierre Robiquet (1788–1840), a pharmacist who was also a phytochemist, made a number of significant discoveries, including codeine (1832). Codeine, an analgesic weaker than but similar to morphine, is a drug widely used to control pain.

Henri Moissan (1852–1907) obtained free fluorine (1886) by electrolytic methods, thus completing the elements in the halogen family of drugs.

Other Influences

Native American Influence

Native Americans have used herbs medicinally for thousands of years. A few selections from particular tribes are cited here as examples:

Native American a person who was an original resident of the Americas

- Algonquins (Northeast United States) used inhalation of burning balsam firs (Christmas trees) to treat colds and respiratory congestion.
- Apaches (Oklahoma) used cayenne to increase blood flow to the skin (as a rubefacient). Cayenne also blocks pain and swelling when rubbed into an arthritic joint.
- Cheyennes (Minnesota) used echinacea for burns, wounds, and fever and to strengthen the immune system.
- Chippewas (North Dakota) used raspberry tea for diarrhea and dysentery.
- Iroquois (New York) used angelica as a poultice for broken bones and for ulcers. Dandelion plants were used for eczema and hives.
- Mohegans (Connecticut) used bayberry for kidney disorders and influenza. Slippery elm was used as a laxative.
- Navajos (Arizona) used alum root to heal sores, wounds, and animal bites.
- Penobscots (Maine) used sarsaparilla for colds and coughs.
- Winnebagos (Nebraska) used bee balm for cane and various skin eruptions.

The selections above were chosen from among numerous Native American tribes and the innumerable herbs used by them. Today more than 200 prescription drugs can be traced back to early Native American remedies. The USP (U.S. Pharmacopeia) has in the past included Native American remedies. Alumroot, used for stomach problems, was included in 1820–1882.

Black cohosh, used as a sedative, was included 1820–1936. Cascara sagrada, currently used as a laxative, has been included since 1890 to the present.

Canadian Influence

A dramatic and lifesaving discovery was made by Frederick Banting (1891–1941) and Charles Best (1899–1978) when they collaborated to discover insulin (1922). The lives of millions of people with diabetes have been saved and enhanced by this major therapeutic breakthrough.

World Health Organization

The World Health Organization (WHO) published the first *International Pharmacopoeia* in Geneva, Switzerland, in 1951. This book was published in English, French, and Spanish and later in German and Japanese. Although not a legal document, it assists in setting internationally acceptable drug standards. Drugs included in any pharmacopoeia are those of proven pharmaceutic and therapeutic value.

Developments in the United States Related to Health Care and Drug Therapy

Hospitals have emerged over the years, from **almshouses** for the sick poor, **asylums** for the care and confinement of orphans and those with mental illnesses, infirmaries for short-term acute care, **hospices** for people with terminal illnesses, and **sanatoriums** for the long-term care of patients with tuberculosis and others with chronic diseases.

almshouse a home for the sick poor and indigent

asylum an institution for the relief or care of orphans and those with mental illnesses, especially those who were insane

hospice an institution that provides a program of palliative and support services to patients with terminal illnesses and their families in the form of physical, psychological, social, and spiritual care

sanatorium an institution for the treatment of chronic diseases, such as tuberculosis or nervous disorders

Nonmilitary Hospitals

Nonmilitary hospitals came into existence in New Amsterdam, New York; Salem, Massachusetts; and Philadelphia, Pennsylvania. Philadelphia General Hospital was started in 1713 by the Quakers as an almshouse to give relief to the sick, the incurable, the poor, orphans, and abandoned infants.

Benjamin Franklin obtained a grant in 1751 to found the first American hospital, known as the Pennsylvania Hospital. Jonathan Roberts was recruited as the apothecary and enjoys the reputation of being the first American hospital apothecary. This institution has had a reputation for excellence from its earliest beginnings. The New York Cornell Medical Center was initially supported by King George III in a charter granted in 1771. The apothecary-in-chief was one of the four administrative officers named in the original charter.

Psychiatric Care

In the United States, the physician Benjamin Rush introduced new methods of treatment for psychiatric patients based on moral principles. His concerns and methods were outlined in a treatise on the topic that he published in 1812.

Dr. Rush was a friend of Benjamin Franklin and cared for people with mental illness at Pennsylvania Hospital. The hospital was a forerunner in the care of such patients in a general hospital, although at that time, psychiatric patients were housed in the lower level of the hospital and separated from the medical treatment areas.

Custodial Care

The nineteenth century continued the manner of dealing with mental patients by separating them from family and society. At the same time, the term *hospital* was substituted for the term *asylum*. The growth in the number and size of mental hospitals after the turn of the century was tremendous. Custodial care (non-medical care provided to persons requiring assistance with activities of daily living) in gigantic facilities became the norm, with half the hospital beds in the United States occupied by patients with mental illness. During the middle of the twentieth century, the trend reversed.

Deinstitutionalization

deinstitutionalization the discharge of people with a history of long-term mental health care in a hospital back to the community

Appropriate use of psychiatric drugs and various psychiatric treatment methods allowed many psychiatric patients to leave custodial care and assume the activities of daily living in society. Under this concept of **deinstitutionalization**, large numbers of persons were discharged to communities and, in some cases, they had to fend for themselves in the streets. The movement received strong support from civil liberty groups. State governments were only too willing to unburden themselves of the financial responsibilities involved in institutional care. What seemed to be a humane approach, however, only served to increase the number of homeless in society. Now efforts are being made by professionals to develop small housing facilities for their care. Some now recognize that continued structural support and care are still required.

Surgical Care

Massachusetts General Hospital in Boston was the first hospital to use general anesthesia in surgery. The first operation was performed in 1842, with anesthesia provided by Dr. Crawford Long. Soon chloroform and ether became standard anesthetic agents, which allowed for more frequent, less painful surgery.

Contemporary Medical Practices

"Miracle drugs" are a major part of the medical fabric of the twentieth century. Numerous researchers in universities, in pharmaceutical firms, and under government sponsorship have made and continue to make drug discoveries that stave off death and improve the quality of life.

Polio Vaccine

Poliomyelitis was a disease that crippled American President Franklin Roosevelt and killed and crippled many children. Eventually, two vaccines were developed: an injectable vaccine (by Jonas Salk, 1955) and an oral vaccine (by Albert Sabin, 1961). These vaccines have practically eliminated the disease commonly known as infantile paralysis.

Streptomycin

Selman Waksman (1888–1973) and his colleagues at Rutgers University in New Jersey began an intensive search to find an antibiotic to treat tuberculosis, known as the Great White Plague, which was claiming numerous lives. Streptomycin, discovered in 1944, was the first antibiotic to be effective against the tubercle bacillus, the infective agent in tuberculosis.

Whole hospital buildings were changed or eliminated as a result of new treatments. For example, tuberculosis sanatoriums and poliomyelitis facilities are examples of treatment centers outmoded by the vaccines developed to prevent those diseases. The famed Willard Parker Hospital of New York was declared obsolete after drug and antibiotic treatments reduced contagion and the need for isolation in hospital buildings. More recently, ambulatory (outpatient) treatment of childhood disease has caused a dramatic reduction in the need for pediatric hospital beds.

Review of Therapeutic Advances Discovered in the Nineteenth and Twentieth Centuries

The first book of drug standards published in the United States is known as the U.S. Pharmacopeia (USP) and in 1975 it was combined with another compendium, the National Formulary (NF), to form the USP-NF. Standards in the combined compendia apply to both manufactured and compounded drug preparations. These standards are enforceable under federal law, and some may also be enforceable under state and local laws.

Drug Standards Set by Pharmacopeias

The first USP was published in Philadelphia in 1820 by the U.S. Pharmacopeial Convention. This convention, founded on the American principle of representation, had physician representatives from all of the existing states. The goal of the convention was to select the "official" drugs and to set up standards for their identity, purity, and assay methods. By 1850, pharmacists and physicians were members of the convention. The pharmacopoeia is revised every 10 years. The first pharmacist to be chairman of the convention was Charles Rice, superintendent of the General Drug Department at Bellevue Hospital in New York. He laid the foundation for the sixth edition of the USP, published in 1882.

Biologicals

immunity the condition of being resistant to a particular disease (e.g., polio)

Serum therapy was initiated with the discovery of germ theory by Robert Koch, Edward Jenner's discovery of vaccination to provide **immunity** (the condition of being resistant to a particular disease), and Emil von Behring's discovery of antitoxins to neutralize microbial toxins. The vaccines, toxoids, and antitoxins, which utilize the clear fluid of the blood, were the first biologicals used in serum therapy. The smallpox vaccine was introduced in the early 1900s, followed by vaccines for typhus, whooping cough, measles, mumps, rubella, diphtheria, tetanus, influenza, and polio. In 1987 a genetically engineered hepatitis B vaccine was marketed.

Hormones

Isolation of human hormones began in 1897 with adrenaline, followed by thyroxine (1916), insulin (1922), cortisone, adrenocorticotropin (ACTH), estrone (1929), and testosterone (1935). These substances are important for replacement therapy and other therapeutic needs. Human insulin (Humulin), a product of genetic engineering, was introduced in 1982.

Anti-Infectives

Anti-infective therapy began with salvarsan (1907) and then prontosil (1935). A major breakthrough occurred with the discovery of penicillin (1928–1940). Other antibiotics soon followed: streptomycin (1944) and chloramphenicol (1947), known as the first broad-spectrum antibiotic.

Synthetics

antianginal a drug used to relieve heart-related chest pain

Synthetic chemicals were rapidly developed, including phenobarbital (1912), Raudixin (1953), Thorazine (1954), lithium (1960), and Valium (1963). **Antianginals**

antiarrhythmic an agent that restores normal heart rhythm

antihypertensive an agent that reduces blood pressure

beta blocker a drug that selectively blocks beta receptors in the autonomic nervous system

vasodilator an agent or drug that causes dilation of the blood vessels; increases the caliber of the blood vessels

immunomodulator an agent that adjusts the immune system to a desired level

(agents that reduce heart-related chest pain), **antiarrhythmics** (agents that restore normal heart rhythms), **antihypertensives** (agents that lower blood pressure), **beta blockers** (agents that block beta receptors in the autonomic nervous system), and **vasodilators** (agents that dilate blood vessels) all improved cardiac and circulatory problems. Drugs were developed to meet problems in the major biologic systems.

Immunomodulators

The most recent category of drugs to be developed is the **immunomodulators** (agents that regulate the immune system). Based on the theory of preserving the integrity of the immune system, immunostimulators are used when there is a deficiency, and immunosuppressants are used to prevent organ transplant rejection and to treat autoimmune diseases. These modulators preserve equilibrium in the second-most complicated biologic system, the immune system. (The most complex is the nervous system.)

Drug Development

The use of medicinal substances is a part of every culture. Plants, minerals, and animal parts were the drug components until the early nineteenth century. Drug therapy was advanced more in the twentieth century than all contributions of ages past, and the United States remains the world's leader in production of vaccines, biologicals, and synthetic drugs.

Today the use of natural products, mainly herbal remedies, is a billion-dollar market. Most pharmacies, while carrying the latest remarkable drugs, are now also including a few shelves of natural products. However, due to inconsistencies in strength and purity, discretion and knowledge are needed for their effective use. The use of alternative medicines, which are often labeled as food supplements, is a growing industry.

Summary

The author hopes that this introductory chapter focusing on the contributions of many persons in many countries over the centuries to the knowledge and use of drugs will lead to an appreciation of the art and science of pharmacy. Even in a profit-oriented culture, professionals still gain a sense of satisfaction for contributing to the relief of human needs. Pharmacy seeks to prevent illness, especially through biologicals, to treat sickness with appropriate drugs and natural products, and to maintain health through education.

TEST YOUR KNOWLEDGE

Multiple Choice

1. Clay tablets found inscribed with names of plants and minerals used as medicinals were found in present-day
   a. Afghanistan.
   b. Romania.
   c. Iraq.
   d. Egypt.

2. The "botanical basis of pharmacy" was written in
   a. China.
   b. Arabia.
   c. Germany.
   d. Egypt.

3. Hippocrates based his pharmacy practice on the concept of homeostasis, which includes
   a. the principle of restoring and maintaining balance in the body.
   b. the practice of treating symptoms with drugs that have the opposite effect.
   c. the treatment of allergic conditions with antihistamines.
   d. all of the above.

4. The "Magna Carta of Pharmacy," which promoted the independence of pharmacy as a profession, was an edict developed and enforced in
   a. the United States.
   b. Great Britain.
   c. Germany.
   d. France.

5. Digoxin, a form of digitalis, is derived from
   a. the poppy plant.
   b. the foxglove plant.
   c. garlic.
   d. frankincense.

Matching

Match the drug to the condition it was used to treat.

1.	______ quinine	a. heart problems
2.	______ arsphenamine	b. malaria
3.	______ streptomycin	c. syphilis
4.	______ digitalis	d. tuberculosis
5.	______ codeine	e. pain control

Match the drugs used in early China with their designated categories.

1.	______ yin drugs	a. colds
2.	______ yang drugs	b. heart conditions
3.	______ red drugs	c. fevers
4.	______ yellow drugs	d. liver conditions

Match the historical figure to what he or she is known for.

1.	______ Hippocrates	a. toxicologist
2.	______ Damian	b. botanist
3.	______ Mithradates	c. patron of pharmacy
4.	______ Theophrastus	d. applied scientific principles to drug therapy

Fill in the Blank

1. Insulin was discovered by ______________ and ______________.
2. Polio vaccines were developed by ______________ and ______________.
3. Penicillin was discovered and developed by ______________ and ______________.
4. The concept of chemotherapy was introduced by ______________.
5. ______________ discovered germ theory.

Suggested Readings

Cichoke, A.J. (2001). *Secrets of Native American herbal remedies*. New York, NY: Avery Trade.

Cowen, D.L., & Helfand, W. H. (1990). *Pharmacy: An illustrated history*. New York, NY: Harry N. Abrams.

Cowie, L. (1986). *Plague and fire*. London, UK: Wayland Publishing.

Donahue, M.P. (2010). *Nursing, the finest art: An illustrated history* (3rd ed.). St. Louis, MO: Mosby.

Dorland's illustrated medical dictionary (31st ed.). (2007). Philadelphia, PA: Saunders.

Dubos, R. (1988). *Mirage of health: Utopias, progress, and biological change*. New Brunswick, NJ: Rutgers University Press.

Garrison, F. H. (1960). *History of medicine* (4th ed.). Philadelphia, PA: Saunders.

Griffin, E. (2005). *Hildegard of Bingen: Selections from her writings*. San Francisco, CA: HarperOne.

Hill, R., Frazier, T., & Horsecapture, G. (2010). *Indian nations of North America*. Washington, DC: National Geographic.

Strehlow, W., & Hertzka, G. (1988). *Hildegard of Bingen's medicine*. Santa Fe, NM: Bear & Company.

Ziegler, P. (2010). *The black death*. New York, NY: Harper Perennial Modern Classics.

CHAPTER

2

Organizational Structure and Function of the Hospital and Pharmacy Department

Competencies

Upon completion of this chapter, the reader should be able to:

1. Explain the primary function of a hospital.
2. List five functions related to patient "processing" activities.
3. Name four treatment services available in a hospital for patient care.
4. Explain the hospital's role in the promotion of health and wellness.
5. Describe the roles of the hospital's governing board.
6. List the functions of the director of a pharmacy department.
7. Identify the major diagnostic and treatment units in the hospital.
8. List major functions of a pharmacy technician in the hospital pharmacy.

Key Terms

board of directors
board of trustees
credentialing
diagnosis
matrix management
product line management
utilization review

Introduction

Hospitals are generally thought of as health care institutions that provide diagnosis and treatment for inpatients. However, many hospitals have expanded their scope of services to include outpatient clinics and services such as wellness centers, community outreach programs, and health education.

When asked to explain what running a hospital was like, an experienced administrator once described it as running the largest hotel in town, the largest restaurant, the largest laundry, the largest laboratory, the largest employment office, the largest cleaning service, and so forth, all wrapped up into one. This scenario, although somewhat amusing, can be particularly helpful in understanding how patient care is delivered and how a hospital functions on a day-to-day basis.

This chapter explores the organizational structure and the functions of a hospital that enable it to maximize optimum therapeutic outcomes for the patients served. It also explores several important topics that impact how pharmacy technicians fit into the hospital environment:

1. The functions of today's modern hospital,
2. How the hospital is organized to achieve those functions,
3. The changing role of pharmacy technicians in hospitals, and
4. The organizational structure and functions of hospital pharmacy departments.

Types of Hospitals and Services

Historically, the meaning of *hospital* was a "place of hospitality." In the United States, hospitals were originally founded and funded by religious groups or charitable individuals and community leaders. Many of today's hospitals still carry names that link back to their founding religious groups: St. Joseph Hospital, Bon Secours Health System, Montefiore Medical Center (New York City), Central Baptist Hospital (Lexington, Kentucky), Methodist Hospital System (Houston, Texas), and many, many more. Although today, hospitals are largely staffed by physicians, pharmacists, nurses, and other health professionals, historically hospital work was performed by members of the founding religious groups or by volunteers.

Today, hospitals are typically funded by the public sector, by for-profit and not-for-profit health organizations, by health insurance companies, or by charities, including direct charitable donations.

During the past 10 to 20 years, many hospitals have joined together to become what is known as *health systems* or *health networks*. In some cases, these hospitals continue to remain somewhat independent and remain "owned" by the community. In other cases, the ownership and governance of the institution are transferred to an umbrella organization, and "ownership" is controlled by a central or corporate organization.

Hospitals are often categorized in different ways to help people understand their position in the community and how they compare to other hospitals. With respect to "ownership," hospitals can be classified as nonprofit, for profit, or government owned. *Nonprofit* (or *not for profit*) generally means that an organization does not have stockholders, and can be thought of as being "owned" by the community. For-profit hospitals, on the other hand, are owned by an individual, a group of individuals, or stockholders who share in the "profits" of the hospital.

Government hospitals are just that: they are "owned" by the city, county, state, or federal government, and are usually supported by tax dollars.

Another way of characterizing hospitals is their mission and scope of service. University teaching hospitals and academic medical centers are usually "owned" by the university identified in the hospital's name and are usually larger in size than community hospitals. The mission of such hospitals is to train physicians, nurses, pharmacists, and other health professionals at the same time they deliver care and treatment to patients. University teaching hospitals usually have a broad scope of services well beyond that usually found in smaller community hospitals, including services such as organ transplants.

Community hospitals are usually smaller than university teaching hospitals, but may range in size from 25 to 500 or more beds. Although many community hospitals are also involved with residency training programs for physicians and pharmacists, their teaching mission is much more limited than that of university teaching hospitals. Some hospitals specialize in treating certain types of patients. Specialized hospitals include trauma centers, rehabilitation hospitals, children's hospitals, psychiatric hospitals, geriatric hospitals, and hospitals for dealing with specific disease categories such as cardiac, oncologic, or orthopedic problems.

Still another way of categorizing hospitals is their geographic location within the state or region. Rural hospitals are so called because they are located in rural areas rather than in cities or metropolitan areas. Some rural hospitals are classified as *critical access hospitals*. These facilities are typically located in rural areas, are generally small, provide limited inpatient and outpatient services, but serve an area that may be 35 miles or more to the next larger hospital. Obviously, these facilities serve a special purpose and, as such, receive some special funding considerations from the state and federal government.

diagnosis the determination of the nature of a disease or symptom through physical examination and clinical tests

Regardless of their size and scope of services, hospitals are complex networks of health care services. These services focus on **diagnosis** (identification of a medical condition), treatment, prevention, and health maintenance of the community that it serves.

Hospital Functions

The primary function of any hospital is to provide resources to assist physicians and other health care professionals in diagnosing and treating patients. In addition, various secondary or support functions must also be provided (e.g., record keeping, billing, discharge planning). This simple breakdown of functions is shown in **Figure 2-1**.

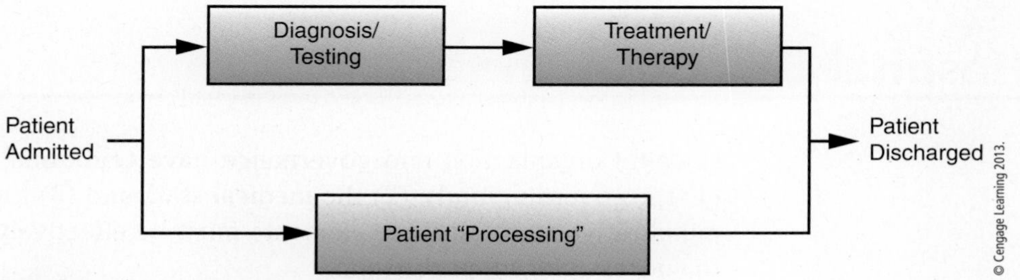

FIGURE 2-1 Simplified diagram of hospital functions.

The "processing" of patients refers to all the functions and paperwork associated with a patient's stay in the hospital. These include the medical records function, utilization review, billing, and discharge planning, to name a few.

Physicians order tests to confirm or identify the patient's diagnosis or medical condition. These tests are carried out in the various departments (e.g., radiology, medical laboratory, cardiopulmonary). Once the diagnosis has been determined, a treatment plan is developed, which may include surgery, physical therapy, respiratory therapy, or drug therapy. Each test or treatment is carried out by the appropriate clinical service. Some departments play an ongoing role in both the diagnosis and treatment functions.

The diagnosis and treatment of a patient is rarely a simple, straightforward process. It is often complicated, involving multiple disciplines within the hospital. In today's aging society, older patients frequently present themselves at the hospital with multiple ailments and complaints; some interrelated to varying degrees, making the diagnosis and treatment functions quite complex. For purposes of understanding the hospital's overall functions, however, it is important to recognize the sequence of diagnosis and treatment, and the corresponding patient "processing" as being of primary significance to the structure and function of the hospital.

Health education and wellness promotion are other functions that hospitals have gradually developed over the past 20 to 30 years. Many hospitals have taken on responsibility not only for helping patients recover good health, but also for helping them maintain good health. To this end, most hospitals have sponsored smoking cessation programs, stress reduction classes, weight loss programs, and instruction in how to identify potential health problems, such as self-examination for breast cancer. Community screening efforts for blood pressure, mammography, cholesterol, and glucose levels are representative of similar efforts to uncover those people at risk of becoming ill before their health actually begins to deteriorate (early detection). In addition, some hospitals have developed support groups for patients and families with such health problems as diabetes, Alzheimer's disease, and cancer. Finally, many hospitals have begun to play a coordinating role in helping whole groups of patients assess their health care needs and gain access to the appropriate health care providers. Senior citizens are one group of people for whom this service is vital.

If we are to superimpose these additional functions onto Figure 2-1, it will now appear as shown in **Figure 2-2**. Anyone who has ever been in a hospital recognizes that there are a great many other things that go on that have not yet been addressed. Clinical nutrition service includes counseling patients about their diets and eating habits, while the food services department involves the preparation and delivery of meals to patients and employees. Housekeeping keeps the hospital clean and plays an integral role in infection control. Plant engineering maintains the facility and provides the necessary heating, air conditioning, water, electricity, and other utilities. Coordination of all of these activities and others is essential to the successful operation of a hospital.

Hospital Organization

Hospital organization and governance have traditionally been characterized by (1) the governing body, (2) the medical staff, and (3) the hospital clinical and administrative staff. All three elements must be effectively integrated for a hospital to successfully support itself.

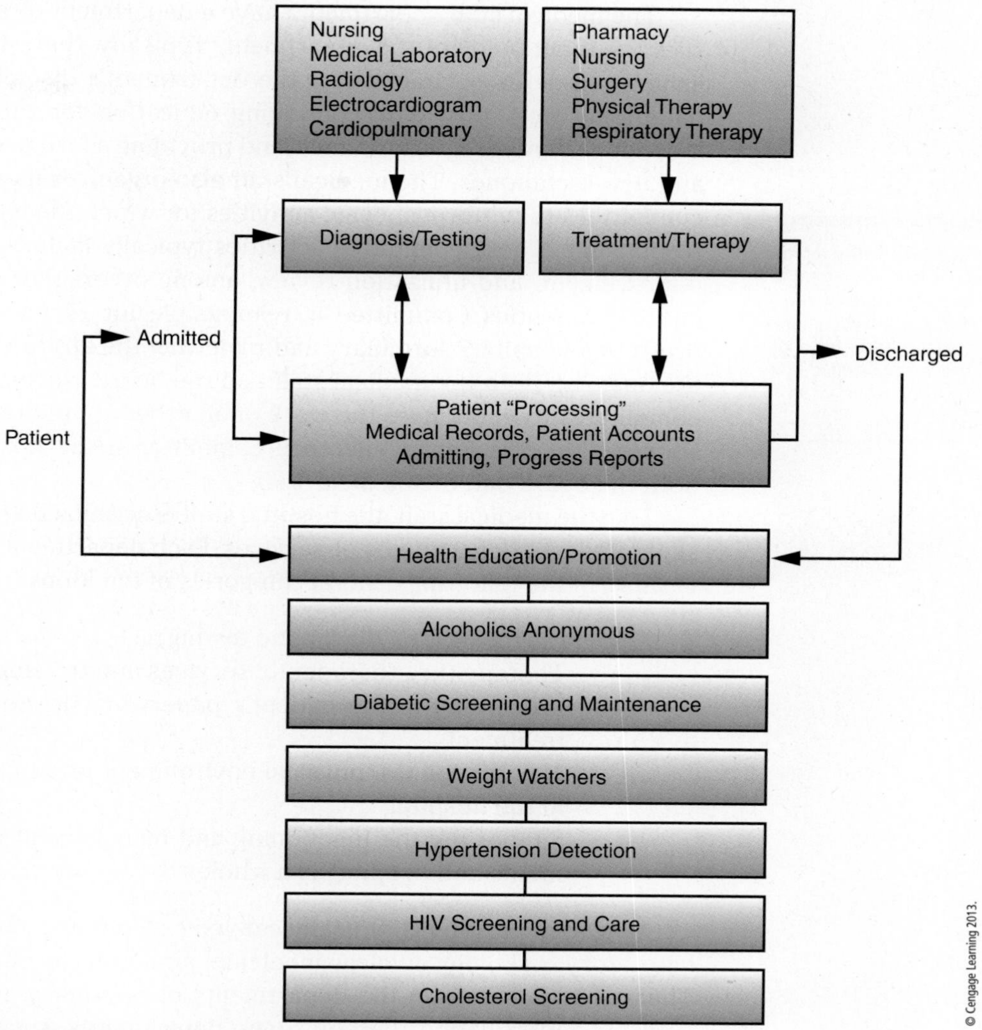

FIGURE 2-2 Expanded diagram of hospital functions.

board of trustees/directors the body responsible for governing the hospital in the community's best interest

The governing body is usually called a **board of trustees** or **board of directors**. (In a government hospital these are sometimes known as a *board of supervisors*.) The board is charged with the ultimate responsibility of governing the hospital in the community's best interest. To this end, the board is ethically, financially, and legally responsible for everything that goes on in the hospital. The board typically organizes itself into various committees to perform the detailed activities required to govern the hospital. These committees usually focus on key elements of the hospital, such as financial activities, community relations, planning, quality assurance, and personnel, as well as a variety of other areas of responsibility.

The medical staff always includes physicians, but may also include dentists, podiatrists, psychologists, physician assistants, nurse practitioners, and sometimes pharmacists, each credentialed in his or her specialty or subspecialty to practice at the hospital. The medical staff is organized into departments such as medicine, surgery, family practice, OB/GYN, psychiatry, and pediatrics, and is further subdivided into subspecialty sections or groups such as cardiology, endocrinology, orthopedics, and neurology. The president of the medical staff functions as the liaison between the medical staff and the hospital administration.

The medical staff departments have a department director or chair who oversees the functioning of the department. Typically, these functions include establishing standards of practice for the department's discipline (medicine, surgery, pathology, etc.), providing continuing education for the discipline, monitoring individual member's performance, and providing a forum for the exchange of ideas and new techniques. The medical staff also organizes itself into multidisciplinary committees to perform specific activities for which the medical staff as a whole is responsible. These committee activities typically include **credentialing**, quality improvement, and utilization review, among others. For example, the Pharmacy and Therapeutics Committee is responsible for reviewing requests for adding drugs to a hospital's formulary and reviewing the appropriate use of drugs within the hospital. Both the medical staff and the board of trustees also have executive committees to coordinate the work of all other committees. They typically share sponsorship of a joint conference committee made up of representatives from both the board and the medical staff.

credentialing a process in which a formal, organized agency recognizes and documents the competencies and abilities performed by an individual or an organization

Like the medical staff, the hospital staff is organized around common functions separated into departments or services. Each department or service performs one or more of the following general categories of functions:

- Diagnosis (i.e., diagnostic testing)
- Therapy (i.e., therapeutic services and treatments)
- Processing of the patient's paperwork or monitoring of the patient's treatment
- Maintaining the physical environment or supporting the patient's stay in the hospital
- Supporting the functioning and management of the individual departments and hospital as a whole.

Diagnostic testing is typically carried out in departments such as the medical laboratory, radiology, nuclear medicine, and EKG (or ECG, electrocardiography). Therapy is provided in the departments of pharmacy, physical therapy, speech therapy, and radiation therapy. Some departments, such as nursing, psychiatry, and respiratory therapy, spend significant amounts of time both determining diagnoses and providing treatments.

Other departments perform "processing" functions that assist the patient throughout the stay without directly affecting diagnosis or treatment. Examples include the medical records, admitting, patient accounts (billing), **utilization review**, and social services departments.

utilization review the work of a committee that determines if the use of resources has met certain established criteria and standards

Another group of departments support the patient's stay either by contributing to the physical environment or by supporting the coordination of services to the patient. Included in this group would be information services (communications), housekeeping, volunteer services, laundry, plant engineering and maintenance, safety and security, and pastoral care. In some hospitals, the dietary department, while providing support to the patient through ongoing nutrition, can also play a therapeutic role and a health education role.

Finally, a variety of departments and services are vital to the overall success of a hospital, but patients may never hear of them while around the hospital. These departments support the ongoing operation of the hospital and the individual clinical departments and services. Examples of these departments include the departments of materials management, human resources, community relations, planning, risk management, and accounting and finance. In addition, clerical personnel support the activities of the medical staff.

Each hospital department or service is generally run by a director, an administrative director, or a section supervisor. These middle managers report to administrators or vice presidents who in turn report to either the executive vice president or directly to the president. Historically, the departments were grouped according to common operating characteristics into four categories: nursing services, clinical services (testing and treatment departments), support services (support and facilities departments), and financial services (accounting, billing, and patient accounts). The organizational chart in **Figure 2-3** reflects this historical division of responsibility.

matrix management an organizational concept that emphasizes the interrelationship among departments and the common areas of decision making

product line management an organizational concept that emphasizes the end product or category of services being delivered

However, hospital organizational structure has changed dramatically over the years and is now tailored specifically to each hospital's activities and the capabilities of its department heads and administrative staff. Although some elements are common to all organizational charts, there is no longer one dominant organizational structure.

Matrix management and **product line management** are just two examples of organizational concepts that can be applied to the rapid technological and service delivery evolution that has taken place in health care. Matrix management structurally emphasizes the overlapping areas of responsibility among departments and the common areas of decision making. Product line management

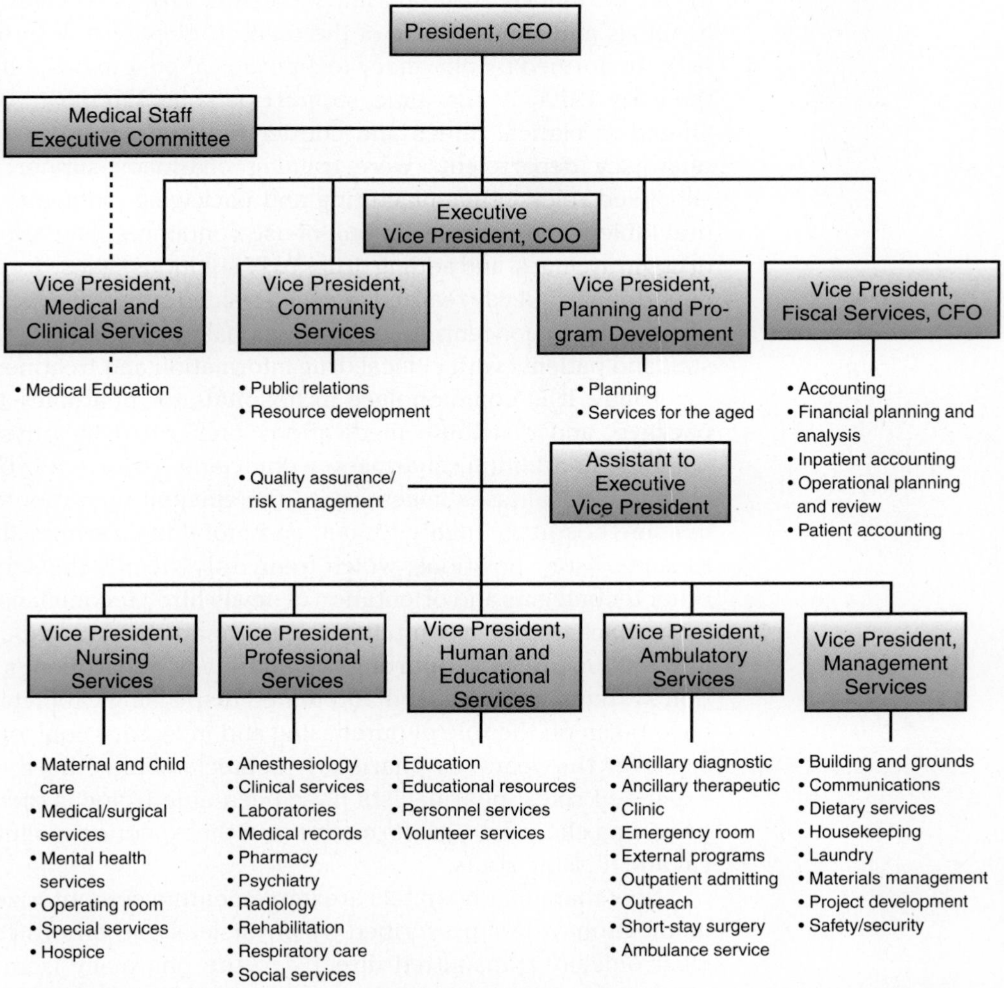

FIGURE 2-3 Hospital organizational chart according to traditional divisions of responsibility.

organizes the hospital not along the lines of comparable operating principles, but by the end product or category of service being delivered.

Fully understanding organizational theory is not essential to appreciate how a hospital functions. What is important is appreciating the great variety of ways in which hospitals are organized and that, in each case, communication and collaboration among departments are vital.

As a way of enhancing communications, the hospital staff, the board of trustees, and the medical staff form committees. Some committees are ongoing, such as safety and quality improvement committees. Many, however, are *ad hoc* working groups brought together to address a specific problem or concern. Once the desired resolution is achieved, these groups disband or form new committees to address different problems and issues. These *ad hoc* committees bring various departments together in a problem-solving situation without dramatically altering the organizational structure of the hospital or interfering with the reporting relationships carefully developed over time. As such, they represent a flexible, informal organizational structure that allows the hospital to get its work done.

Hospital Pharmacy Technicians: A Changing Role

It can be argued that pharmacy "technicians" were first recognized in military hospitals and clinics. Some of the earliest references describing the broad range of tasks performed by pharmacy technicians appear in hospital pharmacy literature of the early 1970s. At that time, support personnel in most hospital pharmacies were limited to clerical duties and courier functions. However, a few forward-thinking pharmacy departments were training pharmacy support personnel to take on expanded roles in manufacturing and packaging ointments and creams, packaging oral tablets and capsules in unit-of-use containers, preparing single-dose injectable drugs in syringes, and adding drugs to IV solutions. Those forward-thinking pharmacy departments quickly realized that well-trained supportive personnel could free up the pharmacist to concentrate on professional functions such as providing the medical staff and patients with clinical drug information and treatment guidance.

Today, it is commonplace in hospitals for pharmacy technicians to prepare, package, and distribute medications prescribed by physicians for hospitalized patients. In addition, pharmacy technicians perform a broad range of the technical and clerical tasks necessary to the efficient operation of a hospital pharmacy. In some hospitals, highly trained and motivated technicians have been promoted to supervisory positions, which frequently include the scheduling and training of other technicians and orientation of newly hired technicians. Pharmacy technicians with a background in computer science or advanced computer skills have migrated into full-time roles supporting the pharmacy department's computerized information systems, robotics, and automated dispensing cabinets. Still other technicians have taken on the role of purchasing and inventory control for the pharmacy.

Over the years, as pharmacy technicians have been assigned more of these expanded roles, pharmacists have been able to focus more on activities such as providing clinical drug information and therapeutic recommendations to the medical and nursing staffs.

Now that most hospitals are implementing computerized order entry systems, medication orders prescribed by physicians and other licensed practitioners are electronically transmitted directly to the pharmacy from all of the patient care units, as well as from remote locations such as a physician's office or even a physician's home. After pharmacists review the orders for appropriateness and perform clinical interventions when applicable, the medication order is processed and technicians assist in preparing the medications for dispensing.

Today the most common method used for preparing and distributing prescribed medications in hospitals is known as *unit-dose drug distribution*. Individual, patient-specific doses of each drug are separately packaged and labeled, ready for administration. These packages also contain a bar code which is used to assist with dispensing and administration. Many commonly used medications are prepackaged in unit-dose form by drug manufacturers so that technicians need only select the right package. When prepackaged unit-doses are not available, technicians must measure or count the prescribed amount from bulk containers and create the packaging with the use of a unit-dose packaging machine. As more and more hospitals implement bar-coded medication administration, pharmacy technicians are playing a larger role in bar-code technology. Information embedded in the medication bar code assists in medication dispensing, and helps ensure that the right patient receives the right drug, in the right dose, by the right route, at the right time. (Refer to Chapter 20 for a review of this topic.)

When unit-doses are to be administered by the injection route, technicians may assist the pharmacist in the transfer of the medication from vials and ampules—using aseptic techniques—to the proper dispensing container. In addition, the technician may assist in the preparation of IV admixtures, adding drugs or nutrients (IV additives) to commercially prepared or compounded intravenous solutions. (See Chapter 17 for information on this topic.) Pharmaceutical calculations must be accurate and checked by a pharmacist, and extreme care must be taken to ensure sterile conditions and aseptic techniques. (Refer to Chapter 15 for information related to this topic.)

Purchasing and inventory control are additional responsibilities for some pharmacy technicians. Technicians keep track of medications and other supplies and prepare orders for additional quantities when stock diminishes. They also receive incoming supplies; reconcile invoices against quantities ordered, received, and billed; and put supplies into the appropriate secured storage areas. (Please refer to Chapter 27 for information on this topic.)

Additional duties performed by pharmacy technicians may include delivering drugs and pharmaceutical supplies to nursing stations (either manually or by utilizing a hospital-wide pneumatic tube transport system); refilling emergency crash cart medications; maintaining automated dispensing and robotic machines; keeping pharmacy work areas well stocked, clean, and orderly; and responding to telephone questions or requests from other hospital personnel.

The hospital pharmacy technician's increasing role, responsibilities, and employment requirements may vary not only from hospital to hospital, depending on the pharmacy department's scope of service, but also from state to state, because the state boards of pharmacy regulations governing the practice of pharmacy vary.

As the need for clinical pharmacists on multidisciplinary hospital care teams increases, the need for, and reliance on, well-trained, highly skilled, and competent technicians will continue to increase. Hence, many states will soon require a formal training program with a competency certification or license examination. Currently, there is a National Pharmacy Technician Certification Board Examination that provides an opportunity for a pharmacy technician to demonstrate that he or she has mastered basic pharmacy knowledge and skills to work in hospital or retail practice settings. (See Chapter 34 for additional information on this topic.)

Structure and Organization of a Pharmacy Department in a Hospital Organization

In hospitals, nursing homes, or assisted living–type facilities, the role of the pharmacy staff has evolved in response to technological, financial, and other operational influences. Typically, the pharmacy director is responsible for the overall operations of the department including staff hiring, scheduling, competency assessment, budgeting, and regulatory compliance. The director participates on committees and other interdisciplinary activities. In larger hospitals and health systems, it is becoming more common to see an individual with greater responsibility than the traditional director of pharmacy. This new role is typically designated chief pharmacy officer and may have a number of directors of pharmacy reporting directly or indirectly to her or him. The chief pharmacy officer may also carry the title of vice president of pharmacy, and be a member of the hospital's executive staff. The chief pharmacy officer role is particularly valuable in health systems consisting of a number of hospitals, community-based clinics, outpatient prescription pharmacies, or a mix of all three.

The role of the pharmacist in hospitals today has expanded well beyond the preparation and distribution of drugs and drug products and the provision of information about medication administration and drug interactions. Note, however, that this role expansion has been possible only because of the increasing and expanding role of pharmacy technicians. All pharmacists today graduate with a doctor of pharmacy (PharmD) degree. Some pharmacists, however, obtain advanced training and education through 1 or 2 years of residency training and are recognized

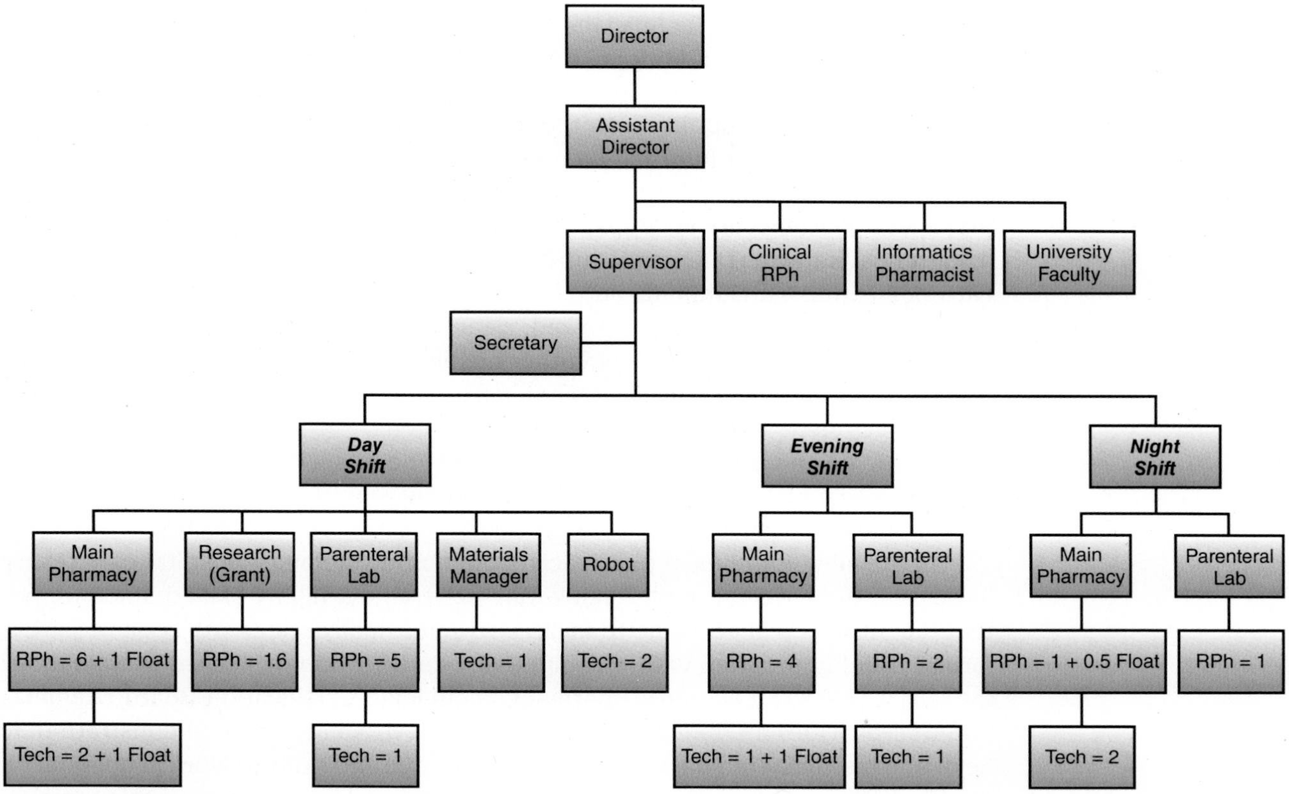

FIGURE 2-4 Hospital pharmacy organizational staffing chart with the pharmacist and technician teams.

as clinical pharmacists or clinical pharmacist specialists. Pharmacy technicians, working alongside pharmacists in the distribution and control functions of the department, create the opportunity for clinical pharmacists to spend much of their time on patient care units, working directly with physicians and nurses, providing guidance on the most appropriate and cost-effective medications available to treat specific conditions (**Figure 2-4**).

Summary

If one conclusion about hospitals' organizational structure and function can be reached, it is that they are continuously changing. New technologies and programs will continue to be developed, and new financial pressures and changing government regulations will continue to force changes to a hospital's organizational structure. New roles are continuously being proposed for the nation's hospitals, and new organizational structures are being developed to meet the challenges that lie ahead. In short, it is far from clear what hospitals will look like in the future or precisely how they will function. In light of the financial crisis hospitals are currently facing, compounded by the technological revolution we are experiencing, we can be sure that hospitals will remain complex organizations that patients depend on to adequately provide the required quality care. We can also be sure that proper and appropriate health care will continue to depend on accurate and precise communication of information and, most importantly, on the skill and dedication of those who staff our hospitals.

TEST YOUR KNOWLEDGE

Multiple Choice

1. The primary functions of a hospital are to provide for which of the following?
   a. diagnosis
   b. treatment
   c. both a and b
   d. none of the above

2. Patient "processing" activities include
   a. the admission process.
   b. utilization review.
   c. discharge planning.
   d. all of the above.

3. Most hospitals provide the following treatment modalities:
   a. surgery.
   b. hypnosis.
   c. acupuncture.
   d. massage therapy.

4. Wellness programs in hospitals typically include
   a. smoking cessation.
   b. Special Olympics.
   c. strength training.
   d. aerobics.

5. The role of the hospital governing board includes responsibility for all the following except
   a. ethical concerns.
   b. hiring supervisory personnel.
   c. legal matters.
   d. financial matters.

Matching

Match the responsible parties with the role they play in the hospital. The answers may be used more than once.

1.	_______ maintains physical environment	a.	board of trustees
2.	_______ establishes medical standards of practice	b.	medical staff
3.	_______ is responsible for overall hospital governance	c.	hospital staff
4.	_______ provides social services		
5.	_______ monitors physician's performance		

Fill in the Blank

1. In the past century, a major development in hospitals were __________ programs.
2. The governing body of the hospital is called the __________.
3. To enhance the communications and efficiencies of the hospital, __________ may be formed.
4. The principal responsibility of __________ is to prepare, package, and distribute medications prescribed by physicians for hospitalized patients.
5. Pharmaceutical __________ must be accurate and checked by a pharmacist, and extreme care must be used to ensure the use of sterile conditions and aseptic techniques.

CHAPTER 3

Home Health Care

Competencies

Upon completion of this chapter, the reader should be able to:

1. Describe the evolution and future of the home health care industry, particularly as related to home infusion therapy and home care pharmacy practice.
2. Explain the difference between home pharmacy services and ambulatory pharmacy services.
3. List at least three different types of organizations that provide home pharmacy services.
4. Describe at least three nontraditional employment opportunities that a pharmacy technician might have in home health care.

Key Terms

durable medical equipment (DME)
durable medical equipment, prosthetics, orthotics, and supplies (DMEPOS)
elastomeric devices
home care
home equipment management services
home health agencies
home health care
home health services
home infusion therapy (HIT)
home medical equipment (HME)
home medical services
National Home Infusion Association (NHIA)
personal care and support services
Safe Medical Devices Act of 1990

Introduction

Home health care in the United States is a diverse and rapidly growing segment of the health care industry. As ambulatory services have largely replaced in-hospital care, the home has become an increasingly important site of health care. Many elderly and infirm Americans, who may experience significant difficulty or hardship when accessing the health care delivery system, may receive a variety of skilled professional services without the need to leave their own home. **Home health care**, or **home care**, may be defined as the provision of health care services to patients in their place of residence. The Centers for Medicare and Medicaid Services (CMS) estimated that in 2004 more than 7.6 million persons in the United States were receiving home care from more than 20,000 providers. By 2010, this number had increased to 33,000 providers caring for 12 million individuals.

home health care provision of health care services to patients at their place of residence

home care care given to patients in their own homes

Evolution of Home Health Care

Home health care is as old as mankind; however, the first home health care agencies were not established until the 1880s. Pharmaceutical services were not a component of these early agencies, which were staffed primarily by nurses, therapists, and home health aides. Retail pharmacies provided medications (primarily oral drugs) to patients in their home by delivering to the home or having the home health care nurse pick up the medications for the patient. Pharmacy's role in home health care at that time then was minor and indistinguishable from community pharmacy practice. Indeed, home health care patients may have received fewer clinical pharmacy services than did their outpatient counterparts because they rarely interacted with the pharmacist.

The first major boom in the number of home health care agencies occurred in 1965 with the enactment of Medicare, which made home health care services available to the elderly and, beginning in 1973, to certain younger Americans with disabilities. Between 1967 and 1985, the number of home health agencies grew by more than threefold, from 1,753 to 5,983. However, pharmacy's role in home health care had increased very little because medications were not a Medicare-covered benefit. In 1983, Medicare initiated a prospective payment system for inpatient hospital care based on diagnosis-related groups (or DRGs) in an effort to reduce health care costs. Because hospitals received a fixed payment according to a patient's diagnosis, this provided economic incentives to discharge patients as early as possible, reducing the patient's length of stay in the hospital. This caused a dramatic shift in the place where care was provided: more and more patients began to receive their care at home.

The role of pharmacy in the growth of home care can be traced back to the birth of home infusion therapy during the early 1970s. Several university-based medical centers demonstrated the feasibility of providing nutrition intravenously (IV), called total parenteral nutrition (TPN), in the home for patients unable to eat orally, or via feeding tubes, called total enteral nutrition (TEN). Technological advances in central venous catheters and smaller more sophisticated infusion pumps made long-term treatment in the home not only possible but sufficiently safe and practical for the patient, their caregivers, and providers. Since Medicare was willing to pay for home TPN at about one-third of the inpatient rate, home infusion therapy (HIT) was born. Once the market for home TPN was established, many companies opened pharmacies to provide TPN and other home infusion services including IV antibiotic therapy and parenteral pain management. Although private insurance carriers were eager to adopt these other HITs over more expensive hospital care, Medicare does not currently cover these therapies at home.

In the United States, the cost for health care is more than in any other country as a percentage of the total economy. For this reason, employers, the U.S. government, and insurance providers are continuously looking for ways to maintain quality care while holding down the cost of that care. One common way to control costs is to manage the provision of the care itself. This concept is called *managed care*. Managed care is designed to direct patients to the most appropriate and most cost-efficient health care setting based on their identified needs. For example, managed care may determine if a patient should be treated at an outpatient clinic, in an inpatient setting, or in the home. An appropriate site of care can reduce costs without reducing the quality of the care provided. For example, home care patients are not exposed to the drug-resistant bacteria that can be found in many hospitals or nursing homes. With many pharmacies providing home care, competition has created incentives for many home care providers to contract with managed care networks.

Despite the tremendous growth of home health care in terms of number of patients and providers, the total cost of home health care is relatively low. Based on CMS data for fiscal year 2009, annual expenditures for home health care represent only 4.2% of their expected payments. This percentage has been fairly constant throughout the past decade. Medicare Part D, the prescription drug benefit became effective in 2006, but did not create a boom for home infusion pharmacy providers due to a lack of reimbursement for costs of infusion-associated supplies and infusion pump rental. These out-of-pocket costs to the elderly may prohibit them from receiving home pharmacy services.

The numbers of patients receiving home care will continue to grow as the population ages. On the basis of satisfaction surveys, most patients prefer home health care to hospital care. One can easily see that delivery of care and services in the home is still a growing market and has not yet reached its peak. Even HIT, which has seen virtually no breakthroughs in technology and new therapies administered in the home in the past few years, is still experiencing a significant annual growth rate. The **National Home Infusion Association (NHIA)**, the trade organization of home infusion providers, estimated in 2011 that 700 to 1,000 home infusion pharmacies would have $9 to $11 billion in sales for the year.

National Home Infusion Association (NHIA) the trade organization for home infusion providers

Home Health Care Services and Providers

home health services the provision of health care services by a health care professional in the patient's place of residence on a per-visit basis

The most frequently provided home care services are **home health services**, defined as the provision of health care services by a health care professional in the patient's place of residence, usually on a per-visit basis. Home health services consist of a wide diversity of services. The dominant form of home health services is nursing. Nursing services can be high tech (e.g., infusion therapy) or low tech (e.g., diabetic teaching and monitoring) on an intermittent visit schedule or as 4- to 12-hour shifts. Other services include those of dietitians, medical social workers, physical therapists, occupational therapists, and speech therapists. Sometimes respiratory therapists, dentists, and physicians are also included in this group. Respiratory therapists are usually associated with the home medical equipment industry rather than with home health agencies. The provision of dental services in the home is relatively new and extremely rare at present. Most people prefer to differentiate physician services in the home, referring to them as **home medical services**. As more bed-bound individuals are cared for in their homes, the need for physicians to make "house calls" has led to creation of a new geriatric subspecialty.

home medical services physician services provided in the home

home health agencies public (governmental) agencies, nonprofit agencies, proprietary agencies, and hospital-based agencies that provide health services in the home

Providers of home health services are called **home health agencies** (HHAs). HHAs can be classified as public (governmental) agencies, nonprofit agencies, proprietary agencies, and hospital-based agencies. Most states require HHAs to be licensed. Approximately 55% of HHAs are Medicare certified. To be Medicare certified, and thus eligible to take care of Medicare patients and receive payment for that care, the organization must meet the Medicare Conditions of Participation (a lengthy list of standards and requirements), have a Medicare provider number, and undergo unannounced inspections by CMS staff or another accrediting body (e.g., The Joint Commission).

Personal Care and Support Services

personal care and support services the provision of nonprofessional services to patients in their place of residence

The second most common form of home care services is **personal care and support services**, defined as the provision of nonprofessional services to patients in their place of residence. These services include homemaking, shopping, food preparation, personal care, and bathing. The individuals who provide these services are called home health aides, homemakers, or personal care attendants. Most personal care and support services are provided by HHAs, although some companies (non–Medicare certified) specialize in this form of care exclusively. One of the growing areas for personal care and support services is private-duty services. Private duty involves the provision of personal care services around the clock or for 8 to 18 hours per day, sometimes by a live-in attendant. These services are generally not reimbursed by Medicare or Medicaid and rarely by insurance, so the payment for personal care services is made by the patients or their families. Home health or nursing services can also be provided on a private-duty basis and that is a rapidly growing area. In 2009 it was estimated that 10% of all home care services were paid for out of pocket.

Home Equipment Management Services

home equipment management services the selection, delivery, setup, and maintenance of equipment and the education of the patient in the use of the equipment, all performed in the home or patient's place of residence

home medical equipment (HME) health-related equipment used at home (e.g., hospital beds, crutches)

durable medical equipment (DME) health-related equipment that is used for long periods of time, is not disposable, and is rented or sold to patients for home care, such as wheelchairs, hospital beds, walkers, canes, and crutches

The third most prevalent form of home care services is **home equipment management services**, also referred to as **home medical equipment (HME)** services or **durable medical equipment (DME)** services. Home equipment management services can be defined as the selection, delivery, setup, and maintenance of equipment and the education of the patient in the use of the equipment—all performed in the patient's place of residence. Medical equipment includes wheelchairs, canes, walkers, beds, and commodes. It also includes higher technology items such as oxygen tanks, oxygen concentrators, ventilators, apnea monitors, phototherapy lights, infusion pumps, enteral pumps, and uterine monitors. Many providers include the sale of medical equipment and supplies (such as ostomy supplies and wound care dressings) in this home care definition. However, the federal government and the accrediting bodies do not include the provision of products without services in their definition of home care. Such sales, without the corresponding services, are considered retail.

Home medical equipment providers are not required to be licensed in most states, although the U.S. Food and Drug Administration and the Department of Transportation require registration for distribution and transportation of oxygen. In 2010, CMS enhanced its **durable medical equipment, prosthetics, orthotics and supplies (DMEPOS)** standards to require accreditation for providers servicing Medicare recipients.

A large number of pharmacies are involved in the provision of home medical equipment services and sales, which may be included in the definition of home care. Many HME organizations also provide clinical respiratory services, which include the professional services of a registered respiratory therapist for performing in-home assessments, monitoring of vital signs (temperature, blood pressure, and pulse rate), oximetry testing (the percent of oxygen saturation in the blood), and administrating therapeutic treatments (e.g., nebulized medications). Pharmacies must be involved in providing the respiratory medications (because these are prescription drugs) either as providers or under contract with the HME provider. There are specialty pharmacy practices that compound only inhaled medications and deliver them, usually by common carrier.

durable medical equipment, prosthetics, orthotics, and supplies (DMEPOS) durable medical equipment is any medical equipment used in the home to aid in a better quality of living; prosthetics are artificial devices that replace a missing body part lost through trauma, disease, or congenital conditions; orthotics are externally applied devices used to modify the structural and functional characteristics of the neuromuscular and skeletal system; and supplies include medical instruments, apparatus, implants, in vitro reagents, and similar or related articles that are used to diagnose, prevent, or treat diseases or other conditions and that do not achieve their purpose through chemical action within or on the body (which would make it a drug)

Home Pharmacy Services

The last major type of home care service is the provision of home pharmacy services. Home pharmacy services do not have a clear and concise definition because of the considerable overlap with retail or community pharmacy practice. However, home care pharmacy generally has the following characteristics:

- All medications are delivered, mailed, or shipped to the patient's home. The patient has never been present in the pharmacy or communicated face to face with a pharmacist (except perhaps in the home).
- The patient may be receiving home health (nursing) services and sometimes medical care in his or her home and may be homebound.
- The pharmacist is usually responsible for monitoring the patient's medication and clinical response on an ongoing basis. If not the pharmacist, then someone else must be responsible (e.g., home health nurse, hospice team, or another pharmacist) for monitoring the patient's drug regimen (**Figure 3-1**).

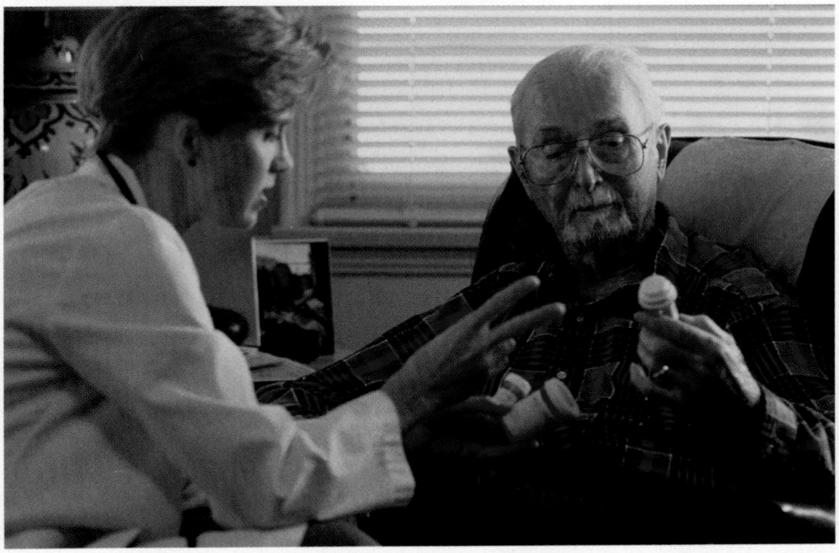

FIGURE 3-1 Home health care, including home pharmacy services, is growing rapidly and can be an area of specialization for pharmacy technicians.

Role of Pharmacy in Home Health Care

More than 90% of home pharmacy services involve home infusion therapy. However, pharmacies that specialize in providing services to hospice patients or hospice pharmacies are also categorized as providing home pharmacy services, as are a growing number of specialized mail-order pharmacies. The dominant specialty areas for such mail-order pharmacies include patients with hemophilia, cystic fibrosis, multiple sclerosis, short stature due to growth hormone deficiency, or respiratory diseases; those who are post-transplant or have some other immune system–compromised state; and those needing various biotech and injectable products. Pharmacists and pharmacy technicians employed in home care have a significant opportunity to develop special skills and knowledge of these disease states and the care of these individuals.

Home Infusion Therapy

home infusion therapy (HIT) intravenous drug therapy provided in the patient's place of residence

According to the U.S. Office of Technology Assessment, **home infusion therapy (HIT)** is described as medical therapy that involves the prolonged (and usually repeated) injection of pharmaceutical products, most often delivered intravenously, but sometimes delivered via other routes (e.g., subcutaneously, intramuscularly, or epidurally) into patients at their place of residence. HIT is generally thought of as comprising three services: pharmacy, nursing (home health), and equipment management services.

Pharmacy Services

Pharmacy services generally involve both compounding and dispensing the intravenous solutions into a ready-to-administer form. In many ways, this is similar to the IV room processes in a hospital pharmacy. Preparation of sterile admixtures for home administration may require special techniques and more stringent environmental controls, however, than a hospital IV admixture room. Unlike hospital care in which a medication is usually prepared within 24 to 48 hours of administration, home care may involve up to 1 month between preparation and administration, thus allowing a greater potential for microbial growth. More extensive quality control and end product testing are also performed on the prepared products for these same reasons. Home infusion pharmacies are required to comply with the U.S. Pharmacopeia (USP) Chapter <797> when compounding sterile preparations.

Home care and hospital pharmacy IV admixtures have significantly different labels. In home care, prescription labels must conform to the requirements for the state pharmacy laws for retail pharmacies and may require more detailed administration instructions. The pharmacy is also responsible for the packaging and delivering of the prepared products to the patient's home. Delivery techniques vary from using one's own delivery vehicles and drivers, to using external contracted delivery services—both local and national (e.g., FedEx), to having the nurse pick up and deliver the medications. Regardless of the delivery method, the pharmacy must always ensure that the product is packed to control the factors that affect the stability of the product (temperature, light, humidity, etc.) during transit to the patient's residence. In some cases, the patient may not live in the same state as the pharmacy. It is then the responsibility of the pharmacist in charge to know and comply with the pharmacy regulations of the state of the patient's residence.

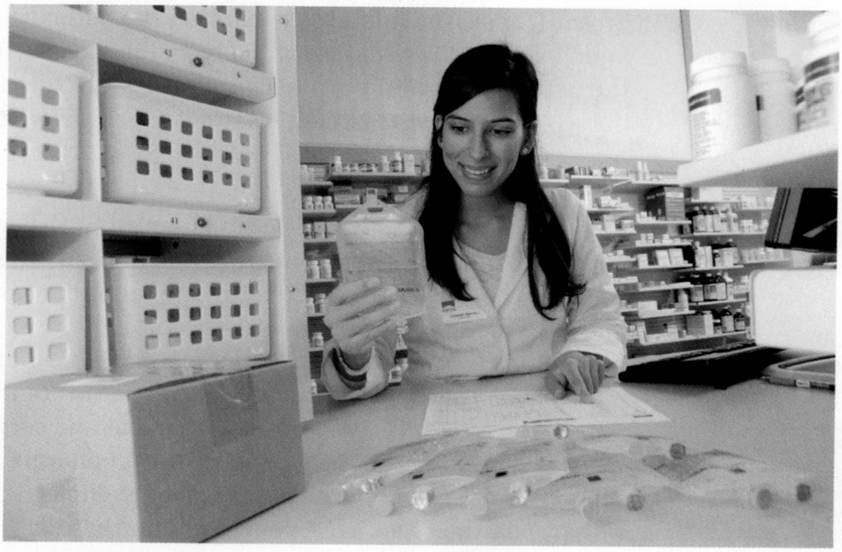

FIGURE 3-2 Pharmacy technicians in home infusion pharmacies are responsible for inventory of supplies, follow-up with the patients to ensure compliance, and other aspects of data collection.

Although the pharmacist is primarily responsible for the pharmaceutical care and clinical monitoring of the patient, many home infusion pharmacies rely greatly on the pharmacy technician to assist the pharmacist in data collection (**Figure 3-2**). For example, the pharmacy technician may be responsible for obtaining copies of laboratory reports, calling the patient for required details (e.g., a patient's weight), and inventorying supplies to assess compliance with prescribed therapies. The pharmacist monitors the drug therapy through evaluation of information received from the patient's nurse, patient, or family member or caregiver, pharmacy technician, delivery driver, and laboratory test results. Frequent and extensive communication regarding the patient may be needed with the physician and nurse, other health care professionals, and the patient or caregiver. The pharmacy maintains not only the normal prescription and dispensing records, but also a clinical record of the patients, called a chart or home care record. In some cases the patient's chart will be an electronic medical record, so few or no paper documents will be available.

The home infusion pharmacy generally operates under outpatient or retail pharmacy laws, although many state boards of pharmacy have either additional or different regulations for home care pharmacies. The pharmacy is often involved in providing the nursing supplies, venous access device, and infusion therapy supplies to patients. These infusion-related supplies and devices are sent with the medications to the patient, for use by the patient, caregiver, or nurse, in the patient's home.

Home Nursing Services

Initially, most patients receiving home infusion therapy will also be receiving home nursing services. Home infusion nurses usually have considerable experience in handling IVs in an acute care setting before they are hired to care for home infusion patients. Major responsibilities of the home care nurse include educating the patient and/or family caregiver regarding administration of the infusion and care of the infusion site, performing dressing and infusion site changes, making in-home physical assessments, and monitoring the patient's health status. Nurses will also administer the medications initially, but in most cases the eventual goal is to train the patient or caregiver to perform this task. Periodic visits are then made by the nurse to monitor the patient's status and response to therapy.

Equipment Management Services

Equipment management services supporting HIT include the selection, delivery, and setup of an infusion control device (i.e., an infusion pump). They also include the separation of clean (patient-ready) and dirty (returned) equipment, cleaning and disinfecting of equipment between patient use, and routine and preventive maintenance of equipment, including inspection and testing. Equipment sent to patients also needs to be tracked at all times in compliance with the **Safe Medical Devices Act of 1990**. Backup equipment and services are needed in case equipment malfunctions. In many home infusion pharmacies, pharmacy technicians are responsible for the routine cleaning and volumetric testing of infusion and enteral pumps and the associated documentation.

Safe Medical Devices Act of 1990 a federal law that requires all facilities that use medical devices (referred to as device-user facilities) to report serious injuries, serious illnesses, and deaths to the U.S. Food and Drug Administration and the manufacturer. The purpose of the act is to protect the public by ensuring that medical devices are not unsafe for their intended use

elastomeric devices a device used to administer therapeutics (e.g., analgesics, antimicrobials, chemotherapy)

As in a hospital or clinic setting, not all home infusion patients will need an infusion pump. Gravity administration of the drug using the rate controller or clamp on the administration set or tubing can be safely used at home for some drugs and administration rates when the patient or caregiver is awake. Special infusion pumps, syringe drivers, and other devices have been developed to meet the needs of home infusion patients. These might require new compounding techniques and skills for pharmacy technicians. Disposable administration devices, such as **elastomeric devices** (e.g., Intermate® and Eclipse®) and small lightweight pumps that do not require an IV pole, are commonly used to make home infusion more comfortable and convenient for the patient. When drug dilution is not required and the administration time is short, some patients may receive their medication as an IV push (a term used when the active ingredient goes directly into the vein). Pharmacy staff must be able to decide whether an infusion device is required and what device or pump is appropriate for the patient, drug, and administration rate and stability of the medication in the system selected.

Types of Home Infusion Providers

Home pharmacy services, as part of home infusion therapy, can usually only be provided by a licensed pharmacy either alone or as part of a broader health care organization. The exception is physician practices, which can provide these services without a pharmacist or pharmacy out of their office under the auspices of their physician's license. Other types of settings where home infusion services are provided include retail or community pharmacies, institutional or long-term care pharmacies, hospital pharmacies, home health agencies, HME-based providers, infusion therapy specialty providers, and ambulatory infusion centers.

Physician-Based Practices

This practice model is most commonly seen in oncology and infectious disease practices. Usually, physicians run an ambulatory infusion center as part of their office. Patients receive cancer chemotherapy, antibiotics, or any type of infusion while they are in the physician's office. Between physician visits, patients may return to the infusion center to receive their IV medications or have them provided through home care. Even in cases when the patient mainly receives care in the infusion center, at times a nurse may need to assist the patient in the home (e.g., leaking IV access on the weekend). Home care is usually provided by the nurses from the physicians' offices and is usually considered a sideline to their office-based practice. In these physician-based practices, nurses—not pharmacy technicians or pharmacists—are usually responsible for compounding and admixing the IV medications.

Sometimes a local pharmacy is contracted to compound and deliver the medications to the physician's office, and occasionally a pharmacist or pharmacy technician is hired by the physician. Whether or not the physician practice employs a pharmacy technician or pharmacist, compliance with USP Chapter <797> is still required.

Retail or Community Pharmacies

Independent retail or community pharmacies are most likely to provide a variety of services including HME, ostomy care products, and diabetic care. Infusion therapy is usually a low-volume component. Pharmacists, and sometimes technicians, usually provide home infusion therapy services in addition to retail and other pharmacy duties. Compounding aseptic isolators (CAI) or "glove boxes" are particularly well suited for community pharmacies since they do not require placement in a controlled air environment or "clean room." Most are "pharmacy-only" providers; however, a few pharmacies hire nurses to help coordinate home infusion therapy services and perhaps provide a limited amount of home health services. Delivery services are provided by nurses or the same delivery mechanism as the retail pharmacy/HME business. Some are part of a franchise in home infusion or participate in a home infusion network. Many are one-owner operations.

Institutional or Long-Term Care Pharmacies

Institutional or long-term care (LTC) pharmacies primarily provide drug distribution services to a large number of nursing homes, independent senior residences, prisons, and other institutional facilities, servicing an average of 4,000 patients daily. Although the primary business is oral medications, many also provide IV therapies to long-term care facilities with subacute units (patients needing more skilled care than a nursing home and less than an acute care hospital). Expanding the provision of IV services from the nursing home to the home care environment is very easy. Thus many LTC pharmacy providers have entered the home care market. However, home infusion therapy is usually a very low percentage of their overall business. These organizations have extensive internal delivery systems (e.g., their own fleet of vans) and usually provide enteral and infusion pumps, and some may also supply other HME. Although these pharmacies may employ a nurse to assist with care coordination and education of the long-term care facility staff, home health services are rarely provided directly by these organizations, which tend to be pharmacy-only operations.

Hospital Pharmacies

HIT may be provided by the pharmacy department in a hospital IV admixture facility or by an outpatient pharmacy utilizing their existing staff. A pharmacist is assigned clinical responsibilities in home care and for interacting with the home health care team. The hospital usually provides a broad array of home health services, although these are operationally in a different department and may not even be on the hospital premises. Infusion pumps are either handled by the biomedical engineering department, home health services department, materials management or pharmacy department, or a combination of these. Delivery services are usually provided by the home care nurses who pick up the medications from the pharmacy. Some hospitals have created separate home infusion pharmacy satellites at another location on their campus. Others with higher volume have created a home infusion division (home health plus pharmacy) that resides off campus, sometimes as a separate corporate entity that functions like an infusion therapy specialty provider.

Home Health Agencies

Some home health agencies (HHAs) have purchased or opened their own pharmacy to supplement their home health services. These are usually large HHAs that provide a wide array of home health services and may have multiple home health offices. The pharmacy may service multiple home health branches and usually looks and operates similar to an infusion therapy specialty provider.

HME-Based Providers

HME providers may also provide home infusion pharmacy services. Usually the primary role of pharmacies is to supply respiratory therapy medications that are needed for the HME and clinical respiratory needs of their patients. The home infusion pharmacy may operate like a retail pharmacy–based infusion program or an infusion therapy specialty provider.

Infusion Therapy Specialty Providers

The infusion therapy specialty provider's sole business is usually providing home infusion therapy. Generally, this organization provides home health services, although most often, the nurses specialize in HIT only. The pharmacy plays the dominant role in this type of organization. Infusion and enteral pumps are usually the only type of medical equipment provided. Maintenance of the infusion and enteral pumps is usually performed by the company's employees, often a pharmacy technician. Infusion therapy specialty providers tend to have their own delivery staff and vans, depending on the size of the organization. This type of provider may service up to 1,000 infusion patients per day. Smaller volume, independent providers in this category also exist.

Ambulatory Infusion Centers

Ambulatory infusion centers (AICs) are usually located in a physician office building. Patients are referred here to receive their infusions in a comfortable setting. The office consists of a series of rooms, each with a relaxing chair, infusion pump, and TV, usually with movies and video games. Nurses manage and run the office and administer the medications. AICs are more cost effective than home care for patients whose infusion requires professional monitoring and may take 2 to 6 hours. In this setting, the nurse may safely care for multiple patients at the same time. AICs are generally licensed as pharmacies and have a pharmacist or pharmacy technician present to prepare the IV admixtures for the nurses to administer. The nursing staff may provide limited home care services to patients treated by the center. As discussed, a nurse will need to visit the patient in the home and provide almost all deliveries. Many ambulatory infusion centers are owned by infusion therapy specialty providers and operate in a similar manner. Others are owned by physicians or health care systems. Only AICs with a physician on the premises may bill Medicare for their infusion therapy.

In all of the preceding cases, the provider can be independent or part of a regional or national chain. Some pharmacies serve patients seen by multiple home health agencies or home medical equipment providers, and service patients in multiple states whose geography is limited only by the areas serviced by overnight delivery services. Others are single-site providers that serve only their local community.

Preparing and Dispensing Medications for Home Care

The preparation and dispensing of medications in home infusion therapy require specialized knowledge and skills. Both pharmacists and technicians from other pharmacy practices (e.g., community, hospital, or long-term care) often take at least a year before they are comfortable with the processes and differences of home care practice.

The pharmacist and technician must first be aware of the differences in pharmacy laws and regulations. In most states, HIT (even if dispensed by the hospital pharmacy) must adhere to retail pharmacy laws and special home care regulations, which are different from those of hospital pharmacy practice. For instance, inpatient pharmacists can often accept verbal orders relayed from a hospital nurse. In outpatient pharmacy regulations, most states prohibit the pharmacist from accepting a verbal prescription from anyone but the physician directly (or the physician's employee agent). When the physician gives medication orders or changes to the home care nurse, the pharmacist must call back the physician to verify the orders or receive a written order or fax directly from the physician. Prescription records and labeling requirements are different from inpatient requirements.

Second, the pharmacist and technician must be aware of the extended stability and beyond-use dates of the products they compound and dispense. In a hospital pharmacy, most parenteral medications are used within 24 hours, which is impractical in home care practice. Special packaging may be required for delivery. Products must often be packed in ice chests or Styrofoam-lined boxes for delivery in extremely hot or cold weather.

Third, pharmacists and technicians need to be aware of special preparation techniques based on the infusion pump the patient will be using. For instance, the use of a fluid-dispensing pump may be needed when preparing drugs in elastomeric devices because of the tremendous pressure needed to fill them. Technicians will need knowledge and training to compound some of the special containers used for ambulatory infusion pumps and other home care friendly devices.

Fourth, home care patients have heightened needs for confidentiality. All infusion staff must be aware of confidentiality requirements and know with whom they can share the patient's protected health information. For example, delivery staff should never leave supplies with a neighbor or other person unless specifically agreed to in advance by the patient.

Sterile compounding practices must adhere to USP Chapter <797>. Many state pharmacy laws also have special requirements for IVs prepared for home use. All pharmacists and technicians involved in compounding sterile preparations must become familiar with these regulations. USP Chapter <797> requirements vary based on the type of compounding performed and risk level or probability of contamination. Although most pharmacies prepare only low- or medium-risk preparations, they must have a primary engineering control, such as a laminar airflow workstation, biological safety cabinet, CAI that maintains an ISO Class 5 air quality (previously called a Class 100 environment since there can be only 100 particles of dust and particulates per cubic foot of air). Training and responsibilities of the people doing the compounding, policies and procedures, beyond-use dating, quality control, and cleaning and disinfection of the compounding environment are some of the other important aspects of USP Chapter <797>.

Most importantly, the timing of preparation and dispensing is critical to ensure that the delivery of a stable, sterile product is coordinated with the needs and dosing regimen of the patient and nurse who may be administering the product. This is considerably more complex and difficult than meeting the delivery needs of inpatients.

Role of Technicians in Home Infusion Therapy

The role of the technician is more varied and is more progressive in home infusion therapy than in almost any other type of pharmacy. It can be challenging and also provides the opportunity for job changes or advancement. Pharmacy technicians are responsible individuals with knowledge and skills that they may adapt to other job functions and responsibilities in home infusion pharmacy practice.

The traditional and key role of the technician in home infusion therapy is in the preparation of sterile products under the supervision of a pharmacist. Some states have more stringent requirements for technician supervision by a pharmacist in outpatient and home care settings (e.g., a pharmacist must be physically present within eyesight of the technician at all times) than in a hospital pharmacy. Some expanded health systems may have a retail or outpatient pharmacy, institutional pharmacy or hospital pharmacy, and clinic or satellite pharmacies in addition to the home infusion pharmacy, making the technician's role more varied and possibly including duties and responsibilities in these other areas as well. Other roles for pharmacy technicians in home infusion therapy include:

- Equipment management technician
- Patient service representative
- Warehouse supervisor/technician
- Purchasing coordinator
- Billing clerk/case manager
- Driver or delivery representative or coordinator.

Equipment Management Technician

Pharmacy technicians who are detail oriented and accustomed to keeping accurate detailed documentation of their work are ideally suited to becoming equipment management technicians. As previously described, the location of all infusion pumps must be known at all times. Additionally, because technicians are used to working with the metric system, syringes, and measuring devices, they can easily learn to operate the infusion pumps and test their volumetric accuracy.

Patient Service Representative

Pharmacy technicians whom enjoy dealing with people can move into the role of the patient service representative or coordinator (PSR or PSC). This person is responsible for telephoning patients to make sure they have an appropriate inventory of ancillary supplies and medications. The PSR is the patient's primary customer service representative and may assist in transmitting the patient's desires and requests to other staff in the organization. They are very helpful to the professional staff by monitoring compliance with therapy and product usage and often identify patient issues before they can become problematic. Pharmacy technicians in this role learn the use of the ancillary supplies and can help the pharmacy effectively manage supply costs. The PSR may also help coordinate deliveries with the warehouse supervisor/technician. This job is less "hands on" and is generally more of a desk job.

Warehouse Supervisor/Technician

Pharmacy technicians who enjoy a challenge and are able to multitask may have the opportunity for promotion to the warehouse supervisor/technician position. This person needs to effectively and efficiently schedule patient medication and supplies deliveries to different locations in a timely manner. Each patient's supplies must be accurately picked and packed to ensure stability and prevent breakage during delivery. With the purchasing coordinator, an appropriate inventory of ancillary supplies must be maintained. The warehouse supervisor may be responsible for ensuring that hazardous materials and wastes are safely stored, handled, and disposed of by a licensed contractor according to law and regulation.

Purchasing Coordinator

Because pharmacy technicians are accustomed to maintaining a sufficient inventory of prescription drugs and dealing with drug manufacturers and wholesalers, they may easily move into an expanded role of purchasing all of the ancillary patient supplies and office supplies required by the pharmacy. This employee may also be responsible for negotiating prices and purchasing contracts and handling drug and product recalls.

Billing Clerk/Case Manager

Pharmacy technicians who have been involved in verifying prescription drug coverage have had an introduction to the reimbursement process. The billing clerk/case manager is responsible for processing patient invoices with insurance companies, Medicare carriers (the organizations responsible for paying the bills for Medicare patients), and/or state Medicaid programs. In addition, this individual may be responsible for verifying a patient's insurance coverage, getting prior authorization from payers, and negotiating prices with insurance company case managers. This individual may also be responsible for the intake process, or obtaining the initial information from the patient and referral source (physician, hospital, insurance company) to admit the patient to service.

Driver or Delivery Representative or Coordinator

The driver or delivery representative transports the products to the patient's home and thus must be competent in infusion pump setup, troubleshooting, and the basics of equipment management; proper storage of the products in the home (i.e., which product must go in the refrigerator); infection control procedures; handling of hazardous materials and wastes; confidentiality; advanced directives and responding in emergency situations; identifying patients who may be abused or at nutritional risk; and so forth. It is important to remember that this individual may be the only employee of the home infusion provider who sees and talks to the patient directly. This individual may have to gather information from the patient or caregiver as well as provide information and care to the patient beyond routine delivery services.

Summary

Home health care is an exciting practice site for pharmacy technicians and other health professionals who received much of their training and experience in acute care or institutional settings. Not every health care provider is ready to take on the challenge of caring for patients in their home. Health care providers should consider the following points before choosing a career in home health care:

- Their interest in personalized patient care
- Their ability to adapt to changing environment
- Previous experience in compounding sterile preparations
- How to communicate with patients on sensitive matters
- Their willingness to participate in a multidisciplinary team.

As inpatient and long-term care (nursing homes) become increasingly more expensive and medical devices become safer for use by nonprofessionals, home health care will continue its rapid growth. For patients to receive the highest quality of services in their homes, health care practitioners of all disciplines—medicine, nursing, pharmacy, and therapies (occupational, physical, and respiratory)—will need to work on creative solutions for patient care delivery. With many of the newly approved medications requiring infusion, there will be an increased need for pharmacy technicians in home health care. The role of the pharmacist and pharmacy technician in home health care is nontraditional, constantly evolving, and a rewarding and challenging career opportunity. There is little doubt that many pharmacy practitioners will transition into home health care in the coming years, and that home health care will become an increasingly important practice site for pharmacy technicians in the future.

TEST YOUR KNOWLEDGE

Multiple Choice

1. How many patients were estimated to be receiving home care in the United States in 2010?
a. 100,000
b. 1,000,000
c. 7,600,000
d. 12,000,000

2. Individuals who are called home health aides are involved in providing which of the following home care services?
a. home health services
b. home infusion therapy
c. home pharmacy services
d. personal care and support services

3. Home care and hospital pharmacy practice differs in which of the following areas?
a. different pharmacy laws
b. packaging products properly for delivery
c. beyond-use dating
d. all of the above

4. Home infusion therapy specialty providers are licensed in many states as
   a. hospital pharmacies.
   b. long-term care pharmacies.
   c. community or retail pharmacies.
   d. home equipment companies.

5. Home infusion therapy services involve the provision of home pharmacy services with
   a. home health services.
   b. home medical equipment.
   c. personal care and support services.
   d. clinical respiratory services.
   e. occupational therapy.

6. Which type of equipment is most frequently used in home infusion therapy?
   a. oxygen cylinders
   b. blood glucose monitors
   c. IV pumps
   d. oximeters

7. The types of pharmacies involved in the provision of home infusion therapy include
   a. retail pharmacies.
   b. hospital pharmacies.
   c. institutional or long-term care pharmacies.
   d. all of the above.

8. The most common form of home infusion therapy is
   a. antibiotics.
   b. TPN.
   c. pain management.
   d. cancer chemotherapy.

Matching

Match the health care provider to the services rendered.

1.	______ monitors vital signs	a. pharmacy technician
2.	______ reviews and monitors drug regimens	b. home health nurse
3.	______ compounds sterile preparations	c. home health aide
4.	______ assists with activities of daily living	d. pharmacist

Fill in the Blank

1. The provision of health care services to patients in their place of residence is called ______________.

2. More than 90% of home pharmacy services are ______________.

3. ______________ is described as a medical therapy that involves the prolonged (and usually repeated) injection of pharmaceutical products, most often delivered intravenously, but sometimes delivered via other routes (e.g., subcutaneously, intramuscularly, or epidurally) into patients in their residence.

4. Pharmacy technicians who are detail oriented and accustomed to keeping accurate detailed documentation of their work are ideally suited to becoming ______________.

5. Pharmacy technicians who enjoy a challenge and are able to multitask may have the opportunity for promotion to the ______________.

Suggested Readings

American Society of Health-System Pharmacists. (2000). ASHP guidelines on quality assurance for pharmacy-prepared sterile products. *American Journal of Hospital Pharmacy, 5*, 1150–1169.

American Society of Health-System Pharmacists. (2007). *Best practices for hospital & health-system pharmacy: Position and guidance documents of ASHP, 2006–2007*. Bethesda, MD: Author.

Buchanan, E. C., & Schneider, P. J. (2009). *Compounding sterile preparations* (3rd ed.). Bethesda, MD: American Society of Health-System Pharmacists.

Catania, P. N., & Rosner, M. M. (Eds.). (1994). *Home health care practice* (2nd ed.). Palo Alto, CA: Markets Research.

Congress, Office of Technology Assessment. (May 1992). *Home drug infusion therapy under Medicare* (OTA-H-509). Washington, DC: Author.

Conners, R. B., & Winters, R. W. (Eds.). (1995). *Home infusion therapy: Current status and future trends.* Chicago, IL: American Hospital Publishing.

U.S. Pharmacopeial Convention. (2012). Chapter <797>: Pharmaceutical compounding—Sterile preparations. In *United States pharmacopeia 36th ed./ National formulary*. Rockville, MD: Author.

Websites

Centers for Medicare and Medicaid Services www.cms.gov

National Association for Home Care (NAHC) www.nahc.org

National Home Infusion Association (NHIA) www.nhia.org

Palmetto GBA, National Supplier Clearing House www.palmettogba.com

CHAPTER 4

Long-Term Care

Competencies

Upon completion of this chapter, the reader should be able to:

1. Define long-term care, as well as who receives care and how the care is provided.
2. Identify the three different types of long-term care facilities by sponsorship, and explain the historical significance of each one.
3. Identify the major sources of funding for the long-term care field.
4. Differentiate between a service pharmacist and a consultant pharmacist.
5. Describe the supportive role of the pharmacy profession to the nursing profession.
6. Discuss the role of the pharmacist and pharmacy technician in the delivery of long-term care.

Key Terms

adult day care facility
assisted living facility
automatic stop order
consultant pharmacist
long-term care (LTC)
medication regimen review (MRR)
not-for-profit facility
nursing home
preferred drug provider (PDP)
proprietary facility
rehabilitation facility
skilled nursing facility (SNF)

Introduction

Society has struggled with the obligation to care for those who can no longer care for themselves. Historically, this obligation fell to immediate family members or people of the same religion, tribe, or national background. The very earliest health care institutions had religious or fraternal philosophies. Individuals not fortunate enough to be taken in by one of these charitable organizations were forced to live on the streets or to seek admission to institutions created by the governing entity (e.g., the county poorhouse, the almshouse, or the local asylum).

In 1965, Congress passed two laws that would have a profound effect on this historical situation. The Medicare and Medicaid programs changed the way America provided for its frail and elderly populations. Under Medicare, the elderly were guaranteed health care and, just as importantly, the children of the elderly were absolved of the legal responsibility of paying for care for their parents. The Medicaid legislation guaranteed payment for those deemed to be indigent. Thus, a new type of medical welfare was created. With these sound sources of income guaranteed, the growth of institutions willing to provide care mushroomed. Just as a generation earlier Social Security had guaranteed a source of income to the elderly and blind, these two pieces of legislation, commonly referred to as Articles 18 and 19, changed the way care was financed and who would ultimately pay the cost.

> **long-term care (LTC)** health care provided in an organized medical facility for patients requiring chronic or extended treatment

Long-Term Care

Long-term care (LTC) is defined as the provision of health and personal care (meeting physical and emotional needs) to individuals over an extended period of time. Long-term care may be required due to traumatic injury, disability, or acute and chronic illness. The need for long-term care may be temporary, spanning a few weeks or months, or ongoing over a period of many years. According to the Administration on Aging, in 2010 about 9 million Americans over the age of 65 needed long-term care services. By 2020 that number will increase to 12 million. Although most people who need long-term care are ages 65 or older, a person can need long-term care services at any age. According to the U.S. Census Bureau, 40 percent of people currently receiving long-term care are adults 18 to 64 years old.

Long-term care may be provided in a number of settings. Most long-term care is provided at home through family members or personal care providers such as home health aides. **Adult day care facilities** provide long-term care that supplements the care an individual may be receiving at home by providing opportunities for socialization and care while the primary caregiver is at work. Individuals who are unable to remain in the home for care but who do not need the level of care provided in nursing homes may reside in **assisted living facilities**. These types of facilities provide a community setting for the residents while having basic needs provided such as meal service, assistance with activities of daily living, and emergency support if necessary. **Nursing homes** or **skilled nursing facilities (SNF)** provide long-term care to individuals who need extensive medical care as well as personal care around the clock. Rehabilitation services are also provided by nursing homes for patients requiring intensive subacute (nonhospital) physical, occupational, and/or speech therapies for return to the community or assisted living environments.

> **adult day care facility** an institution for adults that provides long-term care that supplements the care an individual may be receiving at home by providing opportunities for socialization and care while the primary caregiver is at work
>
> **assisted living facility** a community-like institution that provides care (such as meal service) for individuals who can no longer remain in their homes, but who do not need the level of care provided in nursing homes
>
> **nursing home** or **skilled nursing facility (SNF)** an institution that provides long-term care to individuals needing extensive medical care as well as personal care around the clock

Business Models for Nursing Homes or Skilled Nursing Facilities

proprietary facility a type of long-term care facility that is owned by one person, a family, a partnership, or a corporation; is run like a corporate business; and makes a profit for its investors

not-for-profit facility a type of long-term care facility that does not pay a profit with its extra income, but rather reinvests the excess revenue back into programs or building improvements for the benefit of the serviced population; these facilities are not obligated to pay taxes and have the ability to raise funds for charitable purposes

The three types of business models for long-term care are government-sponsored facilities, **proprietary facilities**, and **not-for-profit facilities**. The smallest percentage of LTC facilities are those institutions run by the government at the federal, state, or county level. These may be veterans' homes and hospitals or county-owned homes run for the benefit of their citizens or some other similar grouping. These are the direct descendents of poorhouses and almshouses. They provide "safety net" services that other facilities are financially unable to provide.

The second type of nursing home is referred to as *proprietary*. This type of long-term care facility is by far the most numerous. These are owned by one person, a family, a partnership, or a corporation. They are run like a corporate business and should make a profit for their investors. The most advanced types of this kind are the large corporations, like Beverly Enterprises, that are traded on the stock market. Proprietary facilities are typically the most financially efficient model for providing services.

The last major type of long-term care facility is referred to as a voluntary or not-for-profit facility. These homes are the direct descendants of those charitable institutions that took care of their own particular followers. The term *voluntary* refers to the composition of the board of directors, who serve without personal benefit, but do so from a wish to benefit society in some fashion. The secondary term, *not for profit*, defines what these institutions do with extra income. Instead of paying a profit or dividend to their shareholders like a for-profit institution rightly does, these facilities are obliged to reinvest the excess revenue back into programs or building improvements for the benefit of the serviced population. These facilities are not obligated to pay taxes and have the ability to raise funds for charitable purposes.

Regulation of Long-Term Care Facilities

The various types of facilities providing long-term care have differing levels of regulations, which makes for a complex system of laws, regulations, directives, and governmental oversight activities at the federal, state, and local municipality levels. Sometimes these regulations are similar, sometimes they are not. The Centers for Medicare and Medicaid Services (CMS) has taken an extremely active role in standardizing these rules, regulations, and directives for the entire nation. Still, each state may create a more stringent set of rules, and the facilities must comply with those higher standards. The length and breadth of these rules, regulations, and directives are so extensive that it has been opined that only the nuclear energy field has more rules.

Regulations related to provision of pharmaceutical care range from prescription transcription (i.e., only a licensed nurse may take a telephone order from an off-site physician) to (most recently) a standardized prescription for all physicians. Additionally, storage must be secure and in some cases must be in a double-locked, permanently affixed cabinet with a certain thickness of construction. Controlled drugs must be counted by both off-going and on-coming licensed nursing personnel before keys are transferred. Proper destruction of unused or expired drugs has its own protocol. Recent regulations further dictate how pain-relieving transdermal patches must be handled. The contents and use of the emergency box (a kit containing medications that can be used in an emergency situation) is also well defined by regulations. Most recently, CMS has issued extensive new regulations concerning gradual dose reductions and tapering of medications and discontinuance of unnecessary medication.

Although many of these rules and regulations are written for the macromanagement of facilities, one example of a very direct rule (with implications every day on every unit on the micromanagement level) is the regulation that the medication nurse has only a 1-hour grace period on either side of the stated medication time to successfully complete his or her medication administration drug pass. The challenge is to administer all of the drugs that must be given to the entire population that must be medicated, with the proper protocols, within this time span. During annual surveys, the medication nurse is closely watched by state inspectors for possible errors. The error rate cannot exceed 5 percent; otherwise the facility receives an unfavorable citation. This margin of error actually creates a de facto threshold of 95 percent for passing—a very high standard to achieve in any field and typical of the regulations that the long-term care industry struggles to meet.

Funding for Long-Term Care

Funding for long-term care can be divided into three primary categories: (1) tax dollars through Medicare and Medicaid, (2) private pay, and (3) third-party payers (**Figure 4-1**). For information related to reimbursement for services, see Chapter 32.

Medicare and Medicaid

Medicare Parts A, B, C, and D account for a large percentage of the dollars spent in health care. Part A usually covers hospital stays and some nursing home time. Part B covers physicians' visits, specialized tests, and supplies. Part C comprises the managed care and/or hospice benefit. Medicare is funded partially by the government through taxes and premiums for individuals and is part of the Social Security benefits package. Medicaid, which is considered the payer of last resort, is an entitlement program paid by federal, state, and local taxes. When all other sources of revenue are exhausted, Medicaid pays for the legitimate costs associated with providing care. In skilled nursing facilities, Medicare coverage is limited to up to 100 days, 80 of which have a significant (approximately 20%) copay requirement. To access this benefit, the patient must be considered to be receiving a "skilled service." Most frail elderly do not qualify and thus do not receive these covered days. **Rehabilitation facilities** (which provide services to patients recovering

rehabilitation facility an institution that provides services to patients recovering from acute or traumatic events on a short-term basis

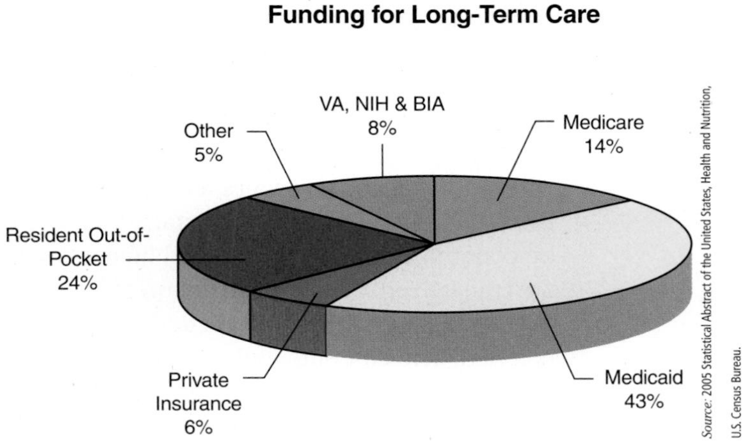

FIGURE 4-1 Funding for long-term care.

from acute or traumatic events on a short-term basis) are more successful in meeting these Medicare eligibility requirements. Many community elderly still are under the assumption that Medicare will pay for long-term care. Medicare functions better for acute or short-term episodes and not continuing care needs.

Medicare Part D is a federal government program that began on January 1, 2006. With this legislation, all individuals who qualify for Medicare Part A or Medicare Part B can purchase drug coverage for their needs. Dually eligible patients who have both Medicare and Medicaid are not subject to copays. The scope of the coverage differs with the plans. Participation is voluntary, copays vary greatly, and as first conceived, gaps exist after certain cost levels are reached (termed "doughnut hole") and before so-termed "catastrophic coverage" begins.

Historically, it is of note that pharmaceutical costs to the long-term care facility under the previous all-inclusive rate system were often as high or higher than the entire food budget for the facility. This was the impetus for restricted formularies, cost containment initiatives, and pressure on the prescribing physicians to be mindful of costs. This latter was only mildly successful, because most physicians were only somewhat aware of drug costs. Suggestions from both the vendor and consultant pharmacy professionals were often ignored or delayed in the day-to-day business of rendering health care.

preferred drug provider (PDP) a gatekeeper between individual and government payers under Medicare Part D

Under Medicare D, all patients are assigned to **preferred drug providers (PDPs)**, which act as gatekeepers between the individual and government payers. Each PDP has its own formulary, and there was much initial confusion about what was the best particular PDP for an individual. Additionally, drugs can be removed or added to these formularies, which could then mandate a switch from one PDP to a different one to obtain optimal coverage. If a nonformulary medication or a noncovered medication is ordered, a prior approval for that medication from the PDP is required. A technician, in consultation with a pharmacist, often assists in collecting the required information from the prescriber to obtain the prior approval. In the first year of use of PDPs, nursing home personnel saw an increase not only in the costs of drugs but in the amount of drugs prescribed.

Private Pay

Individuals who have assets (wealth) to pay for the care they receive until such time that their resources are low enough to be eligible for Medicaid are classified as *private pays*. As stated previously, however, these individuals may qualify for some coverage under Medicare if they are receiving a skilled service. Since the Medicare program is essentially an insurance program, one's level of wealth would not prohibit benefiting from this coverage. However, when the allotted Medicare days are used up, the patient would have to pay with his or her own resources.

Third-Party Payers

This category of nongovernmental payers includes insurance companies that have sold long-term care policies or health maintenance organizations (HMOs) that offer Medicare supplemental/managed care coverage. These managed care companies usually negotiate a price for those patients they are obligated to care for. In many instances these agreements cover all services, so it is important that the rate is sufficient to cover costly items such as prostheses and pharmaceuticals. These entities watch costs very closely and often dictate what drug can be used by means of a restricted formulary. Additionally, these organizations require extensive documentation from the provider periodically during the patient's stay to justify continued treatment.

Nursing Home Operation

For the most part, the challenge to those who operate nursing homes is to balance the rules, regulations, and efficient practices against the need to recognize these patients as people who need to continue to participate in society and enjoy what life has to offer them. Because government policy and funding have created an impetus to admit skilled care patients, the population of today's nursing home does not resemble the population of 10 or 20 years ago. Today's facilities operate at much the same level of intensity as a small community hospital. Floor staffing in the modern long-term care facility consists of, most commonly, a charge nurse, possibly a second nurse on busy shifts, and several certified nursing assistants. Physicians, therapists, and consultants will all be at the facility briefly, but the great bulk of the work is carried out by the nursing staff.

A model nursing unit will have 40 to 45 patients, each of whom will receive an average of nine prescriptions daily (with some drugs given several times a day). This brings the minimum total to about 400 doses daily that the charge nurses must administer. The challenge for the pharmacist and the pharmacy technician working with these types of facilities is to communicate the proper information so that the drug achieves the desired effect. Being mindful that long-term care facilities care for residents 24 hours a day, 7 days a week, it is likely that many different individuals will perform the same function. The labeling of medications must be clear to avoid misinterpretations by staff members.

Nurses are charged with the responsibility of properly administering medication to the residents. One popular medication system that is an effective aid for the charge nurse is the unit-dose system. In this system, individual pills are packaged in blister packs on a 30-day calendar card so that the nurse can check at any time to verify that the dosage has been given (**Figure 4-2**).

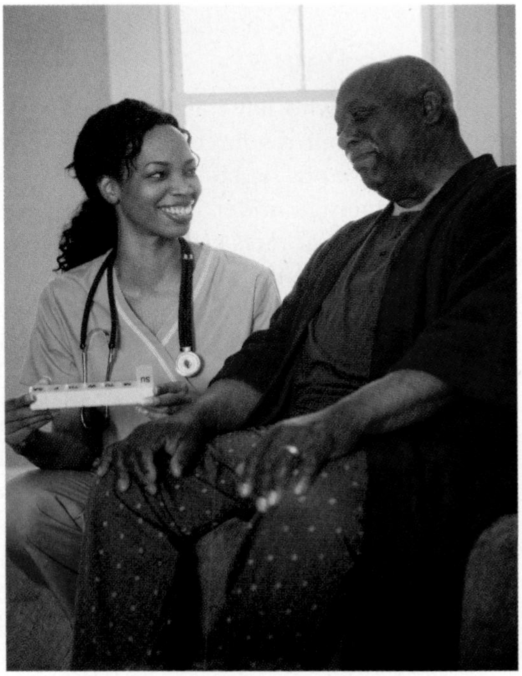

FIGURE 4-2 The nursing staff is responsible for properly and effectively administering medications to patients.

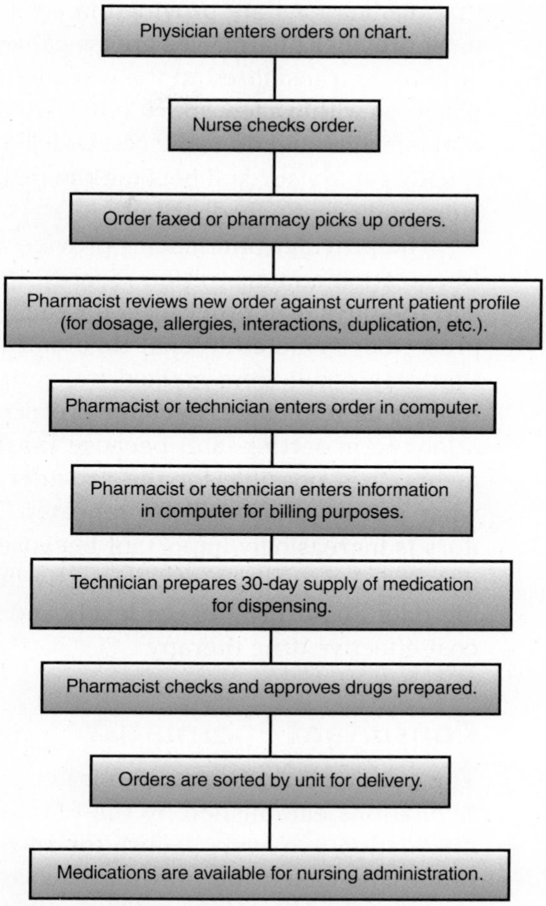
Physician enters orders on chart.
Nurse checks order.
Order faxed or pharmacy picks up orders.
Pharmacist reviews new order against current patient profile (for dosage, allergies, interactions, duplication, etc.).
Pharmacist or technician enters order in computer.
Pharmacist or technician enters information in computer for billing purposes.
Technician prepares 30-day supply of medication for dispensing.
Pharmacist checks and approves drugs prepared.
Orders are sorted by unit for delivery.
Medications are available for nursing administration.

FIGURE 4-3 A medication order-entry flowchart.

automatic stop order a requirement for particular drugs that ensures the proper monitoring of drug usage; mandates that a patient's drug response be reevaluated after specific time intervals; a medical decision is then made to continue the drug, change the dosage, or discontinue the drug

The medical staff, in coordination with the pharmacy consultant, should develop policies for an **automatic stop order** for particular drugs (e.g., antibiotics and steroids). These drugs and others require that the patient's drug response be reevaluated after specific time intervals (e.g., 1 week, 10 days, or 1 month). At that time a medical decision is made to continue the drug, change the dosage, or discontinue the drug. This method is designed to ensure the proper monitoring of drug usage.

Any procedure or helpful practice that enables the pharmacist or pharmacy technician to assist the nurse in providing a safe medication delivery system is of great value (**Figure 4-3**). In the future, an automated dispensing machine may be used to blend nursing's need for access with pharmacy's need to control.

Pharmaceutical Personnel in Long-Term Care

Concerning the business aspects of securing prescriptions, long-term care facilities use several types of arrangements to obtain the prescriptions their residents require. Larger facilities may have an in-house pharmacy staffed by registered pharmacists and pharmacy technicians. Most small to moderate-sized facilities, however, find it more feasible to obtain medications from a vendor or service pharmacy, commonly referred to as a *provider pharmacy.* In an effort to ensure that medications are provided in a timely manner to the long-term care facility, most provider pharmacies are available 24 hours a day, 7 days a week. Physicians' orders are transmitted to the provider pharmacy, and the filled prescriptions are delivered within a few hours, often two to three times a day, depending on the need of the facility and its residents. Drugs are then usually distributed to the units by the RN supervisor and become the responsibility of the charge nurse to properly store and eventually distribute.

The provider pharmacies provide an additional service by printing the MAR (medication administration record), the TAR (treatment administration record), and the physician order form for each resident, which saves both the nurse and prescriber some additional time and helps reduce potential medication errors that may result from manual transcriptions. They also produce administrative reports as requested. Because prescriptions must be renewed every 30 days in a long-term setting, and because most of the prescriptions are for chronic ailments, it is possible for the provider pharmacy to forecast, to a large extent, what prescriptions will be repeated. The database maintained by these vendors is increasingly important because it can be used to meet the government's demands for quality assurance activities. It can also be used for preparing trending data about drug usage levels and pharmaceutical cost data for monitoring cost-effective drug therapy.

Consultant Pharmacist

> **consultant pharmacist** individual responsible for monitoring drug usage and drug therapy of residents in skilled nursing facilities
>
> **medication regimen review (MRR)** the process established by the CMS to provide appropriate drug therapy for patients; it requires a licensed pharmacist to review medication use every month for all residents in a skilled nursing facility

The **consultant pharmacist** is necessary to the long-term care facility. Federal regulations established by the CMS require that a licensed pharmacist review medication use every month for all residents in a skilled nursing facility. This process is called the **medication regimen review (MRR)**. The need for or extent of the MRR in other LTC facilities, such as assisted living facilities or individual residence alternatives, varies from state to state. These reviews are usually performed on site so that the pharmacist can easily access the resident's medical chart. The chart contains information such as laboratory values, physician and nursing notes, and MARs. All this information is helpful for identifying a medication problem. The consultant pharmacist reports his or her findings to the medical director, director of nursing, administrator, and the attending physicians (**Figure 4-4**).

In December 2006, revisions were made to the regulations involving the medication regimen review and the role of the consultant pharmacist. These revisions put greater emphasis on closely evaluating whether each medication prescribed is necessary and the consideration of tapering and/or eliminating unnecessary drug consumption. Special attention is given to the use of certain medications known to be a problem in the elderly. In some situations, the consultant pharmacist is now required to perform the MRR more often than once a month.

In addition to the medication regimen reviews, oversight of all pharmacy services is the responsibility of the consultant pharmacist. This careful supervision helps ensure the safe and effective use of medications as well as control of and accountability for the medications throughout the facility. This may include working on policies and procedures, nursing unit inspections, and in-service education to nursing personnel. The consultant pharmacist also works with administration and the medical and nursing staff to help control medication costs and on preparation for annual surveys and the proper disposition of prescription medication. While the actual MRR must be performed by a licensed pharmacist, a technician can be helpful with these other activities.

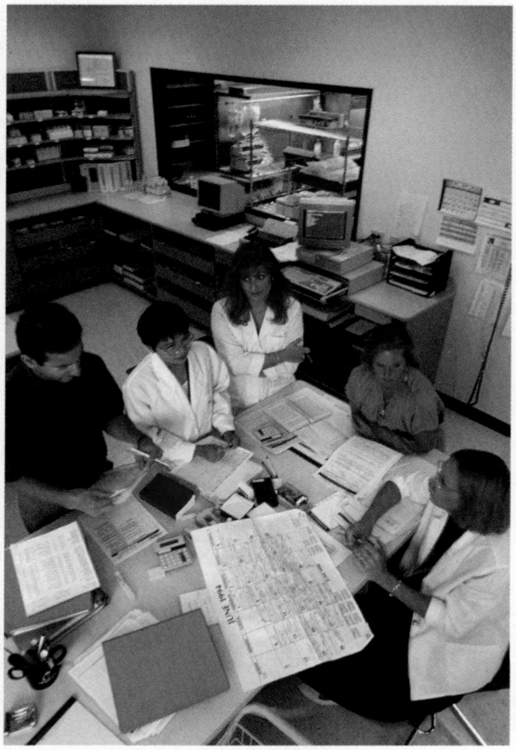

FIGURE 4-4 The consultant pharmacist reports quarterly to the Pharmaceutical Services Committee to provide guidance relating to pharmacy services and unnecessary medications, and to ensure safe administration and education for staff members.

Role of the Pharmacy Technician in a Long-Term Care Pharmacy

When pharmacy technicians began working in the long-term care setting back in the late 1970s, their roles were very much undefined. They provided a "supportive role" to the pharmacist; however, their particular duties varied from facility to facility. They were considered to be in direct competition with pharmacists because they were, in fact, replacing some pharmacist positions and, hence, were not very welcomed by established pharmacies and other health-related facilities such as LTC settings and hospitals.

Over time, especially during the 1980s, the role of the pharmacist expanded and transitioned into the role of the "medication expert." Pharmacists who worked in these settings found themselves now performing MRRs and were now active members of clinical committees such as the pharmacy and therapeutic committee, quality improvement, cost containment, and so forth. They also made rounds with physicians and other clinical disciplines as needed and frequently intervened when medication-related issues arose. Finally, they found themselves consistently on the phone answering questions related to medication therapy management from nurses, physicians, and other disciplines.

As the role of pharmacists expanded and evolved into other areas, the medication orders themselves still needed to be filled. The medications still needed to be prepared, labeled, and delivered. The role of the pharmacy technician now developed into a perfect fit in the LTC setting. These valuable individuals were now able to fill the void left by the pharmacist as the pharmacy technician stepped in to perform and complete the manual work needed to prepare, label, and deliver medications. This freed up the pharmacist from performing the manual job functions.

Let's take a look at some of the job functions now performed by the pharmacy technician in the LTC setting.

Procurement (Ordering of Medications)

Today, almost all pharmacies order medications online from their respective wholesalers. Pharmacy technicians are trained in not only ordering medications, but in maintaining stocking and par (periodic automatic replenishment) levels as they relate to prescription and over-the-counter (OTC) medications as well as other areas such as surgical supplies.

Medication Preparation

Pharmacy technicians play a vital role in the preparation of medications. Their role varies from facility to facility, however it can start with entering the prescription into the computer system, retrieving the medication from stock, labeling the medication, and delivering the medication to the nursing unit or patient. All of this is performed under the supervision of a pharmacist.

Unit Inspections

In the LTC setting, medications are stored within the medication room and medication cart with access provided and afforded to the nurse. These medications must be checked at least once monthly by a member of the pharmacy department. Some of the parameters include ensuring the following:

- The prescription and OTC medications are within the manufacturer's expiration date.
- Internal and external medications are separated on different shelves or cabinets.
- Appropriate auxiliary labels are affixed to medications as needed (i.e., "For External Use Only").
- The refrigerator temperature is maintained according to USP standards (36° to 46° C).
- All multidose vials (e.g., insulins and purified protein derivatives) are dated once opened, then discarded within 28 days of opening.
- The emergency box is sealed and secured and medications are within the manufacturer's expiration date.
- Controlled substances are stored in a double-locked cabinet and are accounted for according to governmental and facility standards.
- Current and appropriate references are available for the unit staff (*Physician's Desk Reference*, *Nursing Drug Handbook*, etc.).

After-Hours Medication Cabinets/Storage Areas

Facilities that utilize the services of an on-site pharmacy are allowed to utilize after-hours medication cabinets/storage areas. The idea is to provide the facility with access to medications for patients 24 hours per day, 7 days per week. Pharmacy technicians are involved in the initial stocking and maintenance of these medication areas. These areas follow a dynamic process in that the medications periodically are updated and removed based on their usage or lack of usage. Pharmacy technicians can track the movement of these medications and recommend which medications should or should not be restocked. The pharmacy technician is also responsible for the replenishment and accountability of the medications stored in the after-hours cabinet.

In the LTC setting, medications are not usually prepared as commonly seen in the community setting where prescription vials are utilized. Medications in the LTC setting are usually dispensed in various dispensing forms:

- Manufacturer/single-dose unit-dose packaging strips
- Prepared unit-dose packaging (i.e., "bingo cards")
- High-speed multidose packaging according to the time of administration
- On-site remote dispensing utilizing real-time dosing administration.

All of these dispensing formulations require the pharmacy technician to be trained and proficient in the operation and maintenance of such equipment and machinery. This can involve on-site training in the pharmacy or LTC setting or even travel to a manufacturer's corporate site for more intensive training and proficiency. The pharmacy technician is the individual who will be called on to operate, maintain, troubleshoot, and maximize the potential of an automated dispensing machine. Automated dispensing machines can dispense medications for any desired time period from 24 hours to 30 days.

Emerging Challenges for the Pharmaceutical and Nursing Professional

Several of the growing concerns in the pharmaceutical field include the somewhat different pharmacokinetics of drug absorption, distribution, metabolism, and excretion of drugs in the elderly. Perhaps one of the most pressing concerns is the sheer number of prescriptions that a typical resident needs and the corresponding direct relationship for potential drug interactions as the number of drugs increases. The changing standard of practice in the treatment of heart disease, for example, currently calls for taking several drugs to control the condition. This is a typical situation in the treatment of many diseases.

This creates a growing problem for the nurse in a long-term care facility. We are rapidly approaching a point where the number of prescriptions for a patient is so large that it becomes physically difficult, if not impossible, for the elderly resident to ingest all of the medications. These residents often have difficulty with swallowing or cannot follow instructions. Increasingly, both State and Federal nursing home surveyors are holding nurses to guidelines listed in the package insert of a prescription. This means that for each prescription, 8 ounces of water should be ingested; a certain time must elapse between administration of certain drugs or between drugs and meals; and so forth. It falls to the pharmaceutical professionals to develop other means of delivering the medication. Long-acting injections (used for certain psychotropics, subdermal implants, and transdermal patches) are just the beginning of what is now the greatest challenge to the delivery of good health care.

Recent legislation now allows hospice providers to serve the dying population in long-term care facilities. Before this change, hospice services were mostly home based. Hospice personnel have developed expertise in pain management. This area is fast becoming not just a concern for the dying, but for all patients who could have a better quality of life if they were able to be more comfortable and less controlled by their medical conditions.

These concerns relating to the number of drugs and patient response present challenges to the consulting and provider pharmacist and medical and nursing personnel, who must be vigilant and work together to provide safe and meaningful drug therapy to the residents in long-term care.

The Future of Pharmacy in Long-Term Care

Pharmacy was probably the first of the caring professions to utilize the computer. Certainly, the logic and structure of the pharmacy is well suited to the strengths of the computer. In the future this natural linkage will become even stronger. With the advent of subacute care in long-term care facilities (with intravenous therapy, as well as a completely new spectrum of high-tech drugs), the need for rational administration and continuous quality improvement will grow. As LTC facilities increase in computer sophistication, information will be rapidly exchanged. Today several computer programs are available that allow physicians to order medications electronically through a computer station or a handheld device. The nurse can review the computer screen and then is able to easily send the vendor pharmacy the computerized order, which can then be immediately produced. The savings in time and the reduction in the potential for errors will be great. Quality assurance and risk management functions can also be set up to shadow these prescribing programs.

On the other end of the spectrum, healthier older adults may gravitate to the assisted living environment—where there is less direct supervision—at a time when their ability to comprehend medication directions may be diminishing. Hence, the challenge will be to package, label, and safeguard the product so that it will be used properly for maximum benefit. A relatively new concept for this market is the color-coded cartridge delivery system. Medications are preloaded into different colored cartridges for different hours of the day. For example, 9 a.m. medications will be in the yellow cartridge, noon meds will be blue, with evening meds being packaged in a different color. This will undoubtedly generate more setup responsibilities for the pharmacy technician, but will also help the elderly maintain independence and safety while getting all of their needed medications.

Cost containment will increase in importance as the managed health care model becomes more popular. Some experts predict that the managed care model will depend more heavily on drug therapy as opposed to more expensive invasive procedures, whereas others maintain that more drugs will become over-the-counter items, a situation that presents a challenge for the dispensing pharmacist to be able to monitor and avoid drug interactions with prescription and nonprescription drugs. Access to databases and "smart cards" that contain entire drug histories for individuals could help in these situations.

Extensive research is being carried out in the use of psychotropic drugs for geriatric (elderly) patients at home. The target goal is to find effective psychotropic drugs with maximum therapeutic benefits and fewer undesirable side effects (e.g., lethargy, apathy, and ataxia). The pharmacist consultant, in conjunction with the medical staff, needs to maintain up-to-date information to provide effective therapy. The future may well see increased use of combination drugs, longer intervals between doses, implants, pumps, disks, or rods. All of these innovations need to be understood, blended for maximum benefit, and tracked for safety. These functions will be within the scope of the pharmacy technicians who understand computers and who stay on the cutting edge of this information explosion.

Summary

Pharmaceutical care provided in long-term care facilities will continue to be a vital service to the care and well-being of the growing elderly population. The challenge will be to provide rational drug therapy that is safe, effective, and affordable. The expanding geriatric population will need help, direction, and counseling to maximize good health. The challenge for the pharmaceutical professional is to make information clear and easily understood for a population with increasing deficits.

TEST YOUR KNOWLEDGE

Multiple Choice

1. Legislation that changed the way long-term care was financed was
  a. Medicare.
  b. Medicaid.
  c. Social Security.
  d. both Medicare and Medicaid.

2. The most common type of long-term care facility is
  a. voluntary, not for profit.
  b. government sponsored.
  c. proprietary.
  d. hospice.

3. The most important goal of a long-term care pharmacist is to
  a. fill the prescription per the physician's order.
  b. write the directions so that no error can be made.
  c. help the nursing personnel properly administer the medication through education and support.
  d. perform all of the above.

4. Drug regimen reviews on each patient are required
  a. upon admission.
  b. upon change of orders.
  c. monthly.
  d. weekly.

5. The consultant pharmacist must report errors and discrepancies to
  a. the medical physician.
  b. the director of nursing services.
  c. the administrator.
  d. all of the above.

6. Technicians will most probably be responsible for
  a. the packaging of the unit-dose cards.
  b. credit on returned drugs.
  c. administrative computer duties.
  d. all of the above.

7. Managed care companies will probably
  a. use more drug therapy than invasive procedures.
  b. become more aggressive in cost-cutting procedures.
  c. exercise greater control over physicians' prescribing habits.
  d. all of the above.

8. To survive in the future, pharmacists and technicians will have to become comfortable with
   a. quality assurance activities.
   b. continuous monitoring/risk identification.
   c. computerization/information sharing.
   d. all of the above.

9. The governmental body driving the standardization of rules and regulations for long-term care facilities is the
   a. Department of Health and Human Services.
   b. Centers for Disease Control and Prevention.
   c. Centers for Medicare and Medicaid Services.
   d. federal Drug Enforcement Agency.

10. Funding for prescription medications is covered under
   a. Medicare Part A.
   b. Medicare Part B.
   c. Medicare Part C.
   d. Medicare Part D.

Fill in the Blank

1. The provision of health and personal care (meeting physical and emotional needs) to individuals over an extended period of time is called _______________.
2. _______________ covers physician visits, specialized tests, and supplies.
3. A gatekeeper between the individual and government payer provided under Medicare Part D is the _______________.
4. _______________ covers hospital stays and some nursing home time.
5. _______________ provide long-term care to individuals needing extensive medical care as well as personal care around the clock.

References

Dean, N.L. (2007, April). *An extra dose of safety.* Health Management Technology. Retrieved from www.healthmgttech.com/features/2007_april/0407extra_dose.aspx

Hagland, M. (2006, September). *Right patient, right dose*. Healthcare Informatics. Retrieved from www.healthcare-informatics.com.

The long-term care state operations manual. HcPro Inc., 483.60 Pharmacy Services. Retrieved from http://www.hcpro.com

U.S. Census Bureau. (2007). *2005 Statistical abstract of the United States, health and nutrition.* Washington, DC: Author.

Websites

National Care Planning Council www.longtermcarelink.net

National Clearinghouse for Long-Term Care Information www.longtermcare.gov

U.S. Department of Health and Human Services Medicare website www.medicare.gov

CHAPTER

5

Community Pharmacy Practice

Competencies

Upon completion of this chapter, the reader should be able to:

1. Define community pharmacy as a branch of ambulatory care.
2. Discuss the knowledge and skills necessary to practice as a pharmacy technician in the community pharmacy setting.
3. Differentiate among available opportunities within community pharmacy.
4. Outline the process of preparing a prescription for dispensing.

Key Terms

ambulatory care
chain pharmacy
collaborative drug therapy agreement
independent pharmacy
medication therapy management (MTM)

Introduction

This chapter provides an overview of community pharmacy practice, highlighting the role of the pharmacy technician. The various types of community pharmacy settings are explored, with an emphasis on the skills and attributes of this popular and rewarding area of practice.

Community Pharmacy Practice

Community pharmacy is a diverse, dynamic, and rapidly evolving practice environment comprised of several different practice settings and offering many opportunities for the pharmacy practitioner. First and foremost, community pharmacy is a practice environment that requires good people skills and excellent communication, because the pharmacy practitioner deals with patients on a daily basis (**Figure 5-1**). Pharmacy technicians play a vital role in the community pharmacy, assisting the pharmacist in preparing prescriptions, collecting information from patients, and performing several important functions that are discussed later in this chapter.

Pharmacists have been at the top of the Gallup poll as the most trusted professionals for years, and many people use their community pharmacist as their sole source of health care information. Most people visit their community pharmacy more often than any other health care setting and look to their community pharmacist for information, advice, and counseling. In the community pharmacy, practitioners can recommend a cough and cold remedy one minute and then help a transplant patient decipher his complex medication regimen in the next. Basically, in the community pharmacy, practitioners have to be ready for anything, and every day offers new and exciting opportunities to assist people in improving their health care and quality of life.

Community pharmacy is a branch of ambulatory care practice. **Ambulatory care** simply means that the patients being treated are not hospitalized or

> **ambulatory care**
> care provided to individuals who do not require either an acute care (hospital) or chronic care (skilled nursing facility) setting; patients come in for treatment and go home the same day; they are not hospitalized

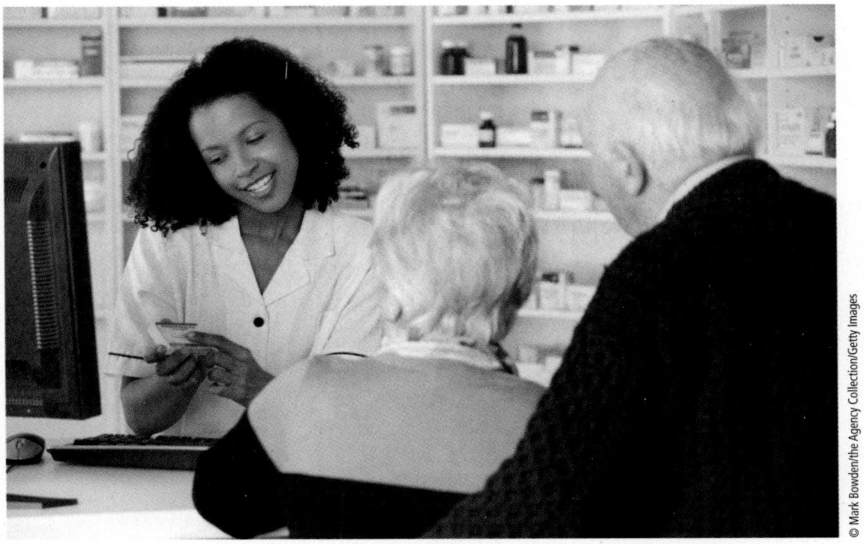
© Mark Bowden/the Agency Collection/Getty Images

FIGURE 5-1 Working in a community pharmacy requires good interpersonal skills.

institutionalized. Other ambulatory care settings include physicians' offices, clinics, and emergency departments. Another term for ambulatory care is *outpatient setting*. When patients are in the hospital or reside in a long-term care facility, they are referred to as *inpatients* because they are living, usually temporarily, in the facility. When they are residing at home, they are referred to as *outpatients*. Community pharmacy is recognized as an outpatient or ambulatory care setting.

The number of prescriptions being filled has increased dramatically during the past few years and is only expected to keep rising. According to CMS, in 2010 alone, $259.1 billion was spent on prescription drugs in the outpatient setting. One of the primary reasons the number of prescriptions is rising is the aging of the population. People are living longer. As they age, their requirements for medications increase and, hence, more prescriptions are needed. In addition to the aging of the population, advances in medicine are allowing physicians to treat patients without putting them in the hospital, adding to the numbers of prescriptions processed in the outpatient or community pharmacy setting. Also, more and more medications become available each year, which results in more prescriptions being generated. These factors, along with an increased access to insurance programs, add up to more prescriptions requiring processing in community pharmacies.

Because of the rapid growth in the number of prescriptions being filled each year, the community pharmacy environment needs to be open to change and adapt to meeting increased needs. One change we are consistently witnessing is the growing role of technology in processing prescriptions (**Figure 5-2**). Virtually all community pharmacies utilize computers and some even use robots to varying degrees in the prescription-filling process.

Besides keeping a computerized patient profile, computers in the pharmacy can be used to screen phone calls, accept refill orders, scan prescriptions to prevent errors, count the units of medication, fill the container, and label the vial. Computers are also used to alert the pharmacist to drug interactions and transmit insurance information to a patient's insurance company. Many pharmacies utilize e-prescribing technology, in which a prescription can be generated at the prescriber's office and electronically transmitted directly into the processing computer

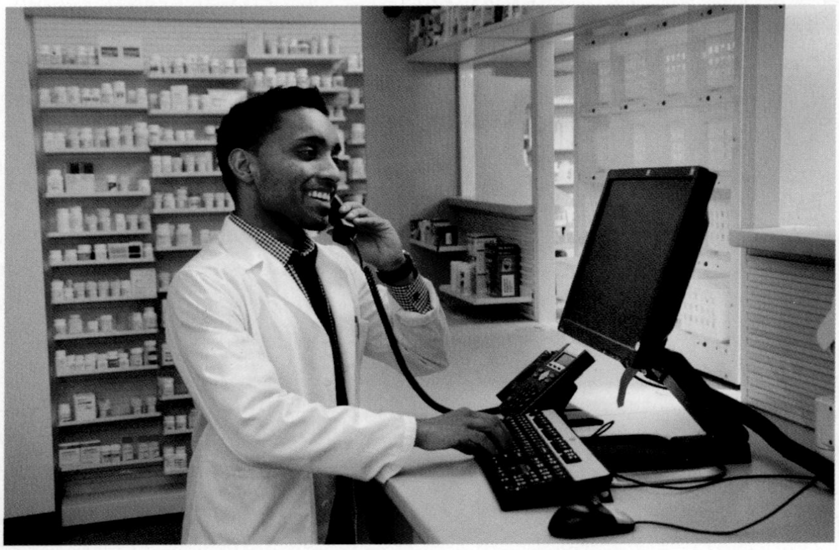

FIGURE 5-2 A solid foundation of computer skills is necessary to work in the community pharmacy.

at the local pharmacy, eliminating the need to enter information from a paper prescription. In the future we may not even be surprised to see various types of medication-dispensing kiosks where consumers can pick up an attached phone and have a video conference with a pharmacist in some remote location off the premises. With the technology available today, some pharmacies have the ability to notify patients when prescriptions need to be refilled and when they are ready for pickup via text messages sent to mobile devices. With prescription volume increasing and the role of the pharmacist changing, this may become more common.

In addition to increasing technology, another expanding area in community pharmacy is the role of pharmacy technicians. Pharmacists are expanding their role as patient care providers and incorporating more patient care activities into their daily practice. With the increasing complexity of drug regimens, pharmacists are spending more time with patients, counseling and educating them on their disease states and medication therapy. Depending on the state in which you practice, pharmacists may provide such services in collaboration with physicians and other health care providers through collaborative drug therapy management (CDTM) and medication therapy management (MTM). CDTM and MTM are discussed further in the *Patient Care* section of this chapter. Providing such services proves to be a difficult task with the increasing volume of prescriptions being handled, so technicians in this area are vital to patient care and maintaining pharmacy workflow. By performing many of the technical functions in support of the pharmacist, pharmacy technicians are enabling patients to spend more time with the pharmacist, receiving care and information that can help them benefit the most from their drug therapy.

Types of Community Pharmacies

The different types of community pharmacies offer varying services to the populations they serve. It is helpful to first break down the pharmacies by definition and then discuss the different services each of the types of pharmacies can provide.

independent pharmacy a retail pharmacy owned and operated by an individual pharmacist or group of individuals, in contrast to chain drug stores

chain pharmacy a retail pharmacy owned by a corporation that consists of many stores in a particular region or across the nation

Independent pharmacies consist of one to four stores owned and operated by an individual pharmacist or group of individuals. They are not part of a large corporation. They vary greatly in size, volume of prescriptions, and services. A benefit of working for an independent pharmacy would be that staff members usually have direct access to the owner or main decision maker, so suggestions can go right to the top. Also, independent pharmacies are sometimes more likely to specialize in one area of pharmacy, such as compounding, durable medical equipment, or home infusion therapy. These types of services are discussed later in the chapter.

Chain pharmacies also vary in size, volume, and services and can be differentiated from one another based on the setting in which they are housed. Chain drugstores are the most common, and although these stores sell mostly traditional drugstore merchandise, many of them carry a large variety of products.

Chain drugstores can be regional, in which the stores are located in one geographic area, or national, with stores spread out all over the country. Examples of national chain drugstores include CVS and Rite-Aid. In addition to chain drugstores, pharmacies can be located in supermarkets and, again, be regional or national in scope. Other types of stores that sometimes house pharmacies are mass merchandisers like Target and WalMart or membership based stores such as Costco. The settings vary greatly and the practices can be quite different from place to place.

Community Pharmacy Services

The services that different types of community pharmacies provide are as diverse as the stores that house them. Customary pharmacy services include prescription processing and basic over-the-counter (OTC) and general merchandise provision. But the services do not have to end there. Many community pharmacies base the services they provide on the population they serve and the demand in the area in which they are located.

Surgical Supply/Durable Medical Equipment

Some community pharmacies provide surgical supplies to patients in their community. Supplies include durable medical equipment such as knee braces, neck collars, hospital beds, canes, walkers, commodes, and other products. A pharmacy specializing in durable medical equipment will have a pharmacist and specially trained staff to assist patients in choosing the best products, fitting patients for products such as braces and orthotic supplies, and obtaining proper reimbursement from insurance providers for these services.

Long-Term Care

Community pharmacies can also provide medications to long-term care facilities in addition to providing prescription processing services to the community. Some long-term care facilities, like nursing homes, have their own pharmacies in the building, but many, because of their size or budget, do not. In these cases the facilities use pharmacies that generally prepare the orders on a daily basis for the inpatients and deliver the medications to the facility. This type of setting combines inpatient and outpatient services into one environment.

Home Infusion

Similar to long-term care provision, some pharmacies provide home care organizations with parenteral medications. These products are prepared in the community pharmacy and then delivered or shipped to the patient's home, where a skilled nurse will administer the medication. Home infusion services are discussed in detail in Chapter 3 of this textbook.

Specialty Compounding Services

Many community and/or compounding pharmacies across the country specialize in compounding pharmaceutical products that are not readily available in a particular dosage form or in the dose necessary for the patient. Compounded pharmaceutical products can take the form of oral suspensions or solutions, intravenous admixtures, capsules, topical preparations, or even the unusual, like lollipops.

Compounding services are an important part of many community pharmacy services. They are especially useful in special patient populations such as children and veterinary practices. Oftentimes children will have illnesses that can be treated only with adult medications. In these cases, the medications may only be available as a tablet or capsule or only in a dosage that would far exceed what would be recommended for a child. The medication needs to be diluted into a child-appropriate dose and possibly into a dosage form that can be taken by a child who cannot swallow tablets or capsules. In these situations, the pharmacist would prepare a solution or suspension by grinding the available tablets into a powder, adding an appropriate amount of water or other diluent, and then flavoring the preparation

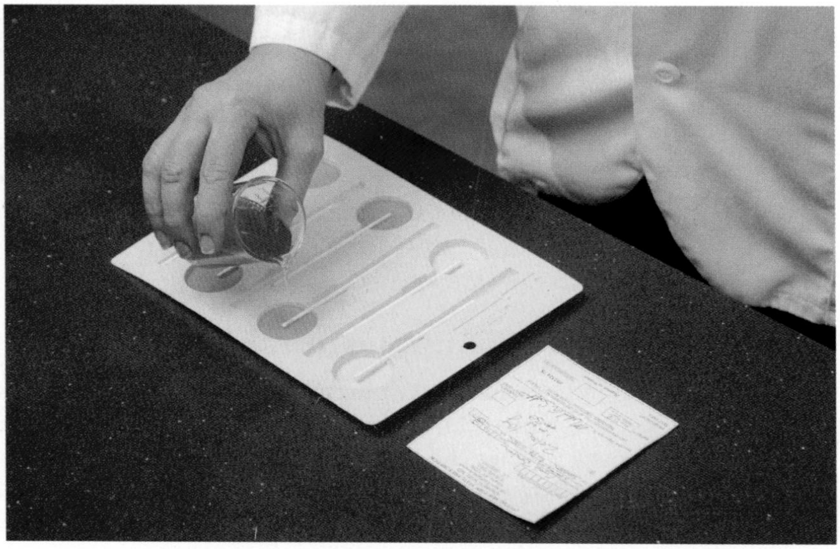

© Cengage Learning 2013

FIGURE 5-3 Some community pharmacies specialize in compounding services for special populations, like these medicinal lollipops being prepared for pediatric use.

to make it palatable (**Figure 5-3**). This is just one example of how pharmacists use compounding services to improve the care offered to patients.

Veterinary practices also use compounding services on a routine basis. Many veterinarians use human medications to treat their animals, but the doses or dosage forms they need are not commercially available. They will then go to a community pharmacy that specializes in compounding veterinary products and use their services to get what they need.

The pharmacy technician offers many types of services to the compounding pharmacist. A technician may be involved in almost every step in the process, from gathering the necessary ingredients to be incorporated to mixing the products together under the supervision of the pharmacist. Some of the skills necessary to participate in compounding services are meticulous attention to detail, knowing how to properly use equipment necessary to weigh and measure wet and dry ingredients, and knowledge of the metric and apothecary system for weights and measures. Extemporaneous compounding is covered in detail in Chapter 16.

Mail-Order Pharmacies and Central Fill Operations

Mail-order pharmacies can be divided into two categories: those affiliated with large pharmacy benefits management (PBM) companies and smaller, independent operations. PBMs are used by employers, or the insurers of employers, to manage and handle pharmacy claims.

Mail-order pharmacies accept new prescriptions from patients through the mail, dispense the prescriptions, and send them back through the mail to the patients. Refills for medication are requested by telephone, e-mail, or a postcard. Sometimes the mail-order pharmacy is located in a state other than the state where the patient lives. The lack of one-on-one contact with a pharmacist and the delay in receiving medication are the main reasons people do not use mail-order pharmacies. However, mail-order pharmacies may be a good option for patients with insurance plans that offer financial incentives to use them. Examples of mail-order pharmacies are Express Scripts, Medco, AdvancePCS, and PharmaCare Direct, and those associated with AARP.

Central fill operations function in a similar manner, but the prepared prescriptions are delivered to an actual pharmacy to be picked up by the patient, allowing for face-to-face interaction with the pharmacist. Pharmacies that use central fill practices are high-volume establishments that need to outsource some of the prescription processing to keep up with the demand. Both mail-order and central fill operations utilize technology to its fullest, most often incorporating robotics into the prescription processing. These types of operations are becoming increasingly popular, as the demand for on-site prescriptions processing increases.

Internet Pharmacy

Recently some Internet or cyberpharmacies have emerged. The first question about these is usually "Are they legal?" They are if they are licensed in the state where they are located and in the states where they are doing business. These pharmacies function much like mail-order pharmacies, with a few exceptions. Some Internet pharmacies establish personal contact between pharmacists and patients via e-mail. They also compile patient profiles, offer OTC products, and provide a wide choice of delivery options including mail, express delivery, or pickup at an affiliated retail pharmacy. Examples of Internet pharmacy services are www.drugstore.com and www.planetrx.com. It is important to know that Internet pharmacy sites that are reputable will have the seal of the National Association of Boards of Pharmacy known as the VIPPS (Verified Internet Pharmacy Practice Site) seal of approval. Sites that do not have this seal of approval should be avoided and the public should be warned against using them.

Telepharmacy

In an effort to provide pharmacy services to patients in areas where pharmacists are not available, such as rural areas, pharmacies are employing telepharmacy operations. Telepharmacy uses computer conferencing technology to allow a pharmacist to oversee and communicate with a technician at another location as the technician processes prescriptions. This area of pharmacy practice is expected to expand in the future.

Outpatient Pharmacies in Hospitals

Some larger hospitals have outpatient pharmacies within the hospital, usually close to the entrance, the clinics, or emergency department. These pharmacies dispense medication to their ambulatory patients. They also fill prescriptions written by physicians on the hospital staff and dispense the first filling of a new prescription for a patient being discharged from the hospital and prescriptions for employees of the hospital. They function much like a regular community pharmacy.

Prescription Processing

The primary activity involved in community pharmacy practice is processing prescriptions and delivering them to a patient or caregiver with provision of appropriate medication information. Although several types of community pharmacy settings offering an array of services exist, this basic function remains consistent across all types.

The process begins when a prescription is presented, either by phone, fax, e-prescribing technology including e-mail, or in person. The prescription is then entered into the computer and cross-checked with the patient's existing profile. If this is the first time the patient is visiting the pharmacy, additional information is collected from the patient and entered into the record.

Once the prescription is entered into the computer, it usually goes on to be processed and filled. If the prescription requires making a clinical decision or

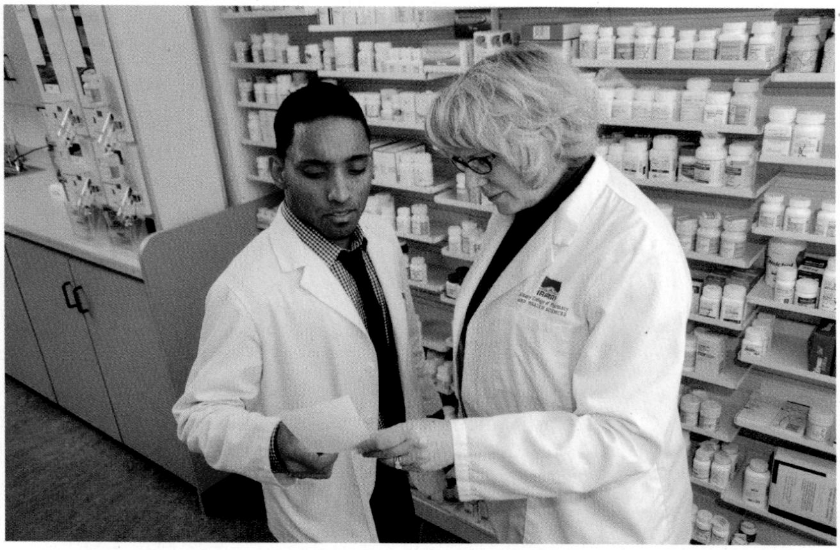

FIGURE 5-4 If the pharmacy technician has a question about a prescription, the pharmacist should be consulted.

some type of pharmacist intervention, the pharmacist needs to be alerted so he or she can resolve the problem (**Figure 5-4**). Once the prescription is deemed adequate to process, the medication is retrieved from the inventory and then the appropriate number of dosing units is counted or measured, placed in a container, and labeled. At this point, the pharmacist will perform one final check to ensure no errors have been made. The prescription is then delivered to the patient or caregiver or put in a location of the pharmacy designated for prescriptions waiting to be picked up. A pharmacy technician can participate in virtually every step of this process, but the laws that outline the tasks that technicians are allowed to perform vary by state. However, when a clinical decision needs to be made, such as how to handle an inappropriate dose or drug interaction, the pharmacist is the only person who should make those decisions. Pharmacists in the community setting routinely make clinical decisions, such as determining the appropriate dose of a medication, modifying prescription regimens to reduce the impact of drug interactions, suggesting the best course of OTC medications to treat a symptom, and choosing therapies to help patients save money on their medications. Making these types of decisions and educating patients about how to best use their medications are the primary clinical functions of the pharmacist in the community setting. Technicians perform vital support functions, which allows pharmacists to concentrate their time on these clinical tasks.

The Pharmacy Technician in the Community Pharmacy

Because of the process just outlined, which comprises most of a community pharmacy technician's time, individuals should possess certain qualifications if they are considering a position as a pharmacy technician in this setting. As previously mentioned, communication and interpersonal skills are a necessity, and potential technicians should pay extraordinary attention to detail because of the nature of their responsibility. Community pharmacies can sometimes be busy, stressful places; and an ability to properly handle situations that may arise is crucial. Maintaining a professional demeanor is of upmost importance. The ability to stay focused among different types of distractions is also necessary. Working in a community pharmacy processing prescriptions also requires knowledge of prescription medications—most importantly, their brand and generic names—as well as computer literacy and an understanding of pharmacy billing and third-party (insurance) reimbursement. Many of these skills can be learned through on-the-job training, but formalized training and technician certification programs are making for higher quality personnel. Many states now have requirements for the training, certification, and registration of pharmacy technicians. Technician certification is discussed in Chapters 33 and 34.

The pharmacy technician is usually the first person the patient encounters at the pharmacy and represents the entire department. As the saying goes, "First impressions are everything." Appropriate attire and appearance are essential in making good first impressions. Some pharmacies may require technicians to wear uniforms, lab coats, or other specific attire. Regardless of requirements, all garments should be conservative, clean, ironed, and neat. Name badges with your designated title should also be visibly worn.

Professionalism is not only demonstrated by attire but also by actions. Technicians are expected to respect not only patients and their right to privacy, but also fellow health care providers. Any issues or difficult situations must be addressed appropriately and in a timely manner.

The pharmacy technician's role in the community pharmacy includes performing the following tasks:

- Greet each patient in a respectful, professional manner—a friendly personality is a great attribute.
- Collect information from the patient to ensure the prescription is processed efficiently and accurately. This includes information such as the patient's name and address, date of birth, individual health information, and insurance information.
- Assist in the technical aspects of prescription preparation. This includes typing information into the computerized database, retrieving medications from stock, counting dosage units, labeling prescription vials, returning items to stock, and keeping the pharmacy department orderly and organized (**Figure 5-5**).

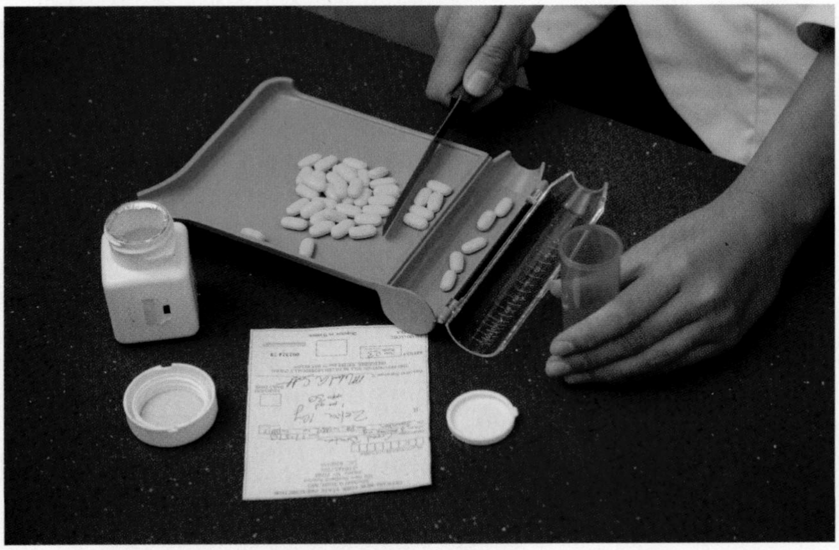

FIGURE 5-5 One aspect of preparing a prescription may be to count the pills to be dispensed.

- Submit electronic claims to insurance providers, and address all issues related to the claims.
- Alert the pharmacist when clinical intervention is necessary.
- Comply with the various federal and state laws governing the practice of pharmacy. The pharmacy technician should be familiar with all laws that govern the practice and aid the pharmacist in complying with those laws.

Patient Care

With the expansion of the pharmacy profession to incorporate more patient care activities into practice, many community pharmacies are offering direct patient care services such as medication therapy management; screenings for conditions such as osteoporosis, diabetes, and high blood pressure; and immunizations. All pharmacists in the community setting provide clinical services to some degree because any prescription being processed in the pharmacy requires some patient-oriented activity. However, some pharmacies are expanding the types of clinical services they provide by offering various patient education programs, disease-state management services, and medication administration services. Technicians may assist in this area by facilitating patient scheduling, obtaining and maintaining proper documentation, and increasing patient awareness of available services. Technicians play a vital role in enrolling patients and ensuring these services are provided and are successful.

The increasing complexity of many medication therapy regimens requires patients to be well educated about their illnesses and the medications being used to treat them. Pharmacists are an excellent source of this information, and many pharmacies offer services to assist patients in managing their illnesses through patient education. The patient education services offered in community pharmacies usually focus on common disease states such as diabetes, asthma, hyperlipidemia, smoking cessation, and hypertension. The pharmacy may offer special counseling sessions with the pharmacist at which patients are taught about their illness, the medications that manage it, and some lifestyle changes they can make to increase their quality of life. This type of program is referred to as **medication therapy management (MTM)**. MTM is defined as a service or group of services that optimizes therapeutic outcomes for an individual patient. The patients and pharmacist meet either on a one-on-one basis or as a group and discuss their disease, monitor their progress, and in many disease management programs, even perform clinical monitoring and make treatment decisions. The results of the meetings are usually reported to the patient's physician, and the pharmacist is part of that patient's treatment team. Some clinical monitoring that takes place in community pharmacies includes cholesterol testing, blood sugar or diabetes testing, and blood pressure screening and monitoring. These types of services go along with the expansion of pharmacy services to more patient-focused activities.

> **medication therapy management (MTM)** pharmacists are reimbursed for nondrug services such as drug therapy management for diabetes, anticoagulation, anemia, hypertension, and renal failure

Another area of involvement for many community pharmacists is immunizations. Pharmacists now routinely provide immunizations as part of their everyday practice and the technician plays a vital role in assisting in the process. Through a collaborative drug therapy agreement with a physician, a pharmacist is given permission to administer an immunization, such as a flu or pneumonia vaccine, to patients who meet defined criteria spelled out in the agreement. Individual state laws regulate which vaccines may be administered and at what age patients may receive vaccinations from pharmacists. The role of the technician in providing immunizations may also vary in each state. Technicians may assist in all steps of the immunization process, including preparing the vaccine, up to the point when the vaccine is actually administered. The pharmacy technician can not administer the vaccination.

collaborative drug therapy agreement an agreement between a physician and a pharmacist that gives the pharmacist expanded prescription authorization regarding management of drug therapy

A **collaborative drug therapy agreement** allows a physician to designate certain responsibilities to a pharmacist. It is a voluntary written agreement between a pharmacist and prescriber that gives expanded authority to the pharmacist, such as the ability to initiate or modify drug therapy or order and perform laboratory tests. The agreements are not limited to the practice of immunizations; we see them being incorporated into programs for diabetes, cholesterol, and anticoagulant therapy.

Because clinical services are directly related to patient care, the pharmacy technician should express the same dedication as pharmacists to caring for patients by offering a courteous, respectful, caring, and professional attitude. The pharmacy technician is frequently the first point of contact with a patient and has the responsibility for generating patient confidence and comfort in the ensuing interaction. A poor greeting and discourteous attitude may create a less-than-favorable situation for the patient, pharmacist, and staff. A pharmacy technician should be committed to providing patient care that goes beyond the customer service found in retail outlets. Individuals presenting to a pharmacy for assistance or to have a prescription filled are considered patients, which means the relationship goes beyond that of a purveyor and customer. The rewards of such patient interactions and the opportunity to develop relationships with patients are some of the most gratifying aspects of becoming a pharmacy technician.

Summary

In summary, community pharmacy is a diverse, fast-paced environment that requires good interpersonal skills and attention to detail. Pharmacy technicians play an increasingly important role in the expansion of pharmacist services to include more patient-focused activities such as medication therapy management. The role of pharmacy technicians will increase in the future as the volume of prescriptions increases. Community pharmacy can be a tremendously rewarding area of pharmacy practice, because practitioners get the opportunity to impact peoples' health and care for patients on a daily basis.

TEST YOUR KNOWLEDGE

Multiple Choice

1. Community pharmacy practice is an example of
   a. long-term care.
   b. acute care.
   c. ambulatory care.
   d. a nuclear pharmacy.

2. In recent years, the number of prescriptions processed in the community pharmacy setting has
   a. steadily increased.
   b. steadily decreased.
   c. remained the same.
   d. varied.

3. The pharmacy technician can perform all of the following tasks in the community pharmacy *except*
   a. counting the correct number of medication units to be dispensed.
   b. labeling the medication container.
   c. receiving the written prescription to be processed from the patient.
   d. counseling the patient on the appropriate use of the medication and side effects.

4. Community pharmacies vary in their services and may provide which of the following?
   a. prescription compounding
   b. durable medical equipment
   c. medication therapy management
   d. all of the above

5. A single pharmacy owned and operated by an individual or group of individuals is an example of
   a. an independent pharmacy.
   b. a chain pharmacy.
   c. a regional pharmacy.
   d. a long-term care pharmacy.

6. Which of the following is an ambulatory care setting?
   a. nursing home
   b. community pharmacy
   c. rehabilitation center
   d. intensive care unit

7. Pharmacy technicians are experiencing an increase in their roles in community pharmacy because
   a. pharmacists are expanding their roles as patient care providers.
   b. technology used in the pharmacy has decreased.
   c. people are living healthier and longer lives.
   d. of an increased need to compound medications.

8. The primary activity of a community pharmacy practice is
   a. preparing medications for inpatients.
   b. processing prescriptions.
   c. managing drug regimens.
   d. delivering medications to patients.

9. The pharmacy technician's role includes which of the following?
   a. counseling patients
   b. making recommendations for over-the-counter products
   c. collecting information from patients
   d. developing drug regimens for patients

10. Types of direct patient care services being offered in the community pharmacy include
    a. medication therapy management.
    b. collaborative drug therapy agreements.
    c. drug reviews.
    d. all of the above.

Fill in the Blank

1. Care provided to patients who walk in and out in the same day is called ______________ care.
2. The primary reason for the increasing number of prescriptions is ______________.
3. A pharmacy owned and operated by a pharmacist or group of pharmacists is called a/an ______________ pharmacy.
4. A pharmacy that is a part of a large business and sells retail items as well as pharmaceuticals is called a/an ______________ pharmacy.
5. One of the primary qualifications for working in a community pharmacy is good ______________ skills.

References

American Pharmacists Association. (2003). White paper on pharmacy technicians: Needed changes can no longer wait. *Journal of the American Pharmacists Association, 43*(1), 93–107.

Centers for Medicare and Medicaid Services. (2012). *National health expenditures 2011 highlights.* http://www.cms.gov/Research-Statistics-Data-and-Systems/Statistics-Trends-and-Reports/NationalHealthExpendData/downloads//highlights.pdf

Gu, Q., Dillon, C.F., & Burt, V.L. (2010). *Prescription drug use continues to increase: U.S. prescription drug data for 2007–2008* (NCHS Data Brief No. 42). Hyattsville, MD: National Center for Health Statistics.

Hagel, H.P., & Rovers J.P. (Eds.). (2002). *Managing the patient-centered pharmacy.* Washington, DC: American Pharmacists Association.

Tindall, W.N., Beardsley, R.S., & Kimberlin, C.L. (Eds.). (2007). *Communication skills in pharmacy practice* (5th ed.). Philadelphia, PA: Lippincott Williams & Wilkins.

Website

National Community Pharmacists Association www.ncpanet.org

CHAPTER

6

Mail-Order Pharmacy Practice

Competencies

Upon completion of this chapter, the reader should be able to:

1. Define a mail-order pharmacy and its place in the patient care continuum.
2. Discuss the different types of mail-order pharmacies.
3. Explain the knowledge and skills necessary to function as a pharmacy technician in the mail-order pharmacy setting.
4. Differentiate between the different roles a pharmacy technician may have in a mail-order pharmacy.

Key Terms

formulary
mail-order pharmacy
payer
pharmacy benefit manager (PBM)
specialty pharmacy

Introduction

This chapter provides an overview of mail-order pharmacy practice, highlighting the role of the pharmacy technician. The various roles for a pharmacy technician in the mail-order pharmacy setting are explored, with an emphasis on the skills and attributes required in this unique and challenging area of practice.

Mail-Order Pharmacy Practice

mail-order pharmacy a pharmacy that fills prescriptions and refills by mail, online, by phone, or via smartphone apps anywhere in the United States; orders are delivered directly to the patient's home

During the past 10 years, **mail-order pharmacies** have represented the fastest growing distribution channel for prescription drugs. Although that tremendous growth has slowed in recent years, the mail-order channel remains second only to chain drugstores in U.S. prescription sales. Mail-order pharmacies also have proven to lower prescription costs, reduce medication errors, and increase medication adherence for those suffering from chronic conditions. Let's first review the different types of mail-order pharmacies that exist, the patient groups they serve, and the types of medication in which they specialize.

Traditional Mail-Order Pharmacies

pharmacy benefit manager (PBM) a provider of prescription drug programs; can be a third-party administrator or part of an integrated healthcare system. Responsibilities include processing and paying prescription drug claims, developing and maintaining the formulary, contracting with pharmacies, and negotiating discounts and rebates with drug manufacturers.

specialty pharmacy a pharmacy that specializes in dispensing expensive injectable medications that require more than just distribution to the patient. In addition to the medication, they generally provide all of the necessary ancillary supplies the patient may need to administer the medication. Patient education is also included and, if necessary, injection training is provided by a nurse either by phone or in person.

Traditional mail-order pharmacies mainly dispense 90-day supplies of maintenance medications to treat chronic disease states like diabetes, heart disease, and depression. These pharmacies specialize in distributing and filling prescriptions efficiently and accurately. They generally offer their customers a variety of ordering options including by mail, phone, and Internet. The large **pharmacy benefit managers (PBMs)** dominate this marketplace. CVS Caremark and Express Scripts, operate several mail-order pharmacy locations that service their membership. The U.S. Department of Veterans Affairs services our veterans by operating several mail-order pharmacy locations throughout the United States. Smaller, independent mail-order pharmacies service the membership of some of the smaller PBMs in the marketplace. Even certain patients of the larger PBMs have chosen to use some of these independent locations. AmeriPharm and DrugSource are independent operators of successful mail-order pharmacy locations. **Figure 6-1** shows pharmacists at work and an assembly line at an Express Scripts location.

Specialty Pharmacies

Specialty pharmacies exploded onto the marketplace as payers demanded more clinical management of complex disease states such as HIV, AIDS, fertility medications and cancers. These types of pharmacies specialize in dispensing expensive injectable medications that require more than just distribution to the patient. In addition to the medication, they generally provide all of the necessary ancillary supplies the patient may need to administer the medication. Patient education is also included and, if necessary, injection training is provided by a nurse either by phone or in person. Because of the cost of these drugs, payers generally limit the quantity to a 30-day supply. All of the big PBMs now operate their own specialty pharmacies, but a number of very successful independent specialty pharmacies have also carved out a niche in this space. Diplomat and ICORE all operate successful specialty pharmacy locations.

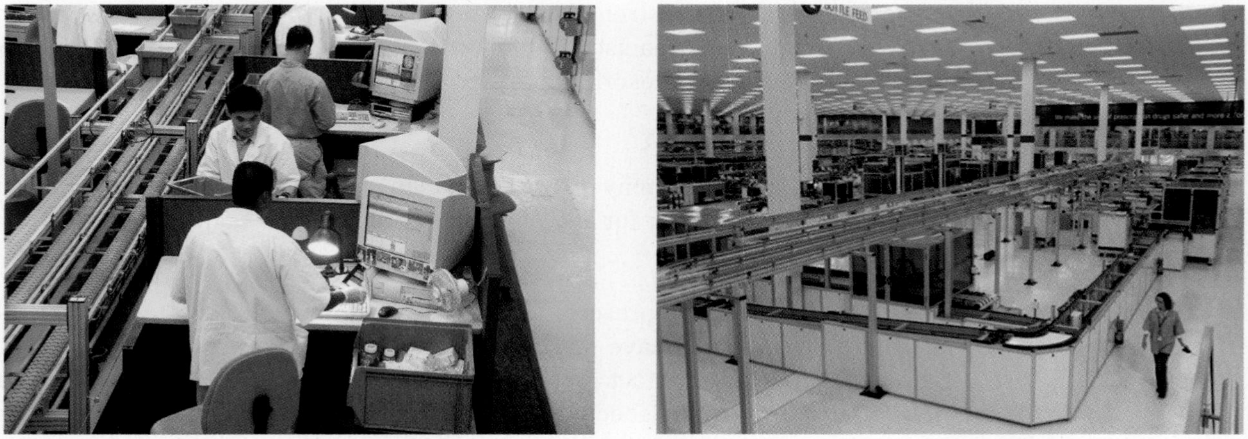

A B

Courtesy of Express Scripts Holding Company

FIGURE 6-1 A. Pharmacists inspecting orders at a mail-order pharmacy. B. Assembly line at a mail-order pharmacy.

Diabetic Supply Pharmacies

It is estimated that 25.8 million children and adults—or 8.3% of the U.S. population—have diabetes. The financial costs of the management and treatment of diabetes are staggering. The American Diabetes Association estimates that $176 billion is spent each year in direct medical costs and an additional $69 billion is spent in indirect costs (disability, work loss, premature mortality). It should be no surprise then that several mail-order pharmacies have built a successful business treating this disease. These pharmacies specialize in dispensing diabetic testing strips and lancets and generally provide the meter and lancing devices for free. They also have expertise in providing insulin pumps and supplies, a service that a number of traditional pharmacies struggle to provide. These businesses have built a niche not only by dispensing medication but also by providing educational materials about the disease, which may include injection training, cookbooks, and tips about physical activity. Liberty Medical, Arriva Medical, and CCS Medical all operate successful pharmacies that provide services to individuals with diabetes.

The Technician's Role

Unlike in a community pharmacy setting where an individual technician or pharmacist facilitates a prescription order to completion, technicians and pharmacists in mail-order pharmacies complete specific tasks within the workflow to prepare a prescription order. One obvious difference between a community pharmacy and mail-order pharmacy setting is that with a mail-order pharmacy you do not interact with the customer face to face. Most patient contact is done over the phone or in some instances via e-mail. For that reason, one of the main attributes needed for a technician to function successfully is clear, concise communication skills (discussed in depth in Chapter 31). Communication is not only important with customers but also with peers and colleagues. In the following sections we walk through each of those tasks where the technician is employed to complete and support the prescription order.

Prescription Entry

In this area, technicians are utilized to interpret and enter prescription orders into computerized fulfillment systems. They are expected to be able to read and interpret prescription orders accurately and efficiently. They must select the correct patient, drug name and strength, directions, quantity, prescriber, and number of refills. Although a pharmacist will review their work, this task is a critical step in delivering an accurate prescription order.

Prescriber Contact

A mail-order pharmacist may direct technicians to contact the prescriber to complete a prescription order for any of a number of reasons, as discussed next.

Refill Authorization

Oftentimes requests for prescription refills called in by patients cannot be filled because they may not have any remaining refills or the prescription may have expired. Technicians contact prescribers to obtain authorization to continue therapy. This can be accomplished via telephone, fax, or electronic prescribing systems.

Prescription Clarification

Written prescriptions sometimes require the pharmacist to contact the prescriber to clarify the order. These clarifications can include the drug name or strength, quantity, or the number of refills prescribed. These clarifications are typically made via phone or fax. Once clarified, notations are either made on the hardcopy prescriptions themselves or annotated on prescription images.

Drug Utilization Evaluation

Drug utilization evaluation questions often arise when attempting to dispense a prescription order. These include drug-drug interactions, drug-age precautions, and over- or underutilization questions about the dose prescribed. This type of clarification is typically made via telephone in conjunction with a pharmacist.

Requests for New Prescriptions

Requests for new prescriptions are often handled by pharmacy technicians. Although most states require a pharmacist to sign off on new prescriptions taken over the phone, technicians may be utilized to reduce the prescription to writing, requiring the pharmacist to merely read back the order to the prescriber and sign off on it.

Failed Claims

payer The pharmacy benefit manager

In today's world of managed medicine, prescription claims must be approved prior to being dispensed. Claims are sent through **payer** networks in real time to check the eligibility of the patient and the drug prescribed. Payers use a sophisticated plan design matrix that checks the drug name, strength, and quantity prescribed within seconds. If approved, the payer will return a paid response to the pharmacy and the prescription may be dispensed. If denied, the payer will return a message indicating why the prescription claim was denied. The returned messages are standard messages prepared by the National Council for Prescription Drug Programs (NCPDP) for use by healthcare payers.

Refill Too Soon

All payers require a certain amount of a prior prescription to be used up before permitting a refill request to be filled. This utilization percentage can be anywhere from 60% to 80%. Any refills attempted prior to that utilization percentage being reached will be denied and the payer will return a message indicating when that refill request may be filled. In a mail-order setting, technicians handle these claims by contacting customers, often this is done via e-mail, to inform them when the prescription may be dispensed and by placing these claims on hold to be dispensed when permitted. Sometimes these claims require intervention with the payer for early refill authorization because of a planned vacation or an increase in dosage.

Prior Authorization Required

formulary a listing of drugs approved by the pharmacy and therapeutics committee of a hospital or a health care system for use within their institution or by health care insurers as determined by the safety, efficacy, effectiveness, and cost of the drugs

Payers create **formularies** that dictate what drugs are covered and what the copayment will be for each drug. Frequently, expensive brand name drugs require prior authorization from the payer before being dispensed. When this occurs in a mail-order setting, technicians work with the patient, prescriber, and payer to attempt to obtain the necessary documentation needed to dispense the prescribed drug. If the patient does not meet the requirements for the originally prescribed drug to be dispensed, a covered alternative may be obtained from the prescriber, or if the patient desires, he may pay the full cost for the originally prescribed drug to be dispensed.

Plan Limitations

Payers often limit the quantity of certain classes of drugs. Drugs used for pain, erectile dysfunction, and others can be limited to a certain quantity over a period of time. When prescriptions are written for drugs and quantities that exceed these limits, technicians are authorized to adjust the quantities prescribed. The patient is notified of the adjustment either electronically or with documentation presented with the prescription.

NDC Not Covered

Some products prescribed are not covered by prescription drug plans. In these instances, technicians will contact patients to provide them with the option of paying the full price for the product or work with the prescriber to obtain an alternative.

Nonmatched Identifier

When prescription claims are submitted to payer systems for approval, at a minimum the member ID and date of birth must match what the payer has on file. If they do not, the payer will return a message indicating such. When this scenario occurs, technicians contact payers and sometimes the patient to verify the information. Once the pharmacy's system matches the payer's, the prescription can be processed and the pharmacy is ensured the claim will be paid.

Filled after Coverage Terminated

When claims are submitted to a payer and the patient has been terminated in the payer's system, payers will return a message indicating that the patient has been terminated. In this scenario, technicians contact payers to verify that the patient's coverage has been terminated. Sometimes, the patient's member ID or group number may have changed and he has coverage under a new ID or group number. If so, the technician will resubmit the claim under the proper member ID to obtain a paid claim. If the patient's coverage termination is confirmed, the technician will contact the patient to see if he has new coverage under a different prescription plan.

Customer Service

Technicians are often employed as customer service agents in a mail-order pharmacy or PBM. Companies that employ technicians in this capacity often market this strategy in an effort to win new business.

Formulary Questions

As mentioned earlier, payers utilize formularies to dictate what drugs are covered and what the copayment will be for each drug. Patients often have questions about what drugs are covered and how much they will cost. Technicians are often employed to answer these questions. They use their knowledge of medication to answer questions about drug coverage.

Place Prescription Orders

Most members of prescription drug plans have many options for having their prescriptions filled. They can select from any retail drugstore or use a mail-order pharmacy for their maintenance prescription needs. Employing technicians in a customer service role can assist in initiating new or refill prescription orders for patients with maintenance medication needs. They can initiate prescriber contact to obtain new prescriptions or transfer prescriptions from another pharmacy.

Adherence Calls

A patient's adherence with medication therapy is a hot button topic in the medical world because it requires vigilance. It is estimated that up to one-half of patients in the United States do not take their medications as prescribed. Such poor medication adherence exacts a heavy toll of unnecessary illness, hospitalizations, disability, and premature death, particularly among patients with chronic disease. In an effort to boost patient adherence, mail-order pharmacies send letters or e-mails to patients who have not ordered refills or who have refills coming due.

Order Clarification

Frequently, patients will be contacted to answer questions about prescription orders during processing. Questions can be about demographic information, allergies, or even the type of diabetic supplies the patient may be using. In addition, most pharmacies set a limit on the amount of patient copayment permitted before an order can be shipped without having credit card information or sufficient payment. They also set limits on the total order copayment even when they do have proper credit card information on file. These types of clarifications are generally performed by pharmacy technicians.

Retail to Mail

As mentioned earlier, members of prescription drug plans have many options when it comes to having their prescriptions filled. When patients are getting maintenance medication filled at local retail pharmacies, and it makes financial sense both for the patient and payer to have those prescriptions instead filled by a mail-order pharmacy, those patients will be targeted to have those prescriptions moved to a mail-order setting.

Formulary Intervention

When prescriptions are presented for either a nonpreferred or higher tier formulary product, interventions are frequently performed in an effort to change the prescription to a preferred product. These can include both brand-to-brand and brand-to-generic interventions. Typically, these interventions are performed by technicians and the interchange must be approved by both the patient and the prescriber. In every case, it must make financial sense for both the patient and the payer before an intervention is performed.

Dispensing

Most mail-order pharmacies have some level of dispensing automation. They generally divide their dispensing pharmacies into several different dispensing areas. Pharmacy technicians are employed to perform specific tasks within each of these areas.

Automation

Several vendors make dispensing automation equipment for tablet and capsule formulations. Mail-order pharmacies also refer to tablet and capsule formulations as oral solids. Each of these automatic machines utilizes either electronic or mechanical counting mechanisms for counting and dispensing oral solids. The medication is generally housed in canisters or cells and technicians refill and maintain these canisters.

Manual Fill

The manual fill dispensing area handles tablets and capsules that cannot be counted accurately by automated means or are not dispensed often enough to warrant automatic dispensing. Medications that are dispensed in their own packaging or unit-of-use medications are also dispensed in this area, as are items such as inhalers, oral contraceptives, creams, and ointments. To dispense prescriptions in this location, technicians retrieve the proper medication from the shelf, count the required quantity, and place the label on the vial or unit-of-use packaging. Often, systems are utilized that require the technician to scan the bar code on the stock bottle before a label is generated. This quality step is necessary to ensure that the proper drug product has been selected.

Bulk Fill

Mail-order pharmacies place prescription orders in totes or containers once filled. Large bulky prescription products may not fit in these containers or totes. For that reason, these items are generally filled last in the dispensing process. Items such as insulin syringes, bulk powders, and refrigerated products are located in this area.

Controlled Substances

Although many controlled substances are not maintenance medications, controlled substances typically account for 3% to 5% of the total prescriptions dispensed in a mail-order setting. Drugs used for ADHD and fibromyalgia are prescribed for 3 months or longer and can be dispensed through the mail. Controlled substances are generally located in separate rooms within a pharmacy to which only certain employees have access. Depending on the volume of prescriptions dispensed by the pharmacy, some level of automation may be used for oral solid Schedule III through V controlled substances. Schedule II narcotics are counted by hand and a perpetual inventory is kept of the specified drug. All controlled substance packages are shipped via traceable methods.

Inventory Control

Mail-order pharmacies work very hard at controlling inventory levels. They want to make sure they have sufficient inventory to fill the volume of prescriptions, but do not want to have too much sitting on their shelves. Technicians frequently order inventory, check it in, and shelve inventory orders when they arrive. Unlike a retail pharmacy, which may only have one or two inventory suppliers, it is not uncommon for mail-order pharmacies to have five or more suppliers of prescription drugs. A mail-order pharmacy may use a wholesaler for the majority of brand products, but it may purchase certain generic drugs directly from a manufacturer.

This is a critical role within a mail-order pharmacy setting and one that is generally held by technicians.

Management Positions

Large mail-order pharmacies can employ upwards of 500 people. To maintain proper workflow and support, layers of supervision are generally required. Department supervisor and even shift manager positions are frequently held by experienced technicians.

Summary

In summary, mail-order pharmacies represent a very important distribution channel for all payers. They offer a high-quality, low-cost option for members of prescription plans to fulfill their prescription needs. It offers pharmacy technicians numerous options for employment in a closed door setting. A number of states that set technician-to-pharmacist ratios have permitted two-to-one and even three-to-one ratios to allow for expansion of the pharmacy technician's role. Whether a technician is interpreting and entering prescriptions into computer systems, assisting members with formulary choices, or filling prescriptions for dispensing, teamwork and good communication skills are required. As stated earlier, unlike a community pharmacy setting where pharmacists and technicians work a prescription to completion, mail-order pharmacies utilize groups of technicians and pharmacists to complete specific tasks within the workflow to prepare prescription orders. Teamwork and communication are paramount to completing prescription orders accurately and efficiently. It is that efficiency that allows a mail-order pharmacy to keep its costs low and offer a high-quality, convenient option to customers.

TEST YOUR KNOWLEDGE

Multiple Choice

1. A mail-order pharmacy that specializes in dispensing medication to treat complex diseases like hepatitis C is called a
   a. specialty pharmacy.
   b. diabetic supply pharmacy.
   c. apothecary.
   d. nuclear pharmacy.

2. An outbound call to remind patients to refill their medication is called
   a. an authorization call.
   b. an adherence call.
   c. a marketing call.
   d. none of the above.

3. Tablet and capsule drug formulations are also known as
   a. unit-of-use drugs.
   b. oral solids.
   c. controlled substances.
   d. sustained-release drugs.

4. Liberty Medical specializes in servicing what disease state?
   a. depression
   b. heart disease
   c. diabetes
   d. cancer

5. One of the jobs a pharmacy technician may perform in a mail-order pharmacy setting is
   a. prescription entry.
   b. customer service.
   c. prescriber contact.
   d. all of the above.

6. Which of the following is true regarding controlled substances in a mail-order pharmacy setting?
   a. They typically represent 3% to 5% of the total prescriptions dispensed.
   b. They cannot be dispensed in 90-day supplies.
   c. They are shipped by any means.
   d. None of the above.

7. Dispensing technicians working in a manual fill area must do what before a prescription label is generated?
   a. Clean the dispensing area with alcohol.
   b. Scan the bar code on the stock bottle.
   c. Select the proper drug for dispensing.
   d. b and c.

8. Technicians performing the prescription entry function must perform all of the following functions *except*
   a. select the proper patient.
   b. select the proper drug and strength.
   c. call the prescriber.
   d. enter the quantity to be dispensed.

9. It is estimated that up to ______________ of patients in the United States do not take their medication as prescribed.
   a. one-third
   b. one–half
   c. 30%
   d. 10%

10. An effort to switch a patient from a nonpreferred to a preferred formulary drug is called
   a. medication therapy management.
   b. a drug utilization evaluation.
   c. a formulary intervention.
   d. polypharmacy.

Fill in the Blank

1. Traditional mail-order pharmacies generally dispense ______________ day supplies.
2. PBMs often target patients who are getting ______________ medications from a retail pharmacy in an effort to move them from a retail to a mail-order channel.
3. It is estimated that ______________ of the U.S. population has diabetes.
4. Drug-drug interactions or drug-age precautions are often examined during drug ______________ reviews.
5. One of the primary qualifications for working in a mail-order pharmacy is good ______________ skills.

Suggested Readings

American Diabetes Association. (2011, January 26). *2011 National diabetes fact sheet.* Retrieved from http://www.diabetes.org/diabetes-basics/diabetes-statistics

IMS Health. (2010). *Top-line market data: Channel distribution dispensed prescriptions (U.S.).* Retrieved from http://www.imshealth.com/portal/site/ims/menuitem.5ad1c081663fdf9b41d84b903208c22a/?vgnextoid=fbc65890d33ee210VgnVCM10000071812ca2RCRD

Pharmaceutical Care Management Association. (2010). As economic recovery sputters, independent pharmacies shouldn't shoulder employers with higher costs. Retrieved from http://www.pcmanet.org/2011-press-releases/as-economic-recovery-sputters-independent-drugstores-shouldn-t-shoulder-employers-with-higher-costs

New England Health Care Initiative. (2011, April). *Improving patient medication adherence: A $100+ billion opportunity.* Retrieved from http://www.google.com/url?sa=t&rct=j&q=&esrc=s&source=web&cd=1&ved=0CCsQFjAA&url=http%3A%2F%2Fadhereforhealth.org%2Fwp-content%2Fuploads%2Fpdf%2FImprovingPatientMedicationAdherence-NPP_Patient_Medication_Adherence_NQF.pdf&ei=7dXuUdG-OuOSiQL7nIGIBQ&usg=AFQjCNGZippAoYl6Wl-9E6-6Or7wDcqXrQ&sig2=J7-njMEdpcr4E_uqKUYilQ&bvm=bv.49641647,d.cGE

Osterberg, L., & Blaschke, T. (2005). Adherence to medication. *New England Journal of Medicine, 353*(5), 487–497.

Websites

American Diabetes Association www.diabetes.org

IMS Health www.imshealth.com

New England Healthcare Institute www.nehi.net

Pharmaceutical Care Management Association www.pcmanet.org

CHAPTER 7

Nuclear Pharmacy Practice

Competencies

Upon completion of this chapter, the reader should be able to:

1. Describe how the practice of nuclear pharmacy differs from standard practices of pharmacy.
2. State the nuclear pharmacy technician's primary job responsibilities in a nuclear pharmacy.
3. State what safety requirements and additional training are required to become a nuclear pharmacy technician.
4. Define the terms for quantifying radioactivity in both the Système International (SI) and American units of measure.
5. Describe the basic principles of how a radiopharmaceutical functions in order to assist in diagnosing and curing disease.
6. List the additional requirements and governing bodies for operating a nuclear pharmacy (licenses, etc.) that differ from those of a standard pharmacy.
7. List the acronym that guides radiation safety and describe the four concepts that allow one to achieve this safety.
8. List the staff members in a typical nuclear pharmacy and describe their roles.
9. List the types of radiation used in a nuclear pharmacy and why it can be used for diagnostic or therapeutic purposes.
10. List four instruments used for radiation detection.
11. Describe a typical compounding scenario from generator elution to quality control.

Key Terms

Agreement State
as low as reasonably achievable (ALARA)
authorized nuclear pharmacist (ANP)
beta particle
dose calibrator
gamma camera
half-life ($t_{1/2}$)
ionizing radiation
isotope
kiloelectron-volt (keV)
nuclear pharmacy
nuclear pharmacy technician (NPT)
Nuclear Regulatory Commission (NRC)
photon (gamma ray)
radiation safety officer (RSO)
radioactive decay
radioactive material (RAM)
radiochemical purity
radionuclidic purity
radiopharmaceutical
RAM license
regulated medical waste (RMW)
restricted area
sodium pertechnetate ($NaTcO_4^-$)
survey meter
target tissue/organ
thin-layer chromatography (TLC)
well counter

Introduction

nuclear pharmacy a specialized pharmacy where radiopharmaceuticals are compounded and dispensed for patient use, usually on the same day they were compounded

A **nuclear pharmacy** is a specialized pharmacy where radiopharmaceuticals are compounded and dispensed for patient use. Radiopharmaceuticals are usually used the same day they are compounded. Radiopharmaceuticals are used in nuclear medicine studies, which are performed on patients in clinics or a hospital's nuclear medicine department. Some radiopharmaceuticals are used as therapeutic agents for treating a particular disease state, but most are used as a diagnostic tool. This type of nuclear medicine study is considered minimally invasive, so it can be used by a physician to determine next steps in care or the effectiveness of an ongoing therapeutic regimen with little or no discomfort to the patient.

Regulatory Standards

Nuclear Regulatory Commission (NRC) U.S. government agency that regulates the use of by-product nuclear material

Agreement State state to which the NRC delegates part of its governing authority in the regulation and safe use and handling of radioactive materials

radioactive material (RAM) a substance that emits radiant energy in the form of alpha, beta, or gamma particles

Nuclear pharmacies belong to a highly regulated industry. They are pharmacies and, as such, are regulated by each individual state's board of pharmacy. But because they use nuclear materials they are also regulated by the **Nuclear Regulatory Commission (NRC)** or, depending on the state, they may be regulated under an Agreement State license. An **Agreement State** is one to which the NRC has delegated parts of its governing authority in the regulation and safe use and handling of **radioactive material (RAM)**.

The storage and use of RAM in the nuclear pharmacy may also result in the release of small amounts of RAM into the atmosphere, prompting the Environmental Protection Agency (EPA) to be involved in regulating what type and how much RAM can be released to the environment. Radiopharmaceuticals are delivered to hospitals and clinics over public roadways, which means that the Department of Transportation (DOT) gets involved. DOT has the right to regulate the safe packaging and transport of RAM (a hazardous material) by establishing guidelines for its packaging, labeling, and transportation. If a nuclear pharmacy ships RAM via an air carrier, the Federal Aviation Administration (FAA) is the department that has the right to regulate the packaging and transport of RAM via commercial or charter flights.

Understanding RAM and the Pharmacy Environment

ionizing radiation radiation that, when interacting with other atoms, ejects an electron, proton, or neutron, changing the ionization state of the atom

The radiation that emanates from an isotope is the result of an unstable isotope releasing energy to become more stable. The type of decay energy released and the rate of decay are two very important properties of RAM used in radiopharmaceuticals. As a particle or photon travels through tissue or any material, it deposits energy in the form of ions, hence the term **ionizing radiation**.

Working Knowledgeably with RAM

The environment within a nuclear pharmacy is one where workers may become "occupationally exposed" to ionizing radiation much like an x-ray technician, dentist, or nuclear medicine technologist would. Nuclear pharmacy technicians are therefore required to work around sources of ionizing radiation utilizing the

as low as reasonably achievable (ALARA) principle used when working with radioactive materials to reduce an individual's exposure to them

radiopharmaceutical substance used as a diagnostic or therapeutic agent to diagnose or treat disease and evaluate organ function and physiological processes

principles of **ALARA**. ALARA stands for "**as low as reasonably achievable**" and is the guiding principle for working safely in a nuclear pharmacy. To work with RAM and keep occupational exposure ALARA, workers employ three mechanisms to reduce their exposure:

- *Time:* The less time spent around a source of ionizing radiation, the less the exposure
- *Distance:* The farther away from a source of ionizing radiation, the less the exposure
- *Shielding:* The greater the shielding between you and the source of ionizing radiation, the less the exposure.

Another just as important mechanism to employ when working around RAM and trying to achieve ALARA doses is *common sense*.

How Radiopharmaceuticals Work

target tissue/organ the tissue or organ of interest in a nuclear medicine study and the one that is the target for a dose of a given radiopharmaceutical

radioactive decay process that occurs when unstable isotopes release energy in the form of waves or particles to achieve a more stable state

isotope any of two or more species of an element with the same atomic number but a different mass number or atomic mass

photon (gamma ray) a particle originating in the nucleus of an atom that is massless and chargeless, similar to light

beta particle a negatively or positively charged electron originating from the nucleus of a neutron-rich (negaton) or proton-rich (positron) radionuclide

kiloelectron-volt (keV) the unit of measurement for energy in an isotope

half-life ($t_{1/2}$) the time an isotope requires to decay by 50% of measured activity

The patient undergoing a nuclear medicine study is injected with or inhales, or ingests the compounded **radiopharmaceutical**. The radiopharmaceutical then circulates throughout the patient's body and localizes in the **target tissue** or **target organ**. Radiopharmaceuticals have two components, a radioactive component (radionuclide) and a pharmaceutical component. The radionuclide emits gamma rays and/or particles through a process called **radioactive decay**. As an unstable isotope undergoes radioactive decay to a more stable state, it emits energy in two ways: in the form of photons (gamma rays), which are then detected by a gamma camera (imaging the patient, nuclear medicine scan) in the nuclear medicine department, or as a particle, which provides therapeutic effects by destroying the nucleus of cells along its path. An **isotope** is any of two or more species of an element with the same atomic number but different mass number or atomic mass.

In other words, **photons (gamma rays)** are used as a diagnostic tool due to the nature of a photon as a type of energy that is similar to light in that it has little effect on tissue. It does, however, deposit energy in living tissue and exposure must be limited to prevent adverse effects. **Beta particles** are released and used as a therapeutic agent because beta particles can damage the nucleus of living cells, causing cellular death. This is effective in cancer therapies. All types of isotopes release photons, particles, or a combination of both at a different energy level (intensity), which also helps identify the isotope. Energy is measured typically in **kiloelectron-volts (keV)**. The rate of decay is called the **half-life ($t_{1/2}$)** and is defined as the time an isotope requires to decay by 50% of measured activity.

Radioactive decay is quantified using the Système International (SI) unit of becquerels or the American unit of curies. A single gamma ray or particle being emitted from an unstable atom is known as a disintegration. One becquerel (Bq) is equal to 1 disintegration per second (dps). One curie is equal to 3.7×10^{10} Bq (37,000,000 dps). Similarly, 1 millicurie (mCi) is equal to 3.7×10^{7} Bq (37 megabecquerels, MBq). The gamma camera translates these detected gamma rays into an image showing both the physiology and functionality of the target organ.

The pharmaceutical component is the component that makes the radiopharmaceutical localize in the tissue, organ, or physiological process of interest. Other common names for radiopharmaceuticals are *radiotracers* and *tracers*. The images are then interpreted by the nuclear medicine physician to determine the current state of the patient's health. The patient images are compared to the normal image, or normal biodistribution, for a given radiopharmaceutical.

Other types of radioactive decay used in nuclear medicine involve an isotope emitting a particle such as a beta or alpha particle. These types of decay are used in a therapeutic role because these particles damage cell nuclei and cause exposed cells to die. These particles do not penetrate well through the patient because most of their energy is deposited in tissue a short distance after being emitted from the nuclide. Gamma-ray emission is ideal for imaging because it is a massless, chargeless particle similar to light that readily penetrates tissue with minimal attenuation (stopping) prior to being absorbed by the gamma camera.

Design of a Nuclear Pharmacy

Nuclear pharmacy does not happen in a typical pharmacy practice setting. Its environment is similar to that of a traditional compounding pharmacy with the added complexity of needing to store, handle, dispense, and dispose of radioactive material on a routine basis. In order for a pharmacy to be a nuclear pharmacy, the facility must possess a radioactive materials license granted by the federal NRC or the state. All aspects of procuring, storing, handling, and disposing of RAM are regulated by the **RAM license**. The RAM license states the type of radionuclides allowed in the pharmacy and the possession limits, chemical forms, and authorized uses of those radionuclides; authorized users and radiation safety officer; conditions for storage and testing of sealed sources; and conditions for storage/disposal and all records associated with radioactive waste.

> **RAM license** license granted to a nuclear pharmacy that regulates the procuring, storing, handling, and disposing of RAM
>
> **restricted area** An area for the preparation and dispensing of compounded sterile products

Based on the RAM used and stored within the facility, the facility is set up to reflect the federal government's definitions of access control. Areas of access are defined as follows:

- *Uncontrolled space:* The public area outside of the four walls of the building is considered uncontrolledspace.
- *Controlled space:* The controlled space generally comprises the administrative/office, break room, bathrooms, and general storage areas.
- *Restricted area:* Within the controlled space is the **restricted area**. This area has additional security measures in place to prevent unauthorized access. This is the area traditionally known as the pharmacy; it is where RAM is stored and used in the compounding of the radiopharmaceuticals.

A typical USP Chapter <797>–compliant nuclear pharmacy has a separate ante and buffer area within the restricted area for the preparation and dispensing of compounded sterile products (CSPs). These areas have specific standards for cleanliness, air handling, personnel training, and testing in order to be compliant with USP Chapter <797> requirements. An ante area is where personnel cleaning and garbing occurs, prior to entering the buffer area where the compounding and dispensing occurs within the restricted area.

> **regulated medical waste (RMW)** used syringes and vials returned from customers

The restricted area is also the area where **regulated medical waste (RMW)** is handled and stored. RMW consists of used syringes and vials that customers have returned and is treated as RAM and biohazardous waste until the isotope fully decays, at which point it is treated solely as biohazardous RMW. All biomedical waste is regulated by federal and state biomedical waste regulations, not the board of pharmacy; however, a nuclear pharmacy technician is often delegated the responsibility of surveying, packaging, and preparing for disposal of this waste.

Typical Staff in a Nuclear Pharmacy

A typical nuclear pharmacy is staffed by a pharmacy manager, staff pharmacists, a radiation safety officer, nuclear pharmacy technicians, and delivery personnel.

Pharmacy Manager

The pharmacy manager (PM) is responsible for the day-to-day operations of the pharmacy from a business and personnel perspective. The PM is usually the pharmacist in charge (PIC) for pharmacy license requirements, and typically an authorized nuclear pharmacist (see next section), but this is not always required. The PM may be just the business manager, with the PIC role delegated to a qualified staff pharmacist who is directly responsible.

Nuclear Pharmacists

Staff nuclear pharmacists who are certified as **authorized nuclear pharmacists (ANPs)** perform compounding, dispensing, and testing functions. An ANP has undergone both classroom training (200 hours) and hands-on training (500 hours) and completed certification to become classified as an authorized user of RAM per NRC requirements.

Radiation Safety Officer

The **radiation safety officer (RSO)** is the individual in charge of the safe use and handling of RAM. This individual must abide by the conditions of the facility's RAM license and has full authority over the nuclear pharmacy and its employees where RAM is concerned. The RSO is typically a nuclear pharmacist but can be an NPT who has completed authorized user training and certification.

Nuclear Pharmacy Technician

The **nuclear pharmacy technician (NPT)** performs tasks delegated by the pharmacist such as dispensing (under the supervision of an ANP), cleaning (compliant with USP Chapter <797> standards), and equipment functionality testing. NPTs can also take prescription orders from customers depending on federal and state law, enter prescriptions into the pharmacy computer system, and perform deliveries to customers as needed. NPT duties are to abide by all federal and state laws, whichever are stricter.

Delivery Personnel

Delivery personnel assist in the wrapping of the dispensed radiopharmaceuticals and packaging of them into delivery cases prior to transporting them in delivery vehicles to the nuclear medicine customer's location.

Administrative Personnel

Administrative personnel work to support the business by performing billing, payroll, and other business functions as required.

authorized nuclear pharmacist (ANP) licensed pharmacist who has undergone NRC required classroom training (200 hours) and hands-on training (500 hours) and completed certification to become classified as an authorized user in the handling of RAM

radiation safety officer (RSO) the individual in charge of the safe use and handling of RAM; abides by the conditions of the facility's RAM license and has full authority over the nuclear pharmacy and its employees where RAM is concerned

nuclear pharmacy technician (NPT) a pharmacy technician who has undergone special training to work in a nuclear pharmacy

Requirements, Licensing, and Testing for the Pharmacy Technician

In addition to having a pharmacy technician license and being certified as a pharmacy technician, further training is required to be an NPT. The American Pharmacy Association (APhA) has published guidelines for nuclear pharmacy technician training programs that provide objectives and competencies for NPT training. In addition, the hiring company will provide on-the-job training and other company-based training (computer training, classes, etc.). Training topics for NPTs include the following:

- Radiation protection/biology/safety
- Shipment/receipt of radioactive materials (DOT regulations)
- Radiation physics and instrumentation
- Mathematics applicable to the practice of nuclear pharmacy
- Radiopharmaceuticals.

NPTs may go further with their training to become authorized users, which expands the scope of practice for an NPT (e.g., radiation safety specialist/radiation safety officer). This training is more intense and defined by the NRC to include 200 hours of didactic training in:

- Radiation physics and instrumentation
- Radiation protection and biology
- Radiopharmaceuticals
- Mathematics of radioactivity.

In addition to the didactic training, 500 hours of on-site practical training in a nuclear pharmacy under the supervision of a licensed authorized nuclear pharmacist is also required. This training includes:

- Ordering, receiving, surveying, and unpacking of radioactive materials
- Calibration of dose calibrators, scintillation detectors, and survey meters
- Calculation, preparation, and calibration of patient doses
- Proper use of syringe shield and other equipment.

NPT Role in Nuclear Pharmacy

As stated previously, a pharmacy technician requires more specialized training to be a nuclear pharmacy technician (NPT), which many companies will provide. Because of the shift in pharmacists' focuses in practice, the demand for NPT support in the daily operations of a nuclear pharmacy has increased. NPTs practice under the direct supervision of a licensed authorized nuclear pharmacist and in compliance with all state laws and regulations.

Some duties that NPTs may perform include:

- Order taking and prescription order entry
- Radiopharmaceutical compounding and dose drawing
- Generator elution (removal of absorbed material using a solvent)
- Quality control of radiopharmaceuticals
- Nonjudgmental tasks related to dispensing.

Order Taking and Prescription Order Entry

Physicians order nuclear medicine studies for patients through nuclear medicine departments. The nuclear medicine technologist will order the appropriate radiopharmaceutical the day prior to the test. Each order received daily at a nuclear pharmacy is considered a new order or prescription, thus pharmacies should comply with state law regarding technicians receiving new prescriptions, whether it is an oral, fax, or electronic order. If the prescription and order entry is completed by a technician, the associated prescription label is then verified by a pharmacist for accuracy.

Radiopharmaceutical Compounding and Dose Drawing

sodium pertechnetate ($NaTcO_4^-$) eluted from a Mo-99/Tc-99*m* generator, it is a radiopharmaceutical used in nuclear medicine alone or bound to a pharmaceutical to diagnose a disease state or to evaluate organ function or a physiological process

Reconstituting reagent kits with **sodium pertechnetate ($NaTcO_4^-$)** is the most common method of radiopharmaceutical compounding, but other methods include using a reactor or cyclotron to create new isotopes for manufacturing radiopharmaceuticals not commercially available. Primarily, NPTs would be involved with the reconstitution of the reagent kits with $NaTcO_4^-$; they would do so under the direct supervision of a licensed authorized nuclear pharmacist. Most nuclear pharmacy companies have internal compounding guidelines, but in the absence of these guidelines, the manufacturer's package insert should be followed for preparation. Furthermore, several factors need to be considered when compounding radiopharmaceuticals that do not generally apply when compounding traditional pharmaceuticals:

- Radiation safety (ALARA)
- Radioactive decay (half-life)
- Compounding requirements (some kits require a boiling water bath).

Typically, pharmacies assign lot numbers to each radiopharmaceutical, as well as to specific concentrations at specific times (calibration times). These lot numbers can be used to guide compounding based on what the need is for a given day. An example of a lot number would be:

- Tc-99*m*-MDP 13135-0015 (40 mCi/mL @ 0600)
  - *Radiopharmaceutical:* Tc-99*m*-MDP
  - *Lot number:* 13135-0015, which indicates the year ("13" for 2013), Julian date (135), and lot (0015)
  - *Concentration and calibration time:* 40 millicuries/milliliter of solution, 6:00 a.m.

Prior to beginning compounding, the technician would wash and don the appropriate garb in the ante area, clean and disinfect the laminar airflow workbench (LAFW) in the buffer area using distilled water followed by 70% isopropyl alcohol (IPA), and then gather the items necessary for compounding (i.e., syringe shields, syringes, 0.9% saline, sterile 70% IPA, prep pads, drug preparation lead shielding, cold drug product). Once the technician has been directed to which radiopharmaceuticals need to be compounded, the kits are set up with their associated labeled lead shield, the pharmacist verifies the cold drug vial, snaps the cap off the drug vial, swabs the septum with a 70% sterile IPA prep pad, and places the drug vial in the lead shield and closes the shield.

Generator Elution

When compounding is to begin, the NPT will perform a generator elution by rinsing normal saline over the generator column and collecting this solution (eluant) in a shielded sterile evacuated vial. Rinsing of a generator column is done in a sterile, closed system, where an evacuated vial pulls sterile 0.9% sodium chloride over the column, rinsing Tc-99*m* with saline off of the column into the evacuated vial, resulting in a solution (eluant) of sodium pertechnetate (Tc-99*m* $NaTcO_4^-$). The Mo-99/Tc-99*m* ratio is then determined, using the dose calibrator. Note that the USP defines a limit of 0.15 µCi Mo-99/1 mCi Tc-99*m* at time of dose injection. The elution information, including generator lot number, time, volume, activity, Mo-99/Tc-99*m* ratio, and concentration of the elution, is recorded on a compounding record. This information is then entered into a pharmacy computer system.

Using this elution, the NPT can begin to compound the radiopharmaceuticals. She then records the compounding information on the compounding record and transfers this information to the pharmacy computer system. This information will include the radiopharmaceutical kit, lot number, concentration, expiration time, current and calibration time activity, total volume of the kit made, elution used, volume of elution used, and the initials of the NPT and pharmacist. It is from these kits that patient-specific unit doses will be drawn using aseptic technique and radiation safety practices.

Quality Control of Radiopharmaceuticals

radionuclidic purity measure of the percentage of the total radioactivity is in the desired form

radiochemical purity measure of the percentage of the total radioactivity is in the desired radiopharmaceutical form

Once prepared, radiopharmaceuticals must undergo quality control tests to determine their **radionuclidic purity** and **radiochemical purity** to ensure they are suitable for diagnostic use. In other words, these tests determine if there was good "tagging" of the drug by the isotope. Radionuclidic purity is a measure of the percentage of the total radioactivity is in the desired form (i.e., Tc-99*m* versus Mo-99, the parent isotope). Radiochemical purity is a measure of the percentage of the total radioactivity is in the desired radiopharmaceutical form (i.e., radionuclide + drug, versus unbound radionuclide). Good labeling of the pharmaceutical by the radionuclide is desired to ensure that the radiopharmaceutical will have the desired actions in the patient and that the image acquired by the nuclear medicine technologist will be free of artifacts and show proper biodistribution. This aids in accurate diagnosis and evaluation. Other quality control tests, including sterility (free from microorganisms) and apyrogenicity (free from fever-producing substances), must be completed on products manufactured, such as PET (positron emission tomography) biomarkets at a PET manufacturing site. Manufacturing is regulated by the FDA, not the board of pharmacy.

thin-layer chromatography (TLC) a method of quality control performed on compounded radiopharmaceuticals

For Tc-99*m*–labeled products, and several others such as In-111 pentetreotide, **thin-layer chromatography (TLC)** is used for QC testing. Using chromatographic paper (Whatman paper, Baker-Flex paper, and separation packs), and solvents (acetone, ethyl acetate, and 0.9% saline), components in the radiopharmaceutical kit can be separated out to determine the percentage of bound drug. The three components being separated are radioactive "bound" drug, radioactive stannous ion, and radioactivity that did not bind, called *free activity*. Minimizing the latter two components as much as possible is desirable because they have a biodistribution in the patient that differs from the biodistribution of the bound drug, which can interfere with the reading and interpretation of the image by the nuclear medicine physician.

A small sample of the prepared radiopharmaceutical will be given to the NPT or designated QC technician in a shielded syringe to perform the testing. A small drop (about 0.1 microliter) of the sample is placed on the chromatography strip at the origin marking, and placed into a developing tank (collection tube, glass jar, etc.) containing the appropriate solvent until the solvent front reaches the top mark on the chromatography strip. Once developing is complete, the strip can be analyzed in various ways:

- With radiochromatography
- With a chromatography system
- By cutting the strip into small segments and counting each segment.

What is being analyzed is the ratio of activity on the strip between the origin line and the solvent front. Based on the chromatograph paper and the solvent, the NPT knows whether a radiopharmaceutical will follow the solvent to the solvent front or remain at the origin (like dissolves like). Whether using a dose calibrator and activity on the segments of the strip, or using a well counter and conducting counts, you can determine percent of drug bound. The USP minimum percent bound is 90% for most radiopharmaceuticals; for some, however, only 80% is required.

Area Wipes and Surveys

Area wipes and surveys must be performed once daily when radioactivity is dispensed and typically completed after the first run. The purpose is to detect radioactive contamination (removable or nonremovable), prevent its spread, and minimize the exposure to those in the area. Removable contamination is easily removed using cleaning solvents and decontaminators and does not require shielding with lead after decontamination and survey. Nonremovable contamination cannot be removed with cleaning solvents and must instead be covered by lead or other methods of shielding until the contamination has decayed to background levels. Both wipes and surveys are done because some activity may be detected by a wipe, but not by a survey meter and vice versa.

Wipes are small pieces of absorbent paper that are used to wipe a 100-cm^2 area that has the potential to have become contaminated and then counted using a scaler. A background measurement is taken in counts per minute (cpm), the wipe is counted (cpm), then the wipe count is subtracted from the background count. The difference has to be below the action limit of 220 cpm, per DOT regulations. If the difference is above the action limit, the wipe is considered contaminated with radioactivity and the area this wipe represents must be decontaminated.

The surveys are performed using a Geiger-Mueller pancake survey meter. The pancake probe is held close to the surface(s) of the specified area, and moved across the surface at a rate of about 3 to 5 inches per second, hence measuring the exposure rate of the area being surveyed. The results are recorded and maintained in the pharmacy.

Equipment Checks

The NPT performs daily tasks that must be accomplished prior to radiopharmaceutical compounding and dose dispensing. For example, quality control tests are performed daily on dose calibrators and scalers. This task utilizes a long-lived isotope (e.g., Cs-137, Co-57) to determine if the equipment can measure a source of activity and exposure, respectively, with a certain degree of reproducibility and repeatedly. It also determines if repair needs to be performed on a given instrument.

Daily Geiger-Mueller survey meter (SM) checks are performed primarily to ensure these units are detecting radiation exposure accurately by using a small check source of a long-lived isotope (e.g., Cs-137, Co-57) attached to the side of the survey meter. At the time of calibration, it is determined what the exposure rate is of this source on the SM and that is the reference point for future tests.

Other tests that may be performed by the NPT include scaler efficiencies, dose calibrator accuracies, linearities, constancies, and geometries. These are instrument quality control tests to ensure the accuracy, reliability, and reproducibility of equipment.

Inventory Management

The NPT plays an active role in inventory management of the pharmacy, and each facility may have its own method of tracking on-hand inventory as well as ordering. One of the easiest methods is to have standing orders in place. With a standing order, specified quantities of particular products are shipped to the pharmacy at specified intervals. The NPT can monitor use of materials, spot-order items, adjust the standing orders, and more.

Waste Management

When spent and unused unit-dose syringes are returned to the pharmacy from nuclear medicine departments, they are considered radioactive waste and must be segregated by half-life and stored for decay in appropriately shielded containers, usually barrels, in compliance with state medical waste regulations. The shielded lead containers are usually lined with a fiberboard drum or another type of sharps container. The waste is left to decay for at least 10 half-lives, after which, upon surveying with a high-level survey meter, the exposure levels at the surface of the barrel must be indistinguishable from background. At this point, the waste is considered biomedical, or medical waste, and can be prepared to be sent for disposal. The waste can be removed from the shielded storage containers, sealed, boxed up, and labeled for shipping, in accordance with state medical waste regulations. Storage information and final survey readings must be recorded on a medical waste record and saved. The technician will participate in proper segregation of the waste by half-life, ensure criteria for disposal are met, prepare the waste for release, and ensure the records for waste and waste release are complete and accurate.

Report Preparation

Governing agencies such as the NRC, DOT, and state boards of pharmacy require records to be kept of many activities that occur in the pharmacy. The NPT may be responsible for preparing and printing these records. The records required to be on location include:

- Generator elution records
- Compounding records
- Dispensing records
- Radiopharmaceutical quality assurance testing records
- Incoming package/outgoing shipping records
- Room wipe records and surveys
- Air monitoring records
- Employee bioassay records
- Employee training documents
- Employee dosimetry reports
- Equipment testing records, both daily and periodic
- LAFW cleaning records
- Laminar flow integrity testing records
- Temperature checks of refrigerator/freezer
- Waste disposal records for hazardous materials and radioactive materials.

Maintenance of Laboratory Cleanliness

Because the pharmacy environment can be a great contributor to microbial and particulate contamination in compounding areas, great attention must be given to minimizing the introduction of microbial and foreign particulate into these areas. USP Chapter <797> describes the cleaning tasks and minimum frequencies associated with these tasks. Their frequency is associated with how likely the area is to play a role in contaminating a sterile product. An example is the surface of a LAFW compared to that of the ceiling of the buffer area. The surfaces of the LAFW are more critical than those of the ceiling because they come into contact with the compounding products. Therefore, they are cleaned and disinfected daily, at the beginning of each shift, between batches, and no longer than 30 minutes following the previous disinfection when ongoing compounding is being performed and more, whereas the ceilings are done monthly. The NPT plays a very active role in that the NPT will perform most of these tasks and do so according to the company's standard operating procedures and USP Chapter <797>.

Commercial nuclear pharmacies have a comprehensive program for maintaining a safe and clean working environment to ensure the quality of the prepared doses. The program is comprised of standard operating procedures developed to provide consistent and compliant practices.

Detecting RAM

The properties of ionizing radiation make it essentially impossible to detect without the use of special equipment. Ionizing radiation is odorless, colorless, and tasteless. It is invisible. The principle of ionizing radiation that allow us to detect it is the deposition of ions in a material as the radiation interacts with it. A typical nuclear pharmacy has **survey meters**, **dose calibrators**, and **well counters** at a minimum. All three instruments work very similarly but have very specific roles in the operation of a nuclear pharmacy.

survey meter radiation detection instrument measuring exposure in millirems per hour; can be gas filled or a scintillation detector

dose calibrator used for compounding and dispensing patient doses; an ionization chamber allowing for the measurement of the amount of radiation present in a source in millicuries or curies

well counter a scintillation detector, used for measuring test tubes housing package and area wipes

The two types of detectors are gas-filled detectors and scintillation detectors. In gas-filled detectors, radiations cause ionization of the gas molecules, which in turn causes ion pairs to collect at electrodes, resulting in a change in voltage across the two electrodes. This provides a measure of exposure in milliroentgens per hour (mR/hr) for Geiger-Mueller counters and millicuries (mCi) and curies (Ci) for dose calibrators.

Scintillation detectors, such as well counters and multichannel analyzers, rely on scintillation events to detect radiation. The detection occurs when sodium iodide (NaI) detectors interact with a particle or photon and emit a light photon. The light electron then strikes a photocathode of a photomultiplier tube, creating a pulse. This pulse is then amplified and sent to the scaler to create a count.

Survey Meter

A survey meter is used to determine radiation levels (in mR/Hr) on the outside of packages and containers, on areas of the skin and clothing, and in a room.

Dose Calibrator

A dose calibrator, which has a gas-filled chamber, is used to determine the amount of radioactivity (mCi, Ci) in a syringe or vial while compounding and dispensing radiopharmaceuticals. It accomplishes this based on the displayed activity of energy of the various isotopes. It can also display the activity at a given time in the future (calibration time). Radiation decays over time, and with a dose calibrator a time in the future or past can be entered and the calibrator will determine decay or back decay to provide the amount of activity in the source being assayed. The decay equation is $A_t = A_o^{-kt}$.The calibration time is the time at which the radiopharmaceutical is to be injected into a patient at a clinic or hospital.

Well Counter

The well counter is highly sensitive and is used to determine contamination levels at a very low level. Depending on the instrument to which the well is connected, it may also determine the type of contamination present. It is used in quality control testing and in determining contamination levels in area wipe testing. It measures counts per minute (cpm).

Gamma Camera

gamma camera camera used in nuclear medicine, along with scintillation detectors, to image patients who ingested, inhaled, or were injected with a radiopharmaceutical

A **gamma camera**, found in nuclear medicine departments, is an instrument used to detect photons emitted from the patient to perform patient nuclear medicine scans. There are two main types:

- Single Photon Emission Tomography (SPECT)
- Positron Emission Tomography (PET)
  - Positron Emission is two identical energy photons emitted from a single decay event simultaneously at 511 KeV
  - Highly specific, works at molecular level for disease state imaging

Summary

Nuclear pharmacy is a specialized pharmacy practice where radiopharmaceuticals, comprised of an isotope or isotope and drug, are compounded and dispensed to nuclear medicine departments for individual patient use for diagnostic or therapeutic purposes. It is also one of the most regulated areas of pharmacy, being governed by state boards of pharmacy and federal law, and other governing bodies which influence the practice including the FDA, NRC, DOT, EPA, and FAA. The pharmacy setting is similar to all compounding pharmacies in that they are USP Chapter <797> compliant, but also include engineering controls to provide radiation protection to be compliant with the As Low As Reasonably Achievable (ALARA) concept. The three concepts used to achieve compliance with ALARA is time, distance, and shielding. Furthermore, instrumentation not seen in a typical pharmacy setting is utilized daily for radiation detection and quantification, including dose calibrators, scalers, and survey meters.

Nuclear pharmacy technicians play a large role in this setting including daily quality assurance on all equipment, USP Chapter<797> cleaning, compounding, quality control testing and drawing of unit dose radiopharmaceuticals, receipt and preparation of radioactive packages, inventory and waste (RMW) management, and report preparation. In addition to having a pharmacy technician license, the American Pharmacist Association (APhA) provides NPT training guidelines including objectives and competencies, companies provide company specific training, and Authorized User programs are available for NPT development. With the Authorized User training, the NPT can further their scope of practice to include roles such as Radiation Safety Officer.

TEST YOUR KNOWLEDGE

Multiple Choice

1. Dosage forms of radiopharmaceuticals include which of the following?
   a. capsule
   b. gas
   c. unit dose syringe
   d. all of the above

2. Which of the following are regulatory agencies governing the practice of nuclear pharmacy (select all that apply):
   a. Nuclear Regulatory Commission
   b. Food and Drug Administration
   c. Department of Transportation
   d. State Board of Pharmacy

3. Regulated medical waste that returns from customers is referred to as ________________ until the isotope fully decays and is then known as ________________.
   a. radioactive and bio-hazardous waste; bio-hazardous RMW
   b. bio-hazardous RMW; radioactive and bio-hazardous waste
   c. spent doses; "cold" trash
   d. returns; decayed-in-storage RMW

4. An NPT may perform the following tasks EXCEPT
   a. daily constancies on dose calibrators.
   b. radiopharmaceutical compounding.
   c. receive oral nuclear medicine orders.
   d. prescription order entry.

5. Quality control of radiopharmaceuticals allows for determination of which of the following:
   a. bound drug
   b. apyrogenicity
   c. sterility
   d. none of the above

6. The USP states the passing rate for radiopharmaceutical quality control is
   a. 60%.
   b. 70%.
   c. 80%.
   d. 90%.

7. Who determines daily and monthly cleaning tasks for the pharmacy clean areas?
   a. Corporate
   b. USP Chapter <797>
   c. State Board of Pharmacy
   d. None of the above

Fill in the Blank

1. All aspects of procuring, handling, storing, and disposing of radioactive material is regulated by the ____________.

2. The area in the pharmacy where RAM is stored is called ____________.

3. Authorized user training requires ____________ hours of didactic and ____________ hours of on-site training.

4. The instrument used to image radiopharmaceuticals is called ____________.

True/False

1. Radiopharmaceuticals can be either diagnostic or therapeutic.
   a. True
   b. False
2. Area wipes and surveys are performed on a bi-weekly basis.
   a. True
   b. False
3. The Molybdenum-99/Technetium-99m ratio does not need to be determined with each elution.
   a. True
   b. False

Short Answer

1. What is the imaging component of most radiopharmaceuticals, and where does it originate?
2. List four radiopharmaceutical routes of administration.
3. List two indications for radiopharmaceuticals.
4. List the four mechanisms used in ALARA to minimize one's exposure to radiation.
5. What is the isotope primarily used in nuclear medicine for imaging?
6. Give four examples of typical staff members in a nuclear pharmacy.

Suggested Readings

Hung, J.C. (2004). Quality control in nuclear pharmacy. In *Radiopharmaceuticals in nuclear pharmacy and nuclear medicine* (pp. 399–450). Washington, DC: American Pharmacists Association.

Wittstrom, K. (2004). The nuclear pharmacy. In *Radiopharmaceuticals in nuclear pharmacy and nuclear medicine* (pp. 381–398). Washington, DC: American Pharmacists Association.

Websites

American Pharmacist Association www.pharmacist.org

American Society of Health-System Pharmacists www.ashp.org

Nuclear Regulatory Commission www.nrc.gov

Pharmacy Technician Information Center www.pharmtechinfocenter.com

PART

II

The Profession of Pharmacy

CHAPTER

8

Regulatory Standards in Pharmacy Practice

Competencies

Upon completion of this chapter, the reader should be able to:

1. Describe the difference between statutes, rules and regulations, and quasi-legal standards.
2. Identify several federal regulatory agencies and their functions and state agencies and their functions and how they differ regarding the practice of pharmacy.
3. Explain the reason for rules, regulations, and practice standards in health institutions.
4. Describe the Food, Drug, and Cosmetic Act, its purpose, how it affects products used for patient care, and the importance of both drugs and medical devices to the practice of pharmacy.
5. Discuss the investigational drug approval process, how it differs from the approval process for medical devices, and the role of the U.S. Food and Drug Administration in these processes.
6. Recognize drugs that are regulated by the Controlled Substances Act and list several requirements of the Controlled Substances Act.
7. Recognize and describe the differences between federal law such as the Food, Drug, and Cosmetic Act and state laws that regulate the practice of pharmacy.
8. Explain the need for safety data sheets (SDS).
9. Cite appropriate categories of drugs requiring patient package inserts.
10. State several basic components of a patient's bill of rights.

Key Terms

abbreviated new drug application (ANDA)
Bureau of Alcohol, Tobacco, Firearms and Explosives (ATF)
Center for Devices and Radiological Health (CDRH)
Center for Drug Evaluation and Research (CDER)
Centers for Medicare and Medicaid Services (CMS)
Consumer Product Safety Commission (CPSC)
Controlled Substances Act (CSA)
covered entities
Department of Justice (DOJ)
Drug Enforcement Administration (DEA)

Key Terms (*Continued*)

Durham-Humphrey Amendment
Environmental Protection Agency (EPA)
False Claims Act (FCA)
false statement
Family Smoking Prevention and Tobacco Control Act
FDA Adverse Event Reporting System (FAERS)
Federal Anti-Kickback Statute
Federal Hazardous Substances Act (FHSA)
Federal Register
Federal Trade Commission (FTC)
Food and Drug Administration (FDA)
Food and Drug Administration Modernization Act of 1997 (FDAMA)
Food, Drug, and Cosmetic Act of 1938 (FDCA)
guidance document
Hazard Communication Standard (HCS)
Health Insurance Portability and Accountability Act (HIPAA)
Homeopathic Pharmacopoeia of the United States
Humanitarian Use Device (HUD)
intended use
interstate commerce
Investigational Device Exemption (IDE)
investigational new drug application (INDA)
Kefauver-Harris Amendments
Medical Device Amendment
medication administration record (MAR)
medication therapy management (MTM)
MedWatch
new drug application (DNA)
Occupational Safety and Health Act of 1970
Occupational Safety and Health Administration (OSHA)
off-label marketing
Omnibus Budget Reconciliation Act (OBRA)
orphan drugs
patent
patient package insert (PPI)
patient's bill of rights
performance improvement (PI)
Poison Prevention Packaging Act
postmarketing surveillance
premarket approval (PMA)
prospective drug review
protected health information (PHI)
Pure Food and Drug Act of 1906
quasi-legal standards
regulation
rule
safety data sheets (SDS)
Schedule I (controlled substance)
Schedule II (controlled substance)
Schedule III (controlled substance)
Schedule IV (controlled substance)
Schedule V (controlled substance)
state board of pharmacy
statute
The Joint Commission
"U.S. Pharmacopeia-National Formulary" (USP-NF)

Introduction

Laws are intended to ensure the orderly and safe functioning of society while protecting and respecting individual prerogatives. Every individual or enterprise is subject to some form of law, whether it is in a business/professional enterprise or in a person's everyday activities, such as crossing a street or parking a car. Laws generally need someone to enforce them, such as the police or in the case of pharmacy practice, the state board of pharmacy. The entity that is responsible for informing people about the requirements of a law, aiding in enforcement, and defining how the law will be implemented may be empowered by the law to enact **rules** and **regulations**. These rules and regulations have the force of law and provide the public with notice as to what is expected of them in order to comply with the law.

rule guideline that dictates particular actions and procedures as issued by a governing body

regulation process or procedure issued by a governing body

Laws and regulations pertaining to health care are intended to provide for the safety and welfare of health care recipients. They provide for the provision of minimum standards by a health care service and are the basis for standards by which to judge reasonable and prudent practice in a court of law. The implementation of new regulations has the overall intent of providing a positive impact on the elevation and expansion of health care services and responsibilities.

The complex U.S. health care system encompasses pharmaceutical and device manufacturers, health care institutions, medical and pharmaceutical practices, insurance companies, governmental reimbursing entities, governmental oversight agencies, and last, but certainly not least, individual patients. Every health care profession, institution, and health care–related business is subject to regulation in some form. The profession of pharmacy with its direct relationship to public health, safety, and welfare is under the watchful eye of various regulatory agencies.

One objective of this chapter is to give the pharmacy technician a broad understanding of laws that affect the delivery of health care products and services in the United States. The second objective is to provide an understanding of some federal and state laws and regulations to which the practice of pharmacy is subject and the regulatory agencies that are empowered to enforce these laws and regulations. The third objective is to provide an appreciation of the relationship of these regulatory standards to the specific activities of the pharmacist and the pharmacy technician in the practice of pharmacy.

Statutes, Rules, Regulations, and Quasi-Legal Standards

statute enacted law

A **statute** is an enacted law. The process of creating a statute generally begins with a bill being introduced into the legislative branch of government. The bill undergoes a series of steps before it finally becomes a law. Federal statutes, for example, are introduced into one of the houses of Congress, either the Senate or the House of Representatives. Sometimes, similar bills may be introduced simultaneously into both bodies of Congress. After the bill goes through a number of committees, debates, and votes, it may be passed by the house of Congress where it was first introduced. The bill then passes to the other house of Congress where a similar process occurs. Finally, after both houses of Congress have voted on the bill (assuming it passed—generally with multiple amendments), it goes to the president of the United States for signature. If signed, the bill becomes law.

This process have many variations, with the preceding discussion being the most simplistic, but it illustrates the general process for purposes of this discussion. A similar process occurs on the state level. States, like the federal government, have three branches of government; the legislature, the executive branch, and the judicial branch. On the state level, after the state legislature passes a bill, the governor of the state signs it so that the bill can become state law.

Federal statutes are sequentially entered into a publication called *Statutes at Large*. This is a listing of laws passed each year. To bring like laws together, they are codified. When this is done, the laws are published in the *United States Code* (*USC*). Oftentimes you will hear a term such as Title 21 or Title 11; this is a reference to the *USC* codification under which the related series of laws are found. The U.S. Food, Drug, and Cosmetic Act of 1938 (FDCA), for example, is found at 21 *USC* 321, *et seq.*

Legislative statutory activity can amend an existing law by removing or modifying a power already found in that law or add new powers to an existing law. Sometimes, a new law is passed that is so expansive that it requires the creation of a regulating body or agency to oversee the implementation and enforcement of the law. Examples of such federal agencies include the **Food and Drug Administration (FDA)**, which administers the FDCA; the **Drug Enforcement Administration (DEA)**, which administers the federal Comprehensive Drug Abuse and Prevention Control Act, more commonly known as the Controlled Substances Act (CSA); the **Centers for Medicare and Medicaid Services (CMS)**, which oversees aspects of the federal medical reimbursement programs; and the **Environmental Protection Agency (EPA)**.

Rules and regulations are implemented by government agencies at the federal, state, and local levels of government. For example, the FDA can implement rules and regulations to enforce the federal Food, Drug, and Cosmetic Act. On the state level, state boards of pharmacy issue detailed regulations to carry out the policies and procedures of the state pharmacy acts.

Federal agencies that wish to establish a regulatory power such as a rule or regulation publish the proposal in a daily publication called the ***Federal Register***. This announcement generally requests comments from interested parties that may be affected by the proposal. After due consideration of all public comments, the proposed rule or regulation may be implemented as originally planned, modified, or abandoned.

Violations of rules and regulations can result in civil and criminal penalties including fines, prison time, and debarment from participation in certain federal and state programs. Federal regulations are codified in a publication known as the *Code of Federal Regulations* (*CFR*).

Quasi means "similar to." **Quasi-legal standards** are established by quasi-governmental or private organizations, such as professional pharmacy organizations. These standards are recognized by the federal government and many state governments and can form the basis of laws and regulations. The American Society of Health-System Pharmacists (ASHP) has developed an extensive series of practice standards covering numerous aspects of institutional pharmacy practice. Practice standards provide a basis for evaluation, review, and goal setting for hospital pharmacy directors and their staffs.

An example of a situation where quasi-legal standards are followed is when contractors who are employed by government agencies inspect health care facilities and manufacturers of pharmaceuticals and medical devices. These third-party inspectors are neither government personnel nor regulators, but they act on behalf of government regulators. Failure to cooperate with them during an inspection or making **false statements** to one of these quasi-governmental inspectors can result in penalties akin to what would have occurred if they were

Food and Drug Administration (FDA) promulgates rules, regulations, and standards; inspects drug and food facilities to ensure public safety regarding drug products

Drug Enforcement Administration (DEA) a federal agency established to enforce the rules and regulations of the Controlled Substances Act (CSA), which was designed to combat controlled substance abuse

Centers for Medicare and Medicaid Services (CMS) a federal agency that administers the Medicare program and works in partnership with state governments to administer Medicaid, the Children's Health Insurance Program, and health insurance portability standards

Environmental Protection Agency (EPA) a federal agency tasked with protecting human health and the environment by writing and enforcing regulations based on laws passed by Congress

Federal Register a publication announcing a new rule or regulation and requesting a public comment period on it

quasi-legal standard recognized standards that are similar to laws

false statement deliberate communication of information that is misleading or incorrect

actually government regulators. Making a false statement to a federal government regulator, investigator, or representative is a violation of federal law and can result in criminal prosecution.

Standards are also important in malpractice lawsuits where a plaintiff must prove that the professional defendant fell ". . . below a standard of care that would be expected of like professionals who practice in that field and in that locale." Expert witnesses testify as to what practice standards require of the professional under the facts of the case. The jury then determines if there was a breach of the duty of care owed by the professional to the patient; that is, whether malpractice occurred. The professional standards applied in these matters are given quasi-legal status and a practitioner who fails to meet them may be found professionally negligent.

Federal versus State and Local Laws

The United States is governed by both federal law and state law. Each state has its own body of laws and regulations, which may differ dramatically from those of neighboring states and the federal government. In addition, many municipalities like New York City, Chicago, Los Angeles, and Dallas have their own laws or ordinances as do many counties and townships.

Those practicing pharmacy have to comply with the laws that exist where they practice. The adage "ignorance of the law is not an excuse" is as valid today as it was when the statement was first coined. Therefore, to determine where you stand in complying with the law, the following guidelines may be of assistance:

1. Pharmacists and pharmacy technicians are responsible for compliance with all applicable federal, state, and local laws and regulations governing their pharmacy practice.
2. The practice of pharmacy is basically regulated by state law and is generally under the auspices of the state board of pharmacy.
3. In addition to the state laws, you may be subject to local laws, such as municipal health codes and privacy laws, which you need to learn and understand.
4. If there is a federal law or regulation that pertains to your practice, it may take precedence over state or local law, especially if Congress has determined that this certain federal law permeates the field or overrides or preempts state or local law.
5. When two or more laws exist in an area (such as federal and state controlled substance laws), generally the best course is to abide by the most stringent law or regulation. Oftentimes, state law or regulation is more stringent than its federal counterpart; however, there may be matters covered in one of the laws that may not have been covered in the other; these differences need to be determined so that noncompliance with a portion of a law does not become an issue.
6. When in doubt seek professional advice from your state's board of pharmacy.

State Regulation of Pharmacy Practice

The practice of pharmacy is primarily regulated by each state, and each state has its own unique structure for the regulation of the education, licensing, and discipline of the profession of pharmacy. Because laws may differ from state to state, boards of pharmacy may have different roles and responsibilities, and the requirements for both the pharmacist and pharmacy technician may vary significantly from state to state.

State Boards of Pharmacy

state board of pharmacy body established to ensure that the public is well served professionally by pharmacists

intended use the stated manner in which a product was created to act and be used

In most states, a major responsibility of the **state board of pharmacy** is to ensure that the public is well served professionally by pharmacists, that the drugs distributed and dispensed by the pharmacy within each state meet that state's standards for purity and potency, and that dispensed medications are properly labeled by the pharmacist for the patient's use. Other responsibilities include, but are not limited to the following:

- Licensing and registering pharmacies
- Dealing with complaints of professional misconduct of pharmacists and pharmacy technicians
- Carrying out disciplinary proceedings
- Developing regulations related to filling and refilling prescriptions
- Substituting generic and therapeutic drugs
- Labeling of medications dispensed by pharmacies
- Performing inspections
- Defining poisons and mandating records to be maintained upon retail sale.

U.S. Food and Drug Administration

Pure Food and Drug Act of 1906 federal law passed by Congress because of concern about the risks to public health and safety associated with unsanitary and poorly labeled foods and drugs

Food, Drug, and Cosmetic Act of 1938 (FDCA) federal law through which the Food and Drug Administration enforces its rules and regulations

Kefauver-Harris Amendments amendments to the federal Food, Drug, and Cosmetic Act that required all new drugs marketed in the United States to be proven safe and effective

Family Smoking Prevention and Tobacco Control Act a federal statute that gives the U.S. Food and Drug Administration the power to regulate the tobacco industry

interstate commerce exchange of goods between states

In contrast to state boards of pharmacy that regulate a profession, the FDA is responsible for ensuring that the products under its jurisdiction are safe and effective for their **intended use**. The FDA has its roots in the Department of Agriculture's chemical division dating from 1862. It became known as the FDA in 1930. From 1953 to 1979 it was under the Department of Health, Education and Welfare. The FDA became part of the Department of Health and Human Services (DHHS) when it was created in 1979. The FDA commissioner reports to the secretary of DHHS.

FDA Enforcement: Past and Present

The first federal statute pertaining to food and drug regulation was the Biologics Control Act of 1902. This was enacted to deal with tetanus-infected diphtheria antitoxin that resulted in the deaths of several children in St. Louis, Missouri. Further, the Department of Agriculture's chemistry division's (early FDA) work on adulterated food led to enactment of the **Pure Food and Drug Act of 1906**. Over the years demand for a complete overhaul of the nation's regulatory system in the area of drugs, cosmetics, mechanical devices, and food resulted in the federal **Food, Drug, and Cosmetic Act of 1938 (FDCA)**. The FDCA has undergone several major amendments over time, such as the **Kefauver-Harris Amendments** of 1962 (in relation to the thalidomide tragedy) and the 1976 medical device amendments. In addition, the FDA has recently been given authority over tobacco products via the **Family Smoking Prevention and Tobacco Control Act** of 2009. Therefore, the FDA regulates pharmaceuticals, medical devices, *in vitro* diagnostic products, cosmetics, food products, animal-derived drugs, and tobacco products that are distributed commercially in the United States and its territories via **interstate commerce**.

FDA Regulatory Oversight

The FDA regulates the labeling, marketing, and manufacturing of the products under its jurisdiction. Manufacturing is regulated through series of regulations called Quality System Regulations (QSRs; formerly called Good Manufacturing Practice

U.S. Pharmacopeia-National Formulary (USP-NF) the official pharmacopeia of the United States, published dually with the National Formulary as the USP-NF; prescription and over-the-counter medicines and other health care products sold in the United States are required to follow USP-NF standards

Homeopathic Pharmacopoeia of the United States one of the three official drug compendia specified in the Federal Food, Drug, and Cosmetic Act

Center for Drug Evaluation and Research (CDER) a federal department that regulates over-the-counter and prescription drugs, including biological therapeutics and generic drugs

Center for Devices and Radiological Health (CDRH) a federal department that is responsible for the premarket approval of all medical devices; also oversees the manufacture, performance, and safety of these devices and the radiation safety performance of nonmedical devices that emit certain types of electromagnetic radiation, such as cellular phones and microwave ovens

investigational new drug application (INDA) the means by which a pharmaceutical company obtains permission to ship an experimental drug across state lines (usually to clinical investigators) before a marketing application for the drug has been approved

new drug application (NDA) vehicle through which drug sponsors formally propose that the Food and Drug Administration approve a new pharmaceutical for sale and marketing in the United States

regulations or cGMPs). Failure to comply with QSRs can result in product recalls, discontinuance, and the shutdown of manufacturing facilities.

The term *drug* is defined in the FDCA as (A) articles recognized in the official **U.S. Pharmacopeia-National Formulary (USP-NF)**, the official **Homeopathic Pharmacopoeia of the United States**, or any supplement to any of them; and (B) articles intended for use in the diagnosis, cure, mitigation, treatment, or prevention of disease in man or other animals; and (C) articles (other than food) intended to affect the structure or any function of the body of man or other animals; and (D) articles intended for use as a component of any article specified in clause (A), (B), or (C).

Pharmacy Compounded Drugs

The FDA regulates the interstate distribution of pharmacy compounded medications. The FDA takes the position that compounded drugs are "new drugs" subject to FDA approval, but because they are dispensed to individual patients pursuant to a prescription, the FDA has exercised "enforcement discretion" to not require compounded prescriptions to undergo regulatory approval as new drugs. The FDA Modernization Act of 1997 (FDAMA) established the parameters under which compounded drugs can be prepared and distributed by pharmacies without having to undergo FDA approval as "new drugs":

1. The compounded drug must be prepared by a pharmacist or physician in response to a valid prescription for an identified patient and in limited quantities.
2. The compounded drug must be made from approved ingredients that meet certain manufacturing and safety standards and that are not on an FDA list of withdrawn or removed drugs as a result of safety or efficacy issues.
3. The compounding practice must not be done in inordinate amounts in relation to commercially available drugs.
4. The drug product must not be identified by the FDA as having demonstrated difficulties for compounding in terms of safety and efficacy.
5. Unless a state has entered into a Memorandum of Understanding with the FDA regarding the distribution of "inordinate amounts" of compounded drugs in interstate commerce by the pharmacy, those pharmacies and physicians may not distribute compounded drugs out of the state in quantities exceeding 5% of that entity's total prescription orders.
6. The prescriptions must be unsolicited and the entity making the compounded drug cannot advertise or promote the compounded drug; however, the pharmacy can advertise to promote the compounding service.

New Drug Development

Two FDA centers of responsibility relevant to the practice of pharmacy are the **Center for Drug Evaluation and Research (CDER)** and the **Center for Devices and Radiological Health (CDRH)**. A pharmaceutical manufacturer wishing to gain FDA approval to manufacture and distribute a drug through interstate commerce will submit an **investigational new drug application (INDA)** to the FDA. CDER reviews the application and after many years and hundreds of million of dollars in research, the manufacturer will apply to the FDA for a **new drug application (NDA)** if the research supports the application. The following subsections discuss some of the steps taken in the conduct of studies needed to gain FDA drug approval.

Preclinical Studies

Preclinical research utilizes animal studies and *in vitro* data to establish a drug's biological and toxicological characteristics. Preclinical studies help to determine the drug's basic pharmacological and pharmacokinetic properties such as drug absorption, distribution, metabolism, and elimination. This information provides the basis for establishing suitable human dosage regimens.

Phase I Clinical Studies

Phase I clinical studies represent the first time a new drug is introduced into human beings. Emphasis is placed on describing the safety of the new agent by defining the pharmacokinetic (absorption, distribution, metabolism, and elimination), toxicological, and pharmacological parameters associated with its use in humans. A minimal number of patients are utilized for Phase I clinical trials.

Phase II Clinical Studies

Phase II clinical studies expand on the activities initiated during Phase I trials. In Phase II, the emphasis is on establishing the activity of the new drug in patients being treated with the experimental drug. Evidence of safety and efficacy must be established before proceeding further with Phase III trials.

Phase III Clinical Studies

Phase III clinical studies provide for broader proof of safety and efficacy and also establish the acceptable use(s) of the drug. Phase III study protocols are often conducted in a number of hospitals concurrently. Hundreds of patients may need to be evaluated before meaningful results can be obtained. Marketing approval via an NDA can be sought only upon completion of all of the aforementioned research.

Postmarketing Surveillance

All FDA-regulated drug and device products are subject to adverse event reporting requirements. Manufacturers of drugs and devices must report adverse events to the FDA whenever the adverse event may have led to or did lead to serious injury or death. This process is called **postmarketing surveillance** and includes the following programs:

- **FDA Adverse Event Reporting System (FAERS):** FAERS is a computerized information database designed to support the FDA's postmarketing safety surveillance program for all approved drug and therapeutic biological products. As a result of findings from the analysis of submitted data, the FDA may take regulatory action to improve product safety and protect the public health, such as updating a product's labeling information, sending out a "Dear Health Care Professional" letter, or reevaluating an approval decision.
- **MedWatch:** The MedWatch program allows health professionals, manufacturers, and the public to report serious reactions and problems (i.e., when the event could have or did lead to serious injury or death) with FDA-regulated medical products. The program helps ensure that new safety information is rapidly communicated to the medical community, which helps to improve patient care. All data contained on the MedWatch form is entered into the FAERS database.

> **postmarketing surveillance** the reporting of adverse events to the FDA by manufacturers of drugs and devices whenever an adverse event may have led to or did lead to serious injury or death
>
> **FDA Adverse Event Reporting System (FAERS)** a computerized information database designed to support the FDA's postmarketing safety surveillance program for all approved drug and therapeutic biological products
>
> **MedWatch** a program that allows health professionals, manufacturers, and the public to report serious reactions and problems related to FDA-regulated medical products

Institutional Review Boards

Institutional review boards (IRBs) are multidisciplinary boards or committees designated by a research institution to objectively review and approve biomedical research involving human subjects in accordance with FDA and other governmental regulations as well as pertinent ethical considerations. The main purpose of the IRB is to ensure that risks to patients are minimized and that written informed consent is obtained from each patient (via a patient consent form). The FDA has issued several **guidance documents** regarding the responsibilities of IRBs in overseeing research involving human subjects that will be submitted to the FDA to support drug or device approval.

guidance documents included under the umbrella title of FDA Information Sheets, these documents represent the Food and Drug Administration's current thinking on protection of human subjects in research

Informed Consent

Clinical studies conducted on humans to support an FDA-regulated product or submission require investigators to obtain informed consent from the patient or the patient's representative for the administration of an experimental drug or for other forms of analyses used to support submissions to the FDA. The informed consent identifies the potential risks, possible benefits, and alternative course(s) of treatment that may be available to persons involved with the clinical study. In addition, many medical and scientific journals require IRB oversight and informed consent in order for a scientific paper that concerns human studies to be accepted for publication. Finally, basic ethical and legal considerations make obtaining informed consent a wise decision.

FDA Advisory Panel Review

The FDA team responsible for reviewing a product submission may call for a panel of experts to review the data submitted in support of an application for a product's approval. The FDA will ask the panel to comment on questions posed to it regarding the submitted data. Ultimately the panel will recommend whether the drug, in their view, is safe and effective for its proposed intended use. The FDA has discretion to accept or reject the panel's recommendation.

Promotion and Marketing

Drug and device manufacturers are limited to marketing their products only for the product's approved intended use. Marketing outside of the approved intended use is called **off-label marketing** and causes the drug or device to be misbranded and adulterated in violation of the FDCA.

off-label marketing providing information regarding the use of a drug for other than its approved and intended use

False Claims Act (FCA) a law that makes it a crime to file a false claim for monetary reimbursement from the government, to withhold overpayments, or to induce someone else to file a false claim

In recent years, the U.S. government has collected billions of dollars in fines and a number of individuals have been prosecuted for promoting products off label. A primary prosecutorial theory employed by the government is that off-label marketing results in the writing of off-label prescriptions and that many of these prescriptions are paid for by the government; therefore, the government and the taxpayer are being defrauded. The law used in such prosecutions is called the federal **False Claims Act (FCA)**, which makes it a crime to file a false claim for monetary reimbursement from the government, to withhold overpayments, or to induce someone else to file a false claim. Filling out false reimbursement claims for prescription drugs dispensed by pharmacies, hospitals, or clinics is a violation of this law.

Neither the practice of medicine nor the practice of pharmacy is regulated by the FDA. It is not illegal for physicians to prescribe drugs for off-label uses, and pharmacists can discuss and dispense medications for off-label uses. Off-label marketing laws apply to those who are regulated by the FDA such as product manufacturers.

patent an exclusive license, provided for in the U.S. Constitution, that provides an inventor with a statutory time period during which the inventor can exclusively market the patented product

Patents and Generic Drugs

A **patent** is an exclusive license provided for in the U.S. Constitution (Article I, sect. 8). It provides an inventor with a statutory time period to exclusively market the patented product. This exclusivity rewards the inventor's ingenuity and provides a means of fostering technological advancement in the country and world (there are also international patents). Once a patent on a drug expires, generic drug manufacturers can file with the FDA to market a generic version of the drug. This application is called an **abbreviated new drug application (ANDA)**. To be granted an ANDA, the generic manufacturer must show that the generic is manufactured in accordance with QSRs and that it is bioequivalent to the patented drug. Bioequivalence is generally demonstrated by the achievement of drug blood levels over time within a set range when compared to the patented product.

abbreviated new drug application (ANDA) a request to create a generic version of a drug or product with an expired patent

Medical Devices

Medical devices distributed through interstate commerce are regulated by the FDA. MRI equipment, cyber knives, CT scanners, *in vitro* diagnostic reagents and kits, hospital beds, thermometers, glucose strips and meters, syringes and needles, latex gloves, and test tubes used to collect specimen samples are all regulated medical devices.

The term *device* in the FDCA

> *. . . means an instrument, apparatus, implement, machine, contrivance, implant, in vitro reagent, or other similar or related article, including any component, part, or accessory, which is:*
>
> 1. recognized in the official USP-NF or any supplement to them,
> 2. intended for use in the diagnosis of disease or other conditions, or in the cure, mitigation, treatment, or prevention of disease, in man or other animals, or
> 3. intended to affect the structure or any function of the body of man or other animals, and which does not achieve its primary intended purposes through chemical action within or on the body of man or other animals and which is not dependent upon being metabolized for the achievement of its primary intended purposes.

Because many medical devices are encountered in the practice of pharmacy, it is important to understand how they are regulated. Devices are classified according to the risk associated with their use: Class I devices present the least risk; Class II, intermediate risk; and Class III, the highest risk. Class I devices include items such as test tubes, hearing aids, and basic chemical reagents; most are exempted by FDA from having to go through a premarket clearance or approval process. Higher risk Class I and Class II devices must get premarket clearance through a procedure called the 510(k) process, in which the applicant must demonstrate that the device is substantially equivalent to a previously FDA cleared device. Most Class III devices have to undergo a **premarket approval (PMA)** that is akin to a drug approval process. Generally, to conduct investigational studies on these devices one files for an **Investigational Device Exemption (IDE)** with the CDRH. This allows the device to be distributed and used in various locales for research purposes. If the FDA approves the product as being safe and effective for its intended use, the product can be marketed under the PMA for that use.

premarket approval (PMA) the process of scientific and regulatory review to evaluate the safety and effectiveness of Class III medical devices; Class III devices are those that support or sustain human life, are of substantial importance in preventing impairment of human health, or present a potential, unreasonable risk of illness or injury

Investigational Device Exemption (IDE) exemption to current law that allows an investigational device to be used in a clinical study in order to collect safety and effectiveness data

Humanitarian Use Devices

Manufacturers of devices that can benefit patients with rare medical conditions (those conditions that affect fewer than 4,000 individuals in the United States

Humanitarian Use Device (HUD) a device that is intended to benefit patients by treating or diagnosing a disease or condition that affects or is manifested in fewer than 4,000 individuals in the United States per year

per year) can apply to the FDA for their device to be classified as a **Humanitarian Use Device (HUD)**. Similar to orphan drugs, which are discussed later in this chapter, the cost of the process is less than the standard review processes, thus fostering development of products for rare conditions.

Risk Evaluation and Mitigation Strategy (REMS) Program

The Food and Drug Administration Amendments Act of 2007 (FDAAA) gave the FDA regulatory authority to implement a program called Risk Evaluation and Mitigation Strategy (REMS). The purpose of the REMS program is to inform patients of the risks associated with certain drug products such as drugs with an addiction potential or other serious side effects. It entails the development and distribution of medical guides and other information to patients on an inpatient and outpatient basis. When a drug has a medication guide, that guide should be dispensed directly to patients or to their caregivers for provision to the patient. In the outpatient setting, the medication guide should be provided the first time a drug is dispensed or whenever the medication guide is materially changed, and any time that a patient or caregiver asks for the guide.

Centers for Medicare and Medicaid Services (CMS)

The CMS, like the FDA, is under the Department of Health and Human Services. The CMS, among other things, has oversight of the government's Medicare and Medicaid reimbursement programs.

Statutes Relevant to CMS-Related Activities

Federal Anti-Kickback Statute 42 USC 1320a-7b illegal payments/bribes that are offered, requested or paid or accepted by any party to influence the sale of a drug, device or other product that is reimbursed under a federal or state program is a felony. Penalties include prison time and monetary fines.

In addition to the False Claims Act, another law regarding reimbursement that carries heavy financial and criminal penalties is called the **Federal Anti-Kickback Statute**. Pursuant to this law, it is illegal to offer or ask, or to pay or receive, directly or indirectly, overtly or covertly, any remuneration of any type, in order to induce the sale, purchase, or lease of a product that is reimbursed under a federal or state reimbursing plan. Many companies have been heavily fined under this law and people, including pharmacists and physicians, have been sent to prison for violating it. Billions of dollars a year in fines are collected by the U.S. government and most companies that sell reimbursed products have decided to no longer offer things of value to those who purchase or prescribe their products.

Various industrial codes of conduct help guide the practices of manufacturers in dealing ethically with health care professionals. Societies such as the Pharmaceutical Research and Manufacturers of America (PhRMA), the Advanced Medical Technology Association (AdvaMed), and the National Electronics Manufacturer's Association's MITA division issue these codes. These ethical codes have gained national and worldwide recognition and have been adopted by a number of states as part of state marketing laws, basically making them quasi-legal laws, as discussed earlier in the chapter. Moreover, the Affordable Care Act has a provision called the Sunshine Act that requires companies that sell FDA-regulated products that are reimbursed by the government to track and report things of value provided to health care practitioners. This act is inspired, in part, by the quasi-legal codes of conduct.

Department of Justice (DOJ) the federal executive department responsible for the enforcement of the law and administration of justice, equivalent to the justice or interior ministries of other countries

Investigation and prosecution for violating the anti-kickback statute and other federal laws are generally conducted by the **Department of Justice (DOJ)**.

Relevant Laws Regarding Pharmacy

A number of federal laws and their amendments relevant to the practice of pharmacy have been enacted over many years. Some of these laws are discussed next.

Pure Food and Drug Act of 1906

As previously noted, the Pure Food and Drug Act of 1906 was passed by Congress because of concerns about the risks to public health and safety associated with unsanitary and poorly labeled foods and drugs. This law prohibited the adulteration and misbranding of foods in interstate commerce. In passing this law, Congress deferred to the National Formulary (NF) and the U.S. Pharmacopeia (USP) for the standards of quality and purity of drugs.

The Food, Drug, and Cosmetic Act of 1938

A major push for the enactment of the Food, Drug, and Cosmetic Act of 1938 was the sulfanilamide elixir tragedy of 1937, which caused 107 deaths. Sulfanilamide elixir, one of the first of the miracle anti-infective sulfa drugs, was mistakenly formulated with diethylene glycol (automobile antifreeze). The 1938 law required that no new drug could be marketed until proven safe for use when used according to directions on the label. The new law also applied to "mechanical devices intended for curative purposes"; false advertising of drugs and foods, and cosmetics; informative product labeling; adulterated products; the operation of factories; and enforcement processes for noncompliance with the law. Drug products marketed prior to 1938 were exempted or "grandfathered" from the law and did not have to be labeled or proven safe under the law. For example, digoxin, nitroglycerin, and phenobarbital were drugs on the market prior to 1938 and were grandfathered from this law.

Durham-Humphrey Amendment of 1951

Durham-Humphrey Amendment an amendment that established two classes of drugs, over-the-counter and prescription, and mandated that labels of prescription drugs include the legend "Caution: Federal law prohibits dispensing without a prescription"

A number of drug products covered by the 1938 FDCA were not safe to use without medical supervision. The **Durham-Humphrey Amendment** (also referred to as the Prescription Drug Amendment) was enacted in 1951 to solve this problem. The amendment established two classes of drugs—prescription and over-the-counter drugs—and provided that the labels of prescription drugs did not have to list "adequate directions for use," but were required to include the legend *"Caution: Federal law prohibits dispensing without a prescription"* on the manufacturer's label. When dispensed by a pharmacist, "adequate directions for use" was satisfied by the pharmacist placing directions written by the prescriber on the label of the dispensed product. These drugs became known as prescription or *legend drugs*. Drugs that did not require medical supervision for their use had to have adequate directions for use on their label and were referred to as over-the-counter or nonprescription drugs.

Kefauver-Harris Amendment of 1962

The Kefauver-Harris Amendment, as mentioned earlier, was adopted as a result of the thalidomide tragedy. Thalidomide was being marketed outside of the United States as a sedative and was used during pregnancy. It was not approved by the FDA for the U.S. market. In 1961 it was confirmed that thalidomide was causing a serious birth defect called dysmelia in thousands of infants in Europe and around the world. The Kefauver-Harris Amendment to the FDCA (also known as the Drug Efficacy Amendment) required that all new drugs marketed in the United States needed to undergo premarket approval where the drug had to be shown to be both safe and effective. This efficacy requirement was made retroactive to all drugs approved between 1938 and 1962.

This amendment also provided for the following:

- The oversight of prescription drug advertising by the FDA
- The establishment of current Good Manufacturing Practices (cGMP) requirements
- Informed consent of patients for clinical drug investigations
- Implementation of reporting of adverse drug reactions.

Medical Device Amendment legislation enacted in 1976 that amended the Food, Drug, and Cosmetic Act; it requires classification of medical devices according to their function and risk

Orphan drugs drugs used for diseases and conditions considered rare in the United States, for which adequate drugs have not yet been developed and do not generate incentives for drug manufacturers to research and develop treatments

Medical Device Amendment of 1976

Congress amended the FDCA in 1976 to provide for more extensive regulation regarding the safety and efficacy of medical devices. The **Medical Device Amendment** requires classification of devices according to their function and risk: Classes I, II, and III as discussed previously.

Orphan Drug Act of 1983

Orphan drugs are used to treat rare diseases. A *rare disease* is one that affects less than 200,000 people in the United States or one that affects more than 200,000 people, but for which there is no reasonable expectation that the cost of developing the drug and making it available will be recovered from the sale of the drug. The law provides various tax and licensing incentives to drug manufacturers to develop and market orphan drugs for the diagnosis, treatment, or prevention of rare diseases or conditions.

Food and Drug Administration Modernization Act of 1997

Food and Drug Administration Modernization Act of 1997 (FDAMA) legislation that streamlined regulatory procedures and encouraged manufacturers to conduct research for new uses of drugs and perform pediatric studies of drugs

Controlled Substances Act (CSA) federal law regulating the manufacture, distribution, and sale of drugs that have the potential for abuse

The **Food and Drug Administration Modernization Act of 1997 (FDAMA)** was passed, in part, to deal with what was felt to be a too-burdensome regulatory system for drug and device approval under the FDCA. This legislation includes:

- Streamlining of regulatory procedures to ensure the expedited availability of safe and effective drugs and devices
- Encouraging drug manufacturers to perform pediatric studies of drugs
- Establishing a safe harbor for pharmacy compounded prescriptions.

The Controlled Substances Act of 1970

The **Controlled Substances Act (CSA)** of 1970 is the major federal law regulating the manufacture, distribution, and sale (dispensing/administration) of certain drugs or substances that are subject to or have a potential for abuse or physical or psychological dependence. These drugs or substances (such as immediate precursors) are designated *controlled substances*.

The Drug Enforcement Administration (DEA) is the federal law enforcement agency charged with the responsibility for combating controlled substance abuse. The DEA was established July 1, 1973. It resulted from the merger of the Bureau of Narcotics and Dangerous Drugs, the Office for Drug Abuse Law Enforcement, and other drug enforcement agencies. The DEA was established to more effectively combat narcotic and dangerous drug diversion and abuse through enforcement and prevention.

TABLE 8-1 Examples of Controlled Substances by Drug Schedule

SCHEDULE I	SCHEDULE II	SCHEDULE III	SCHEDULE IV	SCHEDULE V
heroin	alfentanil	acetaminophen with codeine (Tylenol with codeine)	alprazolam (Xanax)	
marijuana		anabolic steroids (Testoderm, Winstrol)	butorphanol (Stadol)	
LSD	amphetamines	butabarbital (Fiorinal)	chloral hydrate	
peyote	cocaine	dronabinol (Marinol)	chlordiazepoxide (Librium)	
mescaline	fentanyl (Sublimaze, Duragesic)	nalorphine (Nalline)	clonazepam (Klonopin)	Robitussin A-C
	hydromorphone (Dilaudid)	thiopental (Pentothal)		diphenoxylate with atropine (Lomotil)
		diethylpropion (Tenuate)		
hallucinogenic substances	levorphanol (Levo-Dromoran)		eszopiclone (Lunesta)	
	meperidine (Demerol)		flurazepam (Dalmane)	
	methadone		midazolam (Versed)	
	methylphenidate (Ritalin, Concerta)			
	morphine (MS Contin)			
	methamphetamine (Desoxyn)		pentazocine (Talwin)	
	oxycodone (OxyContin)		phenobarbital	
	pentobarbital (Nembutal)		propoxyphene (Darvon, Darvocet)	
	phenmetrazine (Preludin)		sibutramine (Meridia)	
	secobarbital (Seconal)		temazepam (Restoril)	
	sufentanil (Sufenta)		triazolam (Halcion)	
	tincture of opium			

Controlled substances are classified into five schedules (**Table 8.1**) and current regulations listing the schedules may be found at 21 *CFR* 1308:

- **Schedule I:** The controlled substances in Schedule I include drugs with a high abuse potential that have no currently approved medical use in the United States and there is a lack of accepted safety for use of the drug or other substance under medical supervision.

Schedule I a controlled substance with a high potential for abuse that currently has no approved medical use

Schedule II a controlled substance with a high potential for abuse, with severe psychological and/or physical dependence liability

Schedule III a controlled substance whose abuse may lead to moderate or low physical dependence or highly psychological dependence

Schedule IV a controlled substance with less abuse potential and limited risk of physical and psychological dependence

Schedule V contains preparations with limited quantities of certain narcotic drugs

- **Schedule II:** The controlled substances in Schedule II include drugs having a high potential for abuse, a currently accepted medical use in treatment in the United States or a currently accepted medical use with severe restrictions, and abuse of the drug or other substances may lead to severe psychological or physical dependence.
  Some drugs included in Schedule II are also found in other schedules when combined with other drugs. The dispensing of Schedule II controlled substances requires affixing an orange label with the caution statement *"Controlled substance, dangerous unless used as directed."* Additionally, this federal transfer warning statement is required: *"Caution: Federal law prohibits the transfer of this drug to any person other than the patient for whom it was prescribed."*
- **Schedule III:** The controlled substances in Schedule III include drugs that have an abuse potential less than those in Schedule I and Schedule II, they have a currently accepted medical use in the United States, and abuse of these drugs may lead to moderate or low physical or high psychological dependence. Any compound, mixture, or preparation containing amobarbital, secobarbital, or pentobarbital, combined with one or more other active ingredients, is listed as a Schedule III drug, as the drug's abuse potential is not great enough to warrant a Schedule II classification.
- **Schedule IV:** The controlled substances in Schedule IV include drugs having an abuse potential less than those listed in Schedule III, an accepted medical use in the United States, and limited physical or psychological dependence as compared to drugs in Schedule III.
- **Schedule V:** The controlled substances in Schedule V include drugs having an abuse potential less than those listed in Schedule IV, an accepted medical use in the United States, and abuse of these drugs may lead to limited physical dependence or psychological dependence as compared to drugs in Schedule IV. Drugs in Schedule V consist mainly of preparations containing limited quantities of certain narcotic drugs (codeine), generally for antitussive indications and others for antidiarrheal indications.

Each commercial container of a controlled substance is required to have on its label a symbol designating the schedule to which it belongs. The symbols for controlled substances are C-I, C-II, C-III, C-IV, and C-V. Alternatively, the symbol may be a C with the schedule designation inside it.

Registration

The Controlled Substances Act requires federal registration of all individuals (except the ultimate user or patient) involved in the purchase, distribution, or dispensing of controlled drugs. Specifically, every individual or firm who manufactures, distributes, conducts instructional activities with, conducts chemical analysis with, conducts research with, exports, imports, prescribes, administers, or dispenses controlled substances or who proposes to engage in the same must register with the federal DEA. Registration for dispensers is presently effective for 3 years. This registration must be displayed prominently in the pharmacy. **Figure 8-1** shows Form 224, an application for registration, which is commonly processed through the DEA's online registration system (www.deadiversion.usdoj.gov).

Form-224

APPLICATION FOR REGISTRATION
Under the Controlled Substances Act

APPROVED OMB NO 1117-0014
FORM DEA-224 (10-06)
Previous editions are obsolete

INSTRUCTIONS

Save time - apply on-line at *www.deadiversion.usdoj.gov*

1. To apply by mail complete this application. Keep a copy for your records.
2. Print clearly, using black or blue ink, or use a typewriter.
3. Mail this form to the address provided in Section 7 or use enclosed envelope.
4. Include the correct payment amount. FEE IS NON-REFUNDABLE.
5. If you have any questions call 800-882-9539 prior to submitting your application.

IMPORTANT: DO NOT SEND THIS APPLICATION **AND** APPLY ON-LINE.

DEA OFFICIAL USE :

Do you have other DEA registration numbers?

☐ NO ☐ YES

FEE FOR THREE (3) YEARS IS $551
FEE IS NON-REFUNDABLE

MAIL-TO ADDRESS Please print mailing address changes to the right of the address in this box.

SECTION 1 APPLICANT IDENTIFICATION ☐ **Individual Registration** ☐ **Business Registration**

Name 1 (Last Name of individual -OR- Business or Facility Name)

Name 2 (First Name and Middle Name of individual - OR- Continuation of business name)

Street Address Line 1 (if applying for fee exemption, this must be address of the fee exempt institution)

Address Line 2

City State Zip Code

Business Phone Number Point of Contact

Business Fax Number Email Address

DEBT COLLECTION INFORMATION

Mandatory pursuant to Debt Collection Improvements Act

Social Security Number (***if registration is for individual***)

Provide SSN or TIN.
See additional information note #3 on page 4.

Tax Identification Number (***if registration is for business***)

FOR Practitioner or MLP ONLY:

Professional Degree : *select from list only*

Professional School :

Year of Graduation :

National Provider Identification:

Date of Birth (*MM-DD-YYYY*): MM-DD-YYYY

SECTION 2 BUSINESS ACTIVITY

Check one business activity box only

☐ Central Fill Pharmacy
☐ Retail Pharmacy
☐ Nursing Home
☐ Automated Dispensing System
☐ Practitioner (DDS, DMD, DO, DPM, DVM, MD or PHD)
☐ Practitioner Military (DDS, DMD, DO, DPM, DVM, MD or PHD)
☐ Mid-level Practitioner (MLP) (DOM, HMD, MP, ND, NP, OD, PA, or RPH)
☐ Euthanasia Technician
☐ Ambulance Service
☐ Animal Shelter
☐ Hospital/Clinic
☐ Teaching Institution

FOR Automated Dispensing System (ADS) ONLY:

DEA Registration # of Retail Pharmacy for this ADS

An ADS is automatically fee-exempt. Skip Section 6 and Section 7 on page 2. You must attach a notorized affidavit.

SECTION 3 DRUG SCHEDULES

Check all that apply

☐ Schedule II Narcotic
☐ Schedule II Non-Narcotic
☐ Schedule III Narcotic
☐ Schedule III Non-Narcotic
☐ Schedule IV
☐ Schedule V

☐ Check this box if you require official order forms - for purchase or transfer of schedule 2 narcotic and/or schedule 2 non-narcotic controlled substances.

NEW - Page 1

FIGURE 8-1 DEA Form-224 for new registration of a retail pharmacy, hospital/clinic, practitioner, or teaching institution.

SECTION 4

STATE LICENSE(S)

Be sure to include both state license numbers if applicable

You MUST be currently authorized to prescribe, distribute, dispense, conduct research, or otherwise handle the controlled substances in the schedules for which you are applying under the laws of the **state** or jurisdiction in which you are operating or propose to operate.

State License Number (required) ______ Expiration Date (required) __/__/__ MM - DD - YYYY

What state was this license issued in? ______

State Controlled Substance License Number (if required) ______ Expiration Date __/__/__ MM - DD - YYYY

What state was this license issued in? ______

SECTION 5

LIABILITY

IMPORTANT

All questions in this section must be answered.

1. Has the applicant ever been **convicted of a crime** in connection with controlled substance(s) under state or federal law, or is any such action pending? YES ☐ NO ☐

   Date(s) of incident MM-DD-YYYY: ______

2. Has the applicant ever surrendered (for cause) or had a **federal** controlled substance registration revoked, suspended, restricted, or denied, or is any such action pending? YES ☐ NO ☐

   Date(s) of incident MM-DD-YYYY: ______

3. Has the applicant ever surrendered (for cause) or had a **state** professional license or controlled substance registration revoked, suspended, denied, restricted, or placed on probation, or is any such action pending? YES ☐ NO ☐

   Date(s) of incident MM-DD-YYYY: ______

4. If the applicant is a **corporation** (other than a corporation whose stock is owned and traded by the public), association, partnership, or pharmacy, has any officer, partner, stockholder, or proprietor been **convicted of a crime** in connection with controlled substance(s) under state or federal law, or ever surrendered, for cause, or had a **federal** controlled substance registration revoked, suspended, restricted, denied, or ever had a **state** professional license or controlled substance registration revoked, suspended, denied, restricted or placed on probation, or is any such action pending? YES ☐ NO ☐

   Date(s) of incident MM-DD-YYYY: ______ *Note: If question 4 does not apply to you, be sure to mark 'NO'. It will slow down processing of your application if you leave it blank.*

EXPLANATION OF "YES" ANSWERS

Applicants who have answered "YES" to any of the four questions above **must provide a statement to explain each "YES" answer.**

Use this space or attach a separate sheet and return with application

Liability question # ______ Location(s) of incident: ______

Nature of incident:

Disposition of incident:

SECTION 6 EXEMPTION FROM APPLICATION FEE

☐ Check this box if the applicant is a federal, state, or local government official or institution. Does not apply to contractor-operated institutions.

Business or Facility Name of Fee Exempt Institution. **Be sure to enter the address of this exempt institution in Section 1.**

______

FEE EXEMPT CERTIFIER

Provide the name and phone number of the certifying official

The undersigned hereby certifies that the applicant named hereon is a federal, state or local government official or institution, and is exempt from payment of the application fee.

Signature of certifying official (**other than applicant**) ______ Date ______

Print or type name and title of certifying official ______ Telephone No. (required for verification) ______

SECTION 7

METHOD OF PAYMENT

Check one form of payment only

☐ Check — Make check payable to: **Drug Enforcement Administration**. See page 4 of instructions for important information.

☐ American Express ☐ Discover ☐ Master Card ☐ Visa

Credit Card Number ______ Expiration Date ___ - ___

Sign if paying by credit card

Signature of Card Holder ______

Printed Name of Card Holder ______

Mail this form with payment to:

U.S. Department of Justice
Drug Enforcement Administration
P.O. Box 28083
Washington, DC 20038-8083

FEE IS NON-REFUNDABLE

SECTION 8

APPLICANT'S SIGNATURE

Sign in ink

I certify that the foregoing information furnished on this application is true and correct.

Signature of applicant (sign in ink) ______ Date ______

Print or type name and title of applicant ______

WARNING: Section 843(a)(4)(A) of Title 21, United States Code states that any person who knowingly or intentionally furnishes false or fraudulent information in the application is subject to imprisonment for not more than four years, a fine of not more than $30,000, or both.

NEW - Page 2

FIGURE 8-1 (Continued)

Maintenance of Controlled Substances

Hospitals and other health care facilities authorized to purchase, possess, and use controlled substances must keep a number of records both within the pharmacy and at the individual nursing units and/or departments to ensure appropriate storage, use, and control of the controlled substances. These records and reports may be manual or computerized such as with the use of automated dispensing units and include the following characteristics:

- An order must be signed by an individual authorized to prescribe, specifying the controlled substance medication for a specifically indicated patient.
- A separate record must be maintained at the pharmacy (the main point of supply) for controlled substances. This record shows the drug strength and dosage form and indicates the dates and amounts of such drugs received, amount stocked in inventory, and amount dispensed. Controlled drugs must be stored in a double-locked, permanently affixed cabinet or safe for those institutions not utilizing an automated dispensing cabinet (ADC) such as Pyxis or Omnicell.
- A record of authorized requisitions in a manual system or for automated dispensing systems, printouts of minimum/maximum inventory levels on hand, must be maintained for each drug distributed. Centralized automated dispensing records must indicate the user ID number, password, and signature of the dispensing pharmacist. A receipt of controlled drugs is recorded by the signature of a person authorized to receive controlled substances for a manual system, and for an automated dispensing unit a record is printed indicating the name and amount of controlled drugs refilled.
- For all controlled drugs located within the institution, a documentation record of use must be maintained. The documentation record lists the controlled substance, strength, and inventory of the number of doses supplied or refilled, amount on hand, and documentation of withdrawal. The controlled drug documentation record also contains the following:
  - Name of the patient
  - Name of the prescribing physician or practitioner
  - Date and hour of administration
  - Quantity of administration
  - Balance on hand after each administration
  - Signature and/or identifying user ID number and password of the administering nurse.
- Additionally, for a manual system, at the end of each shift (or at the end of the day for controlled drug activities), two nurses must verify the controlled substances inventory on hand. A perpetual inventory is automatically maintained for all controlled substances in an automated dispensing system, with a physical inventory performed, at a minimum, on a weekly basis.
- Upon administration of the controlled substance, an entry must be made in the patient's **medication administration record (MAR)**. The entry includes the name of the administering nurse and the date and hour of administration. Partially used doses, contaminated, or nonused (e.g., if patient refuses them) controlled drugs must have wastage documented by the administering nurse and another nurse (or by another health care practitioner as dictated by hospital policy) as a witness.

medication administration record (MAR) a record maintained by the nursing staff containing information about the patient's medication and its frequency of administration

Ordering Controlled Substances

Under the Controlled Substances Act, a federal triplicate order form (DEA-222) is necessary for the ordering of controlled substances in Schedules I and II and is required for transfer of Schedule I and II products from one pharmacy to another and for returns to the wholesaler or manufacturer (**Figure 8-2**).

DEA forms may be requisitioned on DEA Form-222a or by contacting any division office or the registration unit of the DEA. Order forms are free of charge. Each order form must be signed and dated by a person authorized to sign an application for registration. Copy 1 (brown) and Copy 2 (green) go to the supplier, and Copy 3 is retained by the purchaser. The forms may also be completed electronically.

BLANK DEA FORM-222
U.S. OFFICIAL ORDER FORM—SCHEDULES I & II

See Reverse of PURCHASER'S Copy for Instructions	No order form may be issued for Schedules I and II substances unless a completed application form has been received, (21 CFR 1305.04).	**OMB APPROVAL NO. 1117-0010**

TO: *(Name of Supplier)*	STREET ADDRESS

CITY and STATE	DATE	**TO BE FILLED IN BY SUPPLIER** SUPPLIERS DEA REGISTRATION No.

TO BE FILLED IN BY PURCHASER

LINE No.	No. of Packages	Size of Packages	Name of Item	National Drug Code	Packages Shipped	Date Shipped
1						
2						
3						
4						
5						
6						
7						
8						
9						
10						

NO. OF LINES COMPLETED	SIGNATURE OF PURCHASER OR HIS ATTORNEY OR AGENT

Date Issued	DEA Registration No.	Name and Address of Registrant
Schedules 2, 2N, 3, 3N, 4, 5		
Registered as a PHARMACY	No. of this Order Form	

DEA Form-222
U.S. OFFICIAL ORDER FORMS—SCHEDULES I & II
DRUG ENFORCEMENT ADMINISTRATION
SUPPLIER'S COPY 1

SAMPLE

Courtesy of U.S. Department of Justice, Drug Enforcement Administration, Office of Diversion Control.

FIGURE 8-2 DEA order form, Form-222, for Schedule I and II level drugs.

Lost or Stolen Order Forms and Drug Theft or Loss

Both federal and state laws have requirements for drug security and regulations for reporting lost or stolen order forms and controlled drug theft or loss. Controlled drug theft or loss must be immediately reported to the DEA diversion field office (using DEA Form-106), and a controlled drug theft should also immediately be reported to the local police.

Inventory Requirements

The Controlled Substances Act requires each registrant to make a complete and accurate record every 2 years of all stocks of controlled substances on hand. The biennial inventory date of May 1 may be changed by the registrant to fit the regular general physical inventory date as long as the date is no more than 6 months from the biennial date that would otherwise apply. The inventory must be maintained at the location appearing on the registration certificate for at least 2 years.

Most hospital pharmacy departments take a physical inventory of their controlled drugs much more frequently than required by federal law. Some departments take manual controlled drug inventories on a daily basis to ensure appropriate accountability and reconciliation. Many departments of pharmacy have automated dispensing cabinets specifically for controlled substances, where an ongoing perpetual inventory is maintained for each controlled drug transaction.

Refer to Chapter 20 for a comprehensive review of automated dispensing technology and the role and responsibilities of the pharmacy technician.

Destruction of Controlled Substances

A DEA form 41 is used to request the destruction of controlled substances. A pharmacy can dispose of any excess, expired, or undesired stocks of controlled substances by:

- Returning them to the manufacturer
- Returning them to the wholesaler
- Contracting with a reverse distributor company for pickup and disposal.

Issuing Prescriptions and Dispensing Controlled Substances

A prescription for a controlled substance may be issued only by an individual practitioner authorized to prescribe controlled substances in the state in which he or she is licensed to practice. An employee of the individual practitioner (a nurse, secretary) may communicate a prescription issued by a practitioner to a pharmacist. Only a pharmacist, or a pharmacy intern under the supervision of a pharmacist, may fill a prescription for a controlled substance. Whether a pharmacy technician may engage in the dispensing of a controlled substance under the supervision of a licensed pharmacist depends on state law.

Controlled drug prescriptions must be dated on the day when written and must include:

- The name and address of the patient
- The drug name, strength, and dosage form
- The quantity prescribed
- Directions for use
- The name, address, and DEA registration number of the prescriber.

The prescription must have the name of the prescriber stamped, typed, or hand printed on it, as well as the signature of the physician.

The responsibility for the proper prescribing and dispensing of controlled substances rests with both the prescriber and the pharmacist who fills the prescription. A prescription ordered by a person knowingly prescribing a controlled substance that is not within the usual course of his or her legitimate practice is not deemed a legal prescription. Individuals prescribing such a prescription and a pharmacist knowingly filling it are in violation of the Controlled Substances Act.

Emergency Situations

An emergency situation is an exception to the requirement that a pharmacist dispense a Schedule II drug only pursuant to a written prescription. Although state regulations may vary, in New York State, a pharmacist may dispense a Schedule II drug on oral authorization of the prescriber under the following emergency circumstances:

- The quantity prescribed is limited only to the amount necessary to treat the patient for the emergency.
- The prescription must be immediately reduced to writing by the pharmacist.
- The prescriber must deliver to the dispensing pharmacist within 7 days a written prescription for the emergency quantity prescribed. The prescription must have written on its face *"Authorization for Emergency Dispensing."* On receipt, the pharmacist must attach this prescription to the oral emergency prescription. Failure of the prescriber to deliver the written prescription within the 7-day period requires the pharmacist to notify the state bureau of controlled substances. Failure of the pharmacist to do so voids the prescription.

Recordkeeping Requirements

Controlled substances records (e.g., inventory, records of receipt, records of disposition, records of theft or loss, prescriptions) must be kept for at least 2 years at the place of registration. Specific states may require controlled drug records to be maintained for longer than the federal requirement of 2 years. For example, New York State's requirement is 5 years.

Penalties for Violations of the CSA

The assessment of criminal and civil penalties under the CSA depends on such things as the schedule of the controlled substance involved, the amounts involved, the nature of the misuse of the controlled substance, the potential for harm to others, and the intent of the violator. Penalties can range from monetary fines up to life imprisonment and even death.

Federal Hazardous Substances Act (FHSA) act that requires hazardous household products to bear cautionary labels to alert consumers of potential dangers and to inform them of measures to take to protect themselves

Consumer Product Safety Commission (CPSC) an independent agency that does not report to, nor is it part of, any other department or agency in the federal government; created to protect the public "against unreasonable risks of injuries associated with consumer products"

Federal Hazardous Substances Act of 1960

The **Federal Hazardous Substances Act (FHSA)** was enacted in 1960. This act requires that certain hazardous household products ("hazardous substances") bear cautionary labeling to alert consumers to the potential hazards that those products present and to inform them of the measures they need to protect themselves from those hazards. The **Consumer Product Safety Commission (CPSC)** enforces this act. The CPSC was created to protect the public "against unreasonable risks of injuries associated with consumer products." The CPSC is an independent agency that does not report to, nor is it part of, any other department or agency in the federal government.

Poison Prevention Packaging Act

Poison Prevention Packaging Act a federal law mandating special packaging requirements that make it difficult for children under the age of 5 to open the package or container

The **Poison Prevention Packaging Act** of 1970 is an amendment to the Federal Hazardous Substances Act. It regulates certain substances defined as "household substances." These are defined in the statute as including:

a. *hazardous substances as defined in the Federal Hazardous Substance Act;*
b. *foods, drugs, or cosmetics defined under section 201 of the FDCA; or*
c. *substances intended for use as a fuel when stored in a portable container and used in the heating, cooking, or refrigeration of a house.*

The act requires that these substances be packaged for consumer use in "special packaging" that will make it significantly difficult for children under the age of 5 to open, but not difficult for adults to open within a reasonable time. The "special packaging" is often referred to as a *child-resistant container.*

Drugs dispensed via prescription or a medical practitioner's order are exempt from the special packaging requirement if the prescribing physician specifies a noncompliant container in the prescription or if the patient or customer receiving the drug requests a noncompliant container. Another exemption is made for over-the-counter items for individuals who are elderly or have a handicap. For the exemption to apply, however, such noncompliant packaging must contain the printed statement *"This package for households without young children."*

The following is a list of substances that are currently required to be sold or dispensed to consumers in the special child-resistant containers:

- Aspirin-containing preparations
- Controlled substances
- Prescription-only (legend) drugs, unless the patient or guardian requests a non–child-resistant container and signs a release to this effect.

Exempt from the special packaging requirement for legend drugs are sublingual nitroglycerin preparations and sublingual and chewable isosorbide dinitrate (e.g., Isordil®) preparations, because these drugs are prescribed for cardiac patients who must be able to quickly get at their medication.

Occupational Safety and Health Act of 1970 federal law that ensures every working man and woman in the nation safe and healthy working conditions; established the Occupational Safety and Health Administration (OSHA)

Occupational Safety and Health Administration (OSHA) organization created to decrease hazards in the workplace, to maintain a reporting system for monitoring job-related injuries and illnesses, and to develop mandatory job safety and health standards

Hazard Communication Standard (HCS) a regulation to ensure that information about hazardous chemicals is communicated to the workers handling them

Occupational Safety and Health Act of 1970

The **Occupational Safety and Health Act of 1970** was passed to ensure every working man and woman in the nation safe and healthy working conditions. Under the act, the **Occupational Safety and Health Administration (OSHA)** was created to decrease hazards in the workplace, to maintain a reporting system for monitoring job-related injuries and illnesses, and to develop mandatory job safety and health standards. OSHA is authorized to conduct workplace inspections to determine whether employers are complying with standards issued by the agency for safe and healthful workplaces. Workplace inspections are performed by OSHA compliance safety and health officers.

Hazardous Drugs and Chemicals

On May 23, 1988, an OSHA regulation became effective that requires employees to know about the hazards associated with any of the chemicals to which they are exposed. The **Hazard Communication Standard (HCS)** is based on the simple concept that employees have both a need and a right to know the identities of the chemicals to which they are exposed when working and any possible hazards. They also need to know what protective measures are available to prevent adverse effects.

The purpose of this standard is to ensure that the hazards of all chemicals are evaluated and that information concerning these hazards is transmitted to affected employees. This transmission of information is to be accomplished by a comprehensive hazard communication program that includes container labeling and other forms of warning, material safety data sheets, and employee training.

Written Hazard Communication Program

Employers must develop and implement a written hazard communications program that includes a list of the hazardous chemicals known to be present in the workplace. They must also obtain from the manufacturers, importers, or distributors of the substance the appropriate **safety data sheets (SDS)**. This is to be done for all toxic/hazardous substances in every department. The SDS must be in English and must contain the following information:

> **safety data sheets (SDS)** documents that provide workers and emergency personnel with procedures for handling or working with a substance in a safe manner; includes information such as physical data (melting point, boiling point, flash point, etc.), toxicity, health effects, first aid, reactivity, storage, disposal, protective equipment, and spill-handling procedures

- Chemical and common names
- If a mixture, chemical and common names of ingredients
- Physical and chemical characteristics, such as flash point and vapor pressure
- Physical hazards, including potential for fire, explosion, and reactivity
- Health hazards, including signs and symptoms of exposure
- Routes of entry into the body
- Precautions for safe handling and use, including hygienic practices and protective measures during repair or maintenance
- Procedures for cleanup of spills and leaks
- Emergency and first aid procedures
- Date of preparation of SDS or date of latest revision
- Name, address, and telephone number of manufacturer, importer, or distributor.

The employer must maintain copies of the required SDS for each hazardous chemical in the workplace and ensure that they are readily accessible to employees during each work shift. Alternatively, the employer may subscribe to a service that will fax an SDS on request of the employee by calling a toll-free telephone number.

Air Contaminants

Employees are to be protected from air contaminants and chemicals that could cause injury or illness with regard to potential carcinogenic agents. OSHA published *Guidelines for Handling Cytotoxic (Antineoplastic) Drugs*, revised in 1995, as a meaningful tool for pharmacy employers and employees handling chemotherapy drugs. The publication provides information regarding personal protective equipment, monitoring, and training. In addition, various groups, institutions, and agencies around the world (e.g., the American Society of Health-System Pharmacists [ASHP], the Oncology Nursing Society [ONS], and the International Society of Oncology Pharmacy Practitioners [ISOPP]) have developed and published guidelines or recommendations for handling antineoplastic agents. Other sources of information include the American Society of Clinical Oncology (ASCO), Canadian Association of Pharmacy in Oncology, AFSCME health and safety fact sheets, and RXMED pharmaceutical monographs.

Radiopharmaceuticals

Please refer to Chapter 7 for a review of this subject and the role and responsibility of the pharmacy technician.

Flammable and Combustible Liquids

Appropriate storage (e.g., vault, cabinet) must be provided for pharmaceuticals such as alcohol, acetone, and flexible collodion.

Portable Fire Extinguisher

A sufficient number of portable fire extinguishers of the appropriate type, depending on the hazards in the department, must be available and immediately accessible.

Omnibus Budget Reconciliation Act of 1990

Omnibus Budget Reconciliation Act (OBRA) mandated three provisions that affect the profession of pharmacy: drug manufacturers are required to provide their lowest prices to Medicaid patients, and pharmacists are to provide drug use reviews and patient counseling

prospective drug review a review of a patient's medication profile by a pharmacist to screen for any drug problems prior to a drug being dispensed

In adopting the federal **Omnibus Budget Reconciliation Act (OBRA)** of 1990, Congress recognized the escalating pressure to expand social programs—particularly those that impact active older citizens—and that the pharmacist could play a key role in improving the effectiveness of drug therapy and reducing the overall costs.

OBRA mandated three main provisions affecting the profession of pharmacy, including the provision that drug manufacturers are required to provide their lowest prices to Medicaid patients, and the provision that drug use reviews and patient counseling are now mandated.

OBRA required states to implement regulations consistent with the objectives of the federal law prior to January 1, 1993. Although the original federal regulations mandated such programs for Medicaid patients only, virtually every state has implemented the new regulations for all patients to ensure all patients a high level of professional service.

Pharmacists are now required to maintain individual patient medication profiles that must contain—in addition to patient demographic information such as name, address, telephone number, gender, and date of birth—information including known allergies and drug reactions, chronic diseases, a comprehensive list of medications and medical devices, and other appropriate information necessary for counseling about the use of prescription and over-the-counter drugs. Utilizing this patient medication profile, pharmacists are expected to conduct a **prospective drug review** before dispensing or delivering a prescription to a patient, or the patient's caregiver, which would include screening for the following:

- Therapeutic duplication
- Drug-drug interactions, including serious interactions with any over-the-counter drugs
- Incorrect drug dosage or duration of treatment
- Drug-allergy interactions
- Clinical abuse or misuse.

After a prospective drug review, regulations require that counseling be provided to each patient and must include all "matters which in the pharmacist's professional judgment, the pharmacist deems significant," including the following:

- The name and description of the medication
- The dosage form, dosage, route of administration, and duration of drug therapy
- Special directions and precautions for preparation, administration, and use by the patient
- Common severe side effects or adverse effects or interactions that may be encountered, including their avoidance and action required if they occur
- Techniques for self-monitoring drug therapy
- Proper storage
- Prescription refill information
- Action to be taken in the event of a missed dose.

For mail-order pharmacies, counseling and patient profile information may be conveyed by toll-free, long-distance telephone and is usually patient initiated.

Although any qualified employee of a pharmacy, such as a technician, may initiate the offer to have the pharmacist counsel a patient, only a pharmacist or a pharmacy intern can provide the actual counseling. The objective of counseling the patient or the patient's caregiver is to improve patient medication compliance, to avoid medication misadventures, and to improve drug therapy outcomes.

Today, with the degree of doctor of pharmacy being conferred on all pharmacy graduates, pharmacists should view these requirements as an opportunity to utilize their education and training in their professional role as drug therapy experts. The public has a need for a readily available professional who will assist them in improving their health care outcomes, and the pharmacist is the most logical professional to meet these needs.

Health Insurance Portability and Accountability Act of 1996

Health Insurance Portability and Accountability Act (HIPAA) an important law that requires the adoption of security and privacy standards in order to protect personal health care information

protected health information (PHI) any individually identifiable health information, with the exclusion of employment records

In 1996 Congress passed the **Health Insurance Portability and Accountability Act (HIPAA)**. The DHHS Office for Civil Rights (OCR) is responsible for enforcing the Privacy and Security Rules. Since 2003, OCR's enforcement activities have resulted in systemic change that has helped to improve the privacy protection of health information for all individuals.

Prior to HIPAA, personal health information could be distributed for reasons having nothing to do with a patient's medical treatment or health care reimbursement. Consequently, HIPAA provisions were made to mandate the adoption of federal privacy protections to protect and guard against the misuse of individually identifiable health information. **Protected health information (PHI)** includes any individually identifiable health information transmitted or maintained in any form, with the exclusion of employment records.

HIPAA is divided into two titles: Title I and Title II. Title I, known as *Insurance Reform*, protects health insurance coverage for workers and their families when they change or lose their jobs. Title II, known as *Administrative Simplification*, has fundamentally changed the way health care facilities handle patient information. Its goal is to improve the efficiency and effectiveness of the American health care system by adopting national standards for electronic health care transactions. The law also requires the adoption of privacy standards (the *Privacy Rule*) and security standards (the *Security Rule*) in order to protect personal health care information.

Definitions

covered entities something to which HIPAA regulations apply; namely, health plans that provide or pay the costs of medical care, health care clearinghouses that facilitate the processing of health information from another entity, and health care providers of medical or health services

HIPAA regulations apply to **covered entities**, which include:

1. A *health plan* that provides or pays the cost of medical care (e.g., group health plan, HMO, Part A or Part B of Medicare, the Medicaid program)
2. A *health care clearinghouse* that facilitates the processing of health information from another entity (e.g., billing service)
3. A *health care provider* of medical or health services (e.g., physicians, chiropractors, dentists; preventive, diagnostic, or therapeutic services; and sellers or dispensers of a drugs [e.g. pharmacies], devices, or equipment).

In addition to covered entities, there is a business associate (BA) who, on behalf of a covered entity, performs or assists in a function or activity involving the use or disclosure of individually identifiable health information.

HIPAA enforcement and penalties were strengthened in a recent law known as HITECH. The Health Information Technology for Economic and Clinical Health (HITECH) Act, enacted as part of the American Recovery and Reinvestment Act of 2009, was signed into law on February 17, 2009, to promote the adoption and meaningful use of health information technology. In-depth information on HIPAA can be found at the DHHS website (www.hhs.gov).

Preexisting Pharmacy Privacy Requirements

American Pharmaceutical Association Code of Ethics for Pharmacists—Principle 2: A pharmacist is dedicated to protecting the dignity of the patient. With a caring attitude and compassionate spirit, a pharmacist focuses on seeing the patient in a private and confidential manner.

American Association of Pharmacy Technicians Code of Ethics for Pharmacy Technicians—Principle VI: A pharmacy technician respects and supports the patient's individuality, dignity, and confidentiality.

New York State Regulations on Unprofessional Conduct—Regents Rules 29.1(b)(8): Unprofessional conduct shall include revealing of personally identifiable facts, data, or information obtained in a professional capacity without the prior consent of the patient, except as authorized or required by law.

Regulatory Standards for Marketed Drugs

The necessary labeling of medications, for both professional and/or patient information, in the form of package inserts is required under the FDCA for the safe and appropriate prescribing and use of medication. The laws and regulations pertaining to marketed drug labeling are under the jurisdiction of the FDA.

Prescription Drug Labeling

Prescription drugs are labeled for the health care professional, not the patient. The following information is required on the manufacturer's commercial label:

- Name and address of the manufacturer, packager, or distributor
- Name of the drug (brand and generic) as applicable
- Ingredients and quantity
- Name of inactive ingredients
- *Quantity in terms of weight or volume (e.g., 1 liter)
- Quantity of the container (e.g., 100 capsules)
- Statement of usual dose or reference to the package insert
- Symbol *"Rx Only"* and/or the legend *"Caution: Federal law prohibits dispensing without prescription"*
- If not for oral use, the route of administration
- Lot or control number
- Expiration date
- Statement directed to the pharmacist (where applicable) specifying the type of container to be used in dispensing the drug (e.g., "dispense in tight, light-resistant container").

Federal Trade Commission (FTC) a federal agency that promotes consumer protection and the elimination and prevention of anticompetitive business practices, such as coercive monopolies

Note that federal regulations define labeling in a much broader sense than the package insert or the label affixed to the product container and include all written materials that accompany the product including marketing materials used in advertising and promotion. This has expanded to include audio and visual advertising. Marketing programs for drugs and devices that do not address FDA-regulated labeling claims are regulated by the **Federal Trade Commission (FTC)**. FTC standards are quite different from FDA regulatory standards, in that the FDA requires strict adherence to the approved labeling claims in regulating product promotion, whereas the FTC standard requires truth in advertising and a fair and balanced approach to marketing.

Unit-Dose Labeling and Packaging

Unit-dose packaging is applicable when a single dosage unit of a drug is packaged and labeled for administration to patients in hospitals, long-term care facilities, and other institutions that use unit-dose systems. This type of packaging is convenient in that it reduces medication errors and diversion and permits the return and crediting of unused, sealed doses. Because of the size of the unit-dose package, the FDA has regulations requiring the label on the unit-dose package to include the following:

- Generic and brand name of the drug, where applicable
- Quantity of active ingredient in each unit-dose package
- Expiration date
- Lot number
- Name of the manufacturer, repackager, or distributor
- Other appropriate information as required (e.g., bar code).

Drug Package Insert

The package insert that accompanies the drug product is derived from the approval process of the drug by the FDA and it comprises part of the drug's labeling. The package insert represents a "license" granted by the FDA so that the drug may be distributed in interstate commerce. The package insert establishes the parameters that mandate what the manufacturer may say about the drug in its marketing. It should also contain all medical information needed for the safe and effective use of the drug by health care professionals. The following information must be contained under the section headings and in the order listed as per federal regulation:

- Generic and proprietary name
- Clinical pharmacology
- Indications and usage
- Contraindications
- Warnings
- Precautions
- Adverse reactions
- Drug abuse and dependence
- Overdosage
- Dosage and administration
- How supplied
- Date of the most recent revision of the labeling.

Patient Package Inserts and Medication Guides

patient package insert (PPI) an informational leaflet written for the lay public describing the benefits and risks of a prescribed medication

FDA regulations require the distribution of **patient package inserts (PPIs)** to educate the patient about the proper use and potential dangers inherent in the use of specific prescription medications. The PPI is an informational leaflet written for the lay public describing the benefits and risks of the medication. PPIs must be provided to patients receiving prescriptions for products such as Accutane® (isotretinoin), as well as those receiving estrogen or progesterone-containing products.

The requirements of the regulation are met if the PPI is provided to the patient before administration of the first dose of the drug and every 30 days thereafter as long as therapy continues. These rules apply to all physicians, community pharmacists, and hospital pharmacists who dispense these drugs. Hospitals and provider pharmacies that provide medications to patients in long-term care facilities are also responsible for providing PPIs to patients (or their families or caregivers) receiving these medications.

As discussed earlier, under the FDA REMS program, manufacturers of certain high-risk medications such as opiates, antidepressants, and other psychotropic drugs are required to put in place a risk management and mitigation plan, a part of which includes patient medication guides. These are to be distributed to patients according to regulation; if a patient is not able to read the guide, a health care professional should be available to discuss matters contained in the guide with the patient, if practicable.

National Drug Code Number

A national drug code (NDC) number is required on all over-the-counter and prescription drug labels. The NDC number assigned to new drugs has 11 digits. The first 5 digits identify the drug manufacturer; the next 4 digits identify the drug entity; and the last two digits identify the drug packaging. The FDA assigns the number for identification purposes, for facilitating the processing of third-party prescription drug claims, and for distributing products between manufacturers, wholesalers, and pharmacies. The FDA requires that all drug labeling include the NDC as a linear bar code to allow health care professionals to scan the bar code to ensure that the right drug, dosage, and route of administration are dispensed and administered to the patient.

Bar Codes

Bar coding of pharmaceuticals (prescription drugs, biologics, and nonprescription drugs) has been mandated by the FDA to help reduce medication errors in hospitals. A bar code consists of a combination of bars and spaces of varying widths that allow encoding of pertinent information concerning a drug product. A scanner is utilized to read the bar code.

Switch of Prescription Drugs to Over-the-Counter Drugs

The FDA has an over-the-counter (OTC) drug review process that provides a mechanism for switching over a prescription drug to OTC status as recommended. If the change is approved, the FDA publishes an OTC drug monograph for this drug.

In some instances the FDA may approve a switch in a drug's OTC status based on a manufacturer's supplemental application to its NDA. This can sometimes be confusing to pharmacists, because approval for one manufacturer's supplemental NDA application does not automatically apply to other manufacturers of the same product. Thus, a product from one manufacturer may be a prescription drug, yet an identical product from another manufacturer may be an OTC drug. Pharmacists and technicians must abide by the label and not sell a legend drug without a prescription, even though the competitor's drug may be OTC.

Orange Book

Every state has enacted generic substitution laws allowing a pharmacist to substitute a generically equivalent drug for the prescribed drug. Pharmacists are responsible for ensuring that the substituted generic drug product is bioequivalent to the prescribed product. To assist pharmacists and technicians in identifying bioequivalent generic medications, the FDA published *Approved Drug Products with Therapeutic Equivalence Evaluations*. This book is often referred to as the *Orange*

Book because of its orange cover. The *Orange Book* can be accessed at the FDA's website (www.fda.gov). The *Orange Book* lists thousands of marketed multisource drugs approved by the FDA as safe and effective.

The FDA uses a two-letter coding system for drug products with therapeutic equivalence evaluations:

- Drug products with the first letter *A* are considered bioequivalent and are therefore therapeutically equivalent to the brand name product. Drug products with the first letter *B* are not considered to be therapeutically equivalent for various reasons.
- The second letter of the code more specifically describes the different dosage forms of the product. For example:
  - AA—bioequivalent drug products in conventional dosage forms
  - AN—bioequivalent solutions and powders for aerosolization
  - AT—bioequivalent topical products.

Handling of Investigational Drugs

The procedures for handling investigational drugs are an important part of hospital drug distribution systems. These procedures will naturally reflect the extent to which an institution is involved with research, the resources available, and the particular needs of the hospital. For most community hospitals, the main activities related to investigational drugs will most likely involve the receipt, storage, dispensing, recordkeeping, and control of investigational drugs. In a large teaching hospital, investigational drug use may result in numerous services and responsibilities requiring full-time personnel.

The basic responsibilities of a hospital pharmacy handling investigational drugs are as follows:

- *Distribution and control of investigational drugs*, including drug procurement, storage, inventory management, packaging, labeling, distribution, and disposition of unused drugs
- *Clinical services*, including pharmacy and nursing staff in-service education and training, perhaps patient education, and the monitoring and reporting of adverse drug reactions
- *Research activities*, which may involve participating in the preparation or review of research proposals and protocols, assisting in data collection and analysis, and serving on the institutional review board (IRB)
- *Clinical study management*, which might involve working on study reports to the research sponsor.

Reporting of Adverse Drug Reactions

One definition of an adverse drug reaction is "any unexpected, or unwanted change in a patient's condition that a physician suspects may be due to a drug, that occurs at doses normally used in humans, and that requires treatment, indicates decrease or cessation of therapy with the drug, or suggests that future therapy with the drug carries an unusual risk in the patient."

Most hospitals have a policy that all suspected adverse reactions to drugs will be brought to the attention of the physician, investigated, documented in the patient's chart; that adverse reactions that could have or did cause serious injury or death will be reported to the FDA; and that any additional requirements of each respective state for reporting severe reactions to the department of health or other agency within the state will be followed.

Upon suspecting that an adverse drug reaction has occurred, hospital procedures should be followed, which may include these steps:

1. Alert the prescribing physician that an adverse drug reaction may have occurred, and initiate appropriate treatment, if necessary.
2. Ensure that the suspected adverse drug reaction is recorded on the patient's chart.
3. Using the hospital's procedures established for reporting an adverse drug reaction, notify the pharmacy of the suspected reaction.

The pharmacy will document and review the drug reaction and, where appropriate, pertinent data will be supplied to the Food and Drug Administration. As discussed earlier, the FDA maintains a voluntary program that allows health care professionals to report adverse drug reactions directly to the FDA. An official reporting form entitled MedWatch (Form FDA 3500) is shown in **Figure 8-3**. This form can be obtained from the FDA by calling 800-FDA-1088 or by writing MedWatch, 5600 Fishers Lane, Rockville, MD 20852-9787. Reports may be telephoned to the same number or faxed to 800-FDA-0718. Reports may also be entered online at the FDA's website (www.fda.gov).

Mandatory Device Reporting

User facilities such as hospitals and nursing homes are legally required to report suspected medical device–related deaths to both the FDA and the manufacturer and serious injuries to the manufacturer or, if the manufacturer is unknown, to the FDA. These reports must be made on Form FDA 3500A, Mandatory Reporting Form. You can download the mandatory form as a PDF document for printing. The FDA website and electronic submission limitations are constantly being updated, so where questions exist regarding electronic submissions, refer to the FDA website at www.fda.gov.

What Is a Serious Adverse Event?

An adverse event is any undesirable experience associated with the use of a medical product in a patient. The event is serious and should be reported to FDA when any of the patient outcomes discussed next occurs.

Death

Report if you suspect that the death was an outcome of the adverse event, and include the date if known.

Life Threatening

Report if you suspect that the patient was at substantial risk of dying at the time of the adverse event, or if use or continued use of the device or other medical product might have resulted in the death of the patient.

Hospitalization (Initial or Prolonged)

Report if admission to the hospital or prolongation of hospitalization was a result of the adverse event. Emergency department visits that do not result in admission to the hospital should be evaluated for one of the other serious outcomes (e.g., life

U.S. Department of Health and Human Services

MEDWATCH

The FDA Safety Information and Adverse Event Reporting Program

For VOLUNTARY reporting of adverse events, product problems and product use errors

Page 1 of ___

Form Approved: OMB No. 0910-0291, Expires: 12/31/2011
See OMB statement on reverse.

FDA USE ONLY

Triage unit sequence #

PLEASE TYPE OR USE BLACK INK

A. PATIENT INFORMATION

1. **Patient Identifier** — In confidence
2. **Age at Time of Event or Date of Birth:**
3. **Sex** — ☐ Female ☐ Male
4. **Weight** — ___ lb or ___ kg

B. ADVERSE EVENT, PRODUCT PROBLEM OR ERROR

Check all that apply:

1. ☐ **Adverse Event** ☐ **Product Problem** *(e.g., defects/malfunctions)*
☐ **Product Use Error** ☐ **Problem with Different Manufacturer of Same Medicine**

2. **Outcomes Attributed to Adverse Event** *(Check all that apply)*
☐ Death: ___ *(mm/dd/yyyy)* ☐ Disability or Permanent Damage
☐ Life-threatening ☐ Congenital Anomaly/Birth Defect
☐ Hospitalization - initial or prolonged ☐ Other Serious (Important Medical Events)
☐ Required Intervention to Prevent Permanent Impairment/Damage (Devices)

3. **Date of Event** *(mm/dd/yyyy)*
4. **Date of this Report** *(mm/dd/yyyy)*

5. **Describe Event, Problem or Product Use Error**

(Continue on page 3)

6. **Relevant Tests/Laboratory Data, Including Dates**

(Continue on page 3)

7. **Other Relevant History, Including Preexisting Medical Conditions** *(e.g., allergies, race, pregnancy, smoking and alcohol use, liver/kidney problems, etc.)*

(Continue on page 3)

C. PRODUCT AVAILABILITY

Product Available for Evaluation? *(Do not send product to FDA)*

☐ Yes ☐ No ☐ Returned to Manufacturer on: ___ *(mm/dd/yyyy)*

D. SUSPECT PRODUCT(S)

1. **Name, Strength, Manufacturer** *(from product label)*
#1 Name:
Strength:
Manufacturer:
#2 Name:
Strength:
Manufacturer:

2. **Dose or Amount** — **Frequency** — **Route**
#1
#2

3. **Dates of Use** *(If unknown, give duration) from/to (or best estimate)*
#1
#2

4. **Diagnosis or Reason for Use** *(Indication)*
#1
#2

5. **Event Abated After Use Stopped or Dose Reduced?**
#1 ☐ Yes ☐ No ☐ Doesn't Apply
#2 ☐ Yes ☐ No ☐ Doesn't Apply

6. **Lot #**
#1
#2

7. **Expiration Date**
#1
#2

8. **Event Reappeared After Reintroduction?**
#1 ☐ Yes ☐ No ☐ Doesn't Apply
#2 ☐ Yes ☐ No ☐ Doesn't Apply

9. **NDC # or Unique ID**

E. SUSPECT MEDICAL DEVICE

1. **Brand Name**
2. **Common Device Name**
3. **Manufacturer Name, City and State**
4. **Model #** — **Lot #**
Catalog # — **Expiration Date** *(mm/dd/yyyy)*
Serial # — **Other #**
5. **Operator of Device**
☐ Health Professional
☐ Lay User/Patient
☐ Other:
6. **If Implanted, Give Date** *(mm/dd/yyyy)*
7. **If Explanted, Give Date** *(mm/dd/yyyy)*
8. **Is this a Single-use Device that was Reprocessed and Reused on a Patient?**
☐ Yes ☐ No
9. **If Yes to Item No. 8, Enter Name and Address of Reprocessor**

F. OTHER (CONCOMITANT) MEDICAL PRODUCTS

Product names and therapy dates *(exclude treatment of event)*

(Continue on page 3)

G. REPORTER ***(See confidentiality section on back)***

1. **Name and Address**
Name:
Address:
City: State: ZIP:
Phone # **E-mail**
2. **Health Professional?** ☐ Yes ☐ No
3. **Occupation**
4. **Also Reported to:**
☐ Manufacturer
☐ User Facility
☐ Distributor/Importer
5. **If you do NOT want your identity disclosed to the manufacturer, place an "X" in this box:** ☐

FORM FDA 3500 (1/09) Submission of a report does not constitute an admission that medical personnel or the product caused or contributed to the event.

FIGURE 8-3 MedWatch form for voluntary reporting by health professionals of adverse events and product problems.

ADVICE ABOUT VOLUNTARY REPORTING

Detailed instructions available at: http://www.fda.gov/medwatch/report/consumer/instruct.htm

Report adverse events, product problems or product use errors with:

- Medications *(drugs or biologics)*
- Medical devices *(including in-vitro diagnostics)*
- Combination products *(medication & medical devices)*
- Human cells, tissues, and cellular and tissue-based products
- Special nutritional products *(dietary supplements, medical foods, infant formulas)*
- Cosmetics

Report product problems - quality, performance or safety concerns such as:

- Suspected counterfeit product
- Suspected contamination
- Questionable stability
- Defective components
- Poor packaging or labeling
- Therapeutic failures (product didn't work)

-Fold Here-

Report SERIOUS adverse events. An event is serious when the patient outcome is:

- Death
- Life-threatening
- Hospitalization - initial or prolonged
- Disability or permanent damage
- Congenital anomaly/birth defect
- Required intervention to prevent permanent impairment or damage (devices)
- Other serious (important medical events)

Report even if:

- You're not certain the product caused the event
- You don't have all the details

How to report:

- Just fill in the sections that apply to your report
- Use section D for all products except medical devices
- Attach additional pages if needed
- Use a separate form for each patient
- Report either to FDA or the manufacturer *(or both)*

Other methods of reporting:

- 1-800-FDA-0178 - To FAX report
- 1-800-FDA-1088 - To report by phone
- www.fda.gov/medwatch/report.htm - To report online

If your report involves a serious adverse event with a device and it occurred in a facility outside a doctor's office, that facility may be legally required to report to FDA and/or the manufacturer. Please notify the person in that facility who would handle such reporting.

-Fold Here-

If your report involves a serious adverse event with a vaccine, call 1-800-822-7967 to report.

Confidentiality: The patient's identity is held in strict confidence by FDA and protected to the fullest extent of the law. FDA will not disclose the reporter's identity in response to a request from the public, pursuant to the Freedom of Information Act. The reporter's identity, including the identity of a self-reporter, may be shared with the manufacturer unless requested otherwise.

The public reporting burden for this collection of information has been estimated to average 36 minutes per response, including the time for reviewing instructions, searching existing data sources, gathering and maintaining the data needed, and completing and reviewing the collection of information. Send comments regarding this burden estimate or any other aspect of this collection of information, including suggestions for reducing this burden to:

Department of Health and Human Services
Food and Drug Administration
Office of Chief Information Officer
1350 Piccard Drive, Room 400
Rockville, MD 20850

Please DO NOT RETURN this form to this address.

OMB statement:
"An agency may not conduct or sponsor, and a person is not required to respond to, a collection of information unless it displays a currently valid OMB control number."

U.S. DEPARTMENT OF HEALTH AND HUMAN SERVICES
Food and Drug Administration

FORM FDA 3500 (1/09) (Back) **Please Use Address Provided Below -- Fold in Thirds, Tape and Mail**

DEPARTMENT OF
HEALTH & HUMAN SERVICES

Public Health Service
Food and Drug Administration
Rockville, MD 20857

Official Business
Penalty for Private Use $300

NO POSTAGE NECESSARY IF MAILED IN THE UNITED STATES OR APO/FPO

BUSINESS REPLY MAIL

FIRST CLASS MAIL PERMIT NO. 946 ROCKVILLE MD

POSTAGE WILL BE PAID BY FOOD AND DRUG ADMINISTRATION

MEDWATCH
The FDA Safety Information and Adverse Event Reporting Program
Food and Drug Administration
5600 Fishers Lane
Rockville, MD 20852-9787

FIGURE 8-3 (Continued)

threatening; required intervention to prevent permanent impairment or damage; other serious medically important event).

Disability or Permanent Damage

Report if the adverse event resulted in a substantial disruption of a person's ability to conduct normal life functions; that is, if the adverse event resulted in a significant, persistent, or permanent change, impairment, damage, or disruption in the patient's body function/structure, physical activities, or quality of life.

Congenital Anomaly/Birth Defect

Report if you suspect that exposure to a medical product prior to conception or during pregnancy may have resulted in an adverse outcome for a child.

Required Intervention to Prevent Permanent Impairment or Damage (Devices)

Report if you believe that medical or surgical intervention was necessary to preclude permanent impairment of a body function, or prevent permanent damage to a body structure, with either situation suspected to be due to the use of a medical product.

Other Serious (Important Medical Events)

Report when the event does not fit the other outcomes, but the event may jeopardize the patient and may require medical or surgical intervention (treatment) to prevent one of the other outcomes. Examples include allergic bronchospasm (a serious problem with breathing) requiring treatment in an emergency department or serious blood dyscrasias (blood disorders) or seizures/convulsions that do not result in hospitalization. The development of drug dependence or drug abuse would also be examples of important medical events.

Drug Quality Reporting System

In addition to the adverse drug reaction program, the FDA maintains a voluntary program through which health care practitioners can report drug quality problems, the Drug Quality Reporting System (DQRS). The FDA encourages pharmacists to report any concerns with a drug product, including poor or improper labeling, the lack of efficacy of an injectable product, particulate matter, abnormal color or taste, and so forth. The FDA receives DQRS reports through the MedWatch program.

Drug Recalls

Drug recalls are mostly voluntary, either manufacturer initiated or FDA requested, and generally occur as the result of reports to the manufacturer from customers such as health professionals. Sometimes, the reports going to FDA alert the agency to a problem. The FDA will then notify the manufacturer that it should institute or consider instituting a recall.

When a company determines that a product has a significant problem, it will generally initiate a recall committee comprised of medical, regulatory, technical, and possibly legal personnel to determine the possible classification of the recall. The company contacts the FDA with its data and recommendation and, working with FDA medical staff, determines the health hazard potential of a product (e.g., subpotent labeling errors, adverse drug reactions, manufacturing issues) and assigns a drug recall classification as follows:

1. *Class I*—There is a reasonable probability that the use or exposure to a product will cause severe adverse health consequences or death.
2. *Class II*—The use of or exposure to a product may cause temporary or medically reversible adverse health consequences.
3. *Class III*—The use of or exposure to a product is not likely to cause adverse health consequences.

The manufacturer is responsible for notifying customers, distributors and sellers of the product about the recall and its conditions, and these entities are responsible for contacting consumers if necessary. The FDA requires that written notices for Class I, Class II, and some Class III recalls be sent by first-class mail with the envelope and letterhead conspicuously marked "URGENT: DRUG RECALL." However, some companies in an effort to be prudent and have a record of notifications send letters by certified mail, return receipt requested. If serious enough, the media can be used to alert the public of the recall.

Once such a notice is received, a pharmacist or technician should immediately retrieve all lot numbers of the recalled medication, supplies, and devices from the facility, and place them in a secure, separate area, following the manufacturer's recommendation to destroy or return the recalled products. A notation on the recall notice should be made noting the date, amount (if any) of the recalled drugs or devices, and their disposition. Note that dispensing a recalled product may violate the FDCA, because the drug is likely adulterated or misbranded.

The company, after notifying the public about the recall has responsibility for monitoring the recall's progress.

A post-recall audit is done by the FDA to verify that manufacturers, wholesalers, pharmacists, or customers have received notification about the recall and have taken appropriate action.

Repackaging of Drugs

Repackaging of drugs in a pharmacy requires the use of a repackaging record. A repackaging record must be maintained that includes the name, strength, lot number, quantity, name of the manufacturer and distributor, the date of repacking, the number of packages prepared, the number of dosage units in each package, the signature of the person performing the repackaging operation, the signature of the pharmacist supervising the repackaging, and other identifying marks added by the pharmacy for internal recordkeeping purposes. In the event of a drug recall, the repackaging record is a source of information referred to in an effort to determine if the recalled drug has been repackaged. Note that those who repackage drugs and devices for commercial distribution through interstate commerce need to register with the FDA as a repackager.

Expiration Dating for Repackaged Drugs

Calculation of the expiration date for a repackaged drug may vary as per state board regulations. In New York State drugs repackaged for in-house use must have an expiration date of 12 months or 50% of the time remaining on the manufacturer's expiration date—whichever is less—from the date of repackaging. The USP Pharmacists' Pharmacopeia states the expiration date shall be 1 year from the date the drug is packaged or the expiration date of the original container, whichever is earlier.

Product Tampering

The FDA promulgated regulations in 1982 requiring that certain OTC drugs and devices be manufactured in tamper-resistant packaging. A tamper-resistant package is defined as "one having an indicator or barrier to entry which, if breached or missing, can reasonably be expected to provide visible evidence to consumers that tampering has occurred."

The U.S. Pharmacopoeia and the National Formulary

The U.S. Pharmacopoeia (USP) and the National Formulary (NF) were founded in 1820. In 1848 the Drug Import Act recognized the USP as an official compendium. During the 1880s and 1890s, states boards of pharmacy began requiring the USP and NF to be maintained in pharmacies. In 1906, the Food and Drug Act utilized the USP and the NF as its standard for drug quality and purity. With the passage of the Food, Drug, and Cosmetic Act in 1938, the USP, NF, and Homeopathic Pharmacopeia became the official compendia of drug standards in the United States.

The USP and NF existed as two separate volumes until 1980 when they became published under one cover. Each chapter of the USP is assigned a number, which appears in brackets along with the chapter name. Chapters 1 to 999 are requirements, as well as official monographs and standards of USP, whereas Chapters 1000 to 1999 are informational.

Chapter <797> of the USP, entitled "Pharmaceutical Compounding: Sterile Preparations," was published on January 1, 2004. The guidelines laid out in this chapter are enforceable by federal and state regulatory agencies. The chapter details the procedures and requirements with which pharmacists, technicians, and other health professionals must comply when they compound sterile preparations. This chapter establishes practice standards that are applicable to all practice settings where sterile preparations are compounded (hospitals, community pharmacies, home infusion services, ambulatory care services, physician offices, nursing homes, etc.). (Refer to Chapter 17 for a comprehensive review of this topic and the role and responsibilities of the pharmacy technician.)

Medicare

The Medicare program was enacted in 1965 to help provide for federal health insurance for those older than 65 years of age and for certain individuals with disabilities, regardless of age. As noted before in this chapter, CMS has the responsibility for Medicare oversight. The law has several components, most notably:

- *Part A*—Provides hospitalization insurance without any charge to eligible beneficiaries. Part A covers inpatient hospital, inpatient skilled nursing facilities, home health care, and hospice care.
- *Part B*—Covers outpatient diagnostic services such as x-rays and laboratory tests, physician services, preventive care, durable medical equipment (e.g., wheelchairs, walkers, oxygen tanks), home health care, and therapy services.
- *Part D*—On December 8, 2003, the Medicare Prescription Drug, Improvement, and Modernization Act, also known as Medicare Part D, was signed into law. In 2006 this law added a voluntary prescription drug

benefit to Medicare. Beneficiaries pay an average $35 monthly premium, a $250 deductible, and a 25% copayment up to $2,250. Coverage then stops for drug costs between $2,251 and $5,100. This is known as the "doughnut hole." After $5,100 in drug expenditures, the plan will pay the greater of either $2 for a generic, $5 for a brand name drug, or a 5% copayment.

medication therapy management (MTM) program in which pharmacists offer nondrug services such as drug therapy management for diabetes, anticoagulation, anemia, hypertension, and renal failure

The law also provides coverage for disease management programs, termed **medication therapy management (MTM)** programs. Pharmacists may receive fees for providing MTM services to patients with chronic diseases who take multiple drugs.

Medicare Advantage allows people to pair private health care insurance with Medicare. Under the Patient Protection and Affordable Care Act (PPACA) and other health care reform measures, Medicare Advantage programs may become a thing of the past because the Medicare system may ultimately be revamped.

Long-Term Care Facility Regulation

A long-term care facility (LTCF) is a facility that is planned, staffed, and equipped to accommodate individuals who do not require hospital care but who are in need of medical, nursing, and related health and social services. Nursing homes that accept federal funds, including Medicare and Medicaid, are required to comply with federal regulations issued by the CMS.

Each nursing home is surveyed annually to determine compliance with the federal regulations. These surveys are enforced through appropriate state agencies, with the majority of the states vesting regulatory power in the state department of health. (Refer to Chapter 4 for a comprehensive review of this topic and the role and responsibilities of the pharmacy technician.)

Tax-Free Alcohol

The federal government's philosophy with respect to the use of tax-free ethyl alcohol is that the alcohol will be used only for specific purposes:

- It will not be used for beverage purposes.
- It is not for resale.
- It is used in accordance with uses stated on the alcohol permit.

Bureau of Alcohol, Tobacco, Firearms and Explosives (ATF) a department of the U.S. Treasury that establishes regulatory standards for procuring, storing, dispensing, and using tax-free alcohol for specific clinical uses

If not used according to stated purposes, a tax will be levied for its procurement and subsequent use. In pursuit of this goal, the **Bureau of Alcohol, Tobacco, Firearms and Explosives (ATF)** is responsible for controlling tax-free alcohol, which has a number of mandated specific federal forms users of tax-free alcohol must complete.

Pharmacies may purchase 95% ethanol, with applicable taxes, for routine compounding of pharmaceutical preparations or for filling prescriptions by using Form ATF-11. Institutions with a need for greater volumes of alcohol may purchase tax-free alcohol, which is much lower in cost than regular alcohol purchases, for which the taxes are quite high. Hospital pharmacies can purchase tax-free alcohol by using Form ATF-1447. Pharmacies purchasing alcohol for use as a beverage must obtain a retail liquor dealer's stamp.

Adequate and secure fire-resistant storage facilities must be available for the prevention of unauthorized access to tax-free alcohol. These facilities must be large enough to hold the maximum quantity of tax-free alcohol that will be on hand at any one time as allowed by the respective institution's tax-free alcohol permit. A bond is required for persons who withdraw more than 1,500 proof gallons of tax-free alcohol per year.

Accurate detailed records of all receipts, shipments, loss, usage, destruction, withdrawal, and use of tax-free alcohol must be kept for easy access by ATF officers. Records must be kept on file for 3 years after the date of each transaction. All records must be kept at the permit premises. A physical inventory must be made of the tax-free alcohol on a semiannual basis. If a loss is incurred, a claim for allowances must be filed with the ATF regional director.

The Joint Commission

The Joint Commission
a not-for-profit organization that sets standards designed to ensure effective quality services (e.g., optimal standards for the operation of hospitals)

The Joint Commission was formed in 1951 as a not-for-profit, private, nongovernmental organization by the American College of Physicians, American College of Surgeons, American Hospital Association, American Medical Association, and later, the American Dental Association, for the purpose of improving the quality of health care provided to the public. The Joint Commission has changed its mission to not only address the quality of patient care, but also patient safety.

The Joint Commission has created a set of standards and National Patient Safety Goals to which health care providers must comply. It then evaluates organizations for compliance with these standards through an on-site inspection called a *survey*. If the organization is in substantial compliance with these standards, the commission awards a certificate of accreditation. To maintain accreditation, the organization is expected to correct any *Recommendation for Improvement (RFI)* and be in continuous compliance. The organization could be surveyed at any time on an unannounced basis, but must be resurveyed at least once every 3 years.

The Joint Commission currently sets standards and accredits the following types of health care providers: hospitals, home health care agencies, home infusion providers and home care pharmacies, long-term care pharmacies, ambulatory infusion centers, home medical equipment and home oxygen providers, ambulatory clinics, ambulatory surgi-centers and office-based surgery practices, community health centers, college and prison health care centers, nursing homes and subacute facilities, assisted living facilities, clinical laboratories, behavioral health organizations, and alcohol and chemical dependency centers, among others.

Accreditation

Accreditation is a voluntary process, and an organization pays to be surveyed and accredited by The Joint Commission. Currently, more than 80% of hospitals are accredited by The Joint Commission, with a significant percentage in other health care areas.

Why do health care organizations seek accreditation? Accreditation signifies achievement of a high level of quality and safety in providing patient care. This brings prestige to the organization, attracting both staff and physicians, and provides a source of pride within the community. Lastly, The Joint Commission has been granted *deemed status* for participation in Medicare. That means that providers accredited by The Joint Commission are "deemed" to meet the Medicare Conditions of Participation and can receive Medicare funding without having separate annual Medicare surveys by state inspectors. Thus, while voluntary in nature, loss of accreditation can mean not only a loss of prestige, but also a loss of significant Medicare and private insurance funding. That is why many hospitals place such importance on preparation for Joint Commission surveys and in adhering to the standards.

The Joint Commission Standards

All standards are published in a *Comprehensive Accreditation Manual* for each of the major accreditation programs (e.g., hospitals, home care, behavioral health, ambulatory, networks, long-term care), which are provided on a complimentary basis to each organization that has applied for accreditation. Most standards related to pharmacy practice fall within the "Medication Use" section of the "Care of the Patient" chapter. However, other chapters often contain standards pertinent to the pharmacy. For example, the requirement for patient education on medications can be found in the education chapter.

Quality Improvement

The Joint Commission is a strong proponent of the principles of continuous quality improvement. This theory requires collection of data to measure, assess, and ultimately improve all processes within the organization. The Joint Commission calls this **performance improvement (PI)**. PI forms the cornerstone of all standards. As a result, the performance improvement coordinator at most hospitals is the key person responsible for coordinating the hospital's accreditation preparation efforts.

performance improvement (PI) is the process of self evaluation whereby the organization can use results of assessments and audits to improve upon areas of practice

Survey Process

Although a Joint Commission survey has a number of components, a pharmacy technician will most likely be involved with visits to patient care settings and tours of the pharmacy. During a typical inpatient hospital unit visit, The Joint Commission surveyor tours the unit to review its overall operation—including appropriate storage of medications—and meets and interviews key unit staff, including physicians, nurses, pharmacists, social workers, dietitians, and possibly even pharmacy technicians. If technicians are interviewed as part of a survey, they need to be able to explain what they do and how they do it, to be knowledgeable about the pharmacy's policies and procedures and about other hospital policies and procedures that describe their responsibilities both within the pharmacy and in their functions in patient care areas.

Survey Results

While the actual final accreditation report of the organization is confidential, The Joint Commission does publicly post a performance report that includes, among other things, the accreditation decision. The final recommendations of the survey team allow the organization to improve its quality and safety of patient care in a positive, nonpunitive environment. For more information about the Joint Commission and the accreditation process, refer to the organization's website (www.jointcommission.org).

Patient's Bill of Rights

Many states have established a **patient's bill of rights** for hospital and health care institutions. This bill of rights ensures that all patients—inpatients, outpatients, and emergency service patients—are afforded their rights. The hospital's responsibility for ensuring patients' rights includes providing patients with a copy of these rights and providing assistance to patients to understand and exercise their rights.

For the purposes of illustration, **Figure 8-4** is an example of New York State Hospital's patient's bill of rights. It is incumbent on all health care workers to be familiar with the bill of rights and to ensure compliance with it.

patient's bill of rights a declaration ensuring that all patients—inpatients, outpatients, and emergency service patients—are afforded their rights in a health care institution

Patients' Bill of Rights

As a patient in a hospital in New York State, you have the right, consistent with law, to:

(1) Understand and use these rights. If for any reason you do not understand or you need help, the hospital MUST provide assistance, including an interpreter.

(2) Receive treatment without discrimination as to race, color, religion, sex, national origin, disability, sexual orientation or source of payment.

(3) Receive considerate and respectful care in a clean and safe environment free of unnecessary restraints.

(4) Receive emergency care if you need it.

(5) Be informed of the name and position of the doctor who will be in charge of your care in the hospital.

(6) Know the names, positions and functions of any hospital staff involved in your care and refuse their treatment, examination or observation.

(7) A no smoking room.

(8) Receive complete information about your diagnosis, treatment and prognosis.

(9) Receive all the information that you need to give informed consent for any proposed procedure or treatment. This information shall include the possible risks and benefits of the procedure or treatment.

(10) Receive all the information you need to give informed consent for an order not to resuscitate. You also have the right to designate an individual to give this consent for you if you are too ill to do so. If you would like additional information, please ask for a copy of the pamphlet "Do Not Resuscitate Orders — A Guide for Patients and Families."

(11) Refuse treatment and be told what effect this may have on your health.

(12) Refuse to take part in research. In deciding whether or not to participate, you have the right to a full explanation.

(13) Privacy while in the hospital and confidentiality of all information and records regarding your care.

(14) Participate in all decisions about your treatment and discharge from the hospital. The hospital must provide you with a written discharge plan and written description of how you can appeal your discharge.

(15) Review your medical record without charge. Obtain a copy of your medical record for which the hospital can charge a reasonable fee. You cannot be denied a copy solely because you cannot afford to pay.

(16) Receive an itemized bill and explanation of all charges.

(17) Complain without fear of reprisals about the care and services you are receiving and to have the hospital respond to you and if you request it, a written response. If you are not satisfied with the hospital's response, you can complain to the New York State Health Department. The hospital must provide you with the State Health Department telephone number.

(18) Authorize those family members and other adults who will be given priority to visit consistent with your ability to receive visitors.

(19) Make known your wishes in regard to anatomical gifts. You may document your wishes in your health care proxy or on a donor card, available from the hospital.

Public Health Law(PHL)2803 (1)(g)Patient's Rights, 10NYCRR, 405.7,405.7(a)(1),405.7(c)

FIGURE 8-4 Patient's bill of rights.

Summary

Numerous statutes, rules, regulations, and quasi-legal standards of practice regulate the pharmacy profession. These requirements have been established to protect the patient and to ensure safe and effective drug therapy. Pharmacists and technicians should be familiar with and ensure compliance with these standards in their daily activities and responsibilities.

LEGAL CITATION FORMAT

Legal terminology, formats, and symbols in legal reading materials are summarized as follows:

- Statutes appearing in the U.S. Code are arranged into titles and divided into sections. For example, the Food, Drug, and Cosmetic Act begins at 21 U.S. Code 321 (Title 21 of the U.S. Code, Section 321).
- Regulations are proposed by federal administrative agencies in the *Federal Register* as discussed earlier. Citations in the *Federal Register* use volume numbers and page numbers, and dates in parentheses. For example, 65 Fed. Reg. 82, 462 (2000).
- Once regulations have been finalized and adopted by the agency, they appear in the *Code of Federal Regulations* (*CFR*). The citations in the CFR refer to title number and section, for example, 21 CFR 120.200.

TEST YOUR KNOWLEDGE

Multiple Choice

1. A patient package insert must be given to all patients who are taking
a. steroids.
b. analgesics.
c. estrogenic drugs.
d. all of the above.

2. Which of the following is considered a controlled substance?
a. Demerol
b. morphine
c. Valium
d. all of the above

3. Laws and regulations affecting pharmacy practice encompass
a. federal and state statutes.
b. state rules and regulations.
c. CSA regulations.
d. all of the above.

4. Which of the following is *not* an approved use of tax-free alcohol?
   a. use in educational organizations for scientific purposes
   b. use in hospitals for medical purposes
   c. laboratory use for scientific research
   d. beverage purposes

5. Which of the following is *not* a responsibility of the Food, Drug, and Cosmetic Act?
   a. the purity of drugs sold in the United States
   b. Consumer Product Safety Commission
   c. the safety and efficacy of drugs and medical devices
   d. over-the-counter drug labeling requirements for safe consumer use

6. Controlled substances are required by federal law to have appropriate safeguards with their use. Which of the following is *not* an issue?
   a. inventory requirements
   b. dispensing records and reports
   c. administration records
   d. patient consent

7. Which of the following are not functions of the FDA?
   a. medical device approvals
   b. regulation of drug marketing
   c. possible drug recalls
   d. enforcement of the anti-kickback statute

8. A Class I recall does *not* generally include
   a. voluntary manufacturer initiation.
   b. the possibility of severe health consequences.
   c. FDA initiation.
   d. assignment of the drug recall classification by the FDA.

9. The function of the Occupational Safety and Health Administration is
   a. to monitor job-related injuries.
   b. to develop job safety and health standards.
   c. to ensure a safe and healthy workplace.
   d. all of the above.

10. Pharmacy practice standards, guidelines, and statements do not include which of the following?
    a. Define reasonable and prudent practices.
    b. Establish minimum standards for the profession.
    c. Improve the delivery of pharmaceutical care.
    d. Establish pharmacist positions.

Matching

Match the legislation with what it enforces.

1. ______ Durham-Humphrey Amendment
2. ______ Orphan Drug Act
3. ______ Controlled Substances Act
4. ______ Poison Prevention Packaging Act
5. ______ Hazard Communication Standard
6. ______ Health Insurance Portability and Accountability Act (HIPAA)

a. Regulates the manufacture, sale, and distribution of drugs that have a high abuse potential.

b. Creates incentives for manufacturers to research and develop drugs to treat rare diseases and disorders.

c. Establishes guidelines to protect patient privacy.

d. Establishes requirements for child-resistant containers.

e. Establishes requirements for prescription versus over-the-counter drugs.

f. Establishes the rights of employees to know the dangers of substances used in the workplace.

Fill in the Blank

1. ______________ and ______________ are administrative enactments implemented by government agencies that meet the intent of statutory policies.
2. The ______________ prohibits the adulteration and misbranding of foods distributed in interstate commerce.
3. A ______________ is submitted to the FDA that contains data to demonstrate that a drug is safe and effective in order for the drug to be legally marketed in the United States.
4. Schedule ______________ drugs have no approved medical use in the United States.
5. The FDA requires distribution of ______________ to educate patients about the proper use of and potential hazards of drugs.

Suggested Readings

Abbod, R. (2005). *Pharmacy practice and the law* (4th ed.). Sudbury, MA: Jones and Bartlett.

American Society of Health-System Pharmacists. (2007–2008). *Best practices for health system pharmacy*. Bethesda, MD: Author.

Berson, S. W., and Flannery, E. J. (2010). *Health care 2010: Managing risks in the new compliance and enforcement environment*. New York, NY: Practicing Law Institute.

Code of Federal Regulations. (2011). Washington, DC: U.S. Government Printing Office.

Dunn, C. W. (1987). *Federal Food, Drug, and Cosmetic Act: A statement of its legislative record*. New York, NY: G. E. Stechert.

Heller, M. A. (2011). *Guide to medical device regulation*. Washington, DC: Thompson Publishing.

Hutt, P. B., & Merrill, R. A. (1991). *Food and drug law: Cases and materials* (2nd ed.). Westbury, NY: Foundation Press.

Joint Commission. (2007). *Comprehensive accreditation manual for hospitals*. Oakbrook Terrace, IL: Author.

Pharmacy law digest (40th ed.). (2009). St. Louis, MO: Facts and Comparisons.

Reiss, B., & Hall, G. (2006). *Guide to federal pharmacy law* (5th ed.). Delmar, NY: Apothecary Press.

Salcido, R.S. (2008). *False Claims Act and the health care industry: Counseling and litigation* (2nd ed.). Washington, DC: American Health Lawyers Association.

Statutes at Large. Washington, DC: U.S. Government Printing Office.

United States Code. Washington, DC: U.S. Government Printing Office.

University of the State of New York, New York State Education Department, & New York State Board of Pharmacy. (2007). *Pharmacy guide to practice.* Albany, NY: Authors.

U.S. Pharmacopeial Convention. (2007). Chapter <797>: Pharmaceutical compounding—Sterile preparations. In *United States pharmacopeia 31st ed./National formulary 26th rev*., second *supplement*. Rockville, MD: Author.

Willig, S.H. (2001). *Good manufacturing practices for pharmaceuticals: A plan for total quality control from manufacturer to consumer* (5th ed.). New York, NY: Marcel Decker.

Relevant Federal Statutes and Regulations

Alcohol Tax Law

Controlled Substances Act of 1970

False Claims Act of 1863 and amendments

Federal Anti-Kickback Statute, 42 U.S.C. 1320a-7b.

Federal Hazardous Substances Act

Food and Drug Administration Modernization Act of 1997

Food, Drug, and Cosmetic Act of 1938 and its amendments

Health Insurance Portability and Accountability Act (HIPAA)

Occupation Safety and Health Act

Poison Prevention Packaging Act of 1970

Social Security Amendments of 1965 (Medicare and Medicaid)

Regulatory Agencies

Bureau of Alcohol, Tobacco, Firearms and Explosives (ATF)

Centers for Medicare and Medicaid Services (CMS)

Consumer Product Safety Commission (CPSC) (Poison Prevention Packaging Act), 16 CFR §§ 1700–1704

Department of Health and Human Services (DHHS)

Department of Justice (DOJ)

Drug Enforcement Administration (DEA)

Federal Trade Commission (FTC)

Food and Drug Administration (FDA)

Internal Revenue Service (Alcohol Tax Law) (IRS)

State boards of pharmacy

Social Security Administration (SSA)

CHAPTER 9

Medication Management: The Foundation of Pharmaceutical Care

Competencies

Upon completion of this chapter, the reader should be able to:

1. State the mission of pharmacy practice.
2. Explain the foundational elements of pharmaceutical care.
3. Briefly describe the elements in the drug use process once the drug is approved by the FDA.
4. Explain how important control is in the medication management process.
4. Describe the role of pharmacists in medication management.
5. Discuss the role of pharmacy technicians in medication management.
6. Discuss the trends in medication management and how these trends may affect the roles of the pharmacist and pharmacy technician.

Key Terms

adverse drug reaction (ADR)
alternative medicine
drug manufacturer
drug wholesaler
group purchasing organization (GPO)
laminar flow hood
medication management system
medication-related problem (MRP)
medication therapy management (MTM)
nonadherence
pharmaceutical care
prescription order form
quality drug therapy
retailer
side effects
unit dose

Introduction

medication management system an organized, complex and controlled system of manufacturing, purchasing, distributing, storing, prescribing, preparing, dispensing, administering, using, controlling, and monitoring a drug's effects and outcomes to ensure that drugs are used safely and effectively

Once a drug is approved for use in the United States, a defined process is employed to distribute the drug product and make it available for use. This organized, complex, and controlled procedure is part of the **medication management system**. Pharmacists and pharmacy technicians are intimately involved in medication management, and they are responsible for controlling parts of the process so the drugs are used safely and effectively and not diverted into the wrong hands.

This chapter describes how drugs make their way to the patient after being made by the manufacturer. It begins with a review of drug distribution; the prescribing, dispensing, and administrating of prescription medication; the self-use of medication; and what it means to provide quality medication therapy. The primary focus is on control of the medication management process and how pharmacists and pharmacy technicians exert that control.

Medication Management System

Once a drug is approved for distribution, medication management encompasses the manufacturing, purchasing, distributing, storing, prescribing, preparing, dispensing, administering, using, controlling, and monitoring of drugs and their effects and outcomes (**Figure 9-1**). In short, the medication management system consists of the steps and procedures used to get a drug to its eventual destination safely, securely, and effectively.

Pharmacy technicians spend most of their time in the ordering, storing, preparing, dispensing, and controlling parts of this process. They should, however, understand the entire medication management system and do what they can to add proper controls as needed.

Manufacturing Drugs

The medication management process begins with the pharmaceutical company or manufacturer that produces the drug. The manufacturer is responsible for manufacturing drugs that are safe and effective for use. Drug research, development, and production are heavily regulated.

drug manufacturer a company responsible for developing, producing, and distributing pharmaceutical products

drug wholesaler a company responsible for delivering medication, medical devices, appliances, and so forth, to pharmacies and retailers

retailer a company responsible for delivering products to patients

Distributing Drugs

The United States has the most complex drug distribution system in the world. Automation, such as bar coding, computerized inventories, and information systems, keeps the products flowing. As drugs flow through the distribution system, the costs of the drugs increase.

Drug manufacturers, wholesalers, and retailers are the major organizations responsible for the supply and distribution of medications in the United States. **Drug manufacturers** develop and produce the pharmaceutical products. **Drug wholesalers** deliver medications, medical devices and appliances, health and beauty aids, and other products to pharmacies and, with the exception of prescription drugs, to other retailers. **Retailers** (like community pharmacies) provide these products to patients.

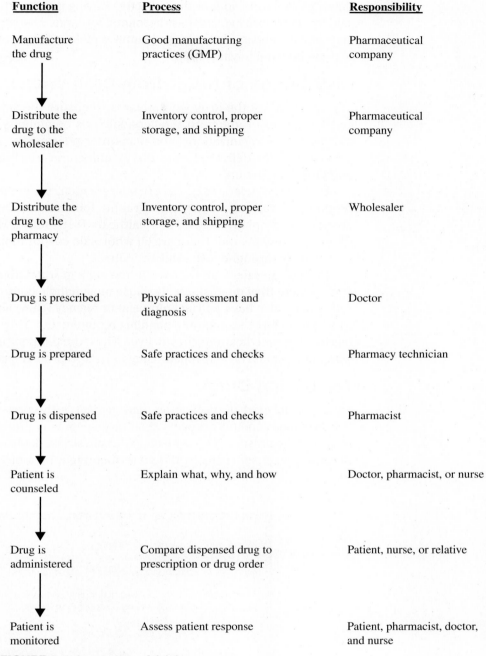

Function	Process	Responsibility
Manufacture the drug	Good manufacturing practices (GMP)	Pharmaceutical company
Distribute the drug to the wholesaler	Inventory control, proper storage, and shipping	Pharmaceutical company
Distribute the drug to the pharmacy	Inventory control, proper storage, and shipping	Wholesaler
Drug is prescribed	Physical assessment and diagnosis	Doctor
Drug is prepared	Safe practices and checks	Pharmacy technician
Drug is dispensed	Safe practices and checks	Pharmacist
Patient is counseled	Explain what, why, and how	Doctor, pharmacist, or nurse
Drug is administered	Compare dispensed drug to prescription or drug order	Patient, nurse, or relative
Patient is monitored	Assess patient response	Patient, pharmacist, doctor, and nurse

FIGURE 9-1 An overview of the drug process.

group purchasing organization (GPO) a group of hospitals or health systems whose collective buying power allows the group to obtain favorable pricing, such as discounts, when making large, ongoing purchases. Pharmaceutical companies ship large quantities of drugs to the warehouses of these hospital buying groups

Distribution of Drugs from Pharmaceutical Manufacturers

Most of the pharmaceutical products made by manufacturers go directly to drug wholesalers and to other major distribution centers. Distribution centers can be set up by chain pharmacies (e.g., CVS, Rite Aid, Walgreens), mass merchandisers (e.g., Kmart, Walmart), supermarket chains that have pharmacies (e.g., Kroger, Stop & Shop), and mail-order pharmacies (e.g., Medco).

Although some hospitals buy directly from the drug manufacturers, most buy their medications through **group purchasing organizations (GPOs)**. Most hospitals are part of a group of hospitals or a health system (e.g., the Catholic Hospital Association, the University Hospital Consortium, the Voluntary Hospitals of America).

These groups form so that the collective buying power of the group can be used to gain favorable pricing, such as discounts, for large, ongoing inventory needs. Pharmaceutical companies ship large quantities of drugs to the buying group warehouses of these hospital buying groups.

Distribution of Drugs from Drug Wholesalers

The basic role of the drug wholesaler is to ensure the smooth, safe, and efficient distribution of products to retailers, such as community pharmacies, hospitals, managed care organizations, and mail-order pharmacies. At the wholesaler, large pallets of drugs delivered from the manufacturer are broken down into smaller units for distribution.

Drug wholesalers (e.g., AmerisourceBergen, Cardinal, and McKesson) store products in various strategic geographic locations so that the products can be quickly sent to pharmacies. The Healthcare Distribution Management Association (HDMA) estimates that there are 60 wholesale corporations that run 225 distribution centers throughout the United States.

Drug wholesalers are licensed in the state in which they are located and in the states where they do business. Because most handle controlled substances, wholesalers must also have a Drug Enforcement Agency (DEA) license. They are required to adhere to strict storage and handling requirements. They must also ensure the integrity of the medications they deliver. Thus, the temperature and humidity in their warehouses must be controlled. They must also protect against theft of a product.

Prescribing Drugs

An important part of medication management is the prescribing of drugs. This involves a more complex process than most people realize. It starts with a patient's need and the prescriber's—for example, a physician, dentist, or midwife—willingness to prescribe. In some states, the prescriber might be a physician assistant or nurse

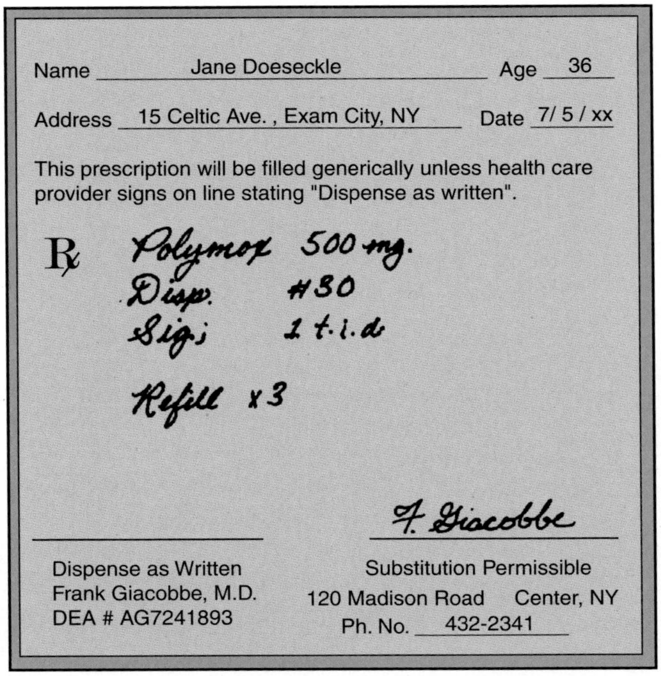
Name Jane Doeseckle Age 36
Address 15 Celtic Ave., Exam City, NY Date 7/ 5 / xx
This prescription will be filled generically unless health care provider signs on line stating "Dispense as written".
℞ Polymox 500 mg.
Disp. #30
Sig: 1 t.i.d
Refill x3
F. Giacobbe
Dispense as Written Substitution Permissible
Frank Giacobbe, M.D.
DEA # AG7241893
120 Madison Road Center, NY
Ph. No. 432-2341

FIGURE 9-2 **A.** Prescription.

practitioner; however, these categories of health care workers have limited prescribing privileges. Veterinarians may also prescribe but only for animals, and certain drugs can be prescribed only by veterinarians and dispensed on the order of a veterinarian.

The details about a medication prescribed for ambulatory patients are written on a prescription (**Figure 9-2A**; see Chapter 12), whereas details about medications prescribed for inpatients are written on a prescription order form (**Figure 9-2B**).

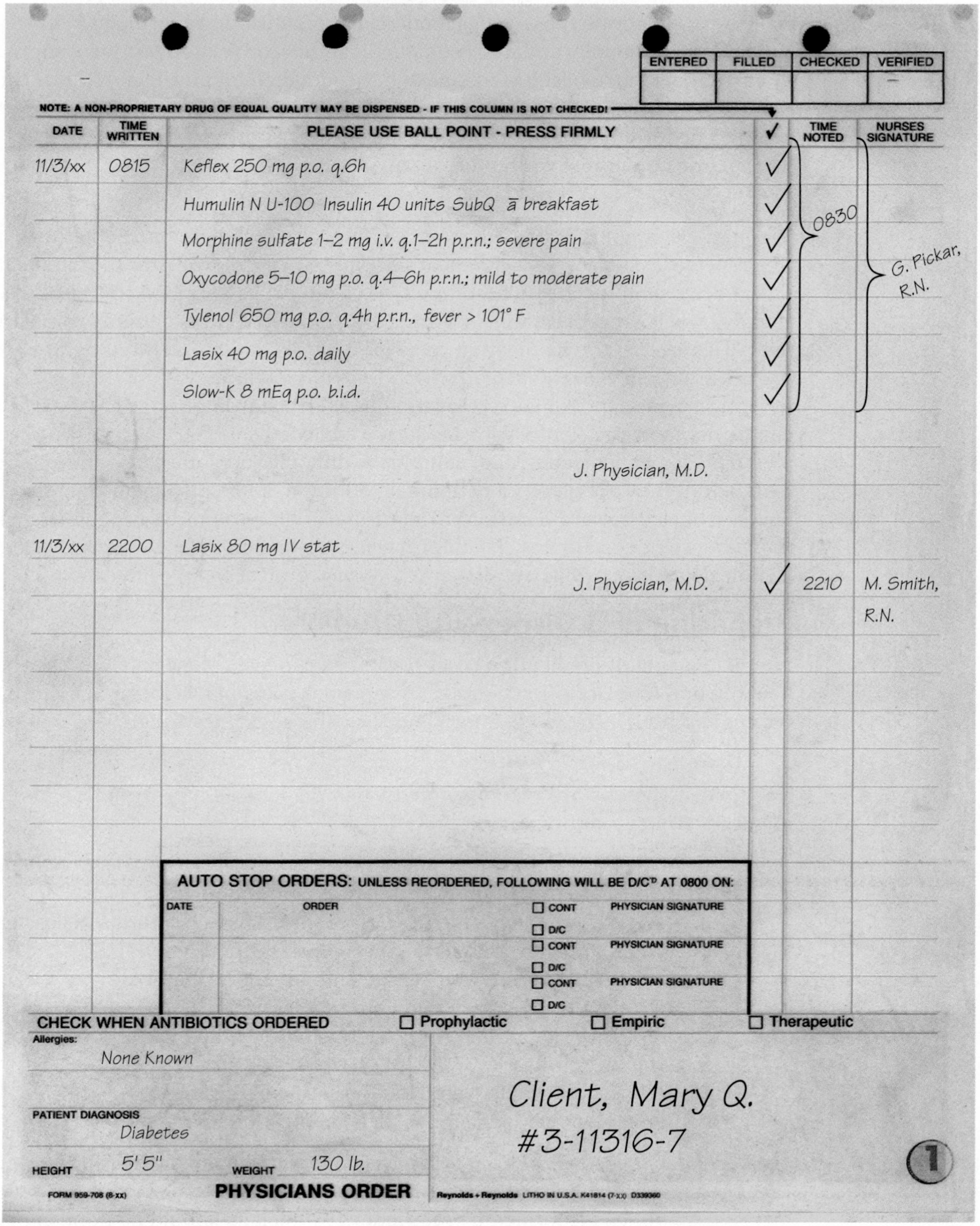

ENTERED	FILLED	CHECKED	VERIFIED
			–

NOTE: A NON-PROPRIETARY DRUG OF EQUAL QUALITY MAY BE DISPENSED - IF THIS COLUMN IS NOT CHECKED!

DATE	TIME WRITTEN	PLEASE USE BALL POINT - PRESS FIRMLY	✓	TIME NOTED	NURSES SIGNATURE
11/3/xx	0815	Keflex 250 mg p.o. q.6h	✓	0830	G. Pickar, R.N.
		Humulin N U-100 Insulin 40 units SubQ $\bar{a}$ breakfast	✓		
		Morphine sulfate 1–2 mg i.v. q.1–2h p.r.n.; severe pain	✓		
		Oxycodone 5–10 mg p.o. q.4–6h p.r.n.; mild to moderate pain	✓		
		Tylenol 650 mg p.o. q.4h p.r.n., fever > 101° F	✓		
		Lasix 40 mg p.o. daily	✓		
		Slow-K 8 mEq p.o. b.i.d.	✓		
		J. Physician, M.D.			
11/3/xx	2200	Lasix 80 mg IV stat			
		J. Physician, M.D.	✓	2210	M. Smith, R.N.

AUTO STOP ORDERS: UNLESS REORDERED, FOLLOWING WILL BE D/C^{D} AT 0800 ON:

DATE	ORDER		PHYSICIAN SIGNATURE
		☐ CONT ☐ D/C	
		☐ CONT ☐ D/C	
		☐ CONT ☐ D/C	

CHECK WHEN ANTIBIOTICS ORDERED ☐ Prophylactic ☐ Empiric ☐ Therapeutic

Allergies: None Known

PATIENT DIAGNOSIS: Diabetes

HEIGHT 5' 5" WEIGHT 130 lb.

Client, Mary Q.
#3-11316-7

FORM 959-708 (8-XX) PHYSICIANS ORDER Reynolds + Reynolds LITHO IN U.S.A. K41814 (7-XX) D339360

1

FIGURE 9-2 **B.** Medication order form.

prescription order form a course of medication therapy ordered by a physician or other health care practitioner in an organized health care setting

A **prescription order form** is a medication order written to a pharmacist by a legal prescriber for an inpatient (an individuals assigned to a bed) at an institution. The differences between a prescription order form and prescription involve the definition, legal status, and how they are written. Legal requirements for a prescription order form exempt the form from having to have all of the information that is required on a prescription, but it does need to have other information that is not on a prescription, such as the patient's location (e.g., room number).

When prescribing drugs in an organized health care setting, the physician normally must prescribe those drugs found in the organization's formulary. A drug formulary is a continually updated list of medications and related products supported by current evidence-based medicine and the judgment of physicians, pharmacists, and other experts in the diagnosis and treatment of disease and preservation of health. The formulary used in the organization is approved by the pharmacy and therapeutic committee within the organization.

Drug Samples

Sometimes patients may receive a sample of a medication. Sometimes they will receive a sample of a medication *and* a prescription for the medication. These drug samples are small quantities of the drugs supplied to the physician, usually by sales representatives of drug companies. The idea behind samples is for the patient to try the medication to see if it works and is tolerated before having the prescription "filled" (slang for *dispensed*) at a pharmacy.

Pharmacists and some regulators, like state boards of pharmacy, health departments, and the Centers for Medicare and Medicaid Services, frown on samples. This is because control of samples is difficult and sometimes they go out of date before they are given to patients. In addition, some physicians feel they may become biased toward a certain drug or start using the most expensive drugs if they are provided samples. Therefore, some physicians refuse to accept samples. It is illegal for a pharmacy to dispense pharmaceutical samples to a customer.

Preparing and Dispensing Drugs

The dispensing of medication is an organized process. Most patients have never been behind a prescription counter to see what takes place. It is much more than "count and pour" (the medication) and "lick and stick" (the label).

The Community Pharmacy

The following steps are recommended when dispensing a prescription in a community pharmacy setting:

1. Accept the prescription and establish the pharmacist-patient relationship.
2. Review the prescription and patient information.
3. Review the patient's medication profile. make updates as necessary.
4. Enter all prescription data into the patient profile.
5. Review the insurance coverage and bill appropriately.
6. Retrieve the drug or ingredients from storage.
7. Prepare or compound (put together) the medication.
8. Label the container.
9. Perform a final check and dispense the medication.
10. Counsel the patients about their medication.

For safety reasons, pharmacy technicians should not be performing duties that encompass clinical judgment or are required by law to be performed by pharmacists. All duties performed by pharmacy technicians should be done under the direct, continuous supervision of a licensed pharmacist.

The Health System Pharmacy

Although some organized health care settings, like hospitals, have outpatient pharmacies that dispense prescribed medications to their ambulatory patients, most of the medication dispensed is for inpatients. Three primary systems are used for dispensing drugs in hospitals and other organized health care settings: floor stock, unit dose, and parental preparations.

Floor Stock System. Medication can be stored on patient care units in the form of a floor stock system. This system, however, is currently being replaced due to innovations in automated dispensing systems. When a floor stock system is used, the number of medications stocked should be limited for safety reasons. A floor stock system offers more opportunity for error because there is no check-and-balance system for avoiding mistakes. The nurse can access floor stock where the medication is stored (usually on a shelf or in a drawer), take out what is needed, and provide it directly to the patient.

The most common drugs in floor stock are narcotics (which are always under lock and key with strict inventory requirements), various intravenous (IV) solutions, and emergency drugs (usually in a kit). Some patient care units, like the emergency department (ED), intensive care unit (ICU), operating room (OR), and recovery room (RR), may have more floor stock than others.

Unit-Dose System. Drugs may also be prepared and dispensed as a unit dose. A **unit dose** is a dose dispensed from the pharmacy in a form and quantity that is ready to be given to the patient—no further dosage preparation, calculation, or manipulation is required. Unit-dose systems are safer than other systems because the opportunity for error is reduced and the check-and-balance system is built in.

unit dose a single-use package of a drug. In a unit-dose distribution system, a single dose of each medication is dispensed prior to the time of administration

In the unit-dose system of medication distribution, two drawers are assigned to each patient. One drawer is in the pharmacy being filled, while the other is on the patient care unit being used by the nurse to give medication to that patient (**Figure 9-3**). Each drawer is usually divided into two sections: one for regularly scheduled medication and the other for PRN (as-needed) medication. The pharmacy allocates enough medication for the patient for the next shift (7 A.M. to 3 P.M., 3 P.M. to 11 P.M., or 11 P.M. to 7 A.M.) or the next 24-hour period. At the end of the shift or 24-hour period, the drawers are exchanged.

The pharmacy receives a copy of the patient's medication orders. Ideally, pharmacy technicians, rather than pharmacists, enter the medication orders into each patient's profile, which is part of the pharmacy computer system. If the hospital has a centralized information system, the orders flow directly from the physician's electronic orders into an electronic version of the patient's pharmacy profile in the computer system. On the patient care unit, the nurses will be able to review the orders for each patient, recognizing what drug to administer, to which patient, and at what time.

Each patient has three types of documentation: the physician's order, the pharmacy patient profile, and the MAR itself. All three should have identical information. The best procedure for checking a patient's unit-dose drawer is for the pharmacist to check the contents of the drawer against the MAR rather than the pharmacy patient profile from which the drawer was filled. If the drawer is not correct, one of three things happened: (1) the drawer was filled improperly, (2) a computer entry error was made in the pharmacy, or (3) a transcription error was made between the physician's order and the nursing record. Which error occurred? The answer can be found by checking the physician's order in the patient's record.

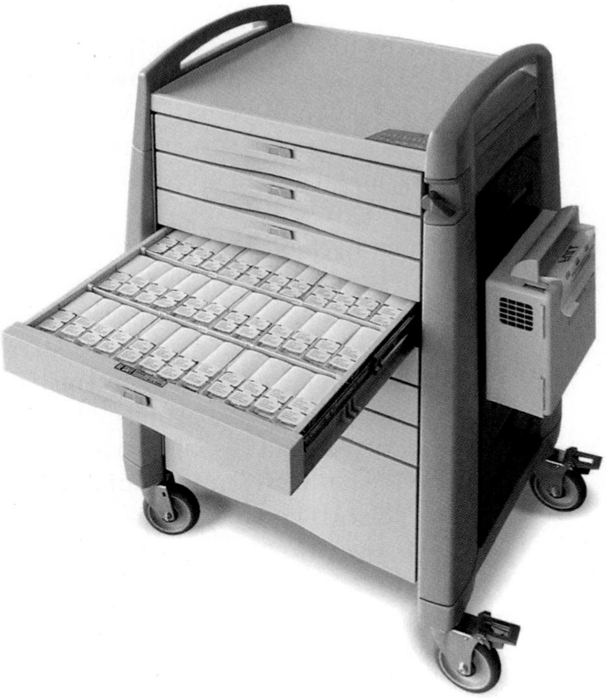

Courtesy of Artomick International, Inc.

FIGURE 9-3 Unit-dose system.

Parenteral Preparation System. The third drug distribution system is used with parenteral preparations. Parenteral preparations are sterile, pyrogen-free liquids (solutions, emulsions, or suspensions) or solid dosage forms containing one or more active ingredients, packaged in either single-dose or multidose containers. The technique of adding medication to IV solutions (compounding) should be carefully performed under ideal aseptic conditions conforming to USP <797> standards (**Figure 9-4**).

USP <797> standards require that parenteral preparations be prepared in a pharmacy using aseptic (germ-free) techniques and a laminar flow or vertical flow hood. A **laminar flow hood** is a sterile work area with a positive-pressure airflow systems that filters the air.

> **laminar flow hood** a sterile work area with a positive-pressure airflow system that filters the air

Pharmacists and pharmacy technicians are trained to prepare IV admixtures properly and should be recertified on how to do this. Once the IV admixtures are prepared, preferably by a pharmacy technician rather than a pharmacist, they should be checked by a pharmacist. When an IV additive solution is contaminated during preparation, the bacteria grow quickly with time and temperature. Therefore, parenteral solutions should be prepared just before they are needed and refrigerated between the time they are prepared and the time they are used. Delivery of IV admixtures to patient care units is usually done by a courier, a pneumatic tube system, or by a robotic delivery system.

Drug preparation and dispensation can be done from a large central pharmacy or from a central pharmacy and smaller, decentralized satellite pharmacies. Decentralized pharmacies are located in strategic locations in the hospital and serve several patient care units. Central pharmacies are more efficient, because they require less inventory and fewer personnel. However, the advantages

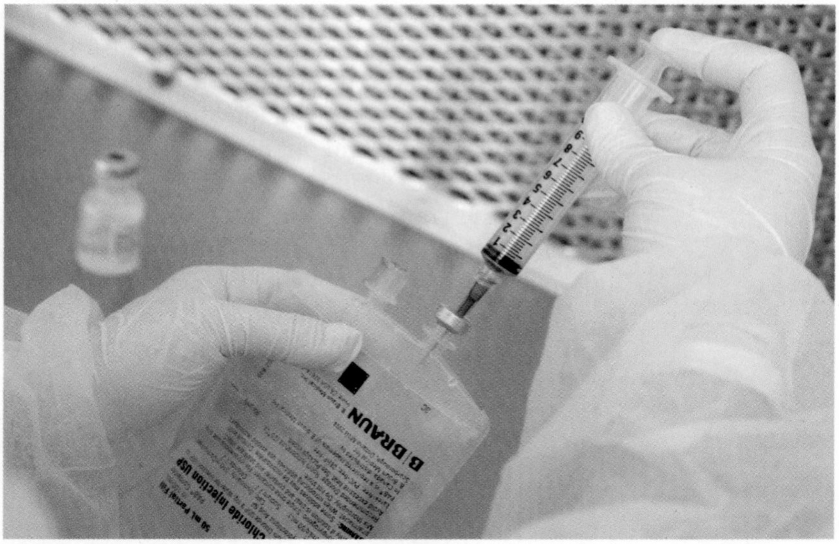

FIGURE 9-4 The pharmacy technician must take care to prepare IV admixtures in a sterile environment.

of decentralized, satellite pharmacies include faster service, more service, and more opportunity for staff pharmacists to deliver pharmaceutical care on the floors.

Counseling Patients

The physician, pharmacist, and nurse are responsible for communicating treatment regimens to the patient. The patient should be made aware of what drug treatments are being prescribed, why they are being prescribed, and how they work. The patient should be encouraged to ask questions about the drug treatments and care being prescribed. It is the patient's right to be informed of therapeutic treatments and to consent to those treatments.

Administering Medications

Patients usually receive medication one of three ways: (1) self-administration; (2) administration by a caregiver, sometimes a friend or relative; or (3) administration by a nurse. Self-administration is the way most medication is taken. It may also be the most dangerous. Unless the physician, nurse, or pharmacist counsels the patient on taking the medication, the chances of the patient taking it correctly decrease. The patient should understand the name of the medication, what it is for, and what to expect from it. Most importantly, the patient needs to understand how to take the medication correctly. Does taking one tablet three times a day mean three times during the waking hours, or spread out over every 8 hours? Does it need to be taken with water, or can it be taken with fruit juice or milk? Can patients stop taking the medication when they feel better, or do they need to take it until it is all gone? If they miss a dose, should they take twice as much next time? How should the medication be stored? What about side effects?

A friend or relative may be called on to administer medication when a patient is sick and at home. This method of medication administration may be safer than self-administration. Most people are more careful when they are responsible for others. They also tend to ask more questions and are afraid to do anything wrong.

Friends and relatives also are better at giving the medication on a schedule or reminding the patient when the medication is due.

Nurse-administered medication is the most accurate medication administration method. Nurses know medication and how to give it, and if they do not, they have been trained to find out how. Nurses pride themselves on this important role. They also have developed ways to administer the medication to the most ornery patient or the youngest child.

No matter who gives the medication, it is easy to make an error like forgetting to give it, giving the wrong drug, giving too much or too little, or giving it at the wrong time. This is unfortunate since patients go to so much effort to make an appointment, see the physician, get a diagnosis and a prescription, and get the prescription filled. Not taking the medication properly can result in an extended illness, going back to the physician, having an adverse reaction, or possibly having to go to the emergency department. All of this results in more time and expense.

Adherence with Taking the Medication as Prescribed

Some people never get their prescription filled or, if it is called in to the pharmacist, never pick it up. How big is this problem? One study evaluated the rate of prescription abandonment in community pharmacies and found that about 3.27% of the prescriptions were never picked up. Prescriptions with a copayment of $40 or higher are 3.4 times or more likely to be abandoned; a new user of a medication is 2.74 times more likely to abandon the prescription than prevalent users, and prescriptions delivered electronically were 1.64 times more likely to be abandoned. Unclaimed prescriptions are also a problem for outpatient pharmacies in hospitals. One proposed solution to this problem is to call the patient as a reminder that the medication is ready for pickup. Fourteen percent to 21% of patients never fill their original prescriptions.

Once a person does pick up a prescription, however, there is no guarantee that he or she will take it as prescribed. Either forgetting or purposely not taking medication as prescribed is called **nonadherence**. Nonadherence is a big problem. There are various means of discovery rates of medication adherence such as urine tests, serum tests, pill counts, patient interviews, and record reviews. As reported in the literature, rates of nonadherence with prescribed therapy vary greatly. The variance is explained by different patient populations, the category of drugs, how many times the medication is to be taken each day, and differences in study design. Medication adherence rates vary significantly for several disease states. It is typically cited that in the United States, the nonadherence rate is 50% to 70%, and the rate of nonadherence is higher with chronic disease because the drug regimen is longer and more complicated.

> **nonadherence** forgetting or purposefully not taking medications as prescribed

The underlying problems associated with medication nonadherence are patient actions (decisions and behaviors). Patients decide whether to take a medication and how often. Reasons for patients not taking their medication or not taking it as prescribed include cost, feeling better, side effects, not realizing the importance of doing so, and forgetting.

The cost of medication nonadherence is high in terms of lives lost, time lost, and added care needed. Poor adherence to medication regimens accounts for substantial worsening of disease, death, and increased health care costs in the United States. Of all medication-related hospital admissions in the United States, 33% to 69% are due to poor medication adherence, with a resultant cost of approximately $100 billion a year. An estimated 125,000 Americans die each year simply because they do not take their medications properly. Another cost is the cost of time, such as having to stay home or leave work or school to seek medical attention. The estimated time cost is a loss of 20 million workdays a year or about $1.5 billion in lost earnings annually in 1990, $100 billion annually in1997, and finally more than $300 billion annually in 2004.

Many individuals and groups of people (e.g., physicians, nurses, pharmacists, AARP, health plans, the Task Force for Compliance, and the National Council on Patient Information and Education) have been working on the problem of medication nonadherence. Much has been learned and more still needs to be done. Each patient not taking medication as prescribed has a different reason or set of reasons for not being in adherence. Thus, the solution for gaining patient adherence differs from one patient to the next.

Pharmacy technicians should learn methods for discovering if a patient has been nonadherent and alert the pharmacist of this problem. Once it has been determined that a nonadherence problem exists, the pharmacist should try to find out why. The most common issues are cost, other needs, fear of the medication not working or causing adverse effects, or forgetfulness.

The most effective way to improve medication adherence is by understanding why the patient is not taking the medication as prescribed and then using a combination of methods specifically designed to address the patient's reasons for not being adherent. Doing this is not only in the patient's best interest, but also in the pharmacist's best interest both clinically and economically.

Monitoring Patients

The pharmacy profession has decided the mission of pharmacy practice is to help patients make the best use of their medication. To do this, pharmacists need to get out from behind their counters and out of the hospital pharmacy and be in direct contact with patients. In other words, pharmacists need to be more concerned about patients than about drug products. This idea is called **pharmaceutical care**, which, according to ASHP, is the direct, responsible provision of medication-related care for the purpose of achieving definite outcomes that improve a patient's quality of life. The definition of pharmaceutical care has evolved during the past 20 years. The most current definition is "a practice in which the practitioner takes responsibility for a patient's drug-related needs and is held accountable for this commitment."

> **pharmaceutical care** the direct, responsible provision of medication-related care for the purpose of achieving definite outcomes that improve a patient's quality of life

There continues to be controversy about the term *pharmaceutical care*. Some pharmacists—mostly community pharmacists—feel the word *pharmaceutical* should be replaced with the words *pharmacy* or *pharmacist* (i.e., pharmacy care or pharmacist care). The rationale is that the word *pharmaceutical* is too closely associated with drug products, and by calling it pharmaceutical care, anyone can provide it. The expression *pharmacy care* or *pharmacist care* avoids these problems. However, most professional pharmacy organizations and schools of pharmacy are still using the original term *pharmaceutical care*.

Elements of Pharmaceutical Care

Regardless of the terminology or definition used, pharmaceutical care encompasses six general principles:

1. *Responsible provision of care.* The pharmacist should accept responsibility for the patient.
2. *Direct provision of care.* The pharmacist must be in direct contact with patients. He or she must see and talk with patients.

3. *Caring.* This virtue, a key characteristic among nurses and physicians, has been the most understated virtue of pharmacy. It is the centerpiece of pharmaceutical care.
4. *Achieving positive outcomes.* Several positive clinical outcomes can occur as a result of taking medication: cure of disease, elimination or decline of a patient's symptoms, arresting or slowing of a disease process, or preventing a disease or a symptom. Negative outcomes may also result from taking medication: the medication may fail to work as expected, it may have nagging side effects, or an adverse drug events can cause moderate patient morbidity (illness), a life-threatening or permanent disability, or death.

   Besides clinical outcomes there are also economic (cost) and humanistic outcomes (functional status, quality of life, and patient satisfaction). Under pharmaceutical care, it is the pharmacists' responsibility to do everything possible to achieve positive patient outcomes and avoid the negative effects of taking medication.
5. *Improving the patient's quality of life.* Everyone has a certain, measurable quality of life. Under the pharmaceutical care model of delivering care, the pharmacist must, along with the patient and the physician, set reasonable treatment goals for each drug prescribed that will improve the patient's functioning and health-related quality of life.
6. *Resolution of medication-related problems.* The task of pharmaceutical care is to resolve medication-related problems. **Medication-related problems (MRPs)** are undesirable events a patient experiences that involve (or are suspected of involving) drug therapy and that actually (or potentially) interfere with a desired patient outcome.

medication-related problem (MRP) undesirable events a patient experiences as a result of drug therapy that interfere with a desired patient outcome

Pharmaceutical care involves identifying potential and actual MRPs, resolving actual MRPs, and preventing potential MRPs. Eight MRPs have been identified:

1. *Needed drug therapy.* The patient has a medical condition that requires introducing new or additional drug therapy.
2. *Unnecessary drug therapy.* The patient is taking drug therapy that is unnecessary given his or her present condition.
3. *Use of wrong drug.* The patient has a medical condition for which the wrong drug is being taken.
4. *Dosage is too low.* The patient has a medical condition for which too little of the correct drug is being taken.
5. *Dosage is too high.* The patient has a medical condition for which too much of the correct drug is being taken.
6. *An adverse drug event.* The patient has a medical condition because of an adverse drug reaction or event.
7. *Not receiving the drug.* The patient has a medical condition for which the patient needs, but is not receiving, the drug.
8. *Drug interaction.* The patient has a medical condition and there is a drug-drug, drug-food, or drug-laboratory test interaction.

Quality Drug Therapy

quality drug therapy safe, effective, timely, and cost-effective drug therapy delivered with care

There is much more to being a pharmacist than making sure the patient receives the drug prescribed and taking actions to ensure the drug is taken as prescribed. Today, pharmacists are trained to help each patient receive quality drug therapy. **Quality drug therapy** is safe, effective, timely, and cost-effective drug therapy delivered with care.

Pharmacists used to fill prescriptions written by physicians and were not allowed to question whether the drug prescribed was the best drug for the patient. This has changed for various reasons. First, drugs are getting more complex, more potent, and more abundant. Second, physicians cannot know everything about every drug. Third, the clinical education of the pharmacist has expanded. And fourth, the scope of practice and legal duty of the pharmacist to help and protect the patient have expanded.

A physician prescribes a drug based on what he or she knows and considers best. A pharmacist may see the patient differently, may know information the physician does not know about the drug, or knows about other drugs that may better benefit the patient. Thus, if the pharmacist thinks the patient may benefit from changing the prescribed drug—its dose, route of administration, or dosage form, or changing to another drug—he or she is obligated to call the physician and discuss it.

Pharmacy technicians should bring forward any problems they suspect in prescriptions and drug orders to the attention of the pharmacist for clarification. This helps the pharmacist and helps protect the patient from harm.

Medication Safety and Drug Misadventures

Although medication can be wonderful—helping to cure an illness or helping a patient feel better—it also has the potential for harm. Harm resulting from medication is called a *drug misadventure.*

Side Effects

side effects known effects of a drug experienced by most people taking the drug; these are usually minor

All drugs have side effects. **Side effects** are the known, usually minor, annoying effects of a drug experienced by most people taking the drug. An example is the drowsiness associated with some antihistamine drugs used for treating hay fever symptoms. Because side effects are expected, minor events, they are not a drug misadventure per se.

Adverse Drug Reactions

adverse drug reaction (ADR) any unexpected, obvious change in a patient's condition that the physician suspects may be due to a drug

Some drugs can cause dangerous conditions, called adverse drug reactions. **Adverse drug reactions (ADRs)** are the unwanted, serious, harmful effects of a drug that are not experienced by every patient taking the drug. They are more serious than side effects. Consider this example of an ADR:

> *Sally is a 34-year-old mother of an 8-year-old and a 5-year-old. She is under stress, both at home and at her law firm, and there is no end in sight. Her stress causes her to be irritable and unable to sleep. After seeing her*

physician, she is told to exercise more and use stress reduction exercises daily. Sally tries these suggestions, but is just too busy to follow them consistently. Sally's friend Sue has had similar problems, so Sue gives Sally a few anti-anxiety pills to try. The drug helps, so Sally pressures her physician to prescribe anti-anxiety medication—5 milligrams three times a day. As the days get more stressful, Sally starts taking the drug three times during the day and once at bedtime. Sometimes during the day she gets drowsy, and sometimes she forgets if she has taken the drug. Driving home one day, she almost falls asleep at the wheel. She wakes up just in time to keep from hitting a car in front of her. When she goes to get a refill of her prescription, the pharmacist tells her that she should still have a week's worth of the drug left, but she has only two tablets.

Allergic Drug Reactions

Patients who are allergic to a drug or an ingredient in a medication, even a color dye, can experience drug reactions that can vary from a minor annoyance to life threatening. It is critical for every pharmacy's patient profile to contain information about each patient's allergies. Here is an example of an allergic drug reaction:

A 45-year-old man with low back pain collapsed 15 minutes after an intramuscular injection of diclofenac (Voltaren). Twenty minutes after successful revival, he went into a coma and never recovered. Before receiving the drug, the patient was asked, "Are you allergic to diclofenac?" The patient said no; however, it was later discovered the patient had a previous reaction to the drug but only knew the drug by its trade name.

Drug-Drug Interactions

Some drugs interact with other drugs, or interact with food or drinks the patient is taking. One drug can make another drug inactive or overactive. The outcome of a drug interaction can range from a minor inconvenience to death. Pharmacists must be vigilant about detecting and preventing these interactions. Here is an example of a drug-drug interaction:

A 47-year-old man was prescribed chlordiazepoxide and haloperidol as part of a supervised alcohol detoxification program. He also received 650 milligrams of acetaminophen twice a day for two days. On the third day the patient experienced disorientation, hallucinations, low blood pressure, jaundice, and a tender liver. He progressively worsened and died on his 28th day in the hospital. His physician suspected a drug interaction between the acetaminophen and alcohol.

Medication Errors

Medication errors rarely occur when considering the millions of prescriptions and doses of medication patients receive yearly. The incidence is a fraction of a percent. However, errors are not acceptable if it happens to you or someone you love. Therefore, the public has zero tolerance for medication errors. That means pharmacists and pharmacy technicians have to be accurate all the time; there is no room for errors. Here is an example of a medication error:

Mike McClave mixed two spoonfuls of prescription medicine he picked up at a pharmacy for his 8-year-old daughter with some clear soda and gave it to her to relieve a raspy, sore throat. The next morning his daughter never woke up. She had received oral morphine, rather than an anesthetic for her sore throat.

Pharmacists have built-in check-and-balance systems—a safety net—for detecting medication errors before they harm patients. However, medication errors occasionally occur within the drug use process. These errors are usually the result of a medication system failure rather than the failure of one person.

Medication Use in the United States

Some surveys have reported that more than half (51%) of American adults were taking two or more medications each day. In addition, almost half of Americans (45%) were taking at least one prescription medication each day, and more than a quarter (28%) were taking multiple prescription medications daily.

The rates of prescription medication use are highest among older Americans. Seventy-nine percent of those ages 65 or older reported taking one prescription medication each day, compared with respondents ages 55 to 64 (63%), ages 45 to 54 (52%), and ages 44 years or younger (28%). Americans ages 65 or older who take prescription medications take an average of four each day.

Among respondents who reported the use of a prescription medication within the past week, the majority (61%) indicated the medication was for a long-term health condition. Twenty-four percent said they were treating a recurring health problem, whereas 10% were treating a short-term, acute health condition.

alternative medicine herbal supplements, megavitamins, and other nontraditional remedies

Besides increased over-the-counter sales in the United States, the use of **alternative medicine** (herbal supplements, megavitamins, and other nontraditional remedies) is increasing dramatically. Overall, 4 out of 10 Americans are trying alternative health treatments. In the ASHP survey, more than one-third (39%) of respondents reported taking an average of four herbal supplements and vitamins in the past week. Forty percent reported taking an average of two herbal supplements or vitamins each day.

Along with more medications being taken, the location where patients are buying their medication is shifting. Although every community pharmacy is filling more prescriptions, the two fastest growing pharmacies are mail-order and grocery store pharmacies, and the slowest growing are independent community pharmacies. In fact, there is some concern that the independent corner drugstore may not be able to survive much longer.

Self-Care and the Role of Over-the-Counter Medication

Pharmacists and pharmacy technicians must understand illness and their patients' reactions to it. Seldom do people go to a physician when they get sick, at least not right away. Most people see how they are feeling and how the illness progresses. Some deny they are ill. Some seek the advice of family or friends. Still others take control and seek out as much information as they can about their problem.

Self-Care

People should be encouraged to take a more active role in their health care. Documentation of increased interest in self-care is witnessed by the many self-help books, TV programs, newspaper articles, the Internet, and talk shows covering health topics. Determining what spawned this self-care revolution is difficult. However, one reason is obvious: consumers are increasingly self-medicating with nonprescription drugs. The Nonprescription Drug Manufacturers Association has surveyed many consumers to learn about their attitudes regarding this practice:

- Almost 7 out of 10 consumers prefer to fight symptoms without taking medication, if possible.
- Among consumers, 85% believe it is important to have access to nonprescription medication.
- About 9 out of 10 consumers realize they should take medication only when necessary.
- Of consumers who ended the use of their nonprescription medication, 90% did so because their medical problems or symptoms resolved.
- Even though a medication may be available without a prescription, almost 95% of consumers agreed that care should be taken when using it.
- Nearly 93% of consumers report that they read instructions before taking a nonprescription medication for the first time.

Over-the-Counter Medication

Some ill patients, and those who experience a health problem, may visit a pharmacy to browse the over-the-counter (OTC) medication aisle for a cure. Many will try reading the labels of various OTC medications to see if the medication will cure what ails them. Pharmacy technicians should watch for this and alert the pharmacist when they see a patient in the OTC area who needs help.

Self-medication is accepted in the United States, and OTC medications are found everywhere—drugstores, convenience stores, supermarkets, and mass merchandisers. If not for this acceptance, we would need many more physicians and health care facilities. A recent survey on patient satisfaction with pharmacy services found that patients' highest awareness of OTCs was for cold cures, vitamins, and dental products, and that satisfaction was high with these products.

Control of the Medication Management Process

The medication management process is extensive and complex. It is also designed with many checks and balances to keep patients from experiencing a preventable drug misadventure. At the center of this control are the pharmacist and pharmacy technician. Although pharmacists have accepted this responsibility and are up to the task, they cannot do it alone. They need the help of pharmacy technicians, other health professionals, and patients who take responsibility for their own health.

Pharmacy technicians are used extensively in the medication management process (drug purchasing, receiving, storage, inventory control, record keeping, and preparation). Although pharmacy technicians are involved extensively in the quick-turnaround world of processing prescriptions and drug orders, they need to think about what they are doing and not make being fast a priority over safety. Finding anything out of the ordinary is cause for concern; that concern should be explored by taking a "safety time-out" to determine if something is wrong. This also holds true when working alongside pharmacists, all of whom occasionally make errors. It is the technician's job to discreetly but forcefully point out that the pharmacist may be making an error. Patient safety should be everyone's number one concern.

Current Issues in the Medication Management Process

Issues that will have a direct impact on the medication management process encompass the "aging of America" and the respective current and projected increase in the numbers of prescriptions that will be generated, along with the continual development and availability of new pharmaceuticals. This, along with the current shortage of pharmacists, will directly affect pharmacists' activities and expand the role of technicians in their collaborative efforts to meet the demands of providing safe and effective drug therapy to their patients.

The Rising Number of Prescriptions and Limited Number of Pharmacists

Due to increased demand and better drugs, the number of prescriptions filled each year is rising at an unprecedented rate. The large "baby boom" generation has started to reach age 65, and these individuals need more medication as they get older. At the same time, the pharmacy profession is being stretched. A shortage of pharmacists has occurred because of their expanded roles and the increased use of medication. This issue is more critical in rural areas, where fewer pharmacies cover larger geographic areas.

The profession's response has been to start more schools of pharmacy. However, from all accounts, this may not be enough. To meet the demands and to preserve or expand the pharmacist's clinical role, the pharmacy profession will need to better use pharmacy technicians, reorganize pharmacies to be more efficient, and increase the use of pharmacy automation and information technology.

Pharmacy Automation

Pharmacy departments are slowly moving toward maximizing the automation available for charting, packaging, labeling, and dispensing medications. The newest technology includes robot dispensing, bar code–enabled medication administration, and electronic prescribing. The cost of equipment in the initial implementation phase is high, and the skills needed must be learned. This is an area where pharmacy technicians can excel. The pharmacist's time can be better utilized in patient care if the technicians can ensure an efficient drug distribution system.

Medication Therapy Management (MTM)

medication therapy management (MTM) a distinct service or group of services that optimize therapeutic outcomes for individual patients; these services are independent of, but can occur in conjunction with, the provision of a medication product

The term **medication therapy management (MTM)** was introduced with the Medicare Prescription Drug, Improvement, and Modernization Act. In 2004, 11 national pharmacy organizations agreed that MTM is defined as "a distinct service or group of services that optimize therapeutic outcomes for individual patients," and that MTM services "are independent of, but can occur in conjunction with, the provision of a medication product." MTM is being provided in various pharmacy settings, such as hospitals, community pharmacies, special pharmacies, and health plans. Since its introduction by the Medicare Part D program, it has been expanded to many employer groups, state Medicaid programs, and others. The role of pharmacists and pharmacy technicians has expanded during the past decade because of the MTM.

Future of Pharmacy Practice

Pharmacy Practice Model Initiative (PPMI)

The ASHP and the ASHP Research and Education Foundation is supporting the hospital and health system Pharmacy Practice Model Initiative (PPMI). The goal of this initiative is to advance meaningfully the health and well-being of patients by developing and disseminating a futuristic practice model that upholds the most effective use of pharmacists as direct patient care providers.

The PPMI has the following objectives:

- Creation of a framework for a pharmacy practice model that ensures provision of safe, effective, efficient, accountable, and evidence-based care for all hospital/health system patients
- Determination of patient care–related services that should be consistently provided by departments of pharmacy in hospitals and health systems and increased demand for pharmacy services by patients/caregivers, health care professionals, health care executives, and payers
- Identification of the available technologies to support implementation of the practice model and identification of emerging technologies that could impact the practice model
- Support for the optimal utilization and deployment of hospital and health system pharmacy resources through development of a template for a practice model that is operational, practical, and measurable
- Identification of specific actions pharmacy leaders and staff should take to implement practice model change including determination of

the necessary staff (pharmacy leaders, pharmacists, and technicians) skills and competencies required to implement this model
- Provision of more advanced and easily accessed training programs for all pharmacy personnel to support the implementation of this model.

Pharmacogenomics

Extensive research is currently being done in the area of *pharmacogenomics*, which is formed by the merging of the words *pharmacology* and *genomics*. Pharmacogenomics is the study of how our genes affect the way our bodies respond to medicines. In the future, drugs may be tailored to our genetic makeup. Instead of the trial-and-error process of trying a new drug for a few weeks to see if it works or if it is tolerated, a drug that works with your body will be identified by using your unique genetic markers.

Health Economic Outcome Research

Medication costs are an important part of overall increasing health care costs in the United States. The high costs of the new specialty medications have made economic outcome research very popular. Researchers are not only looking for drugs that work, but also for drugs that make the most economic sense to use.

Summary

The medication management process is complex and involves the manufacture, distribution, prescribing, preparation, storing, dispensing, administering, monitoring, and review of drugs and their use. The process is controlled, and at the center of this control are various checks and balances, regulations, and pharmacists and pharmacy technicians. Even with control, the system is not perfect and thus needs constant attention and improvement.

Note: Content contained in this chapter has been adapted with permission from Kelly, W. (2011). *Pharmacy: What it is and how it works* (3rd ed.). Boca Raton, FL: Taylor & Francis Group.

TEST YOUR KNOWLEDGE

Multiple Choice

1. The societal purpose of pharmacy practice is to
  a. dispense medication.
  b. provide drug information.
  c. help people make the best use of their medication.
  d. prepare drugs.

2. The drug use process can be described as
   a. what happens when people abuse drugs.
   b. the methods used to prepare drugs.
   c. the steps involved in getting drugs to their final destination.
   d. how drugs are managed.

3. What is drug use control?
   a. Any method used to reduce the improper use of a drug
   b. Federal drug enforcement regulations
   c. A method to accurately measure who uses drugs
   d. FDA manufacturing rules

4. Why is control needed in the drug use process?
   a. To protect patients from harm
   b. To satisfy FDA requirements
   c. To keep drugs from being illegally diverted
   d. a and c

5. Which of the following is *not* a drug use control method?
   a. formulary
   b. laws, rules, and regulations
   c. policies and procedures
   d. all of the above

6. Which of the following is *not* considered a medication misadventure?
   a. errors
   b. adverse reactions
   c. side effects
   d. drug interactions

7. What primary duty do pharmacists perform for society?
   a. Prepare medication for patients.
   b. Help patients use their medication safely.
   c. Supply drugs.
   d. Price prescriptions accurately.

8. Pharmacy technicians will legally perform their duties as long as they
   a. check everything they do in the pharmacy.
   b. read all labels at least three times before dispensing the drug.
   c. have all labels and products checked by the pharmacist.
   d. are certified.

9. A major change transforming pharmacy into a true clinical profession is
   a. the use of automation.
   b. the use of more pharmacy technicians.
   c. pharmaceutical care.
   d. all of the above.

10. How will the changes in Question 9 affect pharmacy technicians?
   a. They will be more involved in running automation.
   b. They will be doing higher level functions.
   c. They may need more education.
   d. All of the above.

Matching

Match the function in drug use control with the party responsible for that function. Answers may be used more than once; some questions may have more than one correct answer.

1. ______________ Manufacture the drug.
2. ______________ Distribute the drug to the wholesaler.
3. ______________ Distribute the drug to the pharmacy.
4. ______________ Prescribe the drug.
5. ______________ Prepare the drug.
6. ______________ Dispense the drug.
7. ______________ Counsel the patient.
8. ______________ Administer the drug.
9. ______________ Monitor the patient.

a. wholesaler
b. patient or family
c. physician
d. pharmacy technician
e. pharmaceutical company
f. pharmacist

Fill in the Blank

1. Drug ______________ develop and produce pharmaceutical products.
2. Drug ______________ deliver medication, medical appliances, and other products to pharmacies.
3. An approved list of medications that may be dispensed ______________.
4. A sterile work area with positive-pressure airflow that filters the air is called a ______________.
5. An unwanted, serious side effect of a drug is a/an ______________.

Suggested Readings

American Pharmaceutical Association (2000). *Handbook of non-prescription drugs.* Washington, DC: Author.

American Society of Health-System Pharmacists (n.d.). Statement on pharmaceutical care. In *Medication therapy and patient care: Organization and delivery of services—Statements* (pp. 243–245). Bethesda, MD: Author.

American Society of Health-System Pharmacists. (2000, December). *Snapshot of medication use in the US.* Retrieved from http://www.ashp.org/s_ashp/docs/files/PR_snapshot.pdf

American Society of Health-System Pharmacists Continuity of Care Task Force (2005). Continuity of care in medication management: Review of issues and considerations for pharmacy. *American Journal of Health-System Pharmacy, 62,* 1714–1720.

Avorn, J. (2004). *Powerful medicines: The benefits, risks, and costs of prescription drugs*. New York, NY: Alfred A. Knopf.

Brodie, D.C. (1967). Drug-use control: Keystone to pharmaceutical service. *Drug Intelligence, 1,* 63–65.

Council on Credentialing in Pharmacy. (2010). Scope of contemporary pharmacy practice: Roles, responsibilities, and functions of pharmacists and pharmacy technicians. *Journal of the American Pharmacists Association, 50,* e35–e69.

Dolder, C., Lacro, J., Dolder, N., & Gregory, P. (2003). Pharmacists' use of and attitudes and beliefs about alternative medications. *American Journal of Health-System Pharmacy, 60*, 1352–1357.

Healthcare Distribution Management Association. (2005). *Healthcare product distribution: A primer.* Retrieved from http://www.healthcaredistribution.org

Japsen, B. (2001, January 26). Saying yes to free drug samples raises concern. *Atlanta Journal.*

Kelly, W.N. (1999). Drug use control: The foundation of pharmaceutical care. *Pharmacy practice for technicians* (2nd ed.). Albany, NY: Delmar.

Kelly, W.N. (2006). *Prescribed medication and the public health: Laying the foundation for risk reduction*. Binghamton, NY: Haworth Press.

Martin, E.W. (1971). The prescription. In *Dispensing of medication* (7th ed.). Easton, PA: Mack Publishing.

McQueen, C.E., Shields, K.M., & Generali, J.A. (2003). Motivations for dietary supplement use. *American Journal of Health-System Pharmacy, 60*, 655.

National Council on Patient Information and Education. (1995). *Prescription medicine compliance: A review of the baseline of knowledge*. Bethesda, MD: Author.

National Council on Patient Information and Education. (2002). *Attitudes and beliefs about the use of over-the-counter medicines: A dose of reality*. Bethesda, MD: Author.

Nonprescription Drug Manufacturers Association. (1992). *Self-medication in the '90s: Practices and perceptions*. Washington, DC: Author.

Salek, M.S., & Sclar, D.A. (1992). *Medication compliance: The pharmacist's pivotal role*. Kalamazoo, MI: Upjohn.

Shrank, W.H., Choudhry, N.K., Fischer, M.A., Avorn, J., Powell, M., Schneeweiss, S., . . . Brookhart, M.A. (2010). The epidemiology of prescriptions abandoned at the pharmacy. *Annals of Internal Medicine, 153*, 633–640.

Task Force for Compliance. (1994, April). *Noncompliance with medications*. Baltimore, MD: Author.

Vermeulen, L.C., Rough, S.S., Thielke, T.S., Shane, R.R., Ivey, M.F., Woodward, B. W., . . . Zilz, D. A. (2007). Strategic approach for improving the medication use process in health systems: The high-performance pharmacy practice framework. *American Journal of Health-System Pharmacy, 64*(16), 1699–1710.

Wertheimer, A. I., & Santella, T. M. (2003). Medication compliance research: Still so far to go. *Journal of Applied Research in Clinical and Experimental Therapeutics, 3*(3), 254–261.

Websites

AARP www.aarp.org

American Society of Health-System Pharmacists, Pharmacy Practice Model Initiative www.ashpmedia.org/ppmi

Centers for Medicare and Medicaid Services, *Exploratory Research on Medication Therapy Management* www.cms.gov/Reports/Downloads/Blackwell.pdf

Health Care Distribution Management Association www.healthcaredistribution.org

National Council on Patient Information and Education www.talkaboutrx.org

World Health Organization, The International Pharmacopoeia http://apps.who.int/phint/en/p/docf/

CHAPTER

10

Ethical Considerations for the Pharmacy Technician

Competencies

Upon completion of this chapter, the reader should be able to:

1. Discuss four concepts presented in the *Code of Ethics for Pharmacy Technicians.*
2. List three ethical principles available to resolve an ethical dilemma.
3. Provide three examples of ethical dilemmas that can occur in pharmacy practice.

Key Terms

autonomy
beneficence
code of ethics
ethical code
ethical dilemma
ethics
fidelity
informed consent
Oath of a Pharmacist
patient confidentiality

Introduction

This chapter focuses on ethical challenges faced by practitioners, pharmacists, and pharmacy technicians in the changing health care environment and with the pharmaceutical care practice model. It describes the nature and importance of ethical codes of behavior, provides guidance on how to approach an ethical dilemma, and presents six ethical principles that may be applied to these dilemmas. Pharmacy technicians are reminded of the responsibilities and risks imposed on them both by state governments and the pharmacists they assist. Practical considerations are raised in the areas of drug distribution and patient communication, and the tools provided should assist pharmacy technicians in making sound ethical evaluations. The key is remembering that final ethical choices about drug therapy remain with the pharmacist.

Codes of Professional Behavior

ethical code a set of standards and responsibilities among members a group that governs interactions with other organizations, patients, colleagues, and society

autonomy the ability to act independently

Self-discipline and self-regulation are essential ingredients of professional behavior. **Ethical codes** set standards and responsibilities among members of a group and govern interactions with other organizations, patients, colleagues, and society. Codes declare the collective conscience of a group and the norms of professional behavior they value. They usually focus on dealing honestly with patients, suppliers, and competitors, respecting individual **autonomy**, recognizing the right to make informed decisions, keeping confidentiality, and promoting just and effective use of resources. The first medical code was the Hippocratic Oath, dating to the fifth century B.C.

World War II and its unethical excesses encouraged the World Medical Association (WMA) to adopt the Geneva Convention of Medical Ethics, followed by the Nuremberg Code, suggesting guidelines for human experimentation and the need for voluntary consent of a patient. Later, the WMA adopted the Declaration of Helsinki, which emphasizes the importance of informed consent and full disclosure to the patient.

Health care professional groups and organizations accept the need to declare to the public the values they consider important and by which they wish to be judged. Albert Jonsen, author of *Clinical Ethics*, believes that professionalism should focus on honesty, integrity, respect for patients, a commitment to patients' welfare, a compassionate regard for patients, and dedication to maintaining competency in knowledge and technical skills.

code of ethics a set of standards and beliefs maintained by a specific group of people

Professional organizations recognize that codes of ethics make clear the primary goals and values of the group, and individuals who join make a moral commitment to uphold the values and duties expressed by the organization. Codes may also focus on inspirational ideals, serve as a statement of organizational principles, and provide rules that govern behavior. When these codes are created and ratified by the membership of a professional organization or profession, they have more societal impact than if they are imposed by the leadership of the organization with little or no member input or acceptance.

The Pharmacist's Code of Ethics

The pharmacist's **code of ethics** has evolved over many generations and reflects behavioral guidelines for pharmacy practice today. Its principles are designed to guide pharmacists in their relationships with patients, health professionals, and

American Pharmaceutical Association
Code of Ethics for Pharmacists (1994)

Preamble. Pharmacists are health professionals who assist individuals in making the best use of medications. This Code, prepared and supported by pharmacists, is intended to state publicly the principles that form the fundamental basis of the roles and responsibilities of pharmacists. These principles, based on moral obligations and virtues, are established to guide pharmacists in relationships with patients, health professionals, and society.

I. A pharmacist respects the covenantal relationship between the patient and pharmacist.

Considering the patient-pharmacist relationship as a covenant means that a pharmacist has moral obligations in response to the gift of trust received from society. In return for this gift, a pharmacist promises to help individuals achieve optimum benefit from their medications, to be committed to their welfare, and to maintain their trust.

II. A pharmacist promotes the good of every patient in a caring, compassionate, and confidential manner.

A pharmacist places concern for the well-being of the patient at the center of professional practice. In doing so, a pharmacist considers needs stated by the patient as well as those defined by health science. A pharmacist is dedicated to protecting the dignity of the patient. With a caring attitude and a compassionate spirit, a pharmacist focuses on serving the patient in a private and confidential manner.

III. A pharmacist respects the autonomy and dignity of each patient.

A pharmacist promotes the right of self-determination and recognizes individual self-worth by encouraging patients to participate in decisions about their health. A pharmacist communicates with patients in terms that are understandable. In all cases, a pharmacist respects personal and cultural differences among patients.

IV. A pharmacist acts with honesty and integrity in professional relationships.

A pharmacist has a duty to tell the truth and to act with conviction of conscience. A pharmacist avoids discriminatory practices, behavior or work conditions that impair professional judgment, and actions that compromise dedication to the best interests of patients.

V. A pharmacist maintains professional competence.

A pharmacist has a duty to maintain knowledge and abilities as new medications, devices, and technologies become available and as health information advances.

VI. A pharmacist respects the values and abilities of colleagues and other health professionals.

When appropriate, a pharmacist asks for the consultation of colleagues or other health professionals or refers the patient. A pharmacist acknowledges that colleagues and other health professionals may differ in the beliefs and values they apply to the care of the patient.

VII. A pharmacist serves individual, community, and societal needs.

The primary obligation of a pharmacist is to individual patients. However, the obligations of a pharmacist may at times extend beyond the individual to the community and society. In these situations, the pharmacist recognizes the responsibilities that accompany these obligations and acts accordingly.

VIII. A pharmacist seeks justice in the distribution of health resources.

When health resources are allocated, a pharmacist is fair and equitable, balancing the needs of patients and society.

Source: American Pharmaceutical Association website (www.pharmacist.com)

FIGURE 10-1 The APhA's *Code of Ethics for Pharmacists*, adopted by the membership of the American Pharmacists Association, then the American Pharmaceutical Association, on October 27, 1994.

OATH OF A PHARMACIST

The revised Oath was adopted by the AACP House of Delegates in July 2007 and has been approved by the American Pharmacists Association. AACP member institutions should plan to use the revised Oath of a Pharmacist during the 2008-09 academic year and with spring 2009 graduates.

"I promise to devote myself to a lifetime of service to others through the profession of pharmacy. In fulfilling this vow:

- I will consider the welfare of humanity and relief of suffering my primary concerns.
- I will apply my knowledge, experience, and skills to the best of my ability to assure ptimal outcomes for my patients.
- I will respect and protect all personal and health information entrusted to me.
- I will accept the lifelong obligation to improve my professional knowledge and competence.
- I will hold myself and my colleagues to the highest principles of our profession's moral, ethical and legal conduct.
- I will embrace and advocate changes that improve patient care.
- I will utilize my knowledge, skills, experiences, and values to prepare the next generation of pharmacists.

I take these vows voluntarily with the full realization of the responsibility with which I am entrusted by the public."

FIGURE 10-2 The AACP's *Oath of a Pharmacist.*

society. The principles include helping patients achieve ideal benefit from medications while maintaining their trust; being caring, compassionate, and discreet; respecting a patient's autonomy and dignity; acting with honesty and integrity; maintaining professional competence; respecting the beliefs and values of colleagues; and allocating health resources in a fair and just manner. A copy of the American Pharmacists Association (APhA) *Code of Ethics for Pharmacists* is shown in **Figure 10-1**. The American Association of Colleges of Pharmacy (AACP) created the ***Oath of a Pharmacist*** (**Figure 10-2**). This oath is taken voluntarily when pharmacists graduate from pharmacy school and declares values that parallel those expressed in the APhA code of ethics.

Oath of a Pharmacist pledge taken by graduating pharmacists to uphold a particular standard of practice

The Code of Ethics for Pharmacy Technicians

The *Code of Ethics for Pharmacy Technicians* was drafted by the American Association of Pharmacy Technicians (AAPT) in 1996 to deal with the particular duties and responsibilities of technicians. A copy of the latest version is shown in **Figure 10-3**. The code has relevance for technicians who are members of the organization, but also has a persuasive impact on all pharmacy technicians, regardless of professional affiliation or work environment. The principles expressed in the technician's code include helping pharmacists provide the best care for patients based on the moral guidelines expressed in the pharmacist's code; supporting honesty and integrity; maintaining competence, knowledge, and expertise; respecting patient confidentiality; avoiding activities that bring discredit to the profession; and meeting standards required by law.

Those pharmacy technicians not separately licensed, registered, or certified serve as agents of a pharmacist and, therefore, are bound by the principles of the APhA's *Code of Ethics for Pharmacists* (see Figure 10-1) because their professional activities derive from the pharmacist's responsibilities.

The American Association of Pharmacy Technicians
www.pharmacytechnician.com
Code of Ethics for Pharmacy Technicians

Preamble

Pharmacy Technicians are healthcare professionals who assist pharmacists in providing the best possible care for patients. The principles of this code, which apply to pharmacy technicians working in any and all settings, are based on the application and support of the moral obligations that guide the pharmacy profession in relationships with patients, healthcare professionals and society.

Principles

- A pharmacy technician's first consideration is to ensure the health and safety of the patient, and to use knowledge and skills to the best of his/her ability in serving patients.
- A pharmacy technician supports and promotes honesty and integrity in the profession, which includes a duty to observe the law, maintain the highest moral and ethical conduct at all times and uphold the ethical principles of the profession.
- A pharmacy technician assists and supports the pharmacists in the safe and efficacious and cost effective distribution of health services and healthcare resources.
- A pharmacy technician respects and values the abilities of pharmacists, colleagues and other healthcare professionals.
- A pharmacy technician maintains competency in his/her practice and continually enhances his/her professional knowledge and expertise.
- A pharmacy technician respects and supports the patient's individuality, dignity, and confidentiality.
- A pharmacy technician respects the confidentiality of a patient's records and discloses pertinent information only with proper authorization.
- A pharmacy technician never assists in dispensing, promoting or distribution of medication or medical devices that are not of good quality or do not meet the standards required by law.
- A pharmacy technician does not engage in any activity that will discredit the profession, and will express, without fear or favor, illegal or unethical conduct of the profession.
- A pharmacy technician associates with and engages in the support of organizations, which promote the profession of pharmacy through the utilization and enhancement of pharmacy technicians.

FIGURE 10-3 The AAPT's *Code of Ethics for Pharmacy Technicians.*

Ethical Reasoning

Organizations and professional associations cannot carry out their policies as a group, but instead rely on individual members to carry out the standards they have adopted. Identifying an ethical question or facing an ethical dilemma is done by an individual, and the actions taken are primarily based on individual moral assumptions or beliefs.

ethics the study of precepts or principles used to assist us in making the correct choice when faced with alternative possibilities in a moral situation

ethical dilemma a difficult moral problem involving two or more mutually exclusive and morally equal courses of action

Ethics is the study of precepts or principles used to assist us in making the correct choice when faced with alternative possibilities for action in a moral situation. Practitioners are encouraged to do right, as if all issues are clearly delineated, focusing on right versus wrong, or good versus evil. Many situations, however, rarely have such clear-cut answers. In reality, we encounter ethical dilemmas and are challenged to come up with acceptable responses. An **ethical dilemma** is a difficult moral problem involving two or more mutually exclusive and morally equal courses of action. We are often asked to choose between the better of two imperfectly acceptable alternatives, or the lesser of two objectionable ones.

The methods we use to determine the correctness of our actions are imprecise and, when placed within a health care setting, have a complexity and impact beyond our personal concerns. How, then, do you handle conflict, make the choices you must, and live with the consequences—as health care practitioners and as individuals? Amy Haddad and her fellow authors say "we utilize ethical judgment skills and apply ethical principles based on our personal and professional value system and the needs of our society and the patient." It is hoped we will be able to recognize when a dilemma exists, define the elements of the dilemma, develop alternative solutions, act on the proper solution, and evaluate the outcome.

Ethical Principles

Ethicists do not agree on the number of ethical virtues and distinct ethical principles used to solve ethical dilemmas. A consensus recognizes the following six ethical virtues: beneficence, truth telling, fidelity, respect, justice, and friendliness.

Beneficence

beneficence the practice of doing good; a kindly action

Beneficence is considered the essential medical virtue: personal caring (compassion) and openness to a real relationship, no matter what the person looks like, their values, their diseases, or their actions. It involves carrying out medical acts according to the highest ethical standard. It requires that we act in a positive way in our dealings with others—that we strive to always do "good." We always believe the patient until proven otherwise.

Truth Telling

Clear communication is the lifeblood of excellent pharmacy/patient relationships. Talking is the verbal expression of benevolence (willingness to help). It is the foundational element of character. As medical personnel, we have a duty to tell the truth in our dealings with others. However, are we bound to do this in every situation, or are there circumstances when it is in no one's best interest to "tell the truth, the whole truth, and nothing but the truth"? The caveat is this: when we speak, we always speak in truth, but not necessarily all the truth, if justified.

Fidelity

fidelity remaining true to a promise; promise keeping

Another word for **fidelity** is faithfulness. All moral people have an obligation to keep the promises they make. However, sometimes even with the best of intentions, we may make promises we are unable to fulfill because circumstances change or the ability to comply is no longer within our control. Fidelity also involves keeping patient confidentiality.

Does promise keeping require us to blindly continue with a promise, no matter what the cost to ourselves or others? The answer is no. The right of confidentiality is not an absolute right. A breach is justified when it is necessary to protect others or when it is in the patient's best interests. So, if a patient is impaired, but is driving an automobile, it is morally right to disclose the impairment to those who are at risk of harm from the patient. If a patient is misusing or abusing a drug, it is morally right to tell family members that a problem exists and how to manage it.

These breaches of confidentiality are never done without first confronting the patient and urging them to take action on his or her own that would remove the need to disclose. Also, the disclosure is always done by providing the least amount of information necessary to protect the patient or others.

Respect

Besides being cognitive, patients are autonomous beings. Therefore, patients have the right to decide for themselves what will be done with their body. People also have the right to live their lives as they see fit within the law. However, autonomy is limited where the rights of one person come in conflict with the rights of another. How do you draw this line?

Pharmacists and technicians need to have a trained attitude to reverence and restraint in witnessing free acts by which patients carry out what they feel is in their best interest. But, how do we do what is in the best interest of the patient, yet respect a patient who chooses to do otherwise? The most common way is to provide options and the ramifications of each option, and let each patient decide his or her course of action.

Justice

The ethical virtue of justice recognizes the belief that all people should receive what is due. At the heart of this virtue is that each person should have convenient access to care. However, it does not guarantee good health—only that we will do everything within our means to help patients achieve that. This ethical virtue is a close companion of respect. A sense of justice leads to the belief that the benefits conferred on one individual should be available to all. However, justice does not mean equal. It does not require that all people be treated exactly alike all the time, but is does mean being treated fairly. As you can see, justice must be tempered with intelligence.

Friendliness

Meeting patients promotes feelings. This happens between pharmacists and patients, and it happens between pharmacy technicians and patients. The key disposition that promotes the right effect is love. This is the deepest foundation of the pharmacy profession. Love of the profession and our healing mission should overcome any initial negative feelings toward a patient. If the love is great, the fruits derived will be great. You know you are on the right track if you feel the patient's vulnerability. A simple exercise is to think of the person you love the most—your mother, father, spouse, child, or grandparent. Now pretend this is the patient you are serving. If you do, you will do your best, you will go the extra mile, and you will fulfill this medical virtue.

Recognizing the presence of competing ethical virtues in a challenging moral situation does not resolve the ethical dilemma. You must decide what medical virtue is dominant in your value system, or what will do the most good—or the least harm—and act accordingly. You have a moral imperative to follow your conscience, regardless of the consequences.

Some Ethical Dilemmas in Pharmacy

Here are some examples of ethical dilemmas that could happen in pharmacy practice:

- A woman calls requesting identification of a small white tablet found in her roommate's jacket pocket Confidentiality should not be breached in this ethical dilemma.
- A man calls requesting verification of the information his physician has given him on the possible adverse effects of beta-blocker therapy. This information is not complete for his situation and you feel the caller should have more information.
- A woman calls and requests information on a diet patch allegedly "approved for weight loss" that she purchased over the Internet. She gives you the product name and ingredients and asks if you agree that these patches are good for weight loss. The patch is not FDA approved.

- A 22-year-old woman calls requesting guidance because she has been taking a drug known to you to be highly teratogenic when taken during the first trimester of pregnancy. She now realizes she is 2 months pregnant. She asks if the drug will harm her baby and says she is thinking about an abortion.
- A woman calls requesting information on drugs that could be taken to interfere with the results of a polygraph test.
- A man calls before his pre-employment physical examination asking how long marijuana is detectable in the urine.

What are the competing ethical virtues in each of these examples?

Ethical Decision Making

When an ethical issue arises in a practice setting, try to understand all the implications of your actions before you act. Following these simple steps may help lessen negative impacts that arise from the decisions you make:

- Look at the ethical issue in the broadest context. Who is involved? Who will it affect? What are the options?
- Decide if you are faced with an ethical question or if you are dealing with an ethical dilemma.
- If you are facing a dilemma, determine the alternative responses you may choose to resolve the situation.
- Look at the risks involved for each response for patients, yourself, your organization or employer, your profession, and society.
- Assess the benefits derived to each group for each alternative.
- Identify the ethical principles present in the situation; see if any are in conflict and determine which principle is most important.
- Make your behavioral decision based on knowledge and evidence, not emotion.
- Afterward, evaluate the effects of your actions and determine if you would select the same choice.
- Realize there will always be unintended consequences to your actions. Just because you make the "right" decision does not mean you will not have to deal with personal, professional, or legal fallout.

Situations that may be a source of ethical conflict for pharmacists and pharmacy technicians fall into two general categories: those related to the drug distribution system, and those involving communication with patients, their families, and other health professionals. How would you handle the situations below?

Some Ethical Dilemmas in Drug Distribution

- What would you do when you feel a prescription presented by a patient seems inappropriate and perhaps harmful, based on the information you possess? Would you be less concerned if the prescription, while inappropriate, was neither harmful nor beneficial?
- How would you handle a patient who asks for a few pills to tide her over until she gets a new prescription? Does it matter how long the patient has been your customer or that the drug involved is habit forming? What about the law?

- Would you dispense a controlled medication to a patient you suspect has a substance abuse problem?
- When is it necessary to confront or report a colleague you believe is diverting drugs?
- If you were approached by a medical retailer to take part in a patient "switch" to their generic drug in return for financial compensation, how would you respond?
- Should you do something if a prescribed drug is not approved for use with a patient's disease?
- Is it important to make sure patient information gathered in the dispensing function is made available to others only on a "need-to-know" basis?
- If you are asked to prepare a medication that contradicts your personal beliefs, ethically or religiously, would you refuse? Are you allowed to refuse?

Some Ethical Dilemmas in Pharmacy Communication

Communication scenarios can also present ethical challenges. Patient involvement and consent to treatment are two of the most basic principles of modern health care. The patient should know what medications he or she is taking, what the side effects may be, what the prognosis is, and what alternative treatments or medications are available.

informed consent giving permission for a specific treatment or action to take place

patient confidentiality the need for all personal information related to patient care to remain between the patient and the health care provider

Everyone agrees patients must provide health professionals with "informed consent." The characteristics of **informed consent** include shared decision making between the patient and his or her provider, based on mutual respect and good communication. Effective communication requires adequate disclosure about an intervention, its risks, and its benefits. Ethical questions arise about how much information is enough, how much is too much, where to draw the line, and who should be making these determinations.

Respecting patients' privacy and maintaining **patient confidentiality** are other ethical minefields for pharmacists and pharmacy technicians. Patients must be able to trust their health care providers so that they will be comfortable continuing treatment. This is true when patients are vulnerable because of their age (e.g., the elderly, a minor child) or their disease (e.g., AIDS, mental illness, sexually transmitted infection). Intentional or unintentional disclosure of information may have a negative impact on patients, their employment status, their finances, or their personal relationships. However, health professionals also have responsibilities to protect the society they serve. How do you distinguish between these competing health needs? Does your answer differ based on the nature of the patient's disease? Can you contemplate a set of circumstances in which you would feel it necessary to keep health information on a child secret from a parent, or information on a husband from a wife?

Other Ethical Dilemmas in Pharmacy

Some ethical dilemmas cross both categories:

- If a prescriber asks you to incorrectly label a prescription because he or she does not want the patient to know the nature of the medication, or that the patient is receiving a placebo, how would you respond?

- When a patient asks what a drug is used for, would you assume the prescriber has not communicated with the patient on the medication and tell the patient everything you know without contacting the prescriber?
- What is your responsibility to your patients and your profession when it becomes clear a colleague is no longer functioning well or acting competently? Would you tell someone? Would you report your colleague anonymously?
- If a medication mistake was made with a patient and you discovered it after the patient had left, how far would you go to rectify the situation? Would you admit the mistake up front and, if so, to whom would you admit the mistake?

We are sure you can easily supply more examples of practice situations where ethical questions are raised and ethical dilemmas faced. You will notice that we did not supply the answers. That is your job. You have been provided some suggestions on the principles to consider and the ways to approach an ethical dilemma. At the end of the day, your value system will determine your response.

Risk/Benefit Response

Any decision brings with it the risk of being judged wrong and having to face the consequences of your actions. Accepting responsibility for your decisions is central to acting professionally. Do not be surprised or caught off guard by one of the examples we have raised. Assess your value system and ask yourself what you would do before being faced with the situation. Be prepared, but always rely on a pharmacist for help.

The extent to which a pharmacy technician may directly experience these situations is dependent on the scope of practice recognized in the state in which the technician is certified to work and the relationship the technician has with the pharmacist he or she assists. If you have made ethical mistakes in the past, you should make time to reflect on what you did and why you did it so you do not repeat the behavior.

As pharmacists become more and more involved in providing pharmaceutical care to patients in all practice settings and as the need for medications continues to expand, the role of pharmacy technicians will expand and the nature of the ethical dilemmas they face will change. Be ready to meet the challenge.

Summary

The changing nature of the health care environment and emerging pharmaceutical care challenges all pharmacy technicians and pharmacists to face each ethical dilemma with diligence based on the principles presented here. This chapter has provided the information and the tools to help you with this important area of pharmacy practice. The two codes of ethics and six ethical virtues present a starting point for your quest to seek solutions to these dilemmas, to minimize risk to your patients and yourself, and to provide the public the benefits of pharmaceutical care.

TEST YOUR KNOWLEDGE

Multiple Choice

1. The earliest known example of an ethical code in medicine was
   a. the Nuremberg Code.
   b. the Hippocratic Oath.
   c. the Declaration of Helsinki.
   d. the Geneva Convention of Medical Ethics.

2. The *Code of Ethics for Pharmacy Technicians* has direct application to the activities of
   a. all pharmacy assistants.
   b. all pharmacy technicians.
   c. all pharmacists.
   d. members of the American Association of Pharmacy Technicians.

3. Which of the following statements is false?
   a. Ethical principles help us make choices between moral alternatives.
   b. Ethical dilemmas always present clear-cut choices between right and wrong.
   c. Our ethical choices sometimes force us to select the lesser of two evils.
   d. Personal and professional values have a place in the ethical decision-making process.

4. The principle of beneficence means you
   a. can do harm.
   b. should do "good."
   c. should treat everyone equally.
   d. should let people do what they want.

5. The ethical decision-making process
   a. can be a complex, time-consuming activity.
   b. takes no time or thought.
   c. never has unintended consequences.
   d. is free of risk.

6. Ethical conflicts in the drug distribution system may include
   a. intentional disclosure of patient information in violation of patient confidentiality.
   b. dispensing of a controlled substance to a patient drug abuser.
   c. not getting "informed consent."
   d. releasing patient information under a public health initiative.

7. Ethical conflicts in the patient communication area may include
   a. finding a colleague who may be diverting drugs.
   b. being asked to prepare a medication whose use conflicts with your religious beliefs.
   c. being asked by a husband about his wife's medication and its purpose.
   d. being asked by a patient to supply a few pills to tide him over.

8. Facing ethical dilemmas will
   a. bring about the same result in every person.
   b. always make you pleased with the results of your decisions.
   c. never subject you to professional or legal consequences.
   d. always be a personal and professional challenge.

Matching

Match the ethical virtue with its description.

1.	__________ honesty	a. Do good.
2.	__________ truth telling	b. All people receive the same benefit.
3.	__________ nonmaleficence	c. Be truthful in dealing with others.
4.	__________ beneficence	d. Do no harm.
5.	__________ respect	e. Do what you say you are going to do.
6.	__________ justice	f. Have the right to do what you see fit.

Fill in the Blanks

1. Self-discipline and self-regulation are essential components of __________.

2. __________ is the study of precepts or principles used to assist us in making the correct choice when faced with alternative possibilities for action in a moral situation.

3. The two primary sources of ethical conflict in the pharmacy setting are __________ and __________.

Suggested Readings

American Society of Health-System Pharmacists. (2003). White paper on pharmacy technicians 2002: Needed changes can no longer wait. *American Journal of Health-System Pharmacy, 60*, 37–51.

Haddad, A.M., Kaatz, B., McCart, G., McCarthy, R.L., Pink, L.A., & Richardson, J. (1993). Report of the Ethics Course Content Committee: Curricular guidelines for pharmacy education. *American Journal of Pharmacy Education, 57*, 34S–43S.

Hepler, C.D., & Strand, L.M. (1990). Opportunities and responsibilities in pharmaceutical care. *American Journal of Health-System Pharmacy, 47*, 533–543.

Jonsen, A.R. (2006). *Clinical ethics*. New York, NY: McGraw-Hill.

National Association of Boards of Pharmacy. (2001). Status of pharmacy technicians. In *Survey of Pharmacy Law*. Park Ridge, IL: Author.

Strandberg, K. (2007). *Essentials of law and ethics for pharmacy technicians*. Boca Raton, FL: CRC Press.

Websites

American Association of Pharmacy Technicians www.pharmacytechnician.com

American Pharmacists Association www.aphanet.org

American Society of Health-System Pharmacists www.ashp.org

CHAPTER

11

Organizations in Pharmacy

Competencies

Upon completion of this chapter, the reader should be able to:

1. Describe the two major issues that have brought about the formation of national pharmacy associations.
2. Identify the major groups in pharmacy that have specialized associations.
3. Explain the historical aspects and identify the first college of pharmacy founded in the United States.
4. Discuss the early problems associated with the issue of drug quality in this country.
5. Match the acronyms to the full names of the various pharmacy associations.

Key Terms

Academy of Managed Care Pharmacy (AMCP)
Accreditation Council for Pharmacy Education (ACPE)
American Association of Colleges of Pharmacy (AACP)
American Association of Pharmacy Technicians (AAPT)
American College of Apothecaries (ACA)
American College of Clinical Pharmacy (ACCP)
American Pharmacists Association (APhA)
American Society of Consultant Pharmacists (ASCP)
American Society of Health-System Pharmacists (ASHP)
National Association of Boards of Pharmacy (NABP)
National Association of Chain Drug Stores (NACDS)
National Community Pharmacists Association (NCPA)
National Pharmacy Technicians Association (NPTA)
Pharmacy Technician Certification Board (PTCB)
Pharmacy Technician Educators Council (PTEC)
reciprocity

Introduction

One of the characteristics of a profession is the organization of the membership into professional associations. Associations act through the collective voice of the members to set standards of practice and conduct for the profession. If the quantity rather than the quality of associations were an indicator of professionalism, pharmacy would certainly be near the top of the list. One of pharmacy's strengths—its diversity of practice environments and opportunities—is also one of its weaknesses. Each group of practitioners formed national associations (and numerous state and local associations) to further their professional objectives. Independent owner pharmacists, hospital pharmacists, long-term care pharmacists, academic pharmacists, and many other groups have formed into associations, each with its own distinctive name and acronym. Selected pharmacy and pharmacy technician organizations and their website are listed at the end of this chapter.

The goal of this chapter is to familiarize the reader with pharmacy associations and the important role they play in the United States. The professional journals that function as the voice of the various associations are also discussed.

Historical Development

Two major issues caused the formation of the first local and national pharmacy associations in the United States: the development of educational standards for practice and the quality of drugs available to the pharmacist for use in preparing prescriptions.

The first issue—education—has continued to be a primary concern of all pharmacy associations, since it affects both current and future practitioners. The formation of the Philadelphia College of Pharmacy in 1821, the first formal educational program in pharmacy, was one result of the organization of the first professional association of pharmacy. Additionally, the Philadelphia College of Pharmacy inspected drugs for quality and acted to arbitrate disputes between members of the college. Following the lead of Philadelphia pharmacists, other associations or colleges of pharmacy were formed in Boston, New York, Baltimore, Cincinnati, and St. Louis. Formal educational programs were not provided in the early years by these other "colleges," but eventually each evolved into a true college of pharmacy, providing a regular curriculum leading to education of pharmacy practitioners.

The issue of drug quality was an important concern to the early practitioners of pharmacy and medicine in the United States, because the drugs available to the physicians and pharmacists of the nineteenth and early twentieth centuries were mostly of natural origin. These animal and vegetable preparations were often imported into the United States. There was no U.S. pharmaceutical industry. The pharmacist would utilize these crude drugs to prepare the medications prescribed by the physician. Because these animal and vegetable products were so costly, it was not uncommon for drug merchants to adulterate (dilute) the desired material with worthless plant or animal by-products. The early pharmacy associations provided inspection committees to examine these imported materials. They also lobbied vigorously for governmental inspection at the major ports of entry. It was not until 1906, with the passage of the Food and Drug Act, that the federal government became involved with ensuring drug quality and purity.

Drug production and drug quality are still major concerns of pharmacy professional associations because of the many sources of drug products now available. The Food and Drug Administration's (FDA's) Medical Products Reporting Program, MedWatch, provides a mechanism for health professionals to report drug-product quality problems to the FDA and, conversely, for the FDA to provide regular feedback to the health care community about safety issues involving medical products. The MedWatch program is supported by over 140 organizations, including all major organizations in pharmacy.

Organizations or associations are a way of life for Americans. The American Society of Association Executives represents more than 10,000 association members serving more than 287 million persons and companies.

Although pharmacy has many organizations, some are of greater importance to the pharmacy technician than others. These include the American Society of Health-Systems Pharmacists (ASHP), formed in 1942, which now has 35,000 members. Housed in its new quarters in suburban Washington, D.C., it has an annual budget of $28 million.

The American Pharmacists Association (APhA) is 150 years old and today has a membership of more than 60,000. APhA provides continuing education programs for pharmacists and technicians and has been the birthplace for many pharmacy associations.

The training and recognition of pharmacy technicians in the United States has been a slowly evolving process that began in the mid-1960s. Although over the years U.S. pharmacists have engaged assistants to carry out ancillary tasks to expedite the preparation and dispensing of medication, European pharmacies have a history of long-established and recognized pharmacy technician education programs.

The first textbook specific to pharmacy technician education was published by Mosby Publishers in 1968 and authored by Durgin and Hanan. Formal technician training programs were established in that same era by Mercy Medical Center in Long Island, New York, and by the Rhode Island Hospital in that state. Throughout the country, formal and informal programs began to emerge to better train technicians who were already on the job. In 1979 the American Association of Pharmacy Technicians (AAPT) was formed. In 1983 the ASHP accredited the first pharmacy technician training program at Thomas Jefferson Hospital in Philadelphia.

National Associations of Pharmacists and Pharmacy Technicians

> **American Pharmacists Association (APhA)** founded in 1852, this is the largest association in pharmacy with more than 60,000 members; formerly known as the American Pharmaceutical Association

The first national association of U.S. pharmacists was the American Pharmaceutical Association, which is now known as the **American Pharmacists Association (APhA)**. APhA represents more than 60,000 practicing pharmacists, pharmaceutical scientists, students pharmacists, pharmacy technicians, and others interested in advancing the pharmacy profession. Formed in Philadelphia in 1852, APhA has grown into the largest of the national associations in pharmacy.

The original objectives of the APhA, written over 100 years ago, addressed the major concerns of the profession then and surprisingly the major concerns now.

They are improvement and regulation of drug supply and quality, inter- and intraprofessional relations, improvement of the scientific knowledge base of the profession and dissemination of that new knowledge through publication, educational standards for practice of the profession, restriction of drug-dispensing functions, and creation of ethical standards of practice. APhA supports voluntary certification of technicians by the pharmacy profession, but opposes licensure, registration, or certification by state law or regulation.

In addition to being the first national professional pharmacy association, APhA is also considered to be the "parent" of many other pharmacy associations. The American Society of Health-System Pharmacists, the National Community Pharmacists Association, the American College of Apothecaries, the American Association of Colleges of Pharmacy, and the American Association of Pharmaceutical Scientists were all initiated by special interest groups that were originally a part of APhA.

APhA is organized into three academies: the Academy of Pharmacy Practice and Management (APPM), the Academy of Pharmaceutical Research (APRS), and the Academy of Student of Pharmacy (ASP). APhA also has a research foundation and a political action committee (PAC). APhA cofounded the Pharmacy Technician Certification Board (PTCB) in 1995 with ASHP, the Illinois Council of Health-System Pharmacists, and the Michigan Pharmacists Association. The PTCB office is located within the APhA association building. PTCB offers certification and recertification exams several times each year. Information on the certification exam process and contents is available on the PTCB website, www.ptcb.org.

APhA was also responsible for the formation of the Board of Pharmaceutical Specialties in 1976 with the following responsibilities: recognize specialties in pharmacy practice, set standards for certification and recertification, objectively evaluate individuals seeking certification and recertification, and serve as a source of information and coordinating agency for pharmacy specialties.

American Society of Health-System Pharmacists (ASHP) a national organization established in 1942; its current membership of 35,000 includes pharmacists in various institutional health care settings and contains a section for pharmacy technicians

National Community Pharmacists Association (NCPA) formed in 1898 to represent the interests of independent pharmacy owners; formerly the National Association of Retail Druggists

The **American Society of Health-System Pharmacists (ASHP)** is a 35,000-member professional association that represents pharmacists who practice in hospitals and other components of the health care system. ASHP currently focuses its programs and resources on a set of 10 practice domains: acute care, ambulatory care, clinical specialists, home care, long-term care, chronic care, managed care, new practitioners, pharmacy practice management, and technicians. ASHP was founded at the 1942 meeting of APhA, and from its founding until 1972, membership in the parent organization (APhA) was required for membership in ASHP.

ASHP has been a vigorous proponent of the role of the pharmacist as the drug-use control expert in organized health care settings. ASHP has taken strong positions regarding education of pharmacists and technicians and has established accrediting standards for pharmacy residencies designed for pharmacy graduates and accreditation of pharmacy technician training programs.

Education has been a hallmark for all organizations in pharmacy, but APhA and ASHP have been exceptionally strong in that area. APhA now provides a framework for specialty certification of pharmacists. Their annual meeting is well organized and of benefit to pharmacists and technicians as well as to the industry.

ASHP holds two large meetings annually. The annual meeting, like the APhA meeting, provides general education. The midyear clinical meeting provides a forum for pharmacists and technicians, but also has special educational programming for clinical specialists.

The **National Community Pharmacists Association (NCPA)**, formerly the National Association of Retail Druggists, developed from the parent APhA's

American Society of Consultant Pharmacists (ASCP) an organization of pharmacists who provide drug therapy management services in long-term care

Academy of Managed Care Pharmacy (AMCP) a professional association of pharmacists and associates who serve patients in the managed health care system environment

American College of Clinical Pharmacy (ACCP) organization with a membership that consists primarily of PharmD clinical practitioners and faculty members of colleges of pharmacy; its mission is to transmit the application of new knowledge in the science of pharmacotherapy

American College of Apothecaries (ACA) a small, selective association of community-based practitioners whose membership is granted only if the pharmacy and practitioners comply with specified pharmacy professional standards

American Association of Pharmacy Technicians (AAPT) professional organization that provides leadership and education to pharmacy technicians; recognizes pharmacy technicians as part of the health care team

National Pharmacy Technicians Association (NPTA) professional organization dedicated to advancing the role of pharmacy technicians in pharmaceutical care by providing education, advocacy, technological support, and leadership training; has practice sites in the community, hospital, home care, long-term care, nuclear sites, military sites, and prison facilities

Section on Commercial Interests as an independent organization in 1898. NCPA has strongly represented the interests of the independent pharmacy owner since its inception and has championed the independent practice alternative to students of pharmacy. In 1991 NCPA created the National Home Infusion Association. A special focus of NCPA has been the training and certification of pharmacists in various areas of "pharmacist care" through the National Institute for Pharmacist Care Outcomes. NCPA also supports a management institute that provides information, training, and resources to improve pharmacy management. NCPA has a reputation for being a vigorous defender of the independent owner's rights on Capitol Hill. NCPA lobbied for over a decade for legislation to make armed robbery a federal offense. The NCPA PAC was also the first in pharmacy and uses the slogan "Get into politics or get out of pharmacy."

The **American Society of Consultant Pharmacists (ASCP)** is an international organization that represents consultant and senior care pharmacists by providing leadership, advocacy, and education to advance the practice of senior care pharmacy. Consultant and senior care pharmacy manages drug therapy management services and medication distribution to older adults and others with chronic illness. ASCP provides health care practitioners with a particular interest in the geriatric patient with education and resources to improve their practice skills.

The **Academy of Managed Care Pharmacy (AMCP)**, representing more than 6,000 members, is a national professional association of pharmacists and other health care practitioners who serve society by using sound medication management principles and strategies to improve health care for all in the managed health care system environment. The goals of AMCP, ASHP, and APhA often overlap, and multiple memberships in these associations are not uncommon.

The **American College of Clinical Pharmacy (ACCP)** is a professional and scientific society that provides leadership, education, advocacy, and resources that enable clinical pharmacists to achieve excellence in practice and research. ACCP's membership includes practitioners, scientists, educators, administrators, students, residents, fellows, and others committed to excellence in clinical pharmacy and patient pharmacotherapy.

The **American College of Apothecaries (ACA)** represents selective associations of community-based practitioners. The mission of ACA is the translation and dissemination of knowledge and recent developments in professional pharmacy practice to benefit pharmacists, pharmacy students, and the public. Membership is granted only if the practitioners and their pharmacy comply with certain standards of professional service and appearance.

In addition to APhA and ASHP, there are two professional associations expressly for pharmacy technicians, the American Association of Pharmacy Technicians and the National Pharmacy Technician Association. Both associations hold annual meetings during the summer months and provide their members with access to educational services.

The **American Association of Pharmacy Technicians (AAPT)** provides leadership and education to pharmacy technicians. It also recognizes pharmacy technicians as part of the health care team. AAPT membership is open to pharmacy technicians and is an active participant in making decisions which affect changes at all levels of our profession. The **National Pharmacy Technicians Association (NPTA)** is dedicated to advancing the role of pharmacy technicians in pharmaceutical care by providing education, advocacy, technological support, and leadership training.

Pharmacy Technician Certification Board (PTCB) established in 1995 to provide a voluntary mechanism for a national certification program for pharmacy technicians

Pharmacy Technician Educators Council (PTEC) an organization with the mission of assisting the profession of pharmacy to prepare high-quality, well-trained technical personnel through education and practical training programs

The **Pharmacy Technician Certification Board (PTCB)** was established in January 1995 through the efforts of APhA, ASHP, the Illinois Council of Health-System Pharmacists, and the Michigan Pharmacists Association. It provides a voluntary mechanism for a national certification program. PTCB offers the certification examination several times each year. To be eligible to take the examination, the candidate must have a high school diploma or GED. The cost for the application fee in 2013 was $129. Recertification every 2 years with 20 hours of continuing education (at least one hour must be in pharmacy law) is required.

The **Pharmacy Technician Educators Council (PTEC)** membership includes the faculty members of formal technician training programs, most often associated with community colleges. PTEC's mission is to assist the profession of pharmacy to prepare high-quality, well-trained technical personnel through education and practical training programs.

The Society for the Education of Pharmacy Technicians (SEPhT) provides educational tools and support for employers, pharmacy technicians, and preceptors. Through educational programming, the role of the pharmacy technician is enhanced and promoted via educational advancement and professionalism.

Other Associations

National Association of Chain Drug Stores (NACDS) an association of corporations represented by chief executive officers, many of whom are not pharmacists; includes chain pharmacies, grocery store pharmacies, department store pharmacies, and discount outlets

American Association of Colleges of Pharmacy (AACP) an organization of pharmacy colleges primarily concerned with education issues, such as curricula and teaching methodologies

Many other national associations in pharmacy represent special segments of the profession. These are discussed next with a brief description of their membership and mission.

The **National Association of Chain Drug Stores (NACDS)** is an organization of corporations, generally represented by their chief executive officers, many of whom are not pharmacists, serving the interest of chain drugstores and their suppliers. The title is misleading because NACDS represents a variety of businesses, not just chain or multiple-outlet pharmacies. Grocery chains, department stores, and a variety of discount outlets that have pharmacies belong to NACDS. The strength of this organization lies in its size and large financial capabilities. Chains are the largest employer of practicing pharmacists. Although nonpharmacy merchandising has been a large concern of NACDS, recent consumer trends have suggested that chains pay more attention to the pharmacy department and the employee pharmacist. The Food Marketing Institute (FMI) represents the food retailing business (supermarkets), including 14,000 pharmacies. Supermarket-located pharmacies are the most rapidly growing sector of retail pharmacy and FMI has a division of programs for this segment of the industry.

The **American Association of Colleges of Pharmacy (AACP)** is an organization of pharmacy colleges and schools. Representation of deans and faculty members is accomplished through membership on their respective councils, which have equal representation in their house of delegates. The AACP is primarily concerned with educational issues, such as curricula and teaching methodologies. Because a minimum of 2 years of pre-pharmacy education is required for entry into the 4-year pharmacy degree program, the PharmD degree is referred to as a 6-year degree program. Presently, more than 50% of all students entering the professional degree program have more than 2 years of pre-professional higher education. The AACP adopted a policy regarding supportive personnel (pharmacy technicians), which states that the training of such personnel be based on sound educational principles. The AACP recommends that its member schools offer their assistance for the development of those objectives.

Accreditation Council for Pharmacy Education (ACPE) the accrediting body for colleges of pharmacy by which high educational standards are established and monitored; formerly known as the American Council of Pharmacy Education

National Association of Boards of Pharmacy (NABP) an organization formed in 1904 to assist member boards in developing pharmacy standards to protect the public health

reciprocity a mutual exchange or interchange between two parties

The **Accreditation Council for Pharmacy Education (ACPE)** is the independent, government-recognized accrediting agency of degree and continuing education programs in pharmacy. Formed in 1932 as the American Council of Pharmacy Education, through the efforts of APhA, AACP, and the National Association of Boards of Pharmacy (NABP), the ACPE has, through its representative membership, proposed and published the standards that schools must meet to obtain accreditation. Criteria such as budget, governance, faculty quality and quantity, admission standards, physical facilities, library, curricula, and student achievement are all considered during the accreditation process. Accreditation is voluntary, but inasmuch as all states require graduation from an accredited school of pharmacy as a prerequisite of licensure, an unaccredited program could not survive. Accreditation is also needed to qualify for a variety of state and federal financial aid programs.

The **National Association of Boards of Pharmacy (NABP)** is an organization of the members of the individual state boards of pharmacy, which are generally charged with the licensure of pharmacies and pharmacists and, in many states, with inspection and law enforcement activities. Since its inception in 1904, the NABP has worked to standardize the requirements for pharmacist licensure while maintaining the posture of individual states' rights. Through its efforts, **reciprocity**—transfer of licensure among most states—has been facilitated and a national licensing exam for pharmacists, the North American Pharmacist Licensure Exam (NAPLEX), is used as a major part of all but a few states' licensing examinations. The NABP makes available the NAPLEX, the Multi-State Pharmacy Jurisprudence Exam, and the Foreign Pharmacy Graduate Equivalency Exam to assist state pharmacy boards in their evaluation of candidates for pharmacy licensure.

The NABP, in conjunction with the ACPE, has set up a continuing education tracking system for pharmacists and pharmacy technicians for participation in accredited programs from ACPE-accredited providers. This service (known as CPE Monitor) will provide state boards of pharmacy with a mechanism for verifying and tracking that licensees and registrants meet their continuing education requirements for the state in which they are licensed or registered. Registration with NABP will provide the registrant with a unique identifier. Paper copies of statements of participation will no longer be required and all ACPE records will be stored in one location.

Association Publications

One of the first actions of a professional association is the publication of a journal for the dissemination of scientific and professional information for the membership and the profession. The founders of the Philadelphia College of Pharmacy were responsible for the publication of the first American pharmacy journal, the *Journal of the Philadelphia College of Pharmacy,* in 1825. In 1835 the title was changed to the *American Journal of Pharmacy*, and it has been published continually to this day. Since that initial effort, the many national associations of pharmacy have continued and expanded on this effort, each with its own journal and newsletter (**Table 11-1**). In addition, several associations—most notably APhA and ASHP—have produced publications providing pharmacists and other health professionals with needed drug information, such as the *Handbook of Nonprescription Drugs* and the *American Hospital Formulary Service.* The ASHP also publishes the *International Pharmaceutical Abstracts,* which is a semimonthly abstracting service of the world's pharmaceutical literature.

TABLE 11-1 Organizational Publications

AACP	*American Journal of Pharmaceutical Education*
AAPS	*Pharmaceutical Research; AAPS PharmSciTech*
AMCP	*Journal of American Pharmacists Association; Pharmacy Today*
ASCP	*America's Pharmacist*
ASHP	*American Journal of Health-System Pharmacists*
APhA	*The Consultant Pharmacist*
NCPA	*Journal of Managed Care Pharmacy*
NPTA	*Today's Technician*
PTEC	*Journal of Pharmacy Technology*

Summary

A number of professional pharmacy organizations have been established to meet the specialty needs of their memberships. Organizations represent members practicing in community, chain, hospital, consulting, and clinical pharmacy practice. Colleges of pharmacy, accrediting agencies, state boards of pharmacy, wholesalers, and more comprise additional specialty membership groups in pharmacy practice.

The various organizations in pharmacy serve to link pharmacists who are engaged in the numerous aspects of the profession. As a result, all pharmacists have the opportunity to enter the mainstream of the constantly evolving growth and development of the profession of pharmacy.

TEST YOUR KNOWLEDGE

Multiple Choice

1. An identifying characteristic of a profession is
   a. the organization of the membership into professional associations.
   b. that all members agree on all professional policies regarding education and other important matters.
   c. that all members have the same professional, academic degree.
   d. that financial objectives are of primary importance.

2. The major issue that prompted establishment of the first national association of pharmacists was
   a. the need for educational standards.
   b. a means of expanding profitability.
   c. the quality and purity of drugs.
   d. a and c.
   e. a, b, and c.

True/False

1. An organization represents the special interests of its membership.
2. The American Society of Health-System Pharmacists has taken a strong position regarding education of pharmacists and technicians.
3. The National Community Pharmacists Association (NCPA) represents the interests of independent retail pharmacy owners.

Matching

1.	__________	ASHP	a.	first national association
2.	__________	NCPA	b.	independent community of retail pharmacists
3.	__________	AACP	c.	health system and hospital pharmacists
4.	__________	APhA	d.	pharmacy colleges and schools
5.	__________	PTEC	e.	pharmacy technician educators

Websites

Academy of Managed Care Pharmacy (AMCP) www.amcp.org

Accreditation Council for Pharmacy Education (ACPE) www.acpe-accredit.org

American Association of Colleges of Pharmacy (AACP) www.aacp.org

American Association of Pharmaceutical Scientists (AAPS) www.aapspharmacetuical.com

American Association of Pharmacy Technicians (AAPT) www.pharmacytechnician.com

American College of Apothecaries (ACA) www.acainfo.org

American College of Clinical Pharmacy (ACCP) www.accp.com

American Pharmacists Association (APhA) www.pharmacist.com

American Society of Consultant Pharmacists (ASCP) www.ascp.com

American Society of Health-System Pharmacists (ASHP) www.ashp.org

American Society of Health-System Pharmacists Technician Forum www.pharmtechinfocenter.com

National Association of Boards of Pharmacy (NABP) www.nabp.net

National Association of Chain Drug Stores (NACDS) www.nacds.org

National Community Pharmacists Association (NCPA) www.ncpanet.org

National Pharmacy Technician Association (NPTA) www.pharmacytechnician.org

Pharmacy Technician Certification Board (PTCB) www.ptcb.org

Pharmacy Technician Educators Council (PTEC) www.ptec.org

PART

III

Professional Aspects of Pharmacy Technology

CHAPTER

12

The Prescription

Competencies

Upon completion of this chapter, the reader should be able to:

1. Describe the various parts of a prescription.
2. Identify the required parts of a prescription.
3. Explain various methods for transmitting prescriptions to pharmacies.
4. Compare the methods of transmitting prescriptions or drug order to pharmacies in community settings to that of institutional settings.
5. List roles for the pharmacy technician in handling and interpreting prescriptions.

Key Terms

automatic substitution
computerized prescriber order entry (CPOE)
dispense as written (DAW)
e-prescribing
formulary
medication order
prescriber
prescription
script
therapeutic interchange

Introduction

Pharmacists are an important part of the health care team, which is made up of physicians, nurses, and many other health care professionals. Unlike many of these, the pharmacist often works in a separate location. For a health care team to function, its members must be able to communicate. The prescription is the primary method of communication. While prescriptions have historically been written, they may also be verbal or, with increasing frequency, electronic. Whatever the format, it is essential for the pharmacy technician to understand the prescription.

The Prescription

prescription permission, granted orally or in writing, from a physician for a patient to receive a certain medication on an outpatient basis that will help relieve or eliminate the patient's problem

script an abbreviated form of the term *prescription*

The **prescription**, or **script** as it is also known, instructs a pharmacist to dispense—select, count, place in an appropriate container, and label—a specific drug in a specific dose and dosage form for a specific patient. Although most prescriptions are for prescription drugs (also called legend drugs), prescriptions may also be written for over-the-counter medications. The prescription is written on a prescription blank that is usually preprinted with frequently used information such as the prescriber's name, phone number, address, and Drug Enforcement Administration (DEA) number (the DEA number is only required on prescriptions for controlled substances). The prescription blank will also have prompts for important information such as the patient's name, address, date of birth, number of refills, and the date the prescription was written. New York State has established an official prescription. It is issued by the state and has a number of safeguards built in to reduce the chance of fraudulent use of the prescriptions to obtain medications illegally. Although its use is only required in New York State, it can serve as a fairly typical example of a prescription and is shown in **Figure 12-1**.

Each state specifies the necessary components of a prescription. Typically, the following items are required on every prescription (the numbers identify the corresponding information in Figure 12-1):

1. *Name, address, and date of birth of the patient.* It is obviously important to identify the patient accurately. While the name may be sufficient to identify the patient, the patient's address and date of birth (DOB) may be necessary in some situations such as for patients with common names (Mary Smith) or if two members of a family share the same or very similar names (Mike and Mickey). The DOB is also important because it helps the pharmacist determine the appropriateness of drug choice, dose, and dosage form for younger and older patients. Prescribers frequently omit the address and DOB of the patient. But this information can often be found in the pharmacy records if the patient has filled prescriptions at the pharmacy previously and, hence, may be added by the pharmacist. If the pharmacy technician receives the prescription from the patient, the technician should ask if the patient has had prescriptions filled at the pharmacy in the past. It may be helpful to ask for the patient's address so it can be added to the prescription. While the specific DOB may be necessary for children, if a patient is an adult it is usually sufficient to note that on the prescription. In other words, a specific DOB is not needed to determine

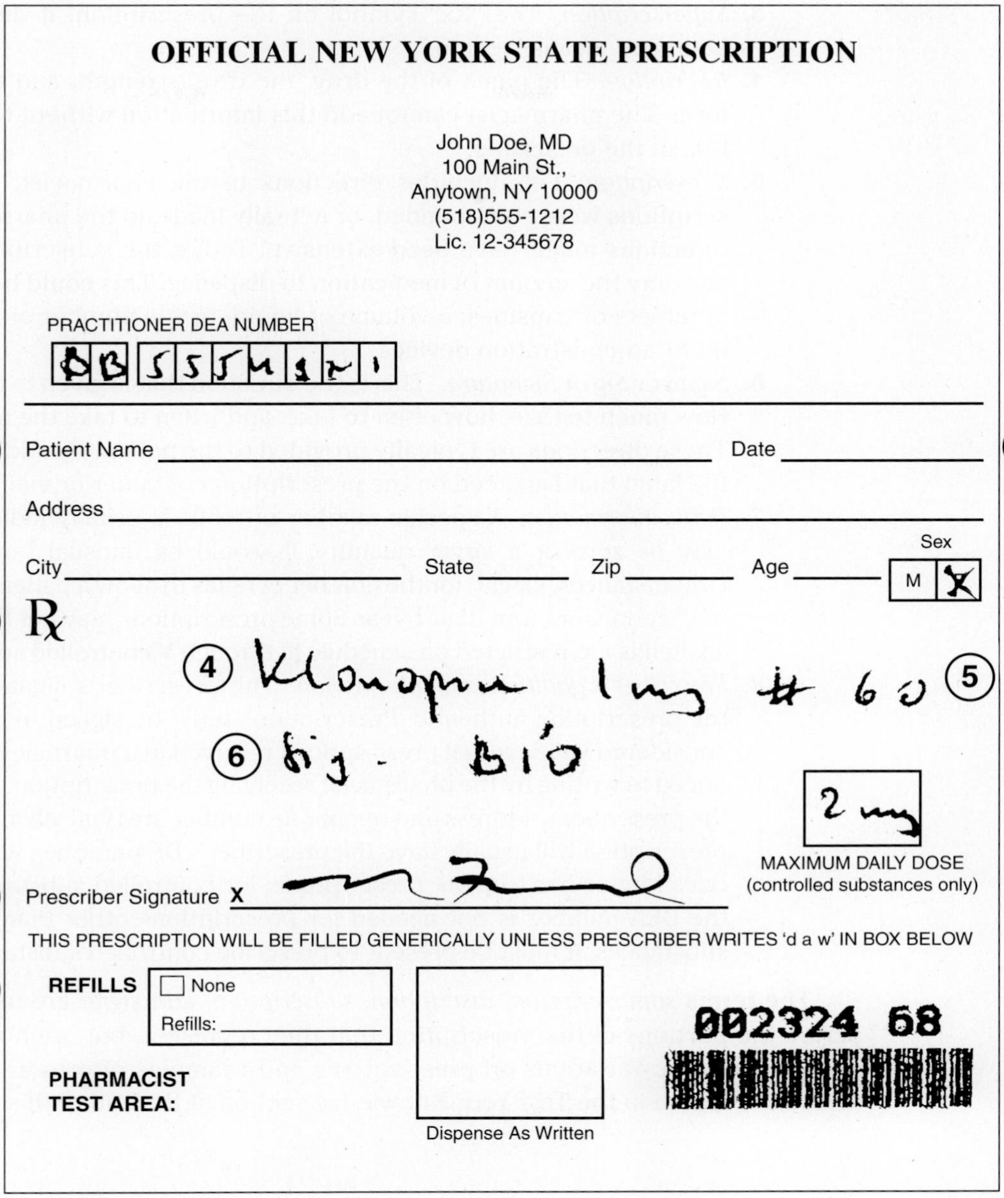
OFFICIAL NEW YORK STATE PRESCRIPTION

John Doe, MD
100 Main St.,
Anytown, NY 10000
(518)555-1212
Lic. 12-345678

PRACTITIONER DEA NUMBER

1 Patient Name ______ Date ______ 2

Address ______

City ______ State ______ Zip ______ Age ______ Sex M F

3 ℞

4 Klonopin 1mg #60 5

6 Sig - BID

2 mg

MAXIMUM DAILY DOSE
(controlled substances only)

8 Prescriber Signature X ______

THIS PRESCRIPTION WILL BE FILLED GENERICALLY UNLESS PRESCRIBER WRITES 'd a w' IN BOX BELOW

7 REFILLS ☐ None
Refills: ______

PHARMACIST
TEST AREA:

Dispense As Written

002324 68

FIGURE 12-1 Prescription.

appropriate doses for an adult. The DOB may still be needed for some adults as a method of identification. Note that the prescriber must have written or provided the patient name. This is not something the pharmacist can add.

2. *Date.* The date that the prescription was written is important. Prescriptions are typically written for a specific purpose, as part of a specific treatment plan and should usually be presented to the pharmacy shortly after the prescription was written. Sometimes, during an annual visit with their physician, patients will receive a prescription for a medication they are currently receiving. These prescriptions may not be filled for a few months as patients wait for their current prescription's refills to be used. The prescriber must have dated the prescription; the pharmacist is not allowed to add the date.

3. *Superscription.* The "Rx" symbol on the prescription. It derives from Latin and means "recipe."
4. *Inscription.* The name of the drug, the drug strength, and the dosage form. The pharmacist cannot add this information without the verification of the prescriber.
5. *Subscription.* This includes directions to the pharmacist. When prescriptions were compounded, or actually made, in the pharmacy, these directions might have been extensive. Today, the subscription is usually only the amount of medication to dispense. This could be a number of tablets or capsules, a volume of liquid, or the number of inhalers or other administration devices.
6. *Signa* or *Sig* or *Signatura.* This is the direction that is given to the patient. How much to take, how often to take, and when to take the medication. These directions are typically provided to the patient by adding them to the label that is placed on the prescription container or vial.
7. *Refill information.* A specific number of refills is usually indicated. This may be zero or a larger quantity. It would be unusual (and in some circumstances, illegal) for the number of refills to allow a patient to receive medication for more than 1 year. Some prescriptions may not be refilled at all. Refills are restricted on schedule III through V controlled substances.
8. *Prescriber signature and information.* The prescriber's signature makes the prescription authentic. Prescriptions must be signed in order to be considered valid. Verbal prescriptions received in a pharmacy may be reduced to writing by the pharmacist receiving the prescription. In addition, the prescriber's address and telephone number are typically present. The prescription will usually have the prescriber's DEA number, which authorizes him or her to write prescriptions for controlled substances. While the DEA number is not needed for prescriptions other than controlled substances, it must be present to prescribe controlled substances.

The terms *superscription*, *inscription*, *subscription*, and *signa* are useful to describe the portions of the prescription that they represent, but are not generally used in practice. Variations on prescriptions and examples of prescriptions with errors are shown in the Test Your Knowledge section at the end of this chapter.

Prescribers

prescriber a licensed person in health care who is permitted by law to order drugs that legally require a prescription; includes physicians, physician assistants, podiatrists, dentists, and nurse practitioners

A licensed **prescriber** is most often a physicians—an MD, doctor of medicine, or DO, doctor of osteopathy—but may also be a dentist, podiatrist, physician's assistant (PA), nurse practitioner, optometrist, or pharmacist. Although each of these nonphysicians may have the right to prescribe, their ability to prescribe is often ethically or legally limited. For example, dentists should only prescribe medications that treat dental concerns; PAs may only prescribe when they have a specific relationship with a physician. Similarly, some states permit pharmacists to prescribe through a process known as collaborative drug therapy management (CDTM), in which the pharmacist has a formal arrangement with specific physicians that allows the pharmacist to prescribe certain drugs for specified conditions under a written agreement between the physician and pharmacist that only applies to that physician's patients. Obviously, the nature of these agreements between nonphysician prescribers and physicians is determined by each state's laws and considerable variation is seen from state to state.

Methods of Receiving a Prescription

When a licensed prescriber determines that a patient requires drug therapy, he or she typically communicates that information to a pharmacist by "writing" a prescription. A written prescription is often given to the patient by the physician, and the patient presents the prescription to the pharmacist. Note, however, that prescriptions may also be given to the pharmacist orally, typically over the telephone. A prescription given orally must convey all of the information listed in the preceding section for a written prescription. The pharmacist is required to immediately transcribe, or write, the oral prescription into written form.

Prescriptions may also be transferred electronically to pharmacies. Perhaps the most common method of doing this is to use a facsimile ("fax") machine, but other methods are continuously being developed. Because of security concerns, e-mail is not considered an acceptable method for transferring prescriptions. However, other technology is available for transmitting prescriptions from prescribers' offices to pharmacies in a safe and secure manner. This is referred to as **e-prescribing**: "a prescriber's ability to electronically send an accurate, error-free and understandable prescription directly to a pharmacy from the point-of-care." The use of this technology is not widespread but it is increasing. Prescription insurance plans that participate in Medicaid will soon be required to use e-prescribing. Other insurance providers may not require e-prescribing, but may offer financial incentives to add that feature.

e-prescribing the ability to digitally send a prescription to the pharmacy

E-prescribing software will include a list of medications available; perform several safety checks, such as for drug interactions and allergies; and allow for prescriptions to be printed as well as electronically transmitted to the patient's pharmacy. Some states may require that printed copies of all electronically transmitted prescriptions be produced and maintained as is done for regular written prescriptions.

Medication Orders

When patients are in institutional settings, such as hospitals or nursing homes, they still require medications, but they obviously do not take prescriptions to the pharmacy to obtain their medications. In these situations, directions to give patients medications are called **medication orders** rather than prescriptions. Medication orders are written on order sheets or may be entered into a computerized physician order entry system. A sample order sheet is shown in **Figure 12-2**. Although prescriptions and medication orders have several differences, some of the more important differences are that multiple drugs may be written on the same medication order and many things other than drugs may be ordered on an order sheet. Thus it is important for the technician to review medication order sheets carefully to identify all of the medications ordered, realizing that all of the drug orders may not be next to one another.

medication order orders for all medications and intravenous solutions; they are written on an order sheet or recorded via computerized physician order entry on a hospital-wide computer system

The requirements for medication orders are usually specified by the hospital or nursing home, but are somewhat similar to those given earlier for prescriptions. Some differences include that a patient is usually identified by medical record number or a room number instead of an address and information about the quantity to dispense and number of refills is not needed. However, in place of listing the quantity to dispense or number of refills, most institutions have automatic stop order policies. These policies specify that medications will be stopped after so many days and must be reordered if they are to be continued. These policies

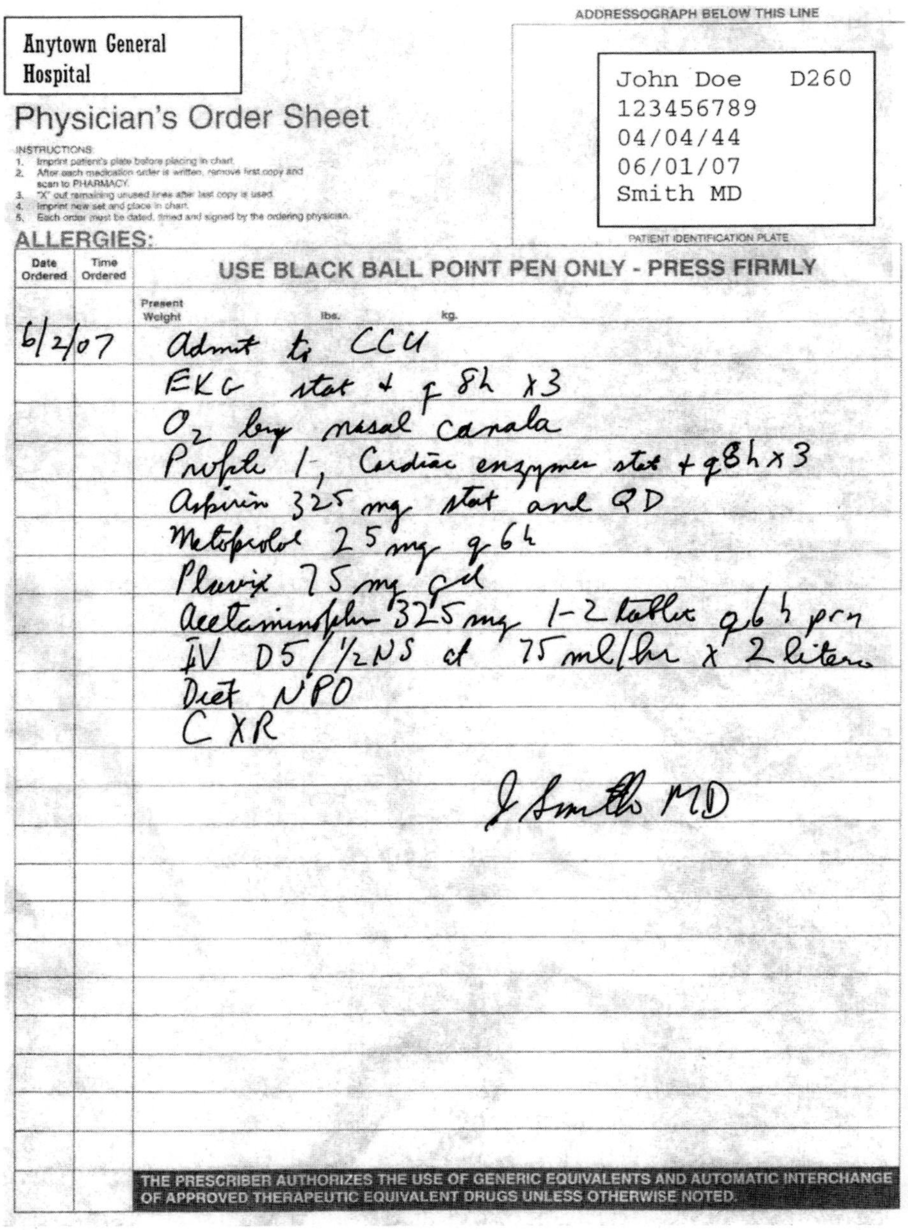
Anytown General Hospital

Physician's Order Sheet

INSTRUCTIONS:
1. Imprint patient's plate before placing in chart.
2. After each medication order is written, remove first copy and scan to PHARMACY.
3. "X" out remaining unused lines after last copy is used.
4. Imprint new set and place in chart.
5. Each order must be dated, timed and signed by the ordering physician.

ALLERGIES:

ADDRESSOGRAPH BELOW THIS LINE

John Doe D260
123456789
04/04/44
06/01/07
Smith MD

PATIENT IDENTIFICATION PLATE

Date Ordered	Time Ordered	USE BLACK BALL POINT PEN ONLY - PRESS FIRMLY
		Present Weight lbs. kg.
6/2/07		Admit to CCU
		EKG stat + q 8h x3
		O_2 by nasal canula
		Profile 1, Cardiac enzymes stat + q8h x3
		Aspirin 325 mg stat and QD
		Metoprolol 25 mg q 6h
		Plavix 75 mg qd
		Acetaminophen 325 mg 1-2 tablets q6h prn
		IV D5/½NS at 75 ml/hr x 2 liters
		Diet NPO
		CXR
		J Smith MD

THE PRESCRIBER AUTHORIZES THE USE OF GENERIC EQUIVALENTS AND AUTOMATIC INTERCHANGE OF APPROVED THERAPEUTIC EQUIVALENT DRUGS UNLESS OTHERWISE NOTED.

FIGURE 12-2 Note the addressograph stamp in the upper right corner of this medication order. These stamps typically contain the patient's name, room number or nursing unit, identification number, date of birth, date of admission, and physician's name. (Opportunities for confusion are obviously present with two names and two dates.) Note also the multiple orders on the sheet, for medications as well as laboratory and other diagnostic tests. The text at the bottom of the order sheet authorizes therapeutic substitutions.

computerized prescriber order entry (CPOE) a drug order entered into a hospital-wide computer system and transmitted to a pharmacy

may also permit prescribers to order therapy for a specific number of days or doses that may exceed the number stated in the stop order policy.

Some institutions have implemented **computerized prescriber order entry (CPOE)**, in which prescribers can directly enter orders, including medications, into an information system. These CPOE systems can perform several safety checks and decrease medication prescribing errors. Depending on the system, a CPOE system may transmit the medication order to the pharmacy electronically.

The pharmacy will then use the electronic information, rather than a paper order, to dispense medication for that patient.

Just a few years ago, such CPOE systems were not in widespread use. Federal legislation has introduced significant incentives to encourage health systems (e.g., hospitals) to implement electronic health records. Included in this legislation are guidelines for incorporating e-prescribing in the institutional setting. This will include CPOE. However, to be compliant with the federal legislation, CPOE systems will need to be enhanced to include the automated review of orders for formulary compliance, drug interactions, allergies, and other concerns. These systems will include an e-prescribing feature as discussed earlier.

formulary a listing of drugs approved by the medical staff for use within an institution as determined by the safety, efficacy, effectiveness, and cost of the drugs

automatic substitution a policy that allows a pharmacist to substitute a formulary drug for the drug ordered without any additional approvals

therapeutic interchange a policy that allows one drug product to be substituted for another that differs in composition but is considered to have the same or very similar pharmacologic and therapeutic activity

dispense as written (DAW) notation on a prescription that means the medication indicated on the prescription may not be substituted with a generic or other brand drug without the authorization of the prescriber

When a prescriber orders medications in an institutional setting, he or she must often consult a **formulary**, or a list of drugs that the institution has in its inventory. For example, a hospital may decide not to have Lipitor (generic name: atorvastatin), a popular cholesterol-lowering drug, in its formulary and instead have the drug Zocor (generic name: simvastatin), a similar cholesterol-lowering drug. If the prescriber fails to check the formulary, many institutions have a policy of **automatic substitution**, which allows the pharmacist to automatically substitute the formulary drug for the drug ordered. When an institution uses CPOE, this formulary check is often done automatically as the order is entered.

In some cases, the ability to order nonformulary drugs is restricted and requires additional, different steps. Committees within the hospital approve such switches and the change is carried out by the pharmacist. This process is called **therapeutic interchange**. If an institution uses therapeutic interchange, a procedure will exist to indicate that the substitution took place. The pharmacy technician should ensure he or she clearly understands this process and realizes that the drugs involved in therapeutic interchange may change in different institutions. In the outpatient setting, brand Name Medically Necessary therapeutic interchange is not routinely used. However, some insurance companies have preferred drugs and will attempt to switch patients to preferred drugs.

The process of therapeutic interchange should not be confused with generic substitution. Generic substitution occurs when a prescription or medication order for one brand name is filled with the same chemical, but one that is sold under either a different brand name or simply by the generic name. In the outpatient or community pharmacy setting, prescriptions may have the notation "**dispense as written**" or "**DAW**" added to prevent generic substitution. In some states, the law may specify that generic drugs must be used unless "DAW" is added to the prescription.

Medication Errors

Historically, the directions to pharmacists were written in Latin, frequently using abbreviations of the Latin instructions and other notations and symbols to indicate quantities. Although the use of these Latin abbreviations and notations persists, the use of many such abbreviations is being strongly discouraged due to the tendency for the abbreviations to be misinterpreted. Misinterpretation occurs because the abbreviations may have two meanings (e.g., MS may mean morphine sulfate or magnesium sulfate) or because the poor handwriting of many prescribers may result in misinterpretation. For example, when written in script, SC, an abbreviation for subcutaneous (an injection given just under the skin) may appear to be SL, an abbreviation for sublingual (under the tongue). A list of frequently misinterpreted abbreviations has been prepared by the Institute for Safe Medication Practices (see **Figure 12-3**). The

Institute for Safe Medication Practices

ISMP's List of *Error-Prone Abbreviations, Symbols,* and *Dose Designations*

The abbreviations, symbols, and dose designations found in this table have been reported to ISMP through the ISMP National Medication Errors Reporting Program (ISMP MERP) as being frequently misinterpreted and involved in harmful medication errors. They should **NEVER** be used when communicating medical information. This includes internal communications, telephone/verbal prescriptions, computer-generated labels, labels for drug storage bins, medication administration records, as well as pharmacy and prescriber computer order entry screens.

Abbreviations	Intended Meaning	Misinterpretation	Correction
µg	Microgram	Mistaken as "mg"	Use "mcg"
AD, AS, AU	Right ear, left ear, each ear	Mistaken as OD, OS, OU (right eye, left eye, each eye)	Use "right ear," "left ear," or "each ear"
OD, OS, OU	Right eye, left eye, each eye	Mistaken as AD, AS, AU (right ear, left ear, each ear)	Use "right eye," "left eye," or "each eye"
BT	Bedtime	Mistaken as "BID" (twice daily)	Use "bedtime"
cc	Cubic centimeters	Mistaken as "u" (units)	Use "mL"
D/C	Discharge or discontinue	Premature discontinuation of medications if D/C (intended to mean "discharge") has been misinterpreted as "discontinued" when followed by a list of discharge medications	Use "discharge" and "discontinue"
IJ	Injection	Mistaken as "IV" or "intrajugular"	Use "injection"
IN	Intranasal	Mistaken as "IM" or "IV"	Use "intranasal" or "NAS"
HS **hs**	Half-strength At bedtime, hours of sleep	Mistaken as bedtime Mistaken as half-strength	Use "half-strength" or "bedtime"
IU**	International unit	Mistaken as IV (intravenous) or 10 (ten)	Use "units"
o.d. or OD	Once daily	Mistaken as "right eye" (OD-oculus dexter), leading to oral liquid medications administered in the eye	Use "daily"
OJ	Orange juice	Mistaken as OD or OS (right or left eye); drugs meant to be diluted in orange juice may be given in the eye	Use "orange juice"
Per os	By mouth, orally	The "os" can be mistaken as "left eye" (OS-oculus sinister)	Use "PO," "by mouth," or "orally"
q.d. or QD**	Every day	Mistaken as q.i.d., especially if the period after the "q" or the tail of the "q" is misunderstood as an "i"	Use "daily"
qhs	Nightly at bedtime	Mistaken as "qhr" or every hour	Use "nightly"
qn	Nightly or at bedtime	Mistaken as "qh" (every hour)	Use "nightly" or "at bedtime"
q.o.d. or QOD**	Every other day	Mistaken as "q.d." (daily) or "q.i.d. (four times daily) if the "o" is poorly written	Use "every other day"
q1d	Daily	Mistaken as q.i.d. (four times daily)	Use "daily"
q6PM, etc.	Every evening at 6 PM	Mistaken as every 6 hours	Use "daily at 6 PM" or "6 PM daily"
SC, SQ, sub q	Subcutaneous	SC mistaken as SL (sublingual); SQ mistaken as "5 every;" the "q" in "sub q" has been mistaken as "every" (e.g., a heparin dose ordered "sub q 2 hours before surgery" misunderstood as every 2 hours before surgery)	Use "subcut" or "subcutaneously"
ss	Sliding scale (insulin) or ½ (apothecary)	Mistaken as "55"	Spell out "sliding scale;" use "one-half" or "½"
SSRI **SSI**	Sliding scale regular insulin Sliding scale insulin	Mistaken as selective-serotonin reuptake inhibitor Mistaken as Strong Solution of Iodine (Lugol's)	Spell out "sliding scale (insulin)"
i/d	One daily	Mistaken as "tid"	Use "1 daily"
TIW or tiw	3 times a week	Mistaken as "3 times a day" or "twice in a week"	Use "3 times weekly"
U or u**	Unit	Mistaken as the number 0 or 4, causing a 10-fold overdose or greater (e.g., 4U seen as "40" or 4u seen as "44"); mistaken as "cc" so dose given in volume instead of units (e.g., 4u seen as 4cc)	Use "unit"
UD	As directed ("ut dictum")	Mistaken as unit dose (e.g., diltiazem 125 mg IV infusion "UD" misinterpreted as meaning to give the entire infusion as a unit [bolus] dose)	Use "as directed"
Dose Designations and Other Information	**Intended Meaning**	**Misinterpretation**	**Correction**
Trailing zero after decimal point (e.g., 1.0 mg)**	1 mg	Mistaken as 10 mg if the decimal point is not seen	Do not use trailing zeros for doses expressed in whole numbers
"Naked" decimal point (e.g., .5 mg)**	0.5 mg	Mistaken as 5 mg if the decimal point is not seen	Use zero before a decimal point when the dose is less than a whole unit
Abbreviations such as mg. or mL. with a period following the abbreviation	mg mL	The period is unnecessary and could be mistaken as the number 1 if written poorly	Use mg, mL, etc. without a terminal period

FIGURE 12-3 Institute for Safe Medication Practices' List of Error-Prone Abbreviations, Symbols, and Dose Designations.

Institute for Safe Medication Practices

ISMP's List of *Error-Prone Abbreviations, Symbols,* and *Dose Designations* (continued)

Dose Designations and Other Information	Intended Meaning	Misinterpretation	Correction
Drug name and dose run together (especially problematic for drug names that end in "l" such as Inderal40 mg; Tegretol300 mg)	Inderal 40 mg Tegretol 300 mg	Mistaken as Inderal 140 mg Mistaken as Tegretol 1300 mg	Place adequate space between the drug name, dose, and unit of measure
Numerical dose and unit of measure run together (e.g., 10mg, 100mL)	10 mg 100 mL	The "m" is sometimes mistaken as a zero or two zeros, risking a 10- to 100-fold overdose	Place adequate space between the dose and unit of measure
Large doses without properly placed commas (e.g., 100000 units; 1000000 units)	100,000 units 1,000,000 units	100000 has been mistaken as 10,000 or 1,000,000; 1000000 has been mistaken as 100,000	Use commas for dosing units at or above 1,000, or use words such as 100 "thousand" or 1 "million" to improve readability
Drug Name Abbreviations	**Intended Meaning**	**Misinterpretation**	**Correction**
To avoid confusion, do not abbreviate drug names when communicating medical information. Examples of drug name abbreviations involved in medication errors include:			
APAP	acetaminophen	Not recognized as acetaminophen	Use complete drug name
ARA A	vidarabine	Mistaken as cytarabine (ARA C)	Use complete drug name
AZT	zidovudine (Retrovir)	Mistaken as azathioprine or aztreonam	Use complete drug name
CPZ	Compazine (prochlorperazine)	Mistaken as chlorpromazine	Use complete drug name
DPT	Demerol-Phenergan-Thorazine	Mistaken as diphtheria-pertussis-tetanus (vaccine)	Use complete drug name
DTO	Diluted tincture of opium, or deodorized tincture of opium (Paregoric)	Mistaken as tincture of opium	Use complete drug name
HCl	hydrochloric acid or hydrochloride	Mistaken as potassium chloride (The "H" is misinterpreted as "K")	Use complete drug name unless expressed as a salt of a drug
HCT	hydrocortisone	Mistaken as hydrochlorothiazide	Use complete drug name
HCTZ	hydrochlorothiazide	Mistaken as hydrocortisone (seen as HCT250 mg)	Use complete drug name
MgSO4**	magnesium sulfate	Mistaken as morphine sulfate	Use complete drug name
MS, MSO4**	morphine sulfate	Mistaken as magnesium sulfate	Use complete drug name
MTX	methotrexate	Mistaken as mitoxantrone	Use complete drug name
PCA	procainamide	Mistaken as patient controlled analgesia	Use complete drug name
PTU	propylthiouracil	Mistaken as mercaptopurine	Use complete drug name
T3	Tylenol with codeine No. 3	Mistaken as liothyronine	Use complete drug name
TAC	triamcinolone	Mistaken as tetracaine, Adrenalin, cocaine	Use complete drug name
TNK	TNKase	Mistaken as "TPA"	Use complete drug name
ZnSO4	zinc sulfate	Mistaken as morphine sulfate	Use complete drug name
Stemmed Drug Names	**Intended Meaning**	**Misinterpretation**	**Correction**
"Nitro" drip	nitroglycerin infusion	Mistaken as sodium nitroprusside infusion	Use complete drug name
"Norflox"	norfloxacin	Mistaken as Norflex	Use complete drug name
"IV Vanc"	intravenous vancomycin	Mistaken as Invanz	Use complete drug name
Symbols	**Intended Meaning**	**Misinterpretation**	**Correction**
ʒ ♍	Dram Minim	Symbol for dram mistaken as "3" Symbol for minim mistaken as "mL"	Use the metric system
x3d	For three days	Mistaken as "3 doses"	Use "for three days"
> and <	Greater than and less than	Mistaken as opposite of intended; mistakenly use incorrect symbol; "< 10" mistaken as "40"	Use "greater than" or "less than"
/ (slash mark)	Separates two doses or indicates "per"	Mistaken as the number 1 (e.g., "25 units/10 units" misread as "25 units and 110" units)	Use "per" rather than a slash mark to separate doses
@	At	Mistaken as "2"	Use "at"
&	And	Mistaken as "2"	Use "and"
+	Plus or and	Mistaken as "4"	Use "and"
°	Hour	Mistaken as a zero (e.g., q2° seen as q 20)	Use "hr," "h," or "hour"

**These abbreviations are included on The Joint Commission's "minimum list" of dangerous abbreviations, acronyms, and symbols that must be included on an organization's "Do Not Use" list, effective January 1, 2004. Visit www.jointcommission.org for more information about this Joint Commission requirement.

ISMP
INSTITUTE FOR SAFE MEDICATION PRACTICES
www.ismp.org

FIGURE 12-3 (Continued)

Joint Commission also publishes a "Do Not Use List"—to print a copy of this list visit www.jointcommission.org. The pharmacy technician should pay particular attention to prescriptions with these abbreviations so that the technician may assist the pharmacist by recalling the potential for misinterpretation. Please see Chapter 30 for a complete review of this topic.

Summary

A prescription is a legal document that communicates the prescriber's medication treatment to the pharmacist. As a legal document, prescriptions are subject to several specific requirements that may vary by state and type of medication. Prescriptions may be written, verbal, faxed, or electronic. In the hospital setting, prescriptions are referred to as medication orders. The pharmacy technician should be able to understand the requirements for each type of prescription and recognize whether they are present in a prescription.

TEST YOUR KNOWLEDGE

Examples of Prescriptions with Errors

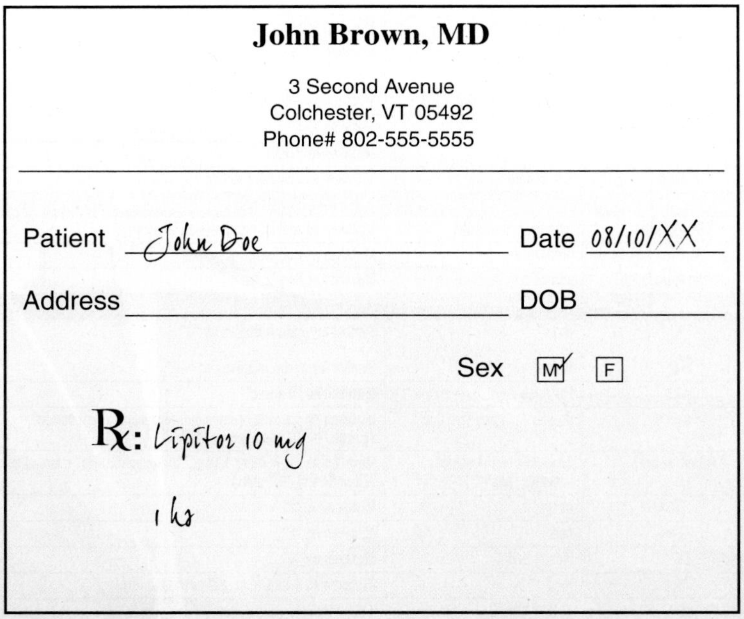

John Brown, MD

3 Second Avenue
Colchester, VT 05492
Phone# 802-555-5555

Patient John Doe Date 08/10/XX

Address ______ DOB ______

Sex [M ✓] [F]

℞: Lipitor 10 mg

1 hs

Prescription 1.

1. What information is missing from this prescription?
2. Are any error-prone abbreviations present?

John Brown, MD

3 Second Avenue
Colchester, VT 05492
Phone# 802-555-5555

Patient John Doe Date

Address DOB

Sex [M ✓] [F]

℞: captopril 25 mg #90

i three times daily

Prescription 2.

1. What information is missing from this prescription?
2. How many days supply of medication is included on this prescription?

John Brown, MD

3 Second Avenue
Colchester, VT 05492
Phone# 802-555-5555

Patient John Doe Date 09/10/12

Address 4 Main St, Milton DOB Adult

Sex [M ✓] [F]

℞: metoprolol 50 mg #180

i twice a day

Prescription 3.

1. What information is missing from this prescription?
2. How many days supply of medication is included on this prescription?

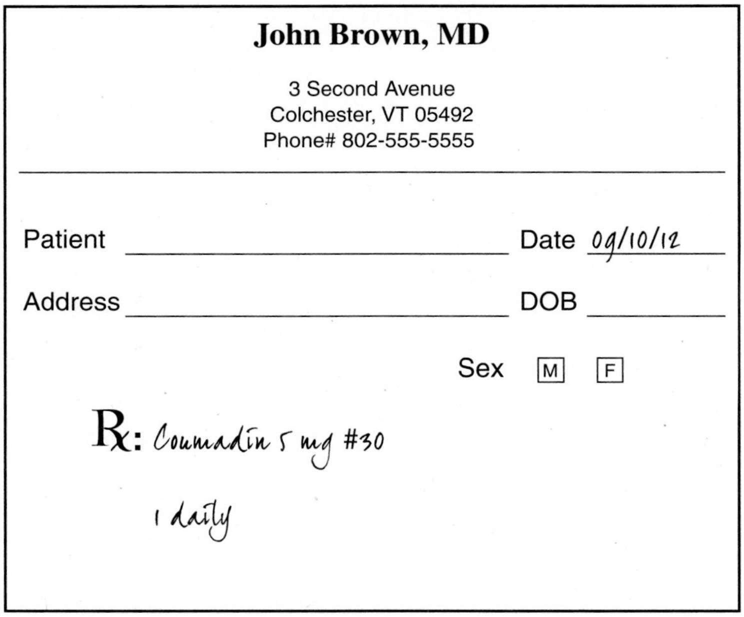

John Brown, MD

3 Second Avenue
Colchester, VT 05492
Phone# 802-555-5555

Patient ____________ Date 09/10/12

Address ____________ DOB ________

Sex [M] [F]

℞: Coumadin 5 mg #30

1 daily

Prescription 4.

1. What information is missing from this prescription?
2. How many days supply of medication is included on this prescription?
3. Could this prescription be filled with a generic drug for Coumadin?

Multiple Choice

1. Which of the following elements cannot be added to a prescription by the pharmacist?
   a. patient name
   b. patient address
   c. patient date of birth
   d. patient allergies
2. Which of the following is not needed to identify the specific patient who will receive a prescription?
   a. patient name
   b. patient address
   c. patient date of birth
   d. indication for drug
3. Which of the following is not an acceptable method of delivering a prescription to a pharmacy?
   a. telephone call from the prescriber
   b. fax from the physician's office
   c. written in an e-mail
   d. delivery of a written prescription by the patient's spouse

4. One difference between a prescription received in a community pharmacy and a medication order received in a hospital pharmacy is
  a. medication orders do not have patient names.
  b. medication orders do not include directions for administration.
  c. medication orders are not required to have patient addresses.
  d. prescriptions will not have lab tests on them.

5. When a pharmacy technician receives a prescription and notices missing information, which of the following should he or she do?
  a. Add the patient's name to the prescription.
  b. Tell the patient that the prescription cannot be filled.
  c. Recommend the patient taken an over-the-counter medication instead.
  d. Bring the missing information to the pharmacist's attention.

Suggested Reading

Centers for Medicare and Medicaid Services. (2013, April 1). *E-prescribing.* Retrieved from http://www.cms.gov/eprescribing

Websites

Institute for Safe Medication Practices www.ismp.org

The Joint Commission www.Joint Commision.org

CHAPTER

13

Medical Terminology and Abbreviations

Competencies

Upon completion of this chapter, the reader should be able to:

1. Identify word element combinations used in medical terminology.
2. Determine the meaning of common medical terms by evaluating the word elements.
3. Define common medical terms related to disease states.
4. Identify common abbreviations and their meanings.
5. Describe the various components of a prescription.

Key Terms

combining form	**root**	**word elements**
prefix	**suffix**	**word root**

Introduction

Understanding the language of medicine or medical terminology is a critical component in the efficient communication with other members of the health care team to facilitate the provision of excellent patient care. The terms used to describe the medical history of a patient will provide you with information about any current transient conditions such as an infection, chronic disease conditions such as hypercholesterolemia, and medical diagnostic or surgical interventions that the patient has undergone such as angiography and angioplasty.

Medical terminology is a growing body of knowledge that has its roots as early as the first-century B.C. and is constantly increasing with the development of new diagnostic methods and the identification of new disease states.

Word Elements

word elements in medical terminology, the parts of a word such as roots, prefixes, and suffixes

root the primary building block of a word; in medical terminology, the core word used to identify fundamental anatomical and physiological nomenclature

combining form a word type that facilitates the attachment of a prefix or suffix; formed when a word root is incorporated into a medical term

prefix a word element attached to the beginning of a word to modify its meaning

suffix a word element attached to the end of a word to create a new word with a specific meaning

Words in the medical vocabulary are constructed with a series of building blocks or **word elements**. The primary building block is the core of the word or the **root**, which identifies the fundamental anatomical or physiological system. The word root is often a Greek or Latin word such as *dermatos* (Greek), meaning "skin," or *renes* (Latin), meaning "kidney."

When the word root is incorporated into the medical term, the word root assumes a **combining form**, which facilitates the attachment of a prefix or suffix. For example, *cardi-/o-* (combining form for the Greek word *kardio*) refers to the heart and is the word root in disease names and diagnostic procedures associated with the heart. The remaining building blocks, the **prefix** (a word element that is not an independent word but is attached to the beginning of a word to modify its meaning) and the **suffix** (a word element that is not an independent word, but is attached to the end of the word to create a new word or grammatical form), are added to the word root to create a word that carries a very specific meaning (see **Figure 13-1**).

For example, the term *electrocardiogram* is composed of the prefix *electro-*, relating to electrical activity; the root *cardio-*, which identifies the organ system as the heart; and the suffix *-gram*, which means a graphical representation. Therefore, *electrocardiogram* means "the graphical representation of the electrical activity in the heart." If the root word changes, as in *electroencephalogram*, the prefix *electro-* and the suffix *-gram* still indicate that the term refers to "a graphic representation of electrical activity," but the organ involved is now the brain because the

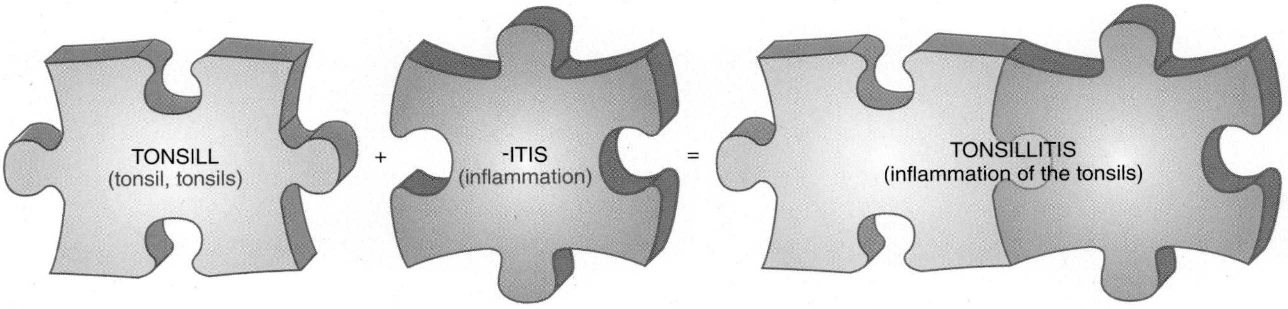

FIGURE 13-1 The word *tonsillitis* is created by adding the suffix *-itis* (the dependent word element added at the end of word) to the root word *tonsil*.

root *encephal-/o-* refers to the brain. Note that a vowel, most commonly an *o*, is inserted to combine the building blocks and make the term easier to pronounce. Root words for some of the major organ structures are presented in **Table 13-1**.

Prefix

The addition of a prefix can modify the root word in many ways. It can indicate time, frequency, the number of parts, or the location/position of body parts or organs, or it can produce a term with the opposite meaning of the root element. For example, the prefix *mono-* means one, whereas the prefix *bi-* means two. Combination of a prefix with the root element *nuclear* (the nucleus of a cell) produces the words *mononuclear* (a cell with one nucleus) or *binuclear* (a cell with two nuclei). Common prefixes that indicate number or measurement such as size are listed in **Table 13-2** and **Table 13-3**.

Prefixes are also used to indicate the position or direction of movement of an organ or body part. The prefix *ab-* means "away from"; for example, *abduction* is a medical term meaning away from the midline. The prefix *pre-* indicates "in front of"

TABLE 13-1 Root Words for Organ Structures

aden-/o-	glands	nas-/o-; rhin-/o-	nose
arteri-/o-	arteries	nephr-/o-	kidneys
arthr-/o-	joints	neur-/o-	nerves
bronch-/o-	bronchial tubes	ocul-/o-	eye
cardi-/o-	heart	oste-/o-	bone
cephal-/o-	head	ot-/o-	ear
cholecyst-/o-	gallbladder	pharyng-/o-	pharynx
col-/o-	colon	pneum-/o-	lungs
cyst-/o-	bladder	pulmon-/o-	lungs
cyt-/o-	cell	splen-/o-	spleen
dermat-/o-	skin	Stomat-/o-	mouth
encephal-/o-	brain	thyr-/o-	thyroid
enter-/o-	intestine	trache-/o-	trachea
esophag-/o-	esophagus	trich-/o-	hair
gastr-/o-	stomach	ur-/o-	urinary
hemat-/o-	blood	uter-/o-	uterus
hepat-/o-	liver	vagin-/o-	vaginal
mamm-/o-	breast	ven-/o-	veins
my-/o-	muscle		

TABLE 13-2 Common Prefixes for Number and Time

mono-	one	re-	again
bi-; di-	two	hemi-	half
tri-	three	multi-; poly-	many
quad-; quadric-; tetra-	four	ante-; pre-	before
nulli-	none	post-	after
pan-	all	neo-	new

TABLE 13-3 Common Prefixes for Measurement

ambi-	both	micro-	small
an-	without	multi-	many
brady-	slow	olig-/o-	few
dipl-/o-	double	pan-	all
hemi-	half	poly-	many
hyper-	above normal; excessive	semi-	partial
hypo-	below normal	super-	above or excess
iso-	equal	tachy-	rapid
macro-	large	ultra-	beyond or excess

TABLE 13-4 Common Prefixes for Position or Direction

a-; ab-	away from	hypo-	under, below
ambi-	both sides	infra-	under, beneath
ante-; antero-	in front of	inter-	among
circum-; peri-	around	intra-	within, inside
de-	down	latero-	side
dextr-/o-	right	medi-; meso-; mid-	middle
di-; per-	through	para-	beside
dorso-	back	postero-	behind
ec-	out, out from	pre-, pro-	in front of
endo-	within, inner	sinistro-	to the left
epi-	upon, over	sub-	below
ex-	out from	super-; supra-	above
exo-	out	sym-; syn-	together
hyper-	over	trans-	across, through

as in *prefrontal* (in front of the frontal bone), and *epi-* is defined as "upon or over," as used in *epigastric* meaning over or above the stomach. Common prefixes that indicate position are listed in **Table 13-4**.

Some prefixes will reverse or produce a term with the opposite meaning of the root element. The importance of these terms is to indicate that an ability of the body has been lost or is not functional. For example, the prefix *a-* means "without" or "away from" such that the addition of *a-* to the root element *phagia* (to eat) creates the word *aphagia*. This term is used to indicate that a patient does not have the capability to eat and specifically is not able to swallow. The prefix *dys-* means "difficult" or "painful." The combination of the root element *lexia* (from the Greek for *word*) with the prefix *dys-* creates the term *dyslexia*, which means an impaired ability to understand the written word. **Table 13-5** lists common prefixes that modify the root element to indicate a lack of ability or poor function or change the root element to mean the opposite of the original meaning.

Other prefixes impart additional information such as color. **Table 13-6** lists prefixes that are related to color.

TABLE 13-5 Common Prefixes for Poor or Lack of Presence or Function

a-	without; away from	im-	not
an-	without	in-	not
anti-	against	mal-	bad; ill
contra-	against	pseudo-	false
counter-	against, opposite	un-	not
dys-	inability or lack of function; difficult; painful		

TABLE 13-6 Prefixes Related to Color

alb-	white	leuk-/o-	white
chlor-/o-	green	melan-/o-	black
cyan-/o-	blue	purpur-/o-	purple
eosin-/o-	rosy	rose-/o-	rose; pink
erythr-/o-	red	xanth-/o-	yellow

Suffix

Like a prefix, the addition of a suffix modifies the meaning of the root word to provide a precise medical term. The addition of a suffix such as *-ac*, *-al*, *-ar*, or *-ic* changes the root word (most commonly a noun) into an adjective meaning *pertaining to* or *resembling*. For example, the addition of *-ac* to the root word *cardio-*, meaning heart, produces the adjective *cardiac* meaning "pertaining to or resembling the heart." Cardiac muscle refers to the muscles of the heart rather than the muscles of the leg or arm. Other suffixes whose addition forms an adjective are *-form*, *-ical*, *-oid*, *-ory*, and *-ous*. Word examples include *multiform*, *neurological*, *anatomical*, *lymphoid*, *sensory*, and *venous*.

A suffix may indicate a condition, disease, or procedure (**Table 13-7**). For example, the root word for blood is *hemat-*. When combined with the suffix meaning a characteristic of the urine, *-uria*, it produces *hematuria*, which indicates the condition in which there is blood in the urine. This symptom is commonly associated with a bacterial infection of the bladder. If the laboratory results confirm the presence of bacteria in the urine, the resulting term is *bacteruria* (from the root *bacter-* or *bacterio-* meaning bacterial organism). The combination of *myo-* (muscle) and *-pathy* (disease) results in *myopathy* or a disease of the muscle characterized by muscle weakness, tenderness, and wasting.

The names of medical procedures indicate the precise type of procedure that is done at a specific anatomical location or to a certain organ. One of the most common suffixes is *-ectomy*, indicating the surgical removal of tissue or an organ such as *gastrectomy* (*gastr-* means stomach), the surgical removal of the stomach. *Dermatoplasty* and *rhinoplasty* both use the suffix *-plasty* to indicate a surgical repair; the former refers to repair of the skin and the latter to repair of the nose. In the same way, diagnostic procedures are constructed using the root word and the appropriate suffix. As discussed earlier, *electrocardiogram* contains the root word *cardio-* and the suffix *-gram* meaning a record of the heart, in this case, the electrical activity (prefix: *electro-*). Common surgical and procedural suffixes are found in **Table 13-8**.

TABLE 13-7 Common Suffixes for Conditions or Diseases

-algia; -dynia	pain	-oma	tumor; mass
-blast	immature; embryonic	-osis	unusual or disease condition
-cele	hernia or protrusion	-pareis	weakness
-ectasis	dilation, expansion	-pathy	disease
-ectopia	displacement	-phobia	abnormal fear
-edema	swelling	-plasm	formation; development
-emesis	vomiting	-plegia	paralysis
-emia	presence in the blood	-ptosis	downward dispalcement; dropping
-genesis	produces; generates	-rrhage; -rrhagia	excessive; abnormal flow
-genic	producing	-rrhea	flow; discharge
-ia	state; condition	-rrhexis	rupture
-iasis	abnormal condition	-sclerosis	hardening
-ism	state; condition	-sis	condition of
-itis	inflammation	-spasm	involuntary muscle contraction
-lysis	disintegration	-stenosis	narrowing
-malacia	abnormal softening	-uria	a particular substance in urine
-megaly	enlargement	-y	condition of

TABLE 13-8 Suffixes for Common Surgical Procedures

-centesis	a puncture or tapping operation	-pexy	fixation (of an organ)
-clasis	to break, surgical fracture	-pheresis	removal of blood components
-desis	binding or fusion (commonly of bone or joint)	-plasty	surgical repair; reconstruction
-ectomy	surgical removal	-rrhaphy	suture
-gram	record or picture	-scope	an instrument for viewing or observing
-graph	instrument for recording	-scopy	observation or viewing
-graphy	process of recording	-stomy; -ostomy	surgical creation of an artificial opening into a hollow organ or the creation of an opening between two hollow organs
-logy	study or science of	-tome	an instrument for cutting
-lysis	destruction; loosening	-tomy	incision
-meter	instrument for measuring	-tripsy	crushing
-metry	process of measuring		
-otomy	cutting into		

Pharmacy-Specific Medical Terminology

Within each discipline in the medical sciences, there is a specific and precise vocabulary. One of the simplest words with a very complex meaning is the term *drug*. A drug may be defined simply as an exogenous substance that alters the function of the body or more specifically in terms of a medical substance as a material for use in the diagnosis, cure, mitigation, treatment, or prevention of disease in man or other animals as defined in the U.S. Food, Drug, and Cosmetic Act [201 U.S.C. 321(g)(1)]. The U.S. Food and Drug Administration (FDA) is the agency of the government responsible for *protecting the public health by assuring the safety, efficacy, and security of human and veterinary drugs, biological products, medical devices, our nation's food supply, cosmetics, and products that emit radiation. The FDA is also responsible for advancing the public health by helping to speed innovations that make medicines and foods more effective, safer, and more affordable; and helping the public get the accurate, science-based information they need to use medicines and foods to improve their health.*

More information on the FDA and the U.S. Food, Drug, and Cosmetic Act can be found on the FDA's website (www.fda.gov).

The medications available in a pharmacy are divided into two dispensing categories. Over-the-counter (OTC) medications have been determined to be safe in the hands of the consumer and do not require a prescription to obtain. Prescription medications require a written order signed by an authorized health care provider in order for these drugs to be dispensed. A second method of categorizing medications is based on use of the terms *generic name* versus *trade, brand,* or *proprietary name*. A generic name is usually a version of the chemical name of the drug and is not capitalized. Trade, brand, or proprietary names are capitalized and are followed by the symbol ® indicating that the name is a registered trademark. Such drugs are protected by a patent and can be manufactured or sold only by the company holding the patent rights. For example, acetaminophen is the generic name for the compound that is an OTC medication to reduce pain and fever; the same medication is also marketed under the trade name of Tylenol®. The same generic name drug may be marketed under different trade or brand names. Note that many drug names, both generic and brand, have spellings that are very close to the same and may sound alike. Extreme caution must be used to ensure that the correct medication is dispensed to the patient.

Most medications fall into one of several categories based on their actions. For example, aspirin is an analgesic, a term that means "to relieve pain," and cortisone is an anti-inflammatory, which means that it reduces inflammation. The major categories of drugs are listed in **Table 13-9**.

TABLE 13-9 Categories of Drugs and Their Actions

CATEGORY	ACTION
adrenergic	mimics the action of epinephrine, an agent in the sympathetic nervous system
analgesic	reduces pain
anesthetic	abolishes the sensation of pain
antiarthritic	relieves the symptoms of arthritis
anticoagulant	prevents blood clotting
anticonvulsant	suppresses or reduces number or intensity of seizures
antidiabetic	prevents or alleviates diabetes
antiemetic	prevents or relieves nausea or vomiting
antihistamine	prevents symptoms of allergy such as running nose
antihypertensive	lowers blood pressure
anti-inflammatory	reduces inflammation and swelling
antineoplastic	prevents the growth of malignant cells
antipruritic	relieves the symptoms of itching

(Continued)

TABLE 13-9 (Continued)

CATEGORY	ACTION
antipyretic	reduces fever
antitoxin	specific agent that neutralizes a poison or toxin
antivenin or antivenom	material used to counteract the action of venoms from snakes and other venomous animals
diuretic	increases formation of urine to reduce swelling and blood pressure
hypnotic, sedative, tranquilizer	induces sleep or partial loss of consciousness
proton-pump inhibitor	reduces or blocks secretion of stomach acid
vaccine	any material that produces active immunization in the formation of antibodies
Anti-Infective Agents	
antiamebic	agent that destroys or suppresses the growth of amebae
antibacterial	anti-infective agent directed against bacteria
antibiotic	agent that inhibits the growth and reproduction of bacteria
antifungal	anti-infective agent directed against fungi
antiparasitic	anti-infective agent directed against parasites
antiviral	anti-infective agent directed against viruses
Cardiac Drugs	
antiarrhythmic	prevents or corrects irregularities in heart rhythm or force of beat
beta-adrenergic blocker	reduces rate and force of heart contraction
calcium channel blocker	slows heart rate, dilates coronary arteries
hypolipidemic	reduces cholesterol (also called statins)
nitrates/antianginal	dilates coronary arteries, lowers blood pressure
Gastrointestinal Drugs	
antidiarrheal	reduces intestinal motility to treat or prevent diarrhea
antiflatulent	reduces intestinal gas
cathartic	produces evacuation of the bowel
emetic	induces vomiting
histamine H_2 antagonist	decreases secretion of stomach acid
laxative	stimulates emptying of large intestine
Psychotropics	
antianxiety agent	alters mental activity, reduces anxiety
antidepressant	raises level of chemicals in the brain to relieve depression
antipsychotic	relieves symptoms of psychoses
Respiratory Drugs	
antitussive	suppresses coughing
asthma maintenance	prevents asthma attacks
bronchodilator	relaxes bronchial smooth muscle to prevent spasm
decongestant	opens the air passages of the nose and lungs
expectorant	induces coughing to remove respiratory secretions
mucolytic	loosens mucus to improve its elimination

Within the pharmacy, a drug can take many different forms and have many different methods of administration. The most common are the solid forms, which include *capsules* (in a gelatin container), *tablets* (solid form), *lozenges* (medicated tablets or disks) and *suppositories* (soft substances molded for insertion through the rectum). Semisolid or liquid forms of medication most often used for *topical* (on the skin) application include creams, ointments, and lotions. Finally, the liquid preparations include *parenteral solutions* (sterile solutions intended for subcutaneous, intramuscular, or intravenous injection or insertion into an IV solution), *aerosols* (medications dispersed in a mist), *elixirs* (sweetened liquids for oral use), *tinctures* (medications dissolved in an alcohol solvent), *emulsions* (mixtures of two liquids that do not disperse into each other), and *suspensions* (fine particles of drug that do not dissolve into the liquid). Due to the lack of dispersal, the last two forms must be shaken well immediately before use.

Methods and Delivery Sites

Pharmaceutics is the study of the delivery, *absorption* (entry into the body through the digestive tract or across another membrane), metabolism, distribution, and elimination of drugs by the body. The form and method of delivery are very important to the efficacy of a treatment. The various methods of medication administration are listed in **Table 13-10**.

TABLE 13-10 Methods of Drug Delivery

hyperalimentation	administration of a nutritionally adequate solution through a catheter into the vena cava; used in cases of long-term coma or severe burns or severe gastrointestinal syndromes
infusion	the slow injection of a solution into a vein or subcutaneous tissue
inhalation	administration by breathing in a nebulizer or aerosol
instillation	introduction through a body cavity such as the ear or eye (liquid)
intradermal	into the skin
intramuscular	into the muscle
intraorbital	into the orbit of the eye
intraspinal	into the spine or vertebral column
intrathecal	into the subdural space of the spinal cord
intravenous	into the vein (most often the antecubital area of the arm or the hand)
iontophoresis	process of introducing medication into the tissue using an electric current
subcutaneous	under the skin
sublingual	under the tongue
topical	applied to the skin
transdermal	absorption through the skin; usually in the form of a patch placed on the surface

Pharmacy Personnel and the Science of Pharmacy

The people who work in the pharmacy and as pharmacy representatives throughout the hospital have a variety of backgrounds. The *pharmacist* is authorized to prepare and dispense the medications ordered for the patient. These individuals have completed a bachelor's degree, master's degree, or *PharmD* (clinical doctorate in pharmacy) program, passed the national examination, and are licensed by the state in which they practice. The role of the PharmD has expanded through the years such that pharmacists are actively involved in the assessment of patients and the development of medication regimens and patient education to achieve the best medical outcome for the patient.

The *pharmacy intern* is a student in a pharmacy program who is preparing to complete the requirements for licensure. The *pharmacy resident* is a graduate pharmacist who is obtaining additional training and expertise often in a specialty such as geriatrics (dealing with elderly patients and their medication issues), *nuclear* or *radiopharmacy* (treatment of disease with radioactive materials), or other disease-specific discipline such as *nephrology* (diseases of the kidney) or diabetes. The *pharmacy technician* is trained and authorized to prepare and dispense medications under the supervision of a registered pharmacist.

The science of pharmacy involves many individuals who study all facets of drug development, delivery, interactions, and use. *Pharmaceutics* is the study of how to prepare a medication (tablet, liquid, injectable, etc.) for use in the body, while *pharmacokinetics* is the study of the concentration of a drug in a patient's body and how the drug is metabolized and cleared from the body. This is very important to the appropriate treatment of the patient because the level of medication in the body is critical to achieve the desired therapeutic outcome for the patient. *Pharmacotherapeutics* is the study of the use of drugs and the effects on the patient's condition. Pharmacotherapeutists also look at patient behavior with respect to medications such as *compliance* (the act of taking medications according to the instructions). *Pharmacology* is a scientific field that investigates how drugs affect the body systems at the biochemical level.

One of the newest areas of interest is *pharmacogenetics*, which is the study of the relationship between the genetic profile of an individual and that individual's response to medication. *Pharmacogenomics* is the biotechnological science that combines the techniques of medicine, pharmacology, and genomics and is concerned with developing drug therapies that are specific for the genetic makeup of an individual patient. The investigation of plants and other natural sources as the origin of new drugs is called *pharmacognosy*.

Medical Vocabulary

Knowledge of medical vocabulary outside the discipline of pharmacy is important to achieve effective communication with other health care providers and to begin to understand which medications are appropriate for each patient's condition. Several common medical terms are presented in **Table 13-11** and are grouped into similar concepts.

TABLE 13-11 Common Medical Terms and Conditions

Medical Assessment	
contraindication	any condition that makes a particular medication or form of treatment undesirable or unsafe (such as an allergy to a medication)
diagnosis	the identification of a disease from its signs and symptoms
etiology	the cause of a disease
prognosis	the expected outcome of the course of a disease
sign	objective evidence of a disease or disorder
symptom	subjective evidence of a disease based on the perception of the patient
syndrome	a group of signs and symptoms that characterizes a particular abnormality
Allergy and Inflammation	
allergen	an agent that causes the body to respond with the symptoms of an allergy
allergist	a physician with a specialty in the diagnosis and treatment of allergies
allergy	a reaction to a particular antigen (allergen). Allergies can include "hay fever," which results in runny or itchy eyes and nose and sneezing and coughing, contact dermatitis or allergic reactions to substances coming in contact with the skin or mucous membranes, or drug allergies (to ingested agents such as sulfa or penicillin), which can be life threatening
anaphylaxis	a hypersensitivity reaction to exposure to an antigen that is immediate; can induce shock-like symptoms and may be fatal
antibody	a product of the immune system in response to an antigen. Each antibody recognizes a specific antigen. Allergens are a specific type of antigen
antigen	an agent that stimulates the body to produce antibodies
eczema	an inflammatory condition of the skin
hives	an itchy skin eruption characterized by weals (a raised mark on the skin) with pale interiors and well-defined red margins; usually the result of an allergic response to insect bites or food or drugs
pruritus	an intense sensation of itching
psoriasis	chronic skin disease characterized by dry red patches covered with scales
urticaria	eruption or rash associated with severe itching
Autoimmune and Inflammatory Conditions	
arthritis	inflammation of the joints
cystitis	inflammation of the urinary bladder and ureters
gastritis	inflammation of the lining of the stomach; nausea and loss of appetite and discomfort after eating
hepatitis	inflammation of the liver
immunity	resistance to infection
infection	invasion and multiplication of microorganisms in body tissues
inflammation	a localized protective response elicited by injury or destruction of tissues, which serves to destroy, dilute, or wall off (sequester) both the injurious agent and the injured tissue; characterized in the acute form by the classical signs of pain (dolor), heat (calor), redness (rubor), swelling (tumor), and loss of function (functio laesa)
meningitis	inflammation of the meninges (the membrane around the brain and spinal cord)
nephritis	inflammation of the nephron (the structure that filters the blood and produced urine) in the kidney
pathogen	any disease-producing microorganism (e.g., bacteria, viruses)
phlebitis	inflammation of the vein (often seen in the legs)
rheumatism	popular name for any of a variety of disorders marked by inflammation, or degeneration, of connective tissue structures of the body, especially the joints and related structures, including muscles, tendons, and fibrous tissue, with pain, stiffness, or limitation of motion
rheumatologist	a physician with specialty training in the diagnosis and treatment of rheumatic disease (those characterized by inflammation such as arthritis)

(*Continued*)

TABLE 13-11 (Continued)

Cardiovascular System	
aneurysm	a sac formed by the dilation of the wall of an artery, a vein, or the heart; it is filled with fluid or clotted blood, often forming a pulsating tumor
arteriosclerosis	any of a group of diseases characterized by thickening and loss of elasticity of arterial walls
atherosclerosis	a common form of arteriosclerosis with formation of deposits of yellowish plaques (*atheromas*) containing cholesterol, in the walls of large and medium-sized arteries
bradycardia	heart rate slower than normal
cardiologist	a physician with specialty training in the diagnosis and treatment of diseases of the heart and vascular system
congestive heart failure	reduced ability or failure of the heart to pump an adequate blood supply to the body
diastolic pressure	the force exerted by the blood on the blood vessels when the heart is at rest (blood is flowing slowly through the vessel)
embolism	the sudden blocking of an artery by a clot or foreign material that has been brought to its site of lodgment by the blood current
fibrillation	rapid, uncoordinated and ineffectual heartbeat
hemorrhage	severe bleeding
hypertension	high blood pressure
hypotension	low blood pressure
myocardial infarction	injury to the heart muscle (myocardium) due to inadequate oxygen supply caused by the occlusion of a coronary artery
occlusion	blockage of a blood vessel
syncope	fainting, a transient loss of consciousness due to inadequate blood flow to the brain
systolic	the force exerted by the blood when the heart is in a state of contraction (blood is flowing rapidly through the vessel)
tachycardia	rapid heartbeat
vasoconstriction	contraction of the smooth muscles surrounding the blood vessels
vasodilation	relaxation of the smooth muscles surrounding the blood vessels
Cancer or Oncology	
ascites	a fluid that accumulates within the abdominal cavity
basal cell carcinoma	the most common type of skin cancer
benign	a description of tissue that is determined to be normal (not cancerous)
carcinogen	any substance that may cause cancer
carcinoma	a malignant new growth made up of epithelial cells tending to infiltrate the surrounding tissues and give rise to metastases
chemotherapy	the use of chemical agents in the treatment or control of disease; most often associated with the treatment of cancer
leukemia	a malignant disease characterized by an increase in white blood cells
lymphoma	a tumor of the tissue in the lymph glands
malignant	a description of tissue that is cancerous and that will grow out of control
mastectomy	removal of a breast
melanoma	a cancer of the skin
metastasis	spreading of disease to another part of the body
neoplasm	a new growth of tissue in which the multiplication of cells is uncontrolled and progressive (also called a tumor)
oncologist	a physician with specialty training in the treatment of cancer
tumor	a new growth of tissue in which the multiplication of cells is uncontrolled and progressive (also called a neoplasm)

TABLE 13-11 (Continued)

Clinical and Anatomical Laboratory Testing	
anemia	a reduction in the number or function of the red blood cells; symptoms include fatigue, weakness, shortness of breath, and pale skin
biopsy	examination of tissues or liquids from the living body to determine the existence or cause of a disease
blood gas	an analysis of the dissolved gases in blood plasma, including oxygen, nitrogen, and carbon dioxide
blood type	a designation of the blood based on normally occurring antigens on the surface of the red blood cell (A, B, O, or AB)
BUN	blood urea nitrogen: nitrogen in the blood, which can be measured to determine kidney function
CBC	complete blood count; an analysis of the blood cells to determine number, type, size, shape, and iron content
clinical laboratory technologist	an individual who has obtained the education and training to perform testing in a clinical diagnostic laboratory
coagulation	the process of blood clotting
creatinine clearance	a test to measure the function of the kidney
cytology	a special area of pathology that studies the structure of cells to determine if they are normal or cancerous
DIC	a condition in which the clotting of blood is out of control and results in bleeding (disseminated intravascular coagulation)
erythrocyte	a red blood cell
heparin	a naturally occurring component of the blood that prevents blood clotting; is often given to prevent stroke in patients whose blood clots too fast
INR	laboratory test used to determine the clotting tendency of blood, in the measure of warfarin dosage
liver profile	a group of chemical tests that indicates the function and health of the liver
pathologist	a physician trained in diagnostic laboratory medicine
pathology	the branch of medical science that studies the causes and nature and effects of diseases
plasma	the fluid portion of the blood
PT and PTT or aPTT	laboratory tests that measure the ability of the blood to clot
serum	the fluid portion of the blood after it has been allowed to clot
Disturbances of Metabolism	
acidosis	a condition in which the blood pH is too acid (<7.4), which impairs body function such as delivery ofoxygen to the tissue
alkalosis	a condition in which the blood pH is too alkaline (>7.4), which impairs body function such as delivery of oxygen to the tissue
diabetes	a chronic disease in which blood glucose does not enter the cells and the blood sugar remains high, causing harm to tissues
diuresis	increased formation of urine, a common symptom of diabetes
glucose tolerance test	a test for diabetes based on the ability of the body to metabolize an induced increase in blood sugar
hypoglycemia	an abnormally low concentration of glucose in the blood
jaundice	yellow appearance of the skin usually associated with a malfunction or strain on the liver
polydipsia	excessive thirst
polyuria	excessive urine formation
Infection	
amebiasis	an infection caused by an ameba or amebae
antiseptic	an agent that inhibits the growth of a microorganism but does not necessarily kill it
bacteriocide	an agent that will kill bacteria

(*Continued*)

TABLE 13-11 (Continued)

Infection	
bacteriostat	an agent that will inhibit the growth of bacteria
decubitus ulcer	a bedsore
febrile	body temperature above normal; fever
impetigo	a very contagious infection of the skin; common in children; localized redness develops into small blisters that gradually crust and erode
incubation	the period between exposure to an infective agent and the appearance of symptoms
pertussis	whooping cough; an acute infectious disease of the respiratory tract
rubella	German measles
sterilization	the process of destroying all microorganisms so that an item is free of contamination
toxin	a noxious or poisonous material
virus	a submicroscopic agent of infectious disease

Common Medical/Pharmacy Abbreviations and Terminology

The medical vocabulary, as in other highly technical fields of science and technology, uses many acronyms or abbreviations in everyday conversation. A familiarity with these terms is important to comprehension and smooth communication. **Table 13-12** lists common medical abbreviations.

TABLE 13-12 Common Medical Abbreviations

A–B			
aa	of equal parts	alb	albumin
AAA	abdominal aortic aneurysm	ALD	alcoholic liver disease
AAD	antibiotic-associated diarrhea	ALL	acute lymphocytic leukemia
AAO	awake, alert, and oriented	amb	ambulatory or mobile
AAPT	American Association of Pharmacy Technicians	AML	acute myelogenous leukemia
ABG	arterial blood gas	amt	amount
ac	before eating	ANDA	abbreviated new drug application
ad lib (*ad libitum*)	as much as one desires	AOB	alcohol on breath
ADH	antidiuretic hormone	AODM	adult-onset diabetes mellitus (type 2)
ADI	American Drug Index	APAP	acetaminophen
adm	admission	APhA	American Pharmacists Association
ADR	adverse drug reaction	aq	aqueous
AED	antiepileptic drug	ARDS	acute respiratory distress syndrome
AFB	acid-fast bacillus	ARF	acute renal failure
AHFS	American Hospital Formulary Service	ASA	aspirin
AIDS	acquired immunodeficiency syndrome	ASAP	as soon as possible
		ASHD	atherosclerotic heart disease
		ASHP	American Society of Health-System Pharmacists

TABLE 13-12 (Continued)

A–B			
BBVD	bloodborne viral infection	BOM	bilateral otitis media (ear infection)
BE	barium enema	BP	blood pressure
bid	twice a day	BPM	beats per minute
biw	twice weekly	BS	breath sounds
BM	bowel movement	BUN	blood urea nitrogen
BM	bone marrow aspiration	BW	body weight
BMR	basal metabolic rate	BX	biopsy

C–E			
c	with	D.D.S.	doctor of dental surgery
CA	cancer	DDx	differential diagnosis
Ca	calcium	diag	diagnosis
CAD	coronary artery disease	DIC	Drug Information Center
cath	catheter	DIC	disseminated intravascular coagulopathy
CBC	complete blood count	Disp	dispense
CC, C/O	chief complaint	DJD	degenerative joint disease
ccu	clean-catch urine	DM	diabetes mellitus
CDC	Centers for Disease Control and Prevention	DNR	do not resuscitate
CF	cystic fibrosis	D.O.	doctor of osteopathy
CHF	congestive heart failure	DOE	dyspnea (shortness of breath) on exertion
CI	cardiac index (heart function)	DPT	diphtheria, pertussis, tetanus vaccine
CMV	cytomegalovirus	DRG	diagnosis-related group (billing)
CNS	central nervous system	DRL	dextrose 5% in Ringer's lactate
CO	cardiac output	DTD	let such doses be given
COPD	chronic obstructive pulmonary disease	dx	diagnosis
CPR	cardiopulmonary resuscitation	D5W	dextrose 5% in water
C&S	culture and sensitivity (for identification of bacteria and the appropriate antibiotics)	D5/0.33	dextrose 5% in 0.33% sodium chloride
CSF	cerebrospinal fluid	D5/0.45	dextrose 5% in 0.45% sodium chloride
CVA	cerebral vascular accident	D5/0.9	dextrose 5% in 0.9% sodium chloride
CXR	chest x-ray	EBL	estimated blood loss
DAW	dispense as written	ECG, EKG	electrocardiogram
D&C	dilatation and curettage; a surgical procedure usually performed under local anesthesia in which the cervix is dilated and the endometrial lining of the uterus is scraped away	EEG	electroencephalogram
		ENT	ears, nose, and throat
		ESR	erythrocyte sedimentation rate
		ETOH	ethanol
		ETT	endotracheal tube

(Continued)

TABLE 13-12 (Continued)

F–I

FBS	fasting blood sugar	Hgb	hemoglobin
FDA	Food and Drug Administration	HIV	human immunodeficiency virus
FFP	fresh frozen plasma	HLA	histocompatibility antigen
FTT	failure to thrive	HO	history of
FU	follow up	HR	heart rate
fuo	fever of unknown origin	HSV	herpes simplex virus
Fx	fracture	HLTV-III	human lymphotrophic virus, type III (AIDS agent, HIV)
g	gram	HTN	hypertension
g, gtt	drops	hx	history
GC	gonorrhea	I&D	incision and drainage
GFR	glomerular filtration rate	I&O	intake and output
GI	gastrointestinal	ID	infectious disease
gr	grain	IM	intramuscular
GSW	gunshot wound	IND	investigational new drug
GTT	glucose tolerance test	IMV	intermittent mandatory ventilation
GU	genitourinary	INF	intravenous nutritional fluid
GYN	gynecology	INH	isoniazid
h, hr	hour	IV	intravenous
HA	headache	IVPB	intravenous piggyback; small volume parenteral
HBP	high blood pressure	IVSS	intravenous soluset; small volume parenteral
HCG	human chorionic gonadotropin		
Hct	hematocrit		
HDL	high-density lipoprotein		

J–M

JODM	juvenile-onset diabetes mellitus (type 1)	LMP	last menstrual period
K	potassium	LOC	loss of consciousness or level of consciousness
KCl	potassium chloride	LP	lumbar puncture
kg	kilogram	LPN	licensed practical nurse
KVO	keep vein open	LR	lactated Ringer's solution
L	liter	LVP	left ventricular pressure
L	left	MAOI	monoamine oxidase inhibitor
lb	pound	MAP	mean arterial pressure
LDH	lactate dehydrogenase (an indicator of cell death)	MAR	medication administration record
LE	lupus erythematosus	MBT	maternal blood type
LIH	left inguinal hernia		

TABLE 13-12 (Continued)

J–M			
mcg	microgram (10^{-6})	MMR	measles, mumps, rubella (vaccine)
MCV	mean cell volume	MOM	milk of magnesia
MD	medical doctor	MRI	magnetic resonance imaging
mEq	milliequivalent	MRSA	methicillin-resistant *Staphylococcus aureus*
mg	milligram	MS	multiple sclerosis
Mg^{++}	magnesium	MSSA	methicillin-sensitive *Staphylococcus aureus*
MI	myocardial infarction; heart attack	mvi	multivitamin injection
mL	milliliter		
mmol	millimole		

N–P			
Na	sodium	OM	otitis media (ear infection)
NAD	no active disease	OPV	oral polio vaccine
NARD	National Association of Retail Druggists	p	para or after
NDA	new drug application	PA	physician assistant
NED	no evidence of recurrent disease	PAP	pulmonary artery pressure
ng	nanogram (10^{-9})	pb	piggyback
ngt	nasogastric tube	pc	after meals
NIDDM	non-insulin-dependent diabetes mellitus	PDR	*Physician's Desk Reference*
NKA	no known allergies	PE	pulmonary embolus/physical examination/pleural effusion
NKDA	no known drug allergies	PFT	pulmonary function tests
NMR	nuclear magnetic resonance	pg	picogram
non rep (nr)	do not repeat	pH	hydrogen ion concentration (measure of acidity or alkalinity)
NPH	neutral protamine Hagedorn insulin	PharmD	doctor of pharmacy
NPO	nothing by mouth	pid	pelvic inflammatory disease
NRM	no regular medications	PMH	previous medical history
NS	normal saline (0.9% sodium chloride)	PO	by mouth
NSAID	nonsteroidal anti-inflammatory drug	POD	postoperative day
NSR	normal sinus rhythm	PP	postprandial (after meals)
NT	nasotracheal	PPD	purified protein derivative (skin test for tuberculosis exposure)
NTG	nitroglycerin	PR	by rectum
n/v	nausea/vomiting	PRN	as needed
O_2	oxygen	PT	prothrombin time (measure of clotting system of the blood)
OOB	out of bed		
OD	doctor of optometry		

(*Continued*)

TABLE 13-12 (Continued)

N–P			
Pt	patient	PUD	peptic ulcer disease
PTH	parathyroid hormone	PVC	premature ventricular contraction
PTT	partial thromboplastin time (measure of blood clotting system)	PVD	peripheral vascular disease
		PZI	protamine zinc insulin

Q–Z			
q	every (e.g., q4h = every 4 hours)	SSE	soap suds enema
QA	quality assurance	SSKI	saturated solution of potassium iodide
qam	every morning	STAT	immediately
qh	every hour	STI	sexually transmitted infection
QID	four times a day	Sx	symptoms
QNS	quantity not sufficient	tab	tablet
qs	quantity sufficient	TB	tuberculosis
r, rt	right	T&C	type and cross (blood for transfusion)
RA	rheumatoid arthritis	TIBC	total iron-binding capacity (blood test for anemia)
rbc	red blood cell	tid	three times daily
RDA	recommended daily allowance	TLC	total lung capacity
RIA	radioimmunoassay	TO	telephone order
RL	Ringer's lactate	TPN	total parenteral nutrition
R/O	rule out	tr	tincture
ROM	range of motion	tw	twice a week
ROS	review of systems	TWE	tap water enema
RRR	regular rate and rhythm	Tx	treatment
RTC	return to clinic	UA	urinalysis
Rx	treatment	UAO	upper airway obstruction
s	without	UC	ulcerative colitis
SBE	subacute bacterial endocarditis	ung	ointment
SDS	same day surgery	USP-NF	U.S. Pharmacopeia-National Formulary
SGA	small for gestational age	ut dict, ud	as directed
s.i.d.	once a day (*semel in dia*)	UTI	urinary tract infection
signa/sig	let it be written or imprinted on the label	VA	Veterans Administration
sl	sublingual (under the tongue)	VC	vital capacity
SLE	system lupus erythematosus	V fib	ventricular fibrillation
sos	if necessary	VO	verbal order
smo	slips made out	VRE	vancomycin-resistant enterococcus
SOB	shortness of breath		
ss	half/semi		

TABLE 13-12 (Continued)

Q–Z			
VS	vital signs	W/U	workup
VSS	vital signs stable	XL	extended release
VT	ventricular tachycardia	XS	excessive
WBC	white blood cells	YOB	year of birth
WDWN	well-developed; well-nourished	Zn	zinc
WNL	within normal limits	ZnO	zinc oxide
WO	written order		

Commonly Used Apothecary Symbols

Apothecary symbols are an important part of the history of the practice of pharmacy (**Table 13-13**). However, many of the symbols have multiple meanings or are easily misinterpreted. Serious medical errors can be caused by the misinterpretation of abbreviations, apothecary symbols, and dose designations; therefore, caution is advised when confronted with information in this format. See Chapter 12 and Chapter 30 for additional information about medication errors.

TABLE 13-13 Apothecary Symbols

ʒ	drachma/dram (1/8 ounce or 60 grains)
℥	ounce
℥ss	half ounce, tablespoon
♏	minim
↑	elevated or increased
↓	depressed or decreased
Δ	change
%	percent
<	less than
=	equals
>	greater than
°	degree
♀	female
♂	male

The Prescription

To provide patients with medications for home use, a physician or other properly licensed medical practitioner must provide a *prescription*, a written or electronic order for a medication or treatment. An *order* to dispense a medication to an inpatient for immediate use in the hospital is not considered a prescription, but is a written instruction that is documented on the patient's chart.

The written or electronic prescription must include the patient's name, name of the medication, the dose and frequency of use, and the number of doses to be dispensed over a period of time. The practitioner's full name, address, and telephone number must be included. Many physicians will use a preprinted or computer-generated form that contains the standard information and blank spaces for the practitioner to hand write or electronically complete the information about the patient, medication desired, and directions for use. If a generic version of the prescribed drug is available (which is most often less expensive), the prescriber should indicate if the medication to be dispensed must be a brand name medication or if the generic version can be substituted. Please see Chapter 12 for more detailed information about prescriptions.

If the prescription is for a controlled substance or narcotic, the practitioner must also provide his or her Drug Enforcement Agency (DEA) number. A valid DEA number consists of two letters; the first identifies the type of practitioner and the second is the first letter of the practitioner's last name. The letters are followed by six numbers and a seventh number or check digit. The check digit is derived by the following calculation:

- Add the first, third, and fifth numbers.
- Add the second, fourth, and sixth numbers and multiply by 2.
- Add the sums together. The check digit is the last number of the sum.

For example, calculation of the check digit for DEA number 568734 would be

$5 + 8 + 3 = 16$

$6 + 7 + 4 = 17$

$17 \times 2 = 34$

$34 + 16 = 50$

The check digit is zero, so the DEA number for Dr. Blake, who is a physician, would appear as CB 5687340. A list of possible first letters for DEA numbers is given in **Table 13-14**.

TABLE 13-14 DEA Number Lettering

FIRST LETTER OF DEA NUMBER	REGISTRANT TYPE
A	Practitioner
B	Hospital/clinic
C	Practitioner
D	Teaching institution
E	Manufacturer
F	Distributer and/or practitioner
G	Researcher
H	Analytical lab
J	Importer
K	Exporter
L	Reverse distributer
M	Midlevel practitioner: nurse practitioner, physician's assistant
N, P, R, S, T, U	Narcotic treatment programs
X	Suboxone/Subutex treatment program

Summary

Medical terminology is a combination of word elements that describe medical history, medical diagnoses, current medical conditions, surgical interventions, and so forth. As such, the pharmacy technician's understanding of this language of medicine is essential to communicate effectively with members of health care teams in the provision of patient care.

TEST YOUR KNOWLEDGE

Multiple Choice

1. The term *tracheotomy* indicates
   a. an injectable solution for the throat.
   b. a surgical procedure that involves cutting into the trachea.
   c. a viral infection of the trachea.
   d. a preparation for topical application.

2. The term *mammography* refers to
   a. a surgical procedure on the chest.
   b. a diagnostic term that indicates a malignancy.
   c. a preparation for topical application.
   d. a diagnostic procedure of the breast.

3. The term *cholecystectomy* refers to
a. a surgical procedure for removal of the gallbladder.
b. a diagnostic procedure on the gallbladder.
c. the condition of having two gallbladders.
d. a solution for irrigation of the gallbladder.

4. The abbreviation *pc* used in an order or prescription refers to ______________, whereas *NPO* indicates ______________
a. patient's compliance; no patient orders.
b. after meals; nothing by mouth.
c. a personal computer; no patient orders.
d. after meals; medication should be taken with meals.

5. If a medication is to be given sublingual, it will be
a. injected under the skin.
b. instilled into the mouth.
c. placed under the tongue.
d. added to an IV preparation.

6. A medication categorized as an analgesic
a. reduces anxiety.
b. stabilizes a patient's blood sugar.
c. reduces pain.
d. increases the heart rate.

7. The term *intravenous* refers to
a. into the spine.
b. into the vein.
c. into the skin.
d. into the mouth.

8. A medication classified as an antibiotic
a. is used to treat a bacterial infection.
b. is used to treat high blood pressure.
c. is used to treat diabetes.
d. is used to treat a heart arrhythmia.

9. If a drug is categorized as an OTC, it
a. is used to treat an ear infection.
b. does not require a prescription for distribution.
c. requires a prescription for distribution.
d. must be shaken thoroughly just before use.

10. The term *myopathy* can be broken into the root word *myo-* and the suffix *-pathy* and means
a. a disease of the inner ear.
b. eye disease.
c. a disease of the brain.
d. muscle disease.

Matching

Match the word part to its meaning.

1. ________ hepato-	a. false
2. ________ -itis	b. red
3. ________ diuretic	c. liver
4. ________ ad lib	d. tumor or mass
5. ________ signa/sig	e. reduces intestinal motility
6. ________ bronchodilator	f. a sterile solution
7. ________ -algia	g. let it be written
8. ________ pneumo-	h. twice a day
9. ________ pan-	i. observation or viewing
10. ________ erythro-	j. lungs
11. ________ anesthetic	k. all
12. ________ bid	l. as much as needed
13. ________ intradermal	m. inflammation
14. ________ parenteral	n. state or condition
15. ________ hyper-	o. pain
16. ________ -ectomy	p. increases urine formation
17. ________ melano-	q. reduces symptoms of allergy
18. ________ antihistamine	r. surgical removal
19. ________ dx	s. black
20. ________ intra-	t. relaxes smooth muscle of the lung
21. ________ -ism	u. one
22. ________ pseudo-	v. study of drug delivery
23. ________ topical	w. over
24. ________ -oma	x. within
25. ________ mono-	y. reduces itching
26. ________ pharmaceutics	z. abolishes the sensation of pain
27. ________ antipruritic	aa. into the skin
28. ________ -scopy	bb. applied to the skin
29. ________ antidiarrheal	cc. below
30. ________ sub-	dd. diagnosis

Calculation

A prescription for a narcotic pain killer is submitted to the pharmacy. The ordering physician is listed as Dr. Thompson with a DEA number of CA 4762343. What is wrong with the number? Determine the correct number.

Suggested Readings

Dorland's Illustrated Medical Dictionary (31st ed.). (2011). Philadelphia, PA: Saunders.

Dorland's Online Dictionary. (n.d.). Available at http://www.dorlands.com/wsearch.jsp

Drug Enforcement Administration. (n.d.). *Decode DEA number information*. Retrieved from http://www.uspharmd.com/student/dea_number

Stedman's Medical Dictionary for the Health Professions and Nursing (7th ed.). (2007). Philadelphia, PA: Lippincott Williams & Wilkins.

CHAPTER 14

Pharmaceutical Dosage Forms

Competencies

Upon completion of this chapter, the reader should be able to:

1. Explain the different interpretations of "dosage form" by the patient, by members of the health care team, and by pharmacists.
2. List four physicochemical properties of a drug.
3. Name four formulation aids used in the preparation of a given dosage form.
4. Describe the advantages and disadvantages of the major classes of pharmaceutical dosage forms: liquids, solids, semisolids, and aerosols.
5. Differentiate the characteristics of a solution and a suspension.
6. List five desirable qualities for an external suspension.
7. Name and define four solid dosage forms currently in use.
8. Explain the differences among compressed tablets, sublingual or buccal tablets, and multiple compressed tablets.
9. Describe an oral osmotic (OROS) drug dosage design and give an example.
10. Outline five advantages of the transdermal patch.

Key Terms

additive
aerosol
anhydrous
anionic
buffer system
capsule
cationic
delayed-release dosage form
density
diluent
dissolution
dosage form
drug
emulsifying agent
emulsion
excipient
extended-release dosage form
fast-dissolving tablet
granule
heterogeneous
homogeneous
hydro-alcoholic
hydrophilic
hydrous
hygroscopic
infusion
intranasal
intraocular
iso-osmotic
isotonic
lacrimal fluid
lipophilic
lotions
medium
molecular form
multiple compressed tablet
ointment
orally dissolving tablet (ODT)
parenteral products
percutaneous
physicochemical properties
polymorphism
preservatives
propellant
pyrogens
radiopaque
receptors
refractory
solution
sublingual
suppository
suspension
tablet
transdermal
volatile
wetting agent

Introduction

dosage form a system or device designed to deliver a drug or other medicinal agent to the biological system at the site of absorption or the site of therapeutic action; dosage forms include capsules, patches, injections, etc.

drug the active ingredient in a medication or pharmaceutical substance intended to cure, prevent, or diagnose a disease or disease process

physicochemical properties the physical and chemical properties of a pharmaceutical

polymorphism the property of a compound to exist in more than one crystalline form

Pharmaceutical dosage forms are drug delivery systems. A **dosage form** is a system or device designed to deliver a drug or other medicinal agent to the biological system at the site of absorption or the site of therapeutic action. A drug or a medicinal agent is seldom administered alone. It is often administered as a dosage form.

Drugs are defined as chemicals of synthetic, semisynthetic, natural, or biological origin. Drugs interact with the biological systems of humans or animals to produce a response. This response may be intended to prevent, cure, or reduce ill effects in the human or animal body, or to detect disease-causing manifestations. In actual practice, a pure drug is rarely used. What is generally administered to obtain the desired effect is a drug delivery system, the dosage form mentioned above. In a dosage form, the active ingredient, referred to as the **drug** is combined with inert or physiologically inactive materials to enable administration of the drug (e.g., administration of the drug in the form of a tablet, capsule, or solution).

In addition to providing the means of delivering a safe, convenient, and accurate dose of the drug, dosage forms are needed for additional reasons. For example, dosage forms protect the drug substance from the destructive influence of the gastric environment after oral administration. They also conceal the bitter, salty, or offensive taste or odor of a drug substance.

The term *dosage form* means different things to different people. To a patient, for instance, the term signifies the gross physical or pharmaceutical form in which the drug is made available for administration or use (e.g., tablet, capsule, solution, injection, ointment). To the members of the health care team, the dosage form of a drug is a drug delivery system. Any alteration in the system (e.g., a change in the amount or type of inert ingredient) may be expected to alter the delivery rate and the total amount of drug delivered at the site of action. The pharmacist, however, uses the term *dosage form* in a more comprehensive manner to include not only the drug delivery system, but also the physicochemical properties of the drug itself. The term **physicochemical properties** refers to both physical as well as chemical properties of the pharmaceutical.

The following are included in the physicochemical properties of a drug:

- *Particle size of the drug powder.* The particle size of the drug powder is important because smaller particles dissolve at a much faster rate than do larger particles. For a drug to be absorbed, it has to be in a solution form at the site of absorption. Faster dissolution of the drug ensures rapid and complete absorption. Drugs that dissolve slowly are more likely to exhibit incomplete or erratic absorption.
- *Salt form of the drug substance.* Most drugs are either weak organic acids (e.g., phenobarbital) or weak organic bases (e.g., tetracycline, morphine, diphenhydramine). These drugs have poor solubility in the biological fluids. The salt forms of these drugs (e.g., phenobarbital sodium, tetracycline hydrochloride, morphine sulfate, diphenhydramine hydrochloride) are generally used because salts dissolve more rapidly in the biological fluids than do weak acids or weak bases.
- *The polymorphic state of the drug substance.* **Polymorphism** means that a compound can exist in more than one crystalline form, called the polymorphic form of the compound. The chemical nature (chemical formula and chemical properties) of all crystalline forms of the substance are identical, but the physical properties (crystal shape, melting point,

boiling point, solubility, etc.) of the crystalline forms may be different. Manufacturers prefer to use the polymorphic form of a drug, which possesses better water solubility and exhibits good stability of the drug.

- *Dissolution characteristics of the drug.* The **dissolution** characteristics of a drug are the rate at which and the extent to which the drug undergoes dissolution. Drugs that dissolve at a faster rate generally exhibit reproducible and complete absorption compared to drugs that dissolve relatively slowly.
- *Formulation aids.* The nature and quantities of various formulation aids (inert ingredients used in the preparation of the given dosage form) employed in the formulation and fabrication of a dosage form can affect the physicochemical properties of the drug. The formulation aids usually used in a dosage form include the following:
    - **Diluents**, also called bulking agents, are used to increase the bulk or gross weight of the dosage form so that an acceptable product can be formulated. Diluents are essential in a solid dosage formulation if the amount of active ingredient is relatively small (e.g., phenobarbital, digoxin, diazepam). Examples of commonly used diluents include lactose, microcrystalline cellulose, and starch.
    - **Excipients** are various formulation aides that must be used to help formulate and prepare the dosage form
    - **Additives** are additional formulation aides which may be essential to the successful formulation and fabrication of a dosage form.
    - **Preservatives**, as the name suggests, are substances that retard, minimize, or prevent the growth of microorganisms in a dosage form.

dissolution breakdown of a drug so that it can be absorbed into the body

diluent an agent that dilutes or reconstitutes a solution or mixture; also called *bulking agent*

excipient an inert substance that is added to a drug to give the drug form or consistency

additive an active ingredient added to a solution that is intended for intravenous administration or irrigation

preservatives substance used to prevent the growth of microorganisms

Classification of Dosage Forms

Although most drugs are synthesized as solid powders or solid crystals, some drugs may exist only in a liquid or gaseous state of matter. A solid drug can be formulated either as a solid dosage form (tablet, powder, or capsule) or as a liquid dosage form (solution, suspension, or emulsion). A drug that exists only as a liquid can only be formulated as a liquid dosage form (solution or emulsion) because it is difficult, if not impossible, to prepare a solid dosage form from a liquid substance. However, if the dose of the drug is extremely small (e.g., a few drops), it may be possible to absorb this small amount of the liquid onto a powder and formulate the mixture as a capsule or tablet dosage form. Similarly, a drug that is gaseous in nature can only be formulated as a gaseous dosage form.

Because of the diverse physical nature of drug substances, their mode of action, and the route of administration used for delivery of drugs, dosage forms are classified in several different ways. However, the major classes of pharmaceutical dosage forms can be broadly categorized into four main classes: (1) liquid dosage forms, (2) solid dosage forms, (3) semisolid dosage forms, and (4) miscellaneous dosage forms.

Liquid Dosage Forms

Biological responses are elicited by the **molecular form** of the drug; that is, the drug's response occurs when molecules of the drug interact with the receptors in the body. The term **receptor** is used to indicate substances in the body that interact with drug molecules and exhibit pharmacological, therapeutic, or toxic effects. Thus, regardless of the state of matter (solid, liquid, or gas) in which the dosage form of a drug is administered, the action at the molecular level will involve

molecular form the drug form that elicits biological responses regardless of dosage form

receptor a cell component that combines with a drug or hormone to alter the function of the cell

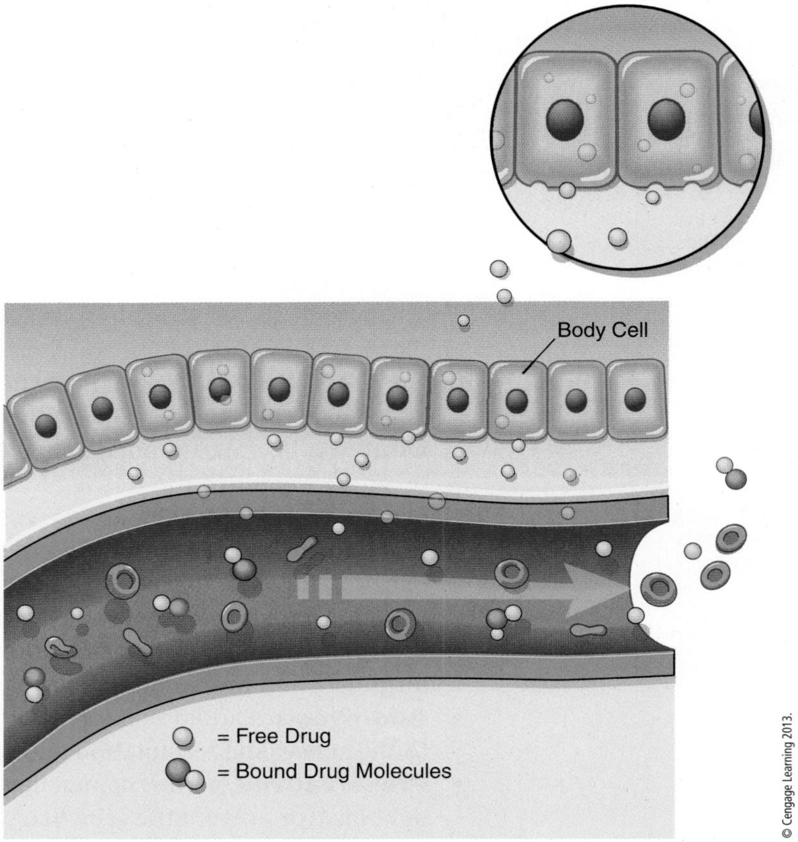

FIGURE 14-1 Drug molecules that attach to plasma proteins in the bloodstream render the drug inactive. Unattached drug molecules are free to leave the bloodstream and act on cells. The cells contain receptors that attract drug molecules to cross the cell membrane and enter the cell. The drug molecules can then act to stimulate or inhibit cell function.

interaction of the biological constituents (receptors) with the individual molecules of the drug. Therefore, for a drug to elicit the desired response, it has to be present in the form of a molecular dispersion (solution) at the site of action (**Figure 14-1**).

Liquid dosage forms are generally classified into two main categories: liquid dosage forms that contain soluble matter and those that contain insoluble matter.

Liquid Dosage Forms That Contain Soluble Matter

solution a homogeneous mixture of one or more substances dispersed in a dissolving solvent; clear liquid with all components completely dissolved

hydrophilic water loving

Liquid dosage forms containing soluble matter are called **solutions**. A solution consists of a solute (substance dissolved) in a solvent (liquid in which the solute is dissolved). A liquid dosage form may consist of one or several soluble substances (solute) dissolved in a suitable solvent (usually water). The solute in a liquid dosage form may be a solid, a liquid, or a gas and the solvent may be any **hydrophilic** liquid. The term *hydrophilic* (*hydro* = water, *philic* = loving) is used for substances that mix or dissolve in water. Hydrophilic solvents are preferred because such a solvent system is safe for the human body and is able to mix with body fluids. Examples of hydrophilic solvents include water, glycerin, ethanol, propylene glycol, and polyethylene glycols. Some of the potential problems that one should be aware of in dealing with the solution dosage forms are described next.

Solvent System Because most drugs are either weak organic acids or weak organic bases, they possess sufficient solubility in organic solvents (e.g., alcohol), but lack adequate solubility in water. Therefore, solutions of such drugs are generally made using a blend (mixture) of solvents. Products intended for

TABLE 14-1 Recommended Alcohol Limits for OTC Oral Products

AGE	ALCOHOL LIMIT
Children under 6 years of age	0.5%
Children 6 to 12 years of age	5%
Children over 12 years of age and adults	10%

hydro-alcoholic a mixture of water and alcohol

oral administration usually utilize a **hydro-alcoholic** solvent system. A hydro-alcoholic (*hydro* = water, *alcoholic* = containing alcohol) solvent system is one that contains both water and alcohol. Some hydro-alcoholic systems contain more than 20% alcohol (e.g., elixirs). Obviously, when a product prepared using a hydro-alcoholic solvent is either diluted with water or combined with a product prepared using only water as the solvent, the mixture is likely to cause precipitation of the poorly water-soluble compound or appear milky due to lack of sufficient alcohol in the system to keep the alcohol-soluble ingredient in solution.

Concern has been expressed over the undesirable pharmacological and potentially toxic effects of alcohol when ingested in pharmaceutical products, particularly by children. The Food and Drug Administration (FDA) has proposed that manufacturers of over-the-counter (OTC) oral products restrict the use of alcohol and include appropriate warnings on their product labels. Note that in the case of neonates ingestion of alcohol (in a pharmaceutical product) can cause some serious problems. For example, alcohol can alter liver function, it can cause gastric irritation, and it can also effect neurological depression. Neurological depression may cause lethargy and poor feeding (reduced formula intake), resulting in unnecessary workup for suspected sepsis. For these reasons the American Academy of Pediatrics Committee on Drugs recommends that, if possible, alcohol should not be included in medicinal products intended for children. The recommended alcohol limits for OTC oral products intended for children are shown in **Table 14-1**.

pH Change In those instances where alcohol should not be used in the solvent system, the manufacturers use a salt form of the drug that, unlike the drug itself, possesses good water solubility. For acidic drugs, the salt form is generally the sodium salt or the potassium salt; and for basic drugs, the commonly used salt forms are the hydrochloride or the sulfate salts. Since the combination of a basic drug with a strong acid (e.g., hydrochloric acid or sulfuric acid) or an acidic drug with a strong base (e.g., sodium hydroxide or potassium hydroxide) results in a strongly acidic or a strongly basic solution, the pH of the resulting solution is far removed from neutrality (pH of 7). Although dilution of these solutions with water does not pose any problems, one must be careful not to mix such solutions. For example, a solution containing the hydrochloride salt of one drug when mixed with a solution containing the sodium salt of another drug is likely to result in the precipitation of both drugs. This is because the hydrochloride and sodium portions mixed together will neutralize each other, resulting in the formation (precipitation) of a poorly water-soluble weakly basic drug or a poorly water-soluble weakly acidic drug.

buffer system used to maintain the pH of a drug solution within the range of optimum stability; when the pH of blood and body fluids is maintained virtually constant although acid metabolites are continually being formed in the tissues or lost in the lungs

Buffer System A number of drug solutions are stable only within a given pH range. To ensure maximum stability of the drug and a longer shelf life for such solutions, a **buffer system** is used to maintain the pH of these solutions within the desirable range. A buffer system helps to resist a change in the pH of the solution when a small amount of an acid or a base is added to the solution. Buffer systems used in pharmaceutical dosage forms generally consist of either a mixture of a weak acid and its corresponding salt with a strong base (e.g., a mixture of citric acid and sodium citrate) or a mixture of a weak base and its corresponding salt with a strong acid (e.g., potassium metaphosphate and potassium phosphate).

Buffer systems maintain the pH of the solution of the dosage form within the range of its optimal or maximal stability. The pH of blood is maintained at 7.4 by four buffer systems: two buffer systems in plasma and two buffer systems in erythrocytes. Note, however, that dilution of a drug product's solution that has been formulated with a buffer system is likely to reduce the capacity (or the strength) of the buffer system and, consequently, diminishes the ability of the buffer to resist the change in pH.

Liquid Dosage Forms That Contain Insoluble Matter

Some drugs are insoluble in solvents that are commonly used in the preparation of liquid dosage forms; therefore, these drugs cannot be formulated as solutions. To derive some or all of the advantages of administering a liquid dosage form, the insoluble solutes may be suspended in a suitable liquid (vehicle). Two common liquid dosage forms of drugs do not possess adequate solubility to be formulated as solutions: suspensions and emulsions.

suspension a liquid containing finely divided drug particles that are uniformly distributed

medium the substance through with another substance is dispersed

Suspensions **Suspension** dosage forms are those dosage forms in which the insoluble solid is suspended or dispersed in a liquid **medium**. The liquid is referred to as the dispersion phase or the external phase. The dispersed solid is generally in a state of fine subdivision, i.e., the solid particles are very small in size. The liquid phase (external phase) in most pharmaceutical suspensions is water and the suspension is called an aqueous suspension.

Suspensions are thermodynamically unstable preparations. Every suspension will ultimately settle or cream. A suspension is said to have settled when the suspended particles settle at the bottom of the container, and a suspension is said to have creamed when the suspended particles rise up and aggregate at the top of the dispersion medium (**Figure 14-2**). Settling occurs when the density of the suspended particles is greater than the density of the liquid medium, and creaming occurs when the density of the suspended particles is less than the density of the liquid in which the particles are suspended. As a rule, smaller particles settle (or cream) more slowly than do larger particles. A good pharmaceutical suspension should not settle (or cream) rapidly, and when it does settle (or cream), it should be easily and rapidly redispersible. If the suspension settles, the settled particles

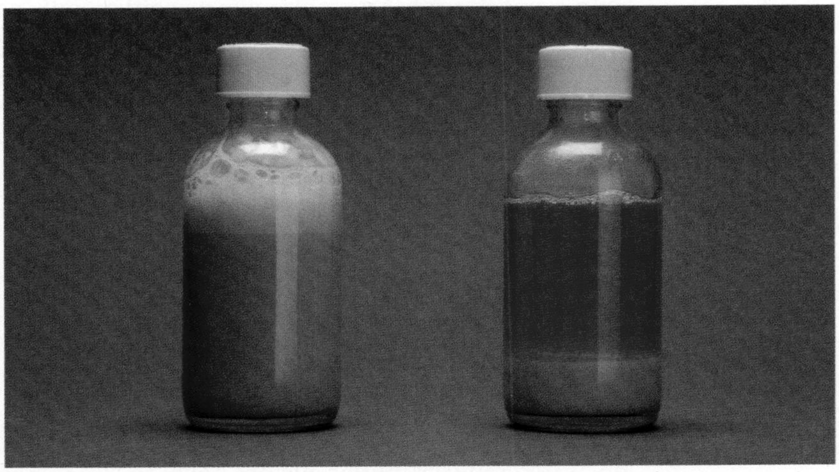

FIGURE 14-2 Suspensions. The suspension on the left is considered "creamed." The suspension on the right is said to have "settled."

can fuse into each other and form a cake that may not break up to allow the suspended particles to redisperse. The concentration of suspended particles of a pharmaceutical suspension is usually expressed in milligrams per teaspoonful.

One common practice to minimize the rate of settling (or creaming) of a suspension is to use a thickening agent. Thickening agents increase the viscosity of the dispersion medium. Examples of viscosity-inducing agents include the following: acacia, bentonite, guar gum, methylcellulose, and sucrose.

A suspension formulation may be preferred over the administration of a solute as a solid dosage form because the solid may have poor solubility. When formulated as a suspension, the solid will generally show a better rate of solubility (dissolution rate) for two reasons: (1) improved wetting of the drug particles and (2) increased surface area of the drug particles due to the very small size of the particles.

Pharmaceutical suspensions may be classified into three groups: (1) orally administered mixtures, (2) externally applied lotions, and (3) injectable preparations.

Orally administered mixtures may supply insoluble and often distasteful substances in a pleasant-tasting liquid dosage form. Examples of oral suspensions are the oral antibiotics which generally contain 250 to 500 mg of the solid material (drug) per 5 mL (teaspoonful) of the suspension. The concentration of the suspended material may be greater in the case of pediatric drops or in antacid preparations and **radiopaque** suspensions. Radiopaque suspensions are generally used for diagnostic purposes. For example, barium sulfate suspension is administered before taking an x-ray of the intestinal tract to determine obstruction in the intestines. Barium sulfate is radiopaque because it does not allow the x-rays to pass through it.

radiopaque having the property of absorbing x-rays

lotion liquid preparation intended for external application

Lotions are suspension dosage forms intended for external application to the skin or mucous membrane. Externally applied lotions provide dermatological materials in a form that is convenient and suitable for external application to the skin. The concentration of the dispersed phase in such formulations may exceed 20% of the total formulation (e.g., calamine lotion).

Injectable suspensions provide an insoluble drug in a form suitable for intramuscular or subcutaneous administration. The concentration of solid particles in these preparations may range from 0.5% to 30%. These preparations are generally of low viscosity (thickness) because viscous liquids are difficult to inject. Particle size is another significant factor in these preparations, since the particle size of the solids affects the availability of the drug, especially in depot therapy (e.g., Procaine Penicillin G or insulin NPH). The term *depot* signifies that the drug is released over a long period of time, so *depot therapy* refers to the slow release of drug over a long period of time to achieve extended therapeutic effect. These injectable preparations are formulated to contain the active ingredient in a relatively minute particle size. This enables the suspension to pass easily through the needle of the syringe.

An acceptable suspension should possess the following desirable qualities:

- Because suspensions, by definition, are unstable dispersal systems, the suspended material should not settle rapidly. The particles that do settle must be readily redispersed into a uniform mixture (suspension) when the container is shaken.
- The suspension must not be too thick and it should pour freely from the orifice of the bottle or through a syringe needle.
- In the case of suspensions intended for external application (e.g., a lotion), the product must be fluid enough to spread easily over the affected area, and yet must not be so mobile that it runs off the surface of application.
- Suspensions intended for external application should dry quickly after application to the affected area

- Suspensions intended for external application should provide an elastic protective film that will not rub off easily
- Suspensions intended for external application should have an acceptable color and odor.

emulsion a heterogeneous system of at least one immiscible liquid intimately dispersed in another in the form of droplets, stabilized by the presence of an emulsifying agent

homogeneous of uniform composition throughout

heterogeneous composed of parts having various and dissimilar characteristics or properties

emulsifying agent a substance used in preparing an emulsion

Emulsions **Emulsions** are liquid preparations consisting of two or more immiscible liquids intimately dispersed into each other in the form of droplets. Emulsions are not homogeneous systems. A **homogeneous** system is one that contains ingredients which are miscible with each other, for example, a solution of sodium chloride in water, or a solution of sucrose in water. Emulsions are **heterogeneous** systems; that is, they contain ingredients that do not mix with each other, for example, a mixture of oil and water. In most emulsions, the droplet size of the dispersed liquid generally ranges from about 0.1 to 10 micrometers in diameter (1 millimeter = 1,000 micrometers , or 1 centimeter = 10,000 micrometers).

Emulsions are also, by definition, unstable dispersions, and the system is stabilized by the presence of one or more **emulsifying agents**. An emulsifying agent is a substance that helps to keep the mixture of immiscible liquids dispersed into each other for a reasonable length of time. Examples of emulsifying agents used in most emulsions include gelatin, acacia, and synthetic substances that reduce tension between the immiscible liquids. The choice of emulsifying agent is governed by the composition of the emulsion and the intended route of administration of the emulsion. Either the dispersed phase or the continuous phase of an emulsion may range in consistency from that of a free-flowing mobile liquid (e.g., emulsions and lotions of relatively low viscosity) to a semisolid (e.g., an ointment).

Emulsions, in general, are considered to be dispersions of oil and water. When an oily substance or an oil is the dispersed phase, the emulsion is called an oil-in-water (o/w) emulsion. When water is the dispersed phase, the emulsion is called water-in-oil (w/o) emulsion. More recent in its origin is a third type of emulsion described as a microemulsion. A microemulsion is also called a transparent emulsion because it possesses the property of transparency due to the very small size of the dispersed droplets (e.g., Haley's M-O). The droplet size in microemulsions is generally 0.05 micrometer or less.

Medicinal emulsions for oral administration are usually of the oil-in-water type and require the use of o/w emulsifying agents. The common examples of oil-in-water emulsifying agents include synthetic nonionic surface active agents (e.g., Tweens and Spans), acacia (also known as gum arabic), tragacanth, and gelatin. A surface active agent is a substance that has the property of reducing surface tension (tension at the surface of a liquid) and interfacial tension (tension at the interface of immiscible liquids).

An oil-in-water emulsion is a convenient means of orally administering oily liquids, especially those that have an unpleasant taste or odor (e.g., mineral oil and castor oil). Because the oil globules are completely surrounded by an aqueous medium, the taste of the oil droplets is almost completely masked and the odor is also markedly suppressed. Also, it has been observed that some oil-soluble compounds (e.g., oil-soluble vitamins) are absorbed more completely when administered as an emulsion than when administered orally as an oily liquid or oily solution. This is because, in an emulsion, the very small globule size of the oily substance renders a large surface area for the oily solution (provided by the oil droplets). That large surface area is made available for contact at the absorption site, which results in better and faster absorption of the oily liquid. Similarly, the use of intravenous emulsions has been studied as a means of maintaining debilitated patients who are unable to assimilate materials administered orally. Radiopaque emulsions have found application as diagnostic agents in x-ray examinations.

Emulsions intended for external application may be either the oil-in-water type or water-in-oil type. An o/w emulsion for external use offers the advantage of being water washable and nonstaining to the clothes. In the preparation of such emulsions, the following emulsifying agents (in addition to the ones already mentioned) are used: triethanolamine stearate, sodium lauryl sulfate, and monovalent soaps (e.g., sodium oleate). The w/o emulsions, which are used almost exclusively for external application, contain one or several of the following emulsifying agents: polyvalent soaps (e.g., calcium palmitate), synthetic nonionic sorbitan esters, wool fat, and cholesterol.

In the pharmaceutical and cosmetic products for external use, emulsification is widely used to formulate dermatological and cosmetic lotions and creams that are better accepted by patients. For example, in the formulation of foam-producing aerosol products, the liquefied gases that propel the emulsion from within the container (called the **propellants**) form the dispersed liquid phase. When the emulsion is discharged from the container, the liquefied gases vaporize. The vaporization of the gases turns the emulsion into a foam.

propellant a substance used to help expel the contents of a pressurized container

Because emulsions are heterogeneous and unstable in nature, they present various stability problems. For example, an improper selection of the emulsifying agent, either in quality or in quantity, may lead to separation of the emulsion during storage. By shaking the container, the emulsion may or may not re-form. When the emulsion does not re-form upon shaking the container, the emulsion is said to have "broken." Once the emulsion is broken, it cannot be re-formed. Therefore, caution must be exercised when an emulsion is to be diluted or mixed with another liquid. An emulsion may be diluted only with a liquid that is miscible with the external phase. Also, dilution of an emulsion may dilute the concentration of the emulsifying agent, leading to the instability or breaking of the emulsion.

If dilution is done with a liquid that possesses characteristics different from those of the external phase of the emulsion, the emulsion can break. The same is true when an emulsion is mixed with another liquid. When two emulsions are mixed, another factor that must be considered is the nature of the emulsifying agent in the two emulsions. If one emulsion contains an **anionic** (carrying a negative charge) emulsifying agent and the other contains a **cationic** agent (carrying a positive charge), the mixture will tend to produce interaction between the positive charges and the negative charges of the emulsifying agents and both emulsions may break.

anionic carrying a negative charge

cationic carrying a positive charge

Some simple methods can be used to determine the type of emulsion (i.e., whether the emulsion is the o/w type or the w/o type). The two commonly used tests are the dilution test and paper test. In the dilution test, the emulsion is diluted with an equal quantity of water and the container is shaken. An oil-in-water emulsion will dilute with water and appear homogeneous. A water-in-oil emulsion will not dilute with water and will have a nonhomogeneous appearance. In the paper test, a drop of the emulsion is placed on a paper towel and allowed to stand for a few minutes. If the emulsion is a water-in-oil emulsion, the drop will sit there and the emulsion will not spread on the paper. If the emulsion is an oil-in-water emulsion, the drop will spread on the paper.

Gels and Jellies

Gels and jellies are also two-phase systems of a solid and a liquid. However, they differ from true suspensions because in these preparations it is difficult to distinguish between the external phase and the internal phase. The particles of the solid phase are interlinked like irregular meshwork; thus, the liquid partly surrounds the interconnected solid particles and is partly occluded by them (e.g., lidocaine gel).

Advantages of Liquid Dosage Forms

Liquid dosage forms (solutions, emulsions, suspensions, etc.) are often the dosage form of choice for the following reasons:

- Liquid dosage forms are effective more quickly than a solid dosage form (tablets or capsules) because the solid form of the drug will have to dissolve in the gastric fluids after administration of the dose.
- They are easier to swallow (especially for pediatric and geriatric patients) than solid dosage forms. Small children and older patients may be afraid that the tablet or capsule will get stuck in the throat.
- Certain substances can be given only in a liquid form because either the character of the remedy or the large dose in any other solid dosage form makes administration of the drug difficult or inconvenient.
- Certain chemical substances may cause pain (e.g., potassium iodide and bromide) or gastric irritation (e.g., aspirin) when administered in a solid state.
- Liquid dosage forms are the dosage forms of choice in certain types of pathological conditions in which absorption of particular ions or molecules is dependent on dissolution of the drug, and the absorption environment is deficient in effecting dissolution. For example, a liquid dosage form provides calcium ions in an absorbable form in patients who lack acidity to dissolve solid calcium compounds (e.g., calcium carbonate powder).

Disadvantages of Liquid Dosage Forms

Although liquid dosage forms offer many advantages, liquid dosage forms also suffer from some disadvantages. The following disadvantages are most common to almost all liquid dosage forms:

- Liquid dosage forms, especially those that contain water, are liable to undergo deterioration and loss of potency much faster than the corresponding solid dosage forms. For example, when aspirin (acetylsalicylic acid) is dissolved in water, it hydrolyses into salicylic acid and acetic acid (vinegar) in a very short period of time. This is one reason aspirin is not available as a solution dosage form.
- Liquid dosage forms present many flavoring and sweetening problems. Some drugs are so bitter that it is almost impossible to mask their bitter taste. Similarly, some drugs have an unacceptable odor and present serious problems when attempting to mask their odor.
- Many instances of incompatibility arise because of interactions between dissolved substances in the liquid dosage form.
- Liquid dosage forms containing water provide an excellent medium for the growth of bacteria and mold. For this reason, substances that prevent or retard the growth of molds and bacteria (called preservatives) are often included in the formulation of such preparations. The most commonly used preservatives in liquid products are methylparaben, propylparaben, benzoic acid, and sodium benzoate. The absence of proper preservatives in liquids containing water results in an excellent medium for bacterial and mold growth.
- The presence of preservatives in a liquid dosage form may present problems of a diverse nature. The U.S. Pharmacopeia-National Formulary (USP-NF) discourages the use of antibacterials in products intended for newborns. Liquid preparations for neonates should not contain

preservatives due to the potential of causing either acute or long-term adverse effects.

- Inaccuracy in various doses may arise due to the patient measuring the dose with a household measuring device (e.g., a teaspoon). A teaspoonful is supposed to be equivalent to 5 mL, but a "standard" teaspoon is not sold as a "standard" measuring device. Some people think that a teaspoon is the smallest spoon in the kitchen, whereas others may think that a teaspoon is an average-sized spoon. A few years ago, a study was conducted by the outpatient department of a hospital to determine the perception of a teaspoonful dose by an average patient. Patients were given a measured amount of a liquid formulation with instructions to take 1 teaspoonful dose twice a day for 10 days and bring the bottle containing unused formulation and also the teaspoon used for measuring the dose back to the hospital. The results demonstrated that the volume of a teaspoonful perceived by the patients ranged from 2 mL (less than ½ teaspoon) to more than 7 mL (almost 1½ teaspoons).
- Oral liquid dosage forms are bulkier and heavier to carry than oral solid dosage forms and necessitate the use of a measuring device (e.g., a teaspoon). Carrying a bottle containing a liquid medication as well as a teaspoon is considered cumbersome by many people, and this may lead to reduced patient compliance in taking the medication.
- Many interactions arise because of changes in solubility produced by mixing solutions or solvent alterations.

Solid Dosage Forms

Solid dosage forms in current use include powders, granules, capsules, and tablets. Powders and granules constitute a very small portion of the solid dosage forms dispensed today. Capsules and tablets have gained popularity for the following reasons:

- They are easy to package, transport, store, and dispense.
- They offer convenience for self-medication.
- They are largely devoid of taste and odor.
- They are more stable than other solid dosage forms.
- They are predivided dosage forms and, therefore, provide an accurate dose.
- They are especially suited for those drugs that are not stable in liquid form and, therefore, provide a longer shelf life for such drugs.
- They are more suited for the formulation of sustained and delayed release of medication because controlled-release techniques are generally more applicable to solid dosage forms than to liquid dosage forms.

Powders

Powders have certain inherent advantages. For example, they give the physician free choice of selecting drugs, amount of drug in each dose, and the amount of powder to be contained in each dose. They permit the administration of a large "bulk" of a medicinal; and they may be administered as a suspension if the patient has difficulty swallowing a tablet or a capsule. However, a powder is not the dosage form of choice for drugs that have an unpleasant taste or unacceptable odor or those are not stable when exposed to atmospheric conditions.

Powders are prescribed for both internal use and external application. When intended for internal use, powders may be prescribed as bulk powders, dispersible powders, or divided powders. Powders prescribed for external use are generally dispensed as dusting powders.

Bulk Powders Bulk powders are supplied as multidose preparations. The dose is measured by the patient. This dosage form is used for drugs that are administered in a relatively large dose, those that have very low toxicity, and those for which a slight variation in the amount of each dose administered does not have a major influence on the therapeutic effect of the drug. These slight variations occur because of the variation in dose weight inherent in domestic methods of measurement (e.g., with a household teaspoon). Also, such measurements are volumetric. Therefore, the weight of powder in each dose will vary with the bulk **density** of the powder and the degree of fill (depending on whether level or heaped measures are used). The bulk density of a powder is a measure of the weight of powder per unit volume.

density weight per unit volume

Antacids are frequently prescribed as bulk powders. Minor differences in the amount of antacid ingested by the patient is of little consequence. Antacids contain substances such as aluminum hydroxide, calcium or magnesium carbonate, magnesium trisilicate, and sodium bicarbonate. Other drugs that may be prescribed as a bulk powder are those for which small variations in the drug dose do not have a major influence on the therapeutic effect of the drug.

Bulk powders may also be used as antiseptics or cleansing agents for a body cavity. For example, tooth powders generally contain a soft soap or detergent and a mild abrasive. Similarly, douche powders are products that are completely soluble and are most commonly intended for vaginal use, although they may also be formulated for nasal (nose), otic (ear), or ophthalmic (eye) use.

Dispersible Powders Dispersible powders are readily wetted by water to form an extemporaneous suspension for oral administration. The quantity contained in a dispersible powder may be enough for a single dose or it may contain a sufficient amount to last 2 to 3 days. Important aspects of a dispersible powder formulation are that the powder, upon suspension in the liquid vehicle, settles slowly and that foam is not produced.

For powders that are not wetted by the liquid easily, a wetting agent may be used. A **wetting agent** is a substance that helps to moisten the particles in a powder. Sodium lauryl sulfate and synthetic surface active agents are generally used as wetting agents. If a wetting agent is used, it must be relatively free from any toxicity.

wetting agent a substance that moistens the particles in a powder

Note that dispersible powders are used for substances that are unstable in the presence of water and, therefore, cannot be formulated as liquid dosage forms.

Dusting Powders Dusting powders are locally applied nontoxic preparations that are intended to have no systemic action; that is, they are not absorbed into blood circulation. They are dispensed in a very fine state of subdivision to enhance their effectiveness and minimize irritation. Commercial dusting powders are available in sifter-top cans, in sterile envelopes, or as an aerosol in a pressurized container. Foot powders, talcum powders, and antiperspirants available as aerosols are generally more expensive than those marketed in nonaerosol containers, but they offer the advantage of protection of the powder from air moisture and contamination, as well as convenience of application.

Absorbent powders are intended to absorb secretions and excretions on the surface of the skin from superficial infections. They usually contain starch, often with zinc oxide, kaolin, or talc.

Antifungal substances, such as salicylic acid and zinc undecylenate, are applied as powders diluted with starch, kaolin, or talc. Insecticides, such as chlorophenothane and benzene hexachloride, are incorporated in dusting powders for the destruction of lice, fleas, ticks, etc.

hygroscopic moisture absorbing

volatile evaporates at low temperature

Divided Powders Divided powders are dispensed in individual doses. To achieve accuracy, each dose is individually weighed, transferred to a powder paper, and the powder paper is folded. Divided powders containing **hygroscopic** and **volatile** drugs are packaged in waxed paper, then double wrapped with a bond paper to improve the appearance of the completed powder. Hygroscopic substances are those substances that absorb moisture when the substance is exposed to humid air. Examples of hygroscopic substances include calcium chloride, ephedrine sulfate, hydrastine, hyoscyamine, lithium bromide, pepsin, phenobarbital sodium, physostigmine, pilocarpine, potassium citrate, and sodium iodide. Volatile substances are those substances that evaporate at very low temperatures, such as room temperature. Examples of volatile substances include alcohol, chloral hydrate, and peppermint oil. Hygroscopic and volatile powders may also be dispensed in metal foils, small heat-seal plastic bags, or other containers that restrict the passage of air through them.

Granules

granule a very small pill, usually gelatin or sugar coated, containing a drug to be given in a small dose

Granules are small, irregular particles. They are used as effervescent granules or they may be marketed for therapeutic purposes. Effervescent granules derive their name from the fact that they produce effervescence when the granules come into contact with water. Effervescent granules are formulated to contain a carbon dioxide–producing combination of a weak acid and a weak base (alkali), in addition to the active therapeutic ingredient(s). On solution in water, carbon dioxide is released as a result of the acid–base reaction causing effervescence, which serves to mask the taste of salty and bitter medications.

The base usually employed in effervescent granules is sodium bicarbonate. The weak acid used in these granules may be citric acid, tartaric acid, or sodium biphosphate. In most effervescent granules a combination of citric acid and tartaric acid is used rather than using either acid alone. When tartaric acid is used alone, the resulting granules readily lose their firmness and crumble. The use of citric acid as the sole acid results in a sticky mixture that is difficult to granulate. The combination of citric acid and tartaric acid results in granules that are neither too sticky nor too soft. Effervescent granules also offer the advantage of quick dissolution of the active ingredient(s) contained in the formulation. Laxative salts, such as magnesium and sodium sulfate, are frequently formulated as effervescent granules.

Capsules

capsule a soluble container enclosing a drug

Capsules are solid dosage forms in which the drug is enclosed in a "shell" of a suitable form of gelatin (**Figure 14-3**). Mothes and Dublanc, two Frenchmen, are generally credited with the invention of gelatin capsules in 1834. The two-piece

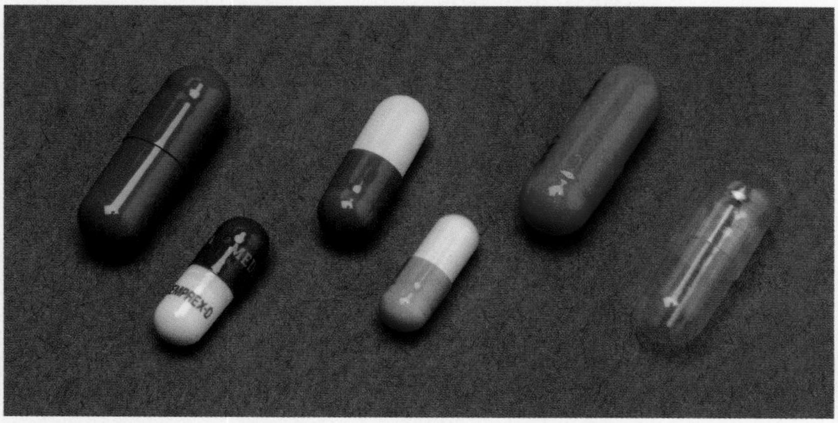

FIGURE 14-3 Hard gelatin capsules.

telescoping capsule was invented by James Murdock of London in 1848 and patented in England in 1865.

Advantages of Capsules Capsule dosage forms offer a wide variety of advantages. Some of these, not necessarily in the order cited, are as follows:

- It is easy to carry the day's supply.
- They are easy to swallow.
- It is easy to identify the product due to the availability of capsules in wide range of colors.
- They are pharmaceutically elegant.
- It is easy to mask undesirable tastes or odors of active ingredients because the shell containing the active ingredient is tasteless.
- They offer flexibility when combining drugs.
- They can be economically produced in large quantities.

Upon administration, the gelatin shell of the capsules softens and begins to partially dissolve within 10 to 20 minutes after the capsule is swallowed, releasing the drug. The capsule shell is eventually digested by proteolytic enzymes and absorbed. Since the capsule shell may not dissolve completely in the gastric fluid, capsules should not be used for substances that may irritate the gastric mucosa or for very soluble compounds. Examples of these compounds include potassium chloride, calcium chloride, potassium bromide, or ammonium chloride. In these cases, when the partially dissolved capsule comes in contact with the stomach wall, the concentrated solution may cause localized irritation and gastric distress.

The capsule dosage form is available as hard gelatin capsules and soft gelatin capsules. Hard gelatin capsules are generally used for dry powders. The contents of these capsules may range from 50 mg to 1 g of powder per capsule (**Figure 14-4**). Some manufacturers prefer to seal their capsules to prevent loss of the drug as a result of accidental opening, to discourage easy removal of the contents, and to safeguard against potential tampering. Soft gelatin capsules, also known as *soft-shell* or *soluble elastic capsules*, have a one-piece construction with the liquid fill material literally wrapped inside a sealed, gelatin matrix. The contents of a soft gelatin capsule range from 1 minim (drop) to almost 3 mL. The capsule may be spherical (pearls) or ovoid (globules) in shape.

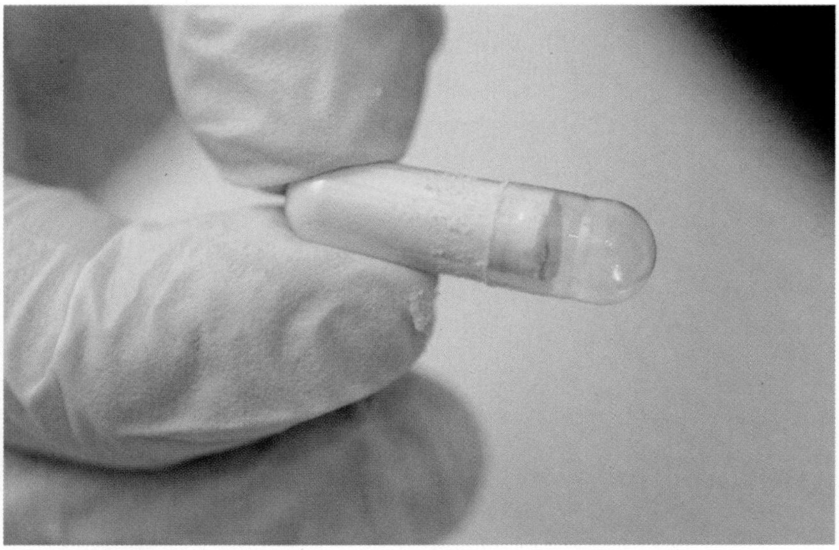

FIGURE 14-4 Hard gelatin capsule after being filled using the punch method.

Hard Gelatin Capsules Hard gelatin capsules are a two-piece capsule manufactured as empty shells (**Figure 14-5**). After manufacture, the capsule shells are filled either mechanically or manually. Historically, hard gelatin capsules for human use have been available in various lengths, diameters, and capacities. Currently, they are available in eight different sizes. These are numbered as follows: 000, 00, 0, 1, 2, 3, 4, and 5 (**Figure 14-6**). Capsule size 000 is the largest and capsule size 5 is the smallest size. Capsule size 000 is generally too large to be conveniently swallowed by a patient. However, this capsule size may be used in cases where the contents of the capsule are emptied and mixed with a liquid (e.g., orange juice) or food (e.g., applesauce). The most commonly employed capsules for humans range in size from size 0 to size 5. Capsule size 00 is the largest size acceptable for swallowing to most patients. This size is used when the required contents of a capsule cannot be accommodated in a smaller capsule. Some patients, especially senior citizens, may find the smaller capsules (size Nos. 5 and 4) somewhat difficult to handle.

The numerical designations of the capsule size are not based on any mathematical or scientific basis, and do not reflect the capacity of the particular capsule. An arbitrary numerical designation was used when the first manufacturer of the empty gelatin capsules marketed its product, and this designation has been used ever since. Eli Lilly and Parke-Davis were the original pioneers in the manufacture of empty gelatin capsules, and both companies have maintained this designation system. In recent years, empty hard gelatin capsules have been marketed by many other manufacturers. Although most of the manufacturers have continued to follow the original numerical designation and almost original capsule volume for each capsule size, some manufacturers have not. Since the empty gelatin capsules are manufactured by various manufacturers, the fill volume of capsules (capacity) of the same designated size is not necessarily identical. Therefore, the volume of powder

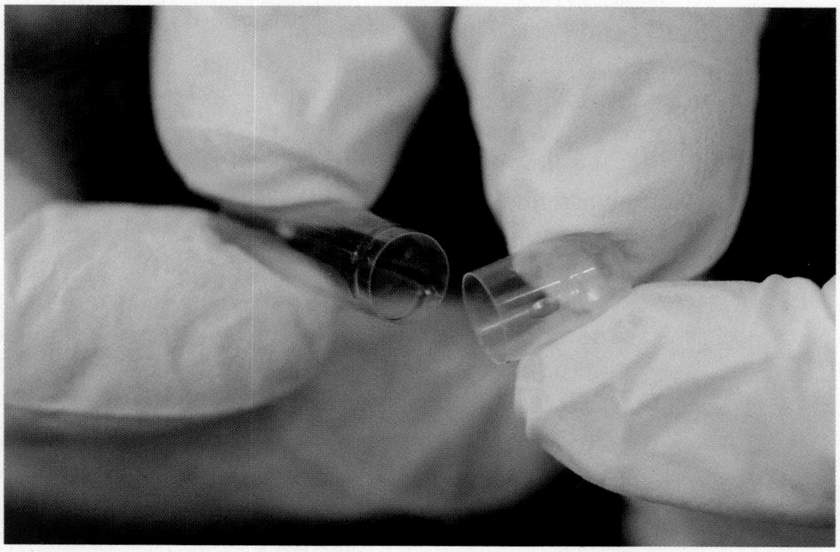

FIGURE 14-5 Notice the two separate pieces of the hard gelatin capsule.

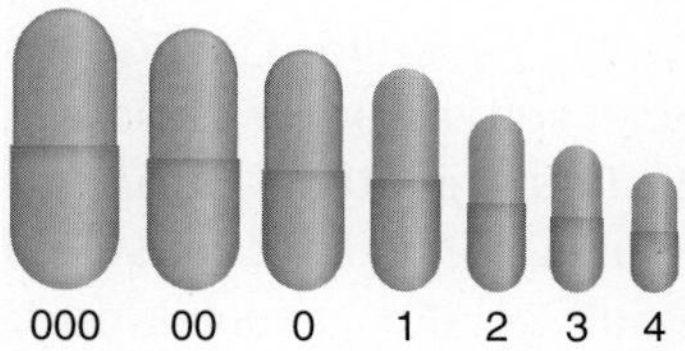

FIGURE 14-6 Various capsule sizes.

TABLE 14-2 Weight of Powder for Different Capsule Sizes

	AVERAGE WEIGHT OF POWDER (MG) IN EACH CAPSULE SIZE							
POWDER	000	00	0	1	2	3	4	5
Acetaminophen	1100	750	540	420	310	240	180	130
Ascorbic acid	1420	980	700	520	400	310	220	130
Aspirin	975	650	490	325	260	195	130	65
Calcium carbonate	1140	790	600	460	350	280	200	120
Calcium lactate	800	570	460	330	260	210	160	110
Corn starch	1150	800	580	440	340	270	200	130
Lactose	1250	850	600	460	350	280	210	140
Sodium bicarbonate	1430	975	715	510	390	325	260	130

that can be found in a given capsule size varies from manufacturer to manufacturer. Note, however, that the weight of powder that can be accommodated in a given capsule size depends on two factors: (1) the density of the powder being placed in the empty capsule and (2) the degree to which the powder can be compacted. A small-sized capsule can accommodate a much larger weight of a dense powder, but it will hold only a smaller weight of a much lighter (less dense) powder.

Empty gelatin capsules for veterinary use are available in three sizes. These are designated No. 10, No. 11, and No.12. Veterinarians refer to No. 10 capsules as 1-oz capsules, No. 11's as 0.5-oz capsules, and No. 12's as 0.25-oz capsules. In recent years, some manufacturers have developed empty gelatin capsules of varying sizes to meet the needs of researchers using small animals (rabbits, guinea pigs, rats, etc.) or doing clinical research involving therapeutic comparative evaluation of two or more drugs.

Table 14-2 shows the weight of different powders that can be used to fill gelatin capsules intended for human use.

The moisture content of a hard gelatin capsule ranges between 10% and 15%. Therefore, hard gelatin capsules should be stored in tight containers and under controlled conditions of relative humidity. Less than 10% moisture in a capsule tends to make the capsules brittle, and moisture content greater than 15% makes them stick to each other.

Empty gelatin capsules are manufactured by dipping thin cylindrical rods in a solution of gelatin in water. The rods are removed quickly and the gelatin solution adhering to the rods is dried. The capsules thus obtained are transparent. Capsules are usually colored by including a dye in the gelatin solution during manufacture of empty capsules. Colored capsules are used either for aesthetic reasons or to make them distinctive. Incorporation of titanium dioxide in gelatin solution makes the capsules opaque. Addition of sucrose in the gelatin solution increases the hardness of the capsule shell, and incorporation of sulfur dioxide results in transparent capsules.

Soft Gelatin Capsules Soft gelatin capsules are used when the ingredient in a capsule is a liquid. The liquid should be nonaqueous because the presence of water can soften and/or dissolve the gelatin shell. Soft gelatin capsules are filled with their liquid contents during the manufacture of the capsules. Unlike hard gelatin capsules, soft gelatin capsules cannot be filled after they have been manufactured.

Soft gelatin capsules do not come in standard sizes. They are more elastic than hard gelatin capsules, and contain a relatively larger moisture content

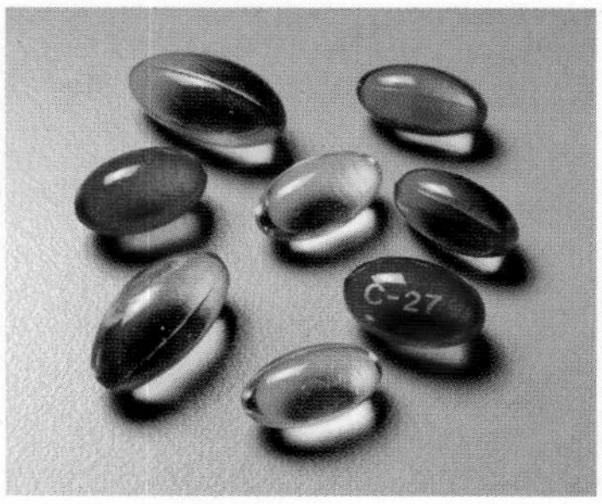

FIGURE 14-7 Soft gelatin capsules.

(**Figure 14-7**). Oil-soluble products, such as vitamin E, or oily solutions of drugs are usually marketed in soft gelatin capsules.

Quality Control All capsule dosage forms must meet USP standards for potency (test for content uniformity), dose contained in each capsule (weight variation test), release of drug from the dosage form (disintegration test), and rate of release of drug from the formulation (dissolution test). If a batch does not meet any one of these tests, the batch cannot be released for sale. In almost all cases, when a batch fails to meet these requirements, the entire batch has to be destroyed.

Tablets

tablet a solid dosage form of varying weight, size, and shape that contains a medicinal substance

Tablets are solid pharmaceutical dosage forms prepared either by compression or by molding. They are the most popular of all the medicinal preparations intended for oral use. They offer the advantages of accuracy and compactness of dosage, portability of the dosage form, convenience of self-administration, and blandness of taste.

Tablets are available in various shapes and sizes. Although most frequently discoid in form, tablets may be round, oval, oblong, cylindrical, or triangular (**Figure 14-8**). Manufacturers generally add a colorant to a tablet formulation either for identification or for aesthetic purposes. Some tablets are scored so that they may be easily broken in halves or in quarters. However, some tablets (e.g., sustained-action, extended-release, or controlled-release tablets) should never be broken or crushed unless directed by the manufacturer to do so. This is because the technology used in the manufacture of such tablets may not warrant their breaking or crushing. A majority of tablet dosage forms are embossed with the name of the manufacturer or a tablet code number.

Classification of Tablets Depending on their method of production, tablets are classified as molded tablets or compressed tablets. Molded tablets were originally

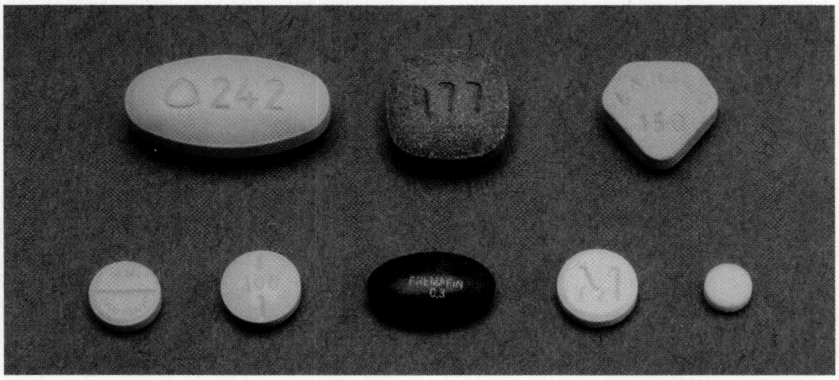

FIGURE 14-8 Various tablet shapes.

made from moist materials on a triturate mold. Later on, molded tablets were made by compression on a tablet machine. Such tablets were intended to be completely and rapidly soluble.

Compressed tablets are formed by compression in a tablet machine and are made from powdered, crystalline, or granular material either alone or in combination with excipients necessary to formulate a tablet. Excipients are inert materials and do not possess any therapeutic activity. Most tablet formulations contain two types of excipients: (1) those that are necessary to formulate a tablet dosage form and (2) those that are included in the formulation for aesthetic purposes or to make the product more acceptable to the patient.

Examples of some of the nonessential ingredients included in a tablet formulation are the following:

- *Colorants* may be added to a formulation to make the tablet attractive in appearance or to impart identification characteristics to the product. Coloring agents used in pharmaceutical preparations must be approved by the FDA.
- *Flavoring agents* or *sweeteners* may be included to make the product more acceptable in, for example, chewable tablets. Flavoring agents may be natural (e.g., mint, lemon, chocolate, vanilla) or artificial (e.g., banana or bubblegum).
- A *polymer coating* may be applied to the finished product to make the tablet look glossy and shiny or to aid in ease of swallowing the tablet. Some tablets are coated with a polymer to resist or prevent the release of drug in the stomach. Such coatings are called *enteric coatings*. Enteric-coatings prevent the release of drug in the stomach. (The term *enteric* means "of or relating to the small intestine.") This is done for those drugs that are either unstable in the gastric environment, or may cause gastric irritation and distress. Ecotrin is an example of an enteric-coated medication containing aspirin.

The essential ingredients in a tablet formulation are those that are necessary for the successful production of the tablet dosage form. These include the following:

- *Drug.* Except for placebo tablets, all tablet formulations must contain the active ingredient.
- *Diluent.* A diluents is an inert ingredient that adds bulk to the tablet formulation. This ingredient is essential for those tablets that contain a very small amount of drug. Without the diluent, the tablet would be so small that it could not be made and could not be handled by the pharmacist or the patient. For example, 1 teaspoonful of diazepam powder contains enough drug to make 1,000 tablets each containing 5 mg of the drug. Examples of drugs that have a very small dose include the following: digoxin, levothyroxine, prednisone, and chlorpheniramine. Examples of diluents used in tablet formulations include lactose, starch, and cellulose esters.
- *Binder.* A binder is a sticky substance that is used to hold (bind) the powders together, so that the powders do not segregate (un-mix) during the process of tablet manufacture. Examples of binders used in a tablet formulation include gelatin, starch, and acacia.
- *Disintegrant.* The function of a disintegrant is to help disintegrate (break down) the tablet when the tablet comes into contact with the body's gastric fluids. It will essentially undo what the binder does to the tablet

formulation. The most commonly used disintegrant is starch. Recently, some manufacturers of tablet dosage forms have begun to use disintegrants that have the ability to disintegrate the tablet in the mouth as soon as it comes into contact with saliva. These tablets have been variously advertised as rapidly disintegrating, quick dissolving, or rapid release.

- *Lubricant.* A lubricant is included in the tablet formulation to facilitate the flow of the tablet formulation through the tablet machine and also to prevent the formulation from sticking to the dies and punches of the machine during tablet compression. Magnesium stearate is the most commonly used lubricant in a tablet formulation. Stearates in general help grease tablet machines to speed up production of the tablets.

Types of Compressed Tablets

Among the various types of compressed tablets currently on the market, the following are the most common:

1. *Standard compressed tablets.* These are the conventional tablets we are all familiar with and are compressed on a tablet machine.
2. *Enteric-coated tablets.* These are compressed tablets coated with a substance (polymer) that resists solution in the gastric fluid, but dissolves in the intestinal fluids, thereby allowing the medication to be released in the intestinal tract. In the manufacture of majority of enteric-coated tablets, a coating of an enteric polymer (a polymer that will not dissolve in the acidic environment of the stomach) is applied to the tablet after the tablet formulation is prepared as a compressed tablet (**Figure 14-9**). Therefore, if the enteric-coated tablet is broken in half or crushed as a powder, the enteric coating is destroyed and the medication is released in the stomach, thereby defeating the purpose of enteric coating.
3. *Sugar-coated tablets.* These are compressed tablets that are coated with sugar after the tablet has been compressed. Sugar coating is used to cover the objectionable taste or odor of a medicinal compound and to protect sensitive materials subject to deterioration due to light, air, oxygen, etc. However, sugar is a hygroscopic substance that can absorb moisture, resulting in tablets sticking to each other if the tablets are stored in humid conditions. Also, the coating operation is very time consuming.
4. *Film-coated tablets.* These are compressed tablets covered with a thin film of a water-soluble polymeric material. Such coverings impart the same general characteristics as a sugar coating and the coating operation is relatively simple, less time consuming, and much more economical.

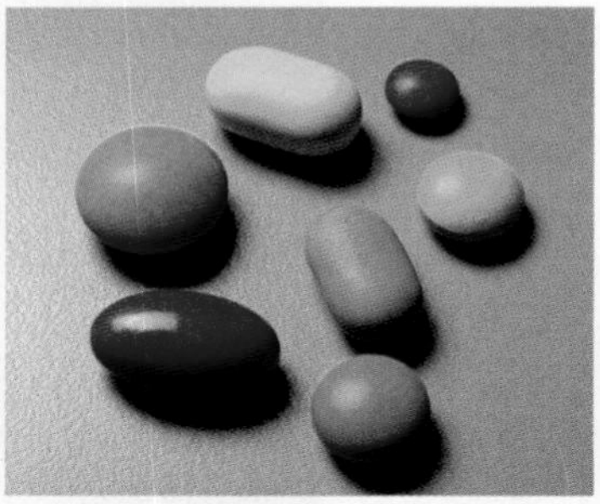

FIGURE 14-9 Enteric-coated tablets.

sublingual under the tongue

multiple compressed tablets tablets that are layered in multiple compression cycles

5. *Sublingual or buccal tablets.* These types of tablets are intended to be inserted below the tongue (**sublingual** tablets as shown in **Figure 14-10**) or in the buccal pouch (buccal tablets) where the active ingredient may be directly absorbed through the oral mucosa. This dosage form is primarily used for those drugs that cannot be administered through the gastrointestinal tract due to stability problems. The drug must dissolve in the mouth quickly and should be absorbed very rapidly. Nitroglycerin is an example of such a drug.
6. *Multiple compressed tablets.* These tablets are made using more than one compression cycle. **Multiple compressed tablets** may be layered tablets or press-coated tablets. Layered tablets are prepared by compressing an additional tablet granulation on a previously compressed tablet. This tablet is in fact a two-layered tablet. The two layers may be of different colors to make the tablet look attractive and for ease of identification of the tablet. Press-coated tablets are prepared by compressing another layer of tablet around a preformed compressed tablet. Press-coated tablets are often referred to as "tablet within a tablet."
7. *Miscellaneous tablets.* Miscellaneous tablets are those that are specially formulated or intended for a specific function. The five common types of miscellaneous tablets are:
   a. *Chewable tablets.* These are compressed tablets that are meant to be chewed rather than swallowed. Some antacid tablets and vitamin C are marketed as chewable tablets. Chewable tablets are often intended for children. They contain a sweetening agent and a flavoring agent to make the product attractive for chewing. Mannitol is generally used as a sweetener because it has a sweet taste and also produces a cooling effect in the mouth.
   b. *Delayed-release tablets.* These are special formulations of tablets in which the active ingredient is released some time after the tablet is ingested. Enteric-coated tablets fall under this category,
   c. *Lozenges.* Also known as *troches* or *pastilles*, these are discoid-shaped solids containing the medicinal agent in a suitable, flavored base. Lozenges are meant to be placed in the mouth where they dissolve slowly, liberating the active ingredient.
   d. *Pellets.* As used currently, the term *pellet* signifies small cylinders that are meant to be implanted under the skin, or in the subcutaneous tissue for prolonged and continuous absorption of potent hormones, such as testosterone or estradiol.

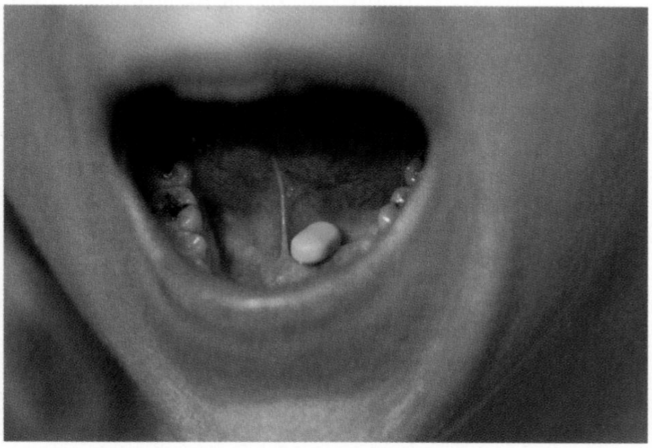

FIGURE 14-10 An example of sublingual tablet administration.

e. *Sustained-release tablets:* These tablets are designed to release their active ingredient for a prolonged period of time. These products are also variously described as *timed release*, *long acting*, *prolonged action*, or some similar term implying an extended period of action for a given drug. **Table 14-3** lists some of the terms (names) that have been used to describe commercial sustained-release dosage forms. The use of some of these terms is no longer very common because the current USP terminology embodies these terms into one term: *extended release*.

Note that, based on the release characteristics of a drug from an oral dosage form, the USP recognizes and defines two terms in solid dosage form technology: (1) immediate-release dosage forms and (2) modified-release dosage forms. Immediate-release dosage forms are those that release their active ingredient soon after ingestion; immediate-release tablets are designed to disintegrate and release their contents almost immediately after the tablet is ingested. These tablets do not contain any special rate-controlling features, such as special coatings or other special techniques that may control the release of active ingredient(s) from the dosage form.

The USP defines modified-release tablets as dosage forms for which the drug-release characteristics (i.e., the time and location of drug release) are chosen to accomplish convenience or therapeutic objectives that are not offered by conventional dosage forms such as solutions or ointments, or dissolving dosage forms such as immediate-release tablets. The USP defines two types of modified-release dosage forms: delayed-release and extended release.

delayed-release dosage form specifically formulated pharmaceutical dosage form in which the active ingredient is released at a constant rate over a specific time period

extended-release dosage form specifically formulated pharmaceutical dosage form in which the active ingredient is gradually released over a predetermined time period

Delayed-release dosage forms are those dosage forms that release their drug at a time other than promptly after administration. Enteric-coated dosage forms are classified as delayed-release dosage forms.

Extended-release dosage forms are formulated in such a manner as to make the contained medicament available over an extended period of time following ingestion. Expressions such as *prolonged action*, *repeat action*, and *sustained*

TABLE 14-3 Some Names Associated with Oral Extended-Release Dosage Forms

Constant release	Prolonged action
Continuous action	Prolonged release
Continuous release	Protracted release
Controlled action	Repeat action
Controlled release	Repository
Delayed action	Retard
Delayed release	Slow acting
Depot action	Slow release
Extended action	Slowly acting
Extended release	Sustained action
Gradual release	Sustained release
Gradual action	Timed coat
Long acting	Timed disintegration
Long-term release	Timed release
Programmed release	

release have also been used to describe such dosage forms. However, the term *extended release* is used for pharmacopeial purposes and designates the pharmacopeial description of such tablets.

The extended-release dosage form allows at least a twofold reduction in dosing frequency as compared to conventional-release (immediate-release) dosage forms. For example, if the frequency of administration of the conventional-release (immediate-release) dosage form is every 4 hours, then the frequency of administration of the extended-release dosage form must not be less than every 8 hours. Compared to conventional-release (immediate-release) dosage forms, extended-release dosage forms offer many advantages, including the following:

- Elimination of peak and valley levels of concentration of drug in blood during chronic administration
- Reduction in adverse side effects because of fewer peak concentrations of the drug
- Reduction in frequency of drug administration
- Enhanced patient convenience
- Enhanced patient compliance due to less frequent administration.

Extended-release tablets can be prepared using a variety of techniques and technologies. Breaking the tablet in half or crushing the tablet to obtain the powder has the potential of destroying the extended-release characteristic of the tablet.

To be a successful extended-release dosage form, the drug should possess the following characteristics:

- It should not be absorbed either very rapidly or very slowly.
- It should be administered in relatively small doses and possess a good margin of safety.
- It should be absorbed uniformly from the gastrointestinal tract.
- It should be used in the treatment of chronic rather than acute conditions.

All tablet dosage forms, immediate release as well as modified release, must conform to the tests indicated in the USP monograph for the particular tablet dosage form. The requirements for each test (content uniformity, weight variation, disintegration test, and dissolution test) depend on the nature of drug and the type of tablet dosage form.

Semisolid Dosage Forms

Semisolid dosage forms are those dosage forms that are too thick or viscous to be considered a liquid dosage form and yet not solid enough to be considered a solid dosage form. The semisolid dosage forms discussed here are intended for topical application. They may be applied to the skin, placed on the mucous membrane of the eye, or used in one of the body cavities (e.g., nasal, rectal, or vaginal). The most commonly used semisolid dosage forms are ointments, pastes, creams, and suppositories.

Ointments, Creams, and Pastes

ointment an oil-based, semisolid, external dosage form, usually containing a medicinal substance

Ointments, creams, and pastes are semisolid preparations used mainly for local application to the skin or mucous membrane. Very few ointments are intended to produce systemic effects due to absorption of the drug into the bloodstream. Nitroglycerin is the most common example of an ointment that is applied to the skin for absorption into the bloodstream. Pastes are similar to ointments and creams, except that pastes contain more solids, and therefore are firmer (thicker) than ointments and creams. Ointments and creams that contain a medicinal agent (therapeutic ingredient) are called medicated ointments or medicated creams. Examples include nitroglycerin ointment, gentamicin sulfate ointment, nystatin cream, lidocaine ointment, and Tinactin cream. They are intended to deliver the drug or a therapeutic agent to the site of application. Some ointments are used for the physical effects they provide, for example, emollients, protectants, or lubricants. Most ointment bases are used unmedicated for their physical effects. Ointment bases are classified according to the relationship of water to the composition of the base used to prepare the ointment or paste. The USP classifies ointment bases into four general groups:

anhydrous containing no water

hydrous combined with water; forming a compound with one or more molecules of water

1. *Absorption bases.* The term *absorption* in absorption bases does not signify absorption of the drug. Absorption bases have the capability of absorbing water or aqueous solutions, hence the name "absorption" bases. There are two types of absorption bases: those that are essentially **anhydrous** in nature and those that are **hydrous**. Anhydrous absorption bases are contain no water. Hydrous absorption bases contain a certain degree of water. Because anhydrous absorption bases do not contain water, they are capable of absorbing more water or aqueous solutions than do hydrous absorption bases. However, both types of bases are insoluble in water and are not water washable. These bases are used when either water or an aqueous solution must be incorporated into an ointment. Examples of anhydrous absorption bases include Aquaphor, Aquabase, lanolin (or wool fat), and Polysorb. Included in the examples of hydrous absorption bases are cold cream, Eucerin, Nivea, and hydrous lanolin (or hydrous wool fat).
2. *Water-removable bases.* These bases are oil-in-water emulsions. Because the external phase of these bases is water, they can be easily washed off of the skin. Hence, they are also referred to as *water-washable bases*. These bases resemble creams in physical appearance. Examples of water-removable bases include hydrophilic ointment USP, Dermabase, Velvachol, and vanishing cream.
3. *Oleaginous bases.* Oleaginous bases contain a mixture of high-molecular-weight and low-molecular-weight hydrocarbons. Hence, they are also termed hydrocarbon bases. High-molecular-weight hydrocarbons are solids, and low-molecular-weight hydrocarbons are liquids. A mixture of these two types of hydrocarbons results into a semisolid product that is useful as an ointment base.

   Hydrocarbon bases are oily in nature, and are insoluble in water. These bases do not contain water, nor do they absorb water. Therefore, these ointment bases are not water washable. Upon application to the skin, they have an emollient effect and protect the escape of moisture from the skin. Therefore, they are effective as occlusive dressings. Because these bases are hydrocarbons in nature, they do not accept aqueous solutions. As a rule, liquids are generally not added to these bases for fear of making the final product too fluid. Examples of oleaginous bases include petrolatum USP, yellow ointment USP, white ointment USP, Plastibase, and Vaseline.
4. *Water-soluble bases.* Water-soluble bases may be essentially anhydrous or they may contain water. In either case, they absorb water to the point of solubility. Thus they are water soluble and completely water washable. Water-soluble bases are often referred to as greaseless bases because they do not contain oily components. Polyethylene glycol ointment NF is an example of a water-soluble base.

Suppositories

suppository a solid dosage form for insertion into a body cavity (e.g., rectum, vagina, urethral), where it melts at body temperature

Suppositories are solid unit dosage forms intended for the application of medication to any of several body orifices, namely, the rectum, vagina, or urethra. These dosage forms may exhibit their therapeutic activity locally or systematically, either by melting at body temperature or by dissolving in the aqueous secretions of the mucous membrane of the body cavity. Suppositories intended for administration via the vagina or the urethra are sometimes referred to as "inserts," particularly when the suppository is made by compression as a specially shaped tablet. Melting or dissolution of suppositories in the secretions of the body cavity usually releases the medication over a prolonged period of time. The commonly used suppository bases can be oleaginous (or oily), water soluble, or hydrophilic (water-loving) solids. Examples of oleaginous bases are cocoa butter (also known as theobroma oil) and mixtures of synthetic triglycerides. Examples of water-soluble bases are glycerinated gelatin, polyethylene, and glycol polymers. An example of a hydrophilic solid is polyethylene sorbitan monostearate, polyoxyl 40 stearate, or a commercial product sold under the trade name Tween 40.

Rectal suppositories for adults are usually between 2.5 and 3.5 cm (1 to 1.4 in.) long. They weigh about 2 g each, and have a tapered shape. The largest diameter of a rectal suppository is about 1.2 to 1.3 cm (about 1/2 in.), usually tapered to about 6 to 7 mm (about 1/4 in.). For pediatric use, the diameter and length are reduced, as is the weight—to about 1 g.

Rectal suppositories are usually prepared using cocoa butter as the suppository base. Upon insertion, cocoa butter melts at body temperature, releasing its active ingredient. Because cocoa butter melts at or near body temperature (37°C or 98°F), suppositories prepared using cocoa butter must be stored in a refrigerator. Examples of suppositories intended for local action include bisacodyl, hydrocortisone, and mesalamine suppositories. Examples of suppositories intended for systemic effect include chlorpromazine, hydromorphone, and promethazine hydrochloride suppositories.

Vaginal suppositories vary in shape from globular or ovoid to modified conical shapes. They weigh between 3 and 5 g and are used primarily for local effects. Vaginal suppositories are usually prepared using polyethylene glycol as the suppository base. Polyethylene glycol is water soluble and it dissolves in vaginal fluids, releasing the therapeutic ingredient into the vaginal environment. Suppositories prepared using polyethylene glycol need not be stored in the refrigerator because the melting point of polyethylene is much higher than that of cocoa butter. When vaginal inserts are prescribed, the pharmacist should instruct the patient to dip the insert into water quickly before insertion to avoid stinging. Examples of vaginal suppositories and inserts include AVC suppositories (sulfanilamide), Monistat 7 suppositories (miconazole), and Semicid vaginal contraceptive inserts (nonoxynol-9).

Urethral suppositories, like vaginal suppositories, are primarily used for local action. These are slender rods, from 3 to 5 mm (less than 0.25 in.) in diameter. The female urethral suppositories range in length from 6 to 7.5 cm (about 2.5 to 3 in.), and the male urethral suppositories range in length between 10 and 15 cm (4 and 6 in.). Although somewhat flexible, urethral suppositories are firm enough for insertion.

Miscellaneous Dosage Forms

The dosage forms considered in this section have been classified miscellaneous for the sake of convenience. The properties associated with these dosage forms are either unique to these dosage forms or represent a combination of the properties of solid and liquid dosage forms.

Aerosols

aerosol a finely nebulized medication for inhalation therapy

Aerosols are systems consisting of a suspension of fine solid particles or liquid droplets in air or in gas. Aerosols are contained in a pressurized container, meaning that the contents contained in the aerosol container are under pressure. Pressure is applied to the aerosol system through the use of one or more propellants. A propellant is a liquid or gas that propels the contents of an aerosol from within the container into the atmosphere. The contents are released when the container is actuated by the valve assembly. The pressure exerted by the propellant(s) forces out the contents of the package through the opening of the valve. Because an aerosol dosage form is a pressurized package, it should be stored away from heat and in a cool place.

Components of Aerosols An aerosol dosage form consists of three components:

1. *Product concentrate.* The product concentrate represents the formulation, which consists of the active ingredient and other ingredients, such as buffers, isotonicity imparting ingredients, antioxidants, and preservatives, that may be necessary to formulate the product.
2. *Container.* The container used in an aerosol dosage form may be made of glass, plastic, or metal. Metal containers may be made of tin, stainless steel, or tin-coated metal. They tend to be relatively more expensive, but they can stand much higher pressures within the container than plastic containers. Plastic containers are relatively cheaper to make, but cannot withstand higher pressures and may adsorb the active ingredient or other formulation ingredients. Glass containers present fewer compatibility problems than plastic or metal containers, but glass containers are fragile and brittle and, hence, can break easily. Tin-coated metal containers are the most widely used metal containers for aerosols.

   The choice of a container for an aerosol product depends on the pressure of the formulation inside the container. The pressure inside the container is expressed in the units of pounds per square inch gauge (psig).The gauge pressure is pressure read on the gauge, which is 14.7 plus the absolute pressure in pounds per square inch (psia), where 14.7 is the absolute pressure of the atmosphere. Thus, psig = 14.7 + psia. Glass and plastic containers can withstand a maximum pressure of about 25 psig, whereas metal containers can withstand pressures of 80 psig.
3. *Propellant.* The propellant in an aerosol container is the driving force that propels the formulation from inside the container into the atmosphere. A propellant may be a gas like carbon dioxide, nitrogen, or nitrous oxide, or it may be a gas that can be liquefied under pressure or by reducing temperature. For many years, chlorofluorocarbons (CFCs; sold under the trade name Freon) were widely used as the propellant in aerosol products. CFCs are gases at room temperature, but can be liquefied by cooling below their boiling point or by compression at room temperature. These propellants have been phased out because the chlorine content in their structure was considered to be responsible for reducing the amount of ozone in the stratosphere, resulting in an increase in the amount of ultraviolet radiation reaching the earth. The increase in ultraviolet radiation has been reported to increase the incidence of skin cancer and other adverse environmental effects.

   The propellants currently used in aerosol packages are fluorocarbons that do not contain chlorine in their structures. They are organic compounds that contain carbon, hydrogen, and fluorine, but

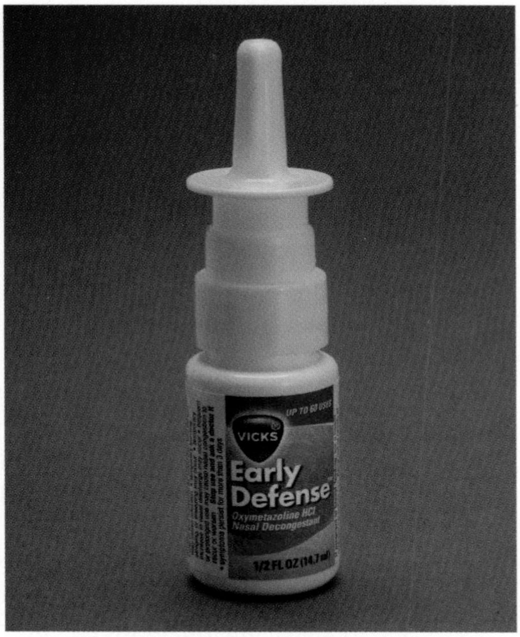

FIGURE 14-11 Nasal sprays are an example of a medicinal aerosol.

no chlorine. The most popular propellant currently in use in aerosol formulation is P-134 (tetrafluoroethane, $C_2 H_2 F_4$).

Types of Aerosols Aerosols may be classified as either pharmaceutical aerosols or medicinal aerosols. Pharmaceutical aerosols are intended for topical administration or for administration into one of the body cavities, such as the nose or the mouth (**Figure 14-11**). The advantage of a pharmaceutical aerosol is that the therapeutic agent can be applied to the desired site without the use of fingertips, making the procedure less messy than with most other types of topical preparations. Medicinal aerosols are intended both for local action in the nasal areas, the throat, and the lungs and for prompt systemic effect when absorbed into the bloodstream (e.g., from lungs—inhalation or aerosol therapy).

Advantages of Aerosols Aerosols offer convenience and ease of application. If the product is packaged under sterile conditions, sterility can be maintained without danger of contamination. The use of aerosols eliminates the irritation produced by the mechanical application of a medicinal, especially over an abraded area. Medication can also be applied to areas that are otherwise difficult to reach.

Inhalation therapy avoids the trauma of injections and reduces the potential risk of orally administered drugs decomposing in the gastrointestinal tract. Examples of drugs delivered by inhalation aerosols include albuterol, cromolyn sodium, ipratropium bromide, metaproterenol sulfate, and triamcinolone acetonide.

The particle size of therapeutic aerosols affects their clinical usefulness. Therefore, it is essential for the aerosol dosage form to be formulated with the most effective particle size. The particle size of the drug contained in aerosols is expressed in micrometers (previously referred to as microns). One centimeter is equal to 10,000 micrometers. Particles larger than 30 micrometers are most likely to be deposited in the trachea. Particles between 10 and 30 micrometers may reach the terminal bronchiole; and those between 3 and 10 micrometers may reach the alveolar duct. Smaller particles can penetrate deeper into the pulmonary tract: those between 1 and 3 micrometers may reach the alveolar sac; and particles less than 0.5 micrometer in size may reach the alveolar sac and be exhaled.

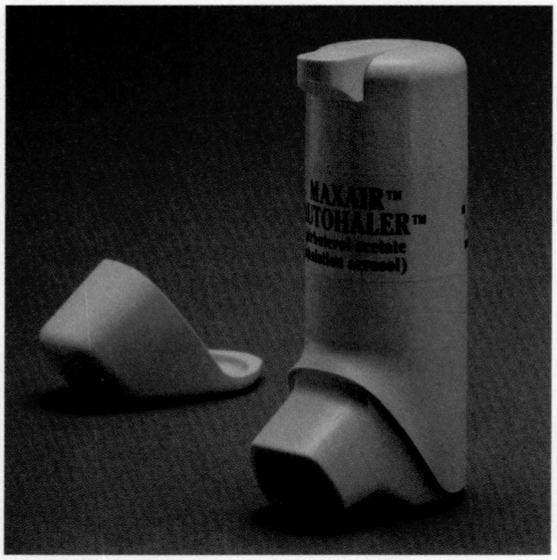

FIGURE 14-12 A metered-dose inhaler.

Metered-Dose Inhalers Metered-dose inhalers are used in inhalation therapy involving potent medications. In these devices, the amount of drug discharged from the inhaler is controlled by an auxiliary valve chamber. A fixed amount of drug is delivered with a single depression of the actuator (**Figure 14-12**). Examples of metered-dose inhalers include Advair, Aerobid, and Ventolin HFA.

A unique translingual (lingual = pertaining to the tongue) aerosol formulation of nitroglycerin (Nitrolingual Spray) permits a patient to spray droplets of nitroglycerin onto or under the tongue for acute relief of an attack of angina pectoris due to coronary artery disease. Two metered spray emissions deliver 0.4 mg of nitroglycerin. Because translingual sprays are intended to deliver the drug on the tongue, Nitrolingual Spray should not be inhaled.

Isotonic Solutions

lacrimal fluid tears
iso-osmotic having the same osmotic pressure
isotonic having the same tone

Body fluids, including blood and **lacrimal fluid** (tears), have an osmotic pressure identical to that of a 0.9% solution of sodium chloride. Thus, a 0.9% solution of sodium chloride is said to be *iso-osmotic* with physiological fluids. The term **iso-osmotic** compares the osmotic pressure of two substances. This term is often used interchangeably with the term **isotonic**, which means "having the same tone." A solution is isotonic with a living cell if there is no net gain or loss of water by the cell, or any other change in the cell, when in contact with that solution. Although most iso-osmotic solutions are isotonic, a solution that is iso-osmotic may not necessarily be isotonic. For example, a solution of boric acid is iso-osmotic with blood and lacrimal fluid; however, it is isotonic only with lacrimal fluids—not with blood. It causes hemolysis of red blood cells because the molecules of boric acid pass freely through the erythrocyte membrane regardless of concentration.

When dealing with isotonic solutions, caution must be exercised because any alteration in the composition of the solution (e.g., mixing it with another solution or diluting it with water) may affect the tonicity of the solution.

Parenteral Products

Some drugs must be administered parenterally because oral administration of these drugs either does not elicit any therapeutic effect, or if a therapeutic effect is elicited, it is less than desirable; that is, they are not therapeutically effective when administered orally. For these drugs the parenteral route of administration is one of the few routes that may be available for drug administration.

parenteral product a dosage form administered by injection

infusion the introduction of a solution into a vein by gravity or by an infusion control device or pump

Parenteral products are dosage forms that are administered by injection. Hence, they are also referred to as injectable products. The most commonly used parenteral products are administered by three routes: (1) intravenously (directly into the bloodstream) either as a rapid bolus (single) dose or as a constant infusion, (2) intramuscularly, and (3) subcutaneously. Examples of parenteral products include lidocaine intravenous injection, warfarin injection, aminophylline **infusion**, chlorpromazine intramuscular injection, and insulin subcutaneous injection (**Figure 14-13**). **Table 14-4** presents the onset of action, peak action, and duration of action of various insulin preparations.

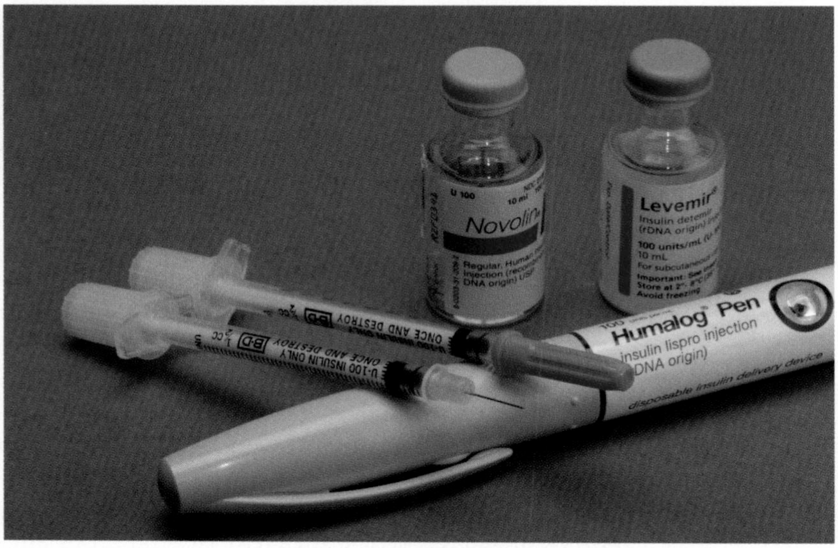

FIGURE 14-13 Insulin injections are a common parenteral product used in all types of pharmacies.

TABLE 14-4 Profiles of Insulin Activity

PREPARATION	ONSET (HR)	PEAK (HR)	DURATION (HR)
Rapid acting			
Insulin Lispro	0.25	0.5–1.0	3
Insulin Aspart	0.25	0.5–1.0	3
Short acting			
Regular insulin	0.5	2–5	5–8
Intermediate acting			
Isophane (NPH) insulin	1–2	6–10	16–20
Insulin zinc (Lente)	1–2	6–12	18–24
Long acting			
Insulin zinc extended (Ultralente)	4–6	10–18	24–28
Insulin glargine	2	None	>24
Mixtures			
Isophane/regular insulin 70/30, 50/50	7–12	16–24	–
NPL/Lispro Mix 75/25	5 min	7–12	1–24

Most parenteral products are manufactured on a large scale by the pharmaceutical industry. Many pharmacists, particularly those working in hospitals, home health care practices, or serving long-term care facilities, routinely handle and manipulate intravenous admixtures and injections. A pharmacist practicing in this specialty area has a special responsibility for understanding and implementing the standards of practice for handling sterile drug products.

Sterility is an absolute term. It means the absence of living microorganisms. A sterile product is completely devoid of living microorganisms. Depending on the nature of the active ingredient(s) and the stage at which the preparation is sterilized, a parenteral product may be sterilized by an established method that ensures the sterility of the product. The USP recognizes the following five methods for sterilization of compendial articles: (1) steam sterilization, (2) dry-heat sterilization, (3) gas sterilization, (4) sterilization by ionizing radiation, and (5) sterilization by filtration. For home-use sterile products, the USP recognizes the following two methods for sterilization: (1) sterilization by filtration and (2) terminal sterilization by moist heat. According to the USP, a home-use sterile product is a drug product requiring sterility that is prepared in and dispensed from a licensed pharmacy for intended administration by the patient or by a family member or other caregiver in a setting other than an organized, professionally staffed health care facility.

> **pyrogen** an agent that causes a rise in temperature; produced by bacteria, molds, viruses, and yeasts

Pyrogens In addition to being sterile, parenteral products must also be pyrogen-free. **Pyrogens** are products of the metabolism of microorganisms. The most potent pyrogenic substances (endotoxins) are constituents of the cell wall of gram-negative bacteria. Endotoxins are high-molecular-weight (about 20,000 daltons) lipopolysaccharides. The presence of pyrogens in parenteral preparations is considered a contamination because pyrogens should not be present in parenteral drug products. Pyrogens can be destroyed by heating at high temperatures. Glassware and equipment can be de-pyrogenated by maintaining a dry heat temperature of 180°F for 4 hours, or 250°F for 45 minutes, or 650°F for 1 minute. The usual autoclaving cycle (moist heat) does not destroy pyrogens.

The presence of pyrogens in parenteral drug products and their subsequent injection into the patient can cause fever, chills, pain in the back and legs, and malaise. The intensity of the pyrogenic response and its degree of severity are determined by the following factors:

1. Medical condition of the patient
2. Potency of the pyrogen injected
3. Amount of the pyrogen injected
4. Route of administration of the pyrogen; intrathecal is the most hazardous route, followed by intravenous, intramuscular, and the subcutaneous route.

Although pyrogenic reactions are rarely fatal, they can cause serious discomfort. In the seriously ill patient, pyrogenic reactions can cause shock-like symptoms that can be fatal.

As with any other route of drug administration, parenteral administration of a drug has some advantages and some disadvantages. In some clinical situations the advantages outweigh the disadvantages, while in other situations, neither the advantage nor the disadvantage may outweigh the other.

Advantages of Parenteral Products Among the many advantages of parenteral administration of drugs, the following are noteworthy:

- Parenteral administration provides a faster physiological or therapeutic response than can be expected by other routes of administration.

- Parenteral administration offers an alternative route of drug administration when a patient is unable to take medication by mouth (e.g., when the patient is unconscious, comatose, or cannot retain medication due to vomiting).
- Parenteral administration offers an alternative route of drug administration to protect the drug from degradation due to inactivation of the drug in the gastrointestinal tract, or first-pass metabolism by the liver.
- Parenteral administration offers an alternative route of drug administration for those drugs that are destroyed or inactivated by gastric secretions such as hydrochloric acid or enzymes.
- Parenteral administration is used to attain local effects for drugs used in dentistry and anesthesiology.
- Parenteral administration offers a route to feed patients who cannot be fed by mouth (e.g., total nutritional requirements may be provided by the parenteral route).

Disadvantages of Parenteral Products Some of the disadvantages associated with parenteral therapy include the following:

- Compared to products administered by nonparenteral routes, parenteral products are more difficult to produce.
- Parenteral products require absolute sterility and must be pyrogen-free.
- Due to stringent sterility and pyrogen-free requirements, parenteral products are much more costly to produce than nonparenteral products.
- Parenteral products require special skills, equipment, devices, and techniques for handling and administration of the product.
- Problems with dose or adverse effects associated with parenteral products may be difficult or impossible to reverse, because, once administered, a parenteral product cannot be removed from systemic circulation.
- Parenteral products may cause discomfort or pain at the site of injection.
- There is always a danger of air embolism by the intravenous route.

Gastrointestinal Therapeutic System

The gastrointestinal therapeutic system (GITS) is based on Alza Corporation's OROS (oral osmosis) design. This dosage form resembles an ordinary tablet, but the characteristics of drug release and drug delivery are very different.

The GITS operates on the principle of osmotic pressure. It consists of a drug-containing core surrounded by a semipermeable polymer membrane that is pierced by a small (0.4 mm) laser-drilled delivery orifice. Upon ingestion of the dosage form, water is osmotically drawn through the membrane from the gastrointestinal tract at a constant and controlled rate, thereby creating a drug solution inside the tablet. The influx (intake) of water pushes the drug solution out of the orifice at a constant rate.

The first product marketed in the United States based on this technology was Ciba-Geigy's Acutrim, an over-the-counter appetite suppressant. Administered once daily, this dosage form delivered 20 mg of phenylpropanolamine initially and then 55 mg released osmotically for approximately 16 hours. Other examples of products using this technology include Glucotrol XL extended-release tablets and Procardia XL extended-release tablets.

> **orally dissolving tablet (ODT)** a tablet that disintegrates rapidly when contact with saliva is made without the need for water; also known as fast dissolving

Orally Dissolving Tablets

Orally dissolving tablets (ODTs) dissolve/disintegrate rapidly in saliva without the need for water. Some tablets are designed to dissolve in saliva within a

fast-dissolving tablet a tablet that disintegrates rapidly when contact with saliva is made without the need for water; also known as orally dissolving

few seconds. These are true orally dissolving or **fast-dissolving tablets**. Others contain ingredients that enhance the rate of tablet disintegration in the mouth, and are more appropriately termed fast-disintegrating tablets. The FDA's Center for Drug Evaluation and Research, in its publication *Approved Drug Products with Therapeutic Equivalence Evaluations* (also called the *Orange Book*), defines an ODT as "a solid dosage form containing medicinal substances, which disintegrates rapidly, usually within a matter of seconds, when placed upon the tongue." The European Pharmacopoeia, however, defines a similar term, *orodisperse,* as a tablet that can be placed in the mouth where it disperses rapidly before swallowing.

Fast disintegrating tablets may take up to 1 minute to completely disintegrate. The current compendial recommendation for fast-dissolving tablets is 30 seconds for complete dissolution of the tablet. For a tablet to be considered fast dissolving or fast disintegrating, it must disintegrate in the saliva, while maintaining a pleasant taste and mouth feel, to allow maximal patient acceptability.

A major claim of some of the fast-dissolving/fast-disintegrating tablet manufacturers is that these tablets exhibit increased bioavailability of the drug compared to the traditional compressed tablets. They offer the following reasons: (1) Quick dispersion of a drug in saliva while the dosage form is still in the oral cavity can result in pregastric absorption from some formulations. Buccal, pharyngeal, and gastric regions are all areas of absorption of the many formulations. (2) Any pregastric absorption avoids first-pass metabolism and can be a great advantage in drugs that undergo a great deal of hepatic metabolism. The major advantage of these formulations is convenience. Pharmacists can expect to see an increase in the number of drug products marketed as ODT formulations. ODTs release drug in the mouth for absorption through oral mucosal tissues and through pregastric (e.g., oral cavity, pharynx, and esophagus), gastric (i.e., stomach), and postgastric (e.g., small and large intestines) segments of the gastrointestinal tract (GIT).

Recent market studies indicate that more than half of the patient population prefers ODTs to other dosage forms and most consumers would ask their physicians for ODTs (70%), purchase ODTs (70%), or prefer ODTs to regular tablets or liquids (>80%). These responses may, in part, be attributed to known ODT advantages such as ease of administration, ease of swallowing, pleasant taste, and the availability of several flavors. ODTs also offer clinical advantages such as improved safety and, in some cases, improved efficacy and other broader indications. In addition, several business needs are driving ODT technology development and the commercialization of new products such as the need for expanded product lines, improved life-cycle management, extended patent life, and marketing advantages.

The ideal characteristics of a drug for dissolution in the mouth and pregastric absorption from an ODT include the following: (1) absence of bitter taste, (2) a lower dose (less than 20 mg), (3) good solubility in water and saliva, and (4) ability to permeate oral mucosal tissue. In contrast, the following characteristics may render a drug unsuitable for delivery as an ODT: (1) It has a short half-life and frequent dosing; (2) it is very bitter or otherwise unacceptable taste because taste masking cannot be achieved, and (3) to be effective, its release must be controlled or sustained.

At present, ODTs are the only quick-dissolving dosage form recognized by the FDA and listed in the *Orange Book*. **Table 14-5** lists some examples of fast-dissolving/fast-disintegrating tablets that are marketed in the United States. ODT products have been developed for numerous indications ranging from migraines (for which a rapid onset of action is important) to mental illness (for which patient compliance is important for treating chronic indications such as depression and schizophrenia).The future possibilities for improvements in ODTs and drug

TABLE 14-5 Examples of Commercial Fast/Rapid-Dissolving Tablets

DRUG	PRODUCT
acetaminophen	Calpol Fast Melts Jr. Tylenol Meltaways
alprazolam	Niravam
aripiprazole	Abilify Discmelt
carbidopa/levodopa	Parcopa
clonazepam	Clonazepam ODT Klonopin Wafers
clozapine	FazaClo
desloratadine	Clarinex RediTabs
diphenhydramine	Benadryl FastMelt UNISOM SleepMelts
donepezil	Aricept ODT
fexofenadine	Allegra-ODT
ibuprofen	Nurofen Meltlets
lamotrigine	Lamictal ODT
lansoprazole	Prevacid SoluTab
loratadine	Alavert Quick Dissolving Tablets Loratadine Redidose Claritin RediTabs
meloxicam	Meloxicam 7.5- and 15-mg Orodispersible Tablets
mirtazapine	Mirtazapine ODT Remeron SolTab
olanzapine	Zyprexa Zydis
ondansetron	Zofran ODT
prednisolone	Orapred ODT
risperidone	Risperdal M-Tab
rizatriptan	Maxalt-MLT
selegiline	Zelapar
zolmitriptan	Zomig-ZMT

delivery are bright, but the technology is still relatively new. Several drug delivery technologies that can help improve ODT drug therapy have yet to be fully realized.

Ocular System

Topical application of drugs to the eye is common for eye disorders. The most prescribed ocular dosage form is the traditional eyedrop solution. But the eyedrop solution is not an efficient drug delivery system because the greater part of the 1 to 2 drops (50 to 100 microliters) of an ophthalmic solution is squeezed out of the eye by the first blink following administration (1,000 microliters = 1 milliliter). The residual volume mixes with the lacrimal fluid (about 7 to 8 microliters), becomes diluted, and is drained away by the nasolacrimal drainage system until the solution volume returns to the normal tear volume of 7 to 8 microliters. The initial drainage results in the loss of about 75% to 80% of the administered dose within 5 minutes of instillation. Then drainage stops and the residual dose declines slowly.

The efficiency of an ophthalmic drug delivery system can be greatly improved by prolonging the time during which the drug is in contact with the corneal surface. To achieve this, various approaches have been used: (1) preparing a suspension of drug particles in pharmaceutical vehicles, (2) adding viscosity-enhancing agents such as methylcellulose to the eyedrop preparation, or (3) providing the drug as an ointment.

In recent years, it has been shown that drug-presoaked hydrogel-type contact lenses prolong the drug–eye contact time. The Bionite lens, for example, is inserted into the eye after being presoaked in the drug solution. Similarly, Sauflon hydrophilic contact lenses are manufactured from a vinyl pyrrolidone acrylic copolymer of high water content. These contact lenses have been shown to improve the delivery of fluorescein, phenylephrine, pilocarpine, chloramphenicol, and tetracycline.

More recently, drug-dispersing ocular inserts have been used for ocular delivery of drugs. The new generation of drug-dispersing ocular inserts consists of a medicated core matrix confined within a pair of flexible, transparent, biocompatible, and tear-insoluble polymer membranes. This polymer membrane provides the required degree of permeability for the drug. When the insert is placed in the conjunctival cul-de-sac between the sclera of the eyeball and the lower lid, the drug is continuously released by diffusion through the membrane as a result of solvation in the lacrimal fluid. Alza Corporation's Ocusert system is a pilocarpine core reservoir sandwiched between two sheets of transparent, lipophilic, rate-controlling membranes. The term **lipophilic** means lipid (or oil) loving; that is, the lipophilic rate-controlling membranes are not readily soluble in the ocular fluids. When placed in the cul-de-sac, the pilocarpine molecules penetrate through the rate-controlling membranes. This controlled pilocarpine-releasing therapeutic system has several advantages over a conventional eyedrop solution. It provides better patient compliance, less frequent dosing, around-the-clock protection for 4 to 7 days, fewer ocular and systemic side effects, and a possible delay in the refractory state. The term **refractory** in ophthalmology implies resistance to treatment or not readily yielding to treatment. Hence, the controlled pilocarpine-releasing therapeutic system enables the use of a significantly smaller dose of pilocarpine for the effective management of **intraocular** pressure (IOP) in the treatment of glaucoma. (IOP is a measurement of the fluid pressure of the aqueous humor inside the eye. The fluid pressure inside the eye is an important aspect in the evaluation of patients with glaucoma.) The administration of one Ocusert Pilo-20 insert, for example, delivers a daily dose of only 0.4 to 0.5 mg compared with the 4 to 8 mg provided by the instillation of 1 to 2 drops of the conventional 2% pilocarpine solution administered four times a day.

> **lipophilic** lipid-loving
>
> **refractory** resistance to treatment or a stimulus
>
> **intraocular** within the eye

Transdermal Drug Delivery System

The **transdermal** drug delivery system is an innovation that employs the skin as a portal of drug entry into the systemic circulation. Using the **percutaneous** route instead of the more conventional oral, parenteral, pulmonary, or rectal routes, this technique is designed to provide systemic therapy for acute or chronic conditions that do not involve the skin.

> **transdermal** entering through the dermis of the skin, as in administration of a drug applied to the skin in ointment or patch form
>
> **percutaneous** through the skin

Transdermal drug delivery systems have several advantages: convenience, uninterrupted therapy, better patient compliance, accurate drug dosage, and regulation of drug concentration. However, percutaneous delivery is more difficult for those drugs that exist as large molecules, for example, those drugs that have a large molecular weight (e.g., insulin) and do not possess adequate lipid and aqueous solubility. Drugs with molecular weights of 100 to 800 and adequate lipid and

TABLE 14-6 Comparison of Nitroglycerin Dosage Forms

	ANTIANGINAL EFFECT		
DOSAGE FORM	DOSE	ONSET	DURATION FORM
Intravenous injection	Variable	Minutes	Minutes
Sublingual tablet	0.15–0.6 mg every 30 min	2 min	Up to 30 min
Oral timed release	2.5–9 mg twice a day	0.5–1 hr	8–9 hr
Topical ointment	1–2 in. every 4 hr	30 min	About 3 hr
Transdermal patch	1 patch every 12–24 hr	30 min	20–24 hr

aqueous solubility can permeate the skin. The ideal molecular weight of a drug for transdermal drug delivery is believed to be less than 400.

Among the most popular and intriguing percutaneously administered drug delivery systems is the transdermal patch. The transdermal patch is formulated to deliver a constant and controlled dose of a drug through the intact skin. The drug enters directly into the bloodstream. Although each manufacturer designs its transdermal system based on the technology developed for its individual product, most delivery systems consist of at least three layers: (1) a backing layer, (2) a drug reservoir, and (3) an adhesive layer that incorporates a priming dose of the drug. The drug is released through the rate-limiting membrane of the patch. It enters the skin and is absorbed into the systemic circulation.

Nitroglycerin is available in various forms—sublingual, oral, intravenous injection, topical ointment, and transdermal preparations (**Table 14-6**). The popular transdermal preparations of nitroglycerin are Searle's Nitrodisc and Key's Nitro-Dur. All nitroglycerin transdermal patches are designed to be applied to the upper arm or chest to provide the drug for 24 hours. Although these patches can be applied anywhere on the body except the distal parts of the extremities, most patients have a tendency to apply these near the thorax, perhaps on the assumption that the medication for the heart should be placed near the heart. Manufacturers do recommend, however, that each patch should be applied at a site different from that used the previous day to avoid irritation.

Transderm-Scop, a scopolamine-containing transdermal delivery system marketed by Ciba-Geigy, is a circular, flat, tan disc, about 2 mm thick and the size of a dime. Each disc contains 1 to 5 mg of scopolamine and is programmed to deliver 0.5 mg of scopolamine directly into the bloodstream over 3 days. According to the manufacturer, this delivery system is more effective than the conventional oral dose, which has been reported to cause excessively rapid heartbeat, confusion, and hallucination. The patch works best when placed behind the ear on a hairless site. The introduction of transdermal drug delivery in pharmaceutical industry started with the FDA's approval of Transderm-Scop in 1981. Since then, many transdermal patches have been introduced in the United States and many other countries.

Since 1981, the FDA has approved 48 patch products, 6 of which have been discontinued. The approved products represent 24 drug molecules, owned or distributed by 26 companies. Fifteen companies manufactured these products. The number of approved drug molecules in patch products approved from 2001 to 2010 was 12, compared to 6 during the 1991–2000 decade, and 2 during the 1981–1990 decade.

Table 14-7 lists the FDA-approved transdermal patch products currently available in the United States. This listing was obtained from the FDA's *Orange Book* as well as from individual product labels. All products listed in Table 14-7 are

TABLE 14-7 Approved Patch Products in the USA

DRUG MOLECULE	NAME OF PRODUCT	DISTRIBUTOR
buprenorphine	Butrans (2010)	Purdue Pharma
capsaicin	Qutenza (2009)	NeurofesX
clonidine	Catapress TTT (1984)	Boehringer Ingelheim
	Clonidine Transdermal System (2009)	Par
	Clonidine Transdermal System (2010)	Mylanr
	Clonidine Transdermal System (2010)	Barr (Teva)
diclofenac epolamine	Flector (2007)	King (Pfizer)
estradiol	Climara (1984)	Bayer
	Estraderm (1986)	Novartis
	Vivelle (1994)	Novartis
	Alora (1996)	Watson
	Vivelle-DOT (1999)	Novartis
	Estradiol Transderm (2000)	Mylan
	Menostar (2004)	Bayer
estradiol/levonorgestrel	Climara Pro (2003)	Bayer
estradiol/norethindrone acetate	Novartis (1998)	
ethinyl estradiol/ norelgestromin	Ortho Evra (2001)	Ortho-McNeil-Jenssen
fentanyl	Duragesic (1990)	Ortho-McNeil-Jenssen
	Fentanyl Transdermal System (2005)	Mylan
	Fentanyl Transdermal System (2006)	Levipharm Labs
	Fentanyl Transdermal System (2007)	Actavis
	Fentanyl Transdermal System (2007)	Watson
	Fentanyl Transdermal System (2008)	Teva
	Fentanyl Transdermal System (2009)	Apotex
	Fentanyl Transdermal System (2011)	Mallinckrodt (Covidien)
granisetron	Sancuso (2008)	ProStrakan
lidocaine	Lidoderm (1999)	Endo
lidocaine/tetracaine	Synera (2005)	ZARS
methyl salicylate/ menthol	Salonpas (2008)	Hisamitsu
methylphenidate	Daytrana (2006)	Noven (Hisamitsu)
nicotine	NicoDerm CQ (1996)	GCK
	Habitrol (1999)	Novartis

(*Continued*)

TABLE 14-7 (Continued)

DRUG MOLECULE	NAME OF PRODUCT	DISTRIBUTOR
nitroglycerin	Nitro-Dur (1995)	Key (Merck)
	Nitroglycerin Transdermal System (1996)	Mylan
	Nitroglycerin Transdermal System (1998)	Hercon Labs
oxybutynin	Oxytrol (2003)	Watson
rivastigmine	Exelon (2007)	Novartis
scopolamine	Transderm-Scop (1981)	Novartis
selegiline	Emsam (2006)	Mylan
testosterone	Androderm (1995)	Watson

available as prescription products except the following three, which do not require a prescription and are sold over the counter: (1) methyl salicylate/menthol patch, (2) NicoDerm CQ patch, and (3) Habitrol patch.

Six patches that were approved by the FDA have since been discontinued by the manufacturers and are no longer available: (1) McNeal's Nicotrol (nicotine patch), (2) Aveva's Prostep (nicotine patch), (3) Novartis's Transderm-Nitro (nitroglycerin patch), (4) Mylan's Nitroglycerin Transdermal System (nitroglycerin patch), (5) UCB's Neupro (rotigotine patch), and (6) Alza's Testoderm (testosterone patch).

Multiple generic patches are available for the following four drug molecules: clonidine, estradiol, fentanyl, and nitroglycerin.

Japan, Europe, and other select countries have approved at least 21 patch products representing at least 12 drug molecules that the United States has not yet approved (**Table 14-8**). Sixteen of these patch products are topical patches. Most are designed for local treatment of pain with various nonsteroidal anti-inflammatory drugs. Psoriatic inflammation (betamethasone valerate) and toenail infection (sertaconazole) are the other topical applications.

Intranasal Drug Delivery

The nasal route for drug delivery is becoming popular because of the need for a route for newly developed drugs that cannot be administered orally because of their lack of stability in the gastrointestinal tract or due to the lack of drug absorption from the gastrointestinal tract due to their molecular weight. Examples of such drugs include newly developed synthetic biologically active peptides and polypeptides. Some drugs that are subject to destruction in the gastrointestinal tract (e.g., insulin) are administered by injection. The **intranasal** route of drug administration is an alternative route for some of these drugs.

intranasal within the nose

The nasal mucosa has been shown to be amenable to the systemic absorption of such drugs as hydralazine, insulin, progesterone, propranolol, and scopolamine. The intranasal bioavailability of those drugs, which are relatively small molecular compounds, appears to be comparable to the bioavailability of the drug administered by injection. Some drugs for intranasal delivery are already on the market, while some drugs are under investigation for intranasal delivery. Examples of drugs under investigation for nasal delivery are butorphanol, calcitonin, desmopressin, insulin, lypressin, oxytocin, progesterone, and vitamin B_{12}.

TABLE 14-8 Patch Products Approved for Use in Countries Other Than the United States

DRUG MOLECULE	NAME OF PRODUCT	COUNTRY
betamethasone valerate	Btasil	Europe
diclofenac diethylammonium	OXA-SAT	India, South America
	Rheumastop	South Korea
diclofenac sodium	Nabol tape	Japan
felbinac	FalzyTape	Japan
	SelTouch	Japan
flurbiprofen	Adofeed	Japan
	TransAct Lat	Europe
ibuprofen	Biatain Ag Patch	Denmark
isosorbide dinitrate	Antup R	Japan
	Frandol Tape-S TDDSs	Japan
ketoprofen	Ketotop Plaster	Asia, Brazil, Japan
	Ketoprofen Patch, Bouty	Europe
	MILTAX PAPax	Japan
	Mohrus Tape/PAP	Asia, Italy, Japan
	TOUCHRON	Japan
loxoprofen sodium dihydrate	Loxonin Tape/PAP	Japan
rotigotine	Neupro	Asia, Europe
sertaconazole	Zalain Nail Pouch	Germany
tulobuterol	Hokunalin tape	China, Japan
	Tulobuterol Tape EMEC	Japan

Summary

Within the past few years, the pharmaceutical industry has made significant progress in the development and manufacture of new dosage forms. The new concepts of bioavailability have made it possible to prepare more efficient delivery systems. The latest developments include such dosage forms as rapid-dissolving tablets, intranasal drug delivery, and metered-dose inhalers. More drugs are being made available as transdermal delivery systems (popularly known as "patches") and as orally dissolving or fast-dissolving/fast-disintegrating tablets and via osmotic pumps and insulin pumps. In the future, one can expect dosage forms containing optimal amounts of active ingredients to provide maximal therapeutic benefits, thus markedly reducing or completely eliminating the side effects associated with therapeutic agents. The current trend appears to be in the direction of development of more efficient and better drug delivery systems rather than the development of new compounds as new drugs.

TEST YOUR KNOWLEDGE

Multiple Choice

1. Drugs are defined as chemicals of
   a. natural origin.
   b. synthetic origin.
   c. semisynthetic origin.
   d. all of the above.
2. Which of the following is not a drug dosage form?
   a. brew
   b. tablet
   c. injection
   d. solution
3. Which of the following are included in drug formulations?
   a. diluents
   b. excipients
   c. preservatives
   d. all of the above
4. For a drug to elicit the desired response, at the site of action it is required to be in the form of
   a. a molecular dispersion.
   b. an isotonic solution.
   c. a soluble gel.
   d. an acidic vehicle.
5. A soluble substance is called
   a. a solvent.
   b. a solute.
   c. a solubilizer.
   d. none of the above.
6. Medicinal emulsions for oral administration are usually
   a. water-in-oil type emulsions.
   b. oil-in-water type emulsions.
   c. microemulsions.
   d. none of the above.
7. Which of the following is not a solid dosage form?
   a. powder
   b. suspension
   c. tablet
   d. granule
8. The most prescribed ocular dosage form is
   a. an eyedrop solution.
   b. a drug-presoaked hydrogel-type contact lens.
   c. an ocular insert.
   d. a Bionite lens.
9. Advantage(s) of transdermal patch include
   a. convenience.
   b. uninterrupted therapy.

c. better patient compliance.
d. all of the above.

10. Which of the following must be sterile?
a. parenteral dosage forms
b. oral dosage forms
c. nasal dosage forms
d. all of the above

11. Which of the following must be pyrogen-free?
a. intramuscular injections
b. subcutaneous injections
c. intravenous injections
d. all of the above

12. Which of the following is the best site of application of a scopolamine patch?
a. on the chest
b. behind the earlobe
c. on the forearm
d. near the deltoid muscle

13. For a tablet to be considered fast dissolving or fast disintegrating, it must dissolve or disintegrate in the saliva in no more than
a. 30 minutes.
b. 15 minutes.
c. 5 minutes.
d. 1 minute.

14. Which of the following are ideal characteristics of an orally dissolving tablet?
a. absence of bitter taste
b. good solubility in water and saliva
c. ability to permeate oral mucosal tissue
d. all of the above

True/False

1. A size 4 capsule holds more aspirin than a size 2 capsule.

2. In actual practice, a "pure" drug is seldom used.

3. Liquid dosage forms are rarely the drug of choice.

4. In an acceptable suspension, the particles never settle down.

5. Emulsions contain at least one immiscible liquid.

6. Capsules should never be chewed before swallowing.

Matching

Match the medication with the form of administration.

7.	______ medicinal aerosol	a.	slowly dissolved in the mouth
8.	______ transdermal patch	b.	implanted subcutaneously
9.	______ Bionite lens	c.	inhaled through nose or mouth
10.	______ lozenge	d.	applied to the skin
11.	______ pellet	e.	inserted into the eye

Suggested Readings

Allen, L.V., Popovich, N.G., & Ansel, H.C. (2011). *Ansel's pharmaceutical dosage forms and drug delivery systems* (9th ed.). Philadelphia, PA: Lippincott Williams & Wilkins.

Das, N., Madan, P.L., & Lin, S. (2010). Development and in vitro evaluation of insulin-loaded buccal Pluronic F-127 gels. *Pharmaceutical Development and Technology, 15*(2), 192–208.

Gennaro, A.R. (Ed.) (2006). *Remington: The science and practice of pharmacy* (21st ed.). London, UK: Mack Publishing.

Madan, P.L. (1985). Sustained release drug delivery systems: I. An overview. *Pharmaceutical Manufacturing, 2*(2), 22.

Madan, P.L. (1985). Sustained release drug delivery systems: II. Preformulation considerations. *Pharmaceutical Manufacturing, 2*(3), 40.

Madan, P.L. (1985). Sustained release drug delivery systems: III. Technology. *Pharmaceutical Manufacturing, 2*(4), 38.

Madan, P.L. (1985). Sustained release drug delivery systems: IV. Oral products. *Pharmaceutical Manufacturing, 2*(5), 40.

Madan, P.L. (1985). Sustained release drug delivery systems: V. Parenteral products. *Pharmaceutical Manufacturing, 2*(6), 50.

Madan, P.L. (1985). Sustained release drug delivery systems: VI. Special devices. *Pharmaceutical Manufacturing, 2*(7), 32.

Madan, P.L. (1990). Sustained release dosage forms. *U.S. Pharmacist, 15*, 39.

Madan, P.L. (2009). Chapter 12 Pharmaceutical Dosage Forms in J. M. Durgin & Z. Hanan (Eds.), *Pharmacy practice for technicians* (4th ed.). Clifton Park, NY: Cengage Learning.

Madan, P.L., & Komotar, A. (1979). Quality control in the pharmaceutical industry. *Drug and Cosmetic Industry, 124*, 66.

Patel, N., Madan, P.L., & Lin, S. (2011). Development and evaluation of controlled release ibuprofen matrix tablets by direct compression technique. *Pharmaceutical Development and Technology, 16*(1), 1–11.

Tiwari, D., Goldman, D., Sause, R., & Madan, P.L. (1999, September 15). Evaluation of polyoxyethylene homopolymers for buccal bioadhesive delivery device formulations. *PharmSci., 1*(3).

Tiwari, D., Goldman, D., Town, C., Sause, R., & Madan, P.L. (1999). In vitro-in vivo evaluation of a controlled release buccal bioadhesive device for oral drug delivery. *Pharmaceutical Research, 16*(11), 1775–1780.

U.S. Pharmacopeial Convention. (2011). *U.S. pharmacopeia/National formulary*. Rockville, MD: Author.

CHAPTER

15

Pharmaceutical Calculations

Competencies

Upon completion of this chapter, the reader should be able to:

1. Interpret a prescription/medication order for calculations and dispensing.
2. Convert quantities stated in apothecary units to their equivalent units in the metric system.
3. Convert quantities within the different systems (e.g., grams to milligrams or ounces to pints).
4. Use proportions to perform calculations for dosing medications.
5. Determine how to dilute ingredients in formulations.
6. Calculate quantities for dosing administered when ordered in fractional doses.
7. Calculate a day's supply or amount to dispense.
8. Calculate dosages for individual patients given the patient's weight and height.
9. Perform calculations necessary for the preparation and infusion of IV medications.
10. Identify techniques to decrease errors in interpreting the name or strength of drugs from the prescription or medication order.

Key Terms

alligation
apothecary system
body surface area (BSA)
grain
gram
International System of Units (SI)
liter
meter
metric system
nomogram
percentage
piggyback
proportion
ratio

Introduction

It is common practice for the pharmacist to calculate and prepare or select the drug dosage form to be administered to a patient. However, this practice does not relieve other health care providers from the legal and professional responsibility of ensuring that the patient receives the correct dose of the correct medication at the correct time in the correct manner. *A pharmacy technician should have every calculation checked by a pharmacist before preparing a prescription or medication order*. This chapter will review the necessary calculations involved in the safe administration of drugs to the patient.

Interpreting the Prescription/Medication Order

The welfare of the patient necessitates proper interpretation of the prescription or medication order. Although this is ultimately the pharmacist's responsibility, the pharmacy technician is often the first person to screen the prescription/medication order. If any doubt or question exists, the pharmacy technician is responsible for confirming the order with the pharmacist before proceeding (**Figure 15-1**).

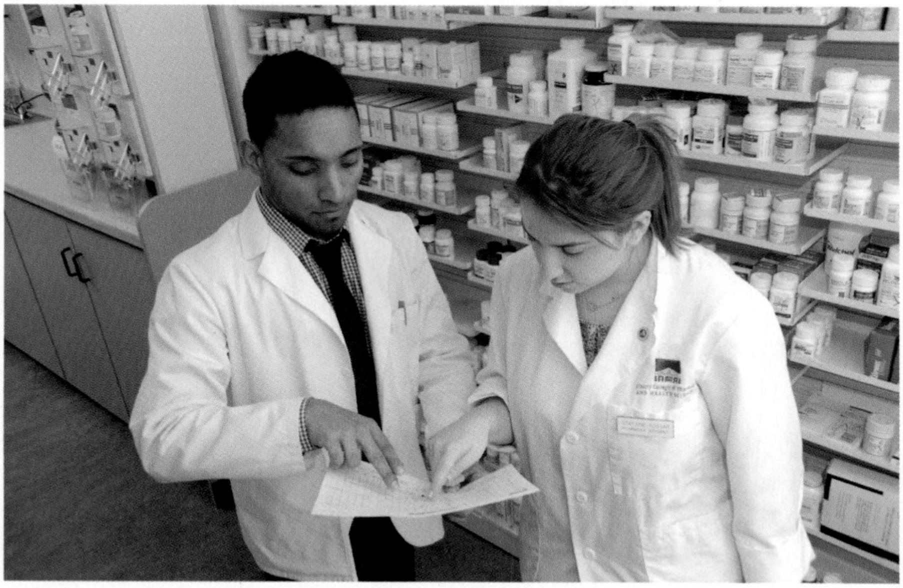

FIGURE 15-1 When in doubt, always verify a prescription with the pharmacist.

Common Abbreviations

Abbreviations derived from Latin are often used by physicians and other prescribers in writing or interpreting drug orders. To reduce errors, however, some of these abbreviations are no longer permitted to be used in certain settings. For a complete list, please refer to the Institute for Safe Medication Practices (ISMP) website listed at the end of this chapter. Also refer to Chapters 13 and 30 for detailed explanation of the ISMP and The Joint Commission Error Prone Abbreviations.

Refer to **Table 15-1** for common abbreviations regarding quantities and dosages seen in drug orders. The pharmacy technician must be able to interpret these abbreviations correctly. Some examples encountered in practice include the following:

TABLE 15-1 Abbreviations Commonly Seen in Drug Orders

ABBREVIATION	ENGLISH
gal	gallon
qt	quart
pt	pint
oz, ℥	ounce
tbsp, ℥ss	tablespoonful
tsp, ʒ, ʒ	teaspoonful
L	liter
mL	milliliter
gtt	drop
lb	pound
gr	grain
kg	kilogram
g	gram
mg	milligram
mcg	microgram
no, #	number
qs	quantity sufficient
$\overline{ss}$ or ṡṡ	one-half

EXAMPLE

Benadryl (diphenhydramine) caps 25 mg po q4h

Interpretation:

Take one 25 mg capsule by mouth every 4 hours.

EXAMPLE

Tylenol (acetaminophen) Elixir ½ tsp po tid and at bedtime

Interpretation:

Take one-half teaspoonful of elixir by mouth three times a day and at bedtime. (Because of the word "**and**" in the directions, this does mean a total of four doses per day.)

EXAMPLE

100 mg Demerol (meperidine) IM stat. 50 mg IM q4h prn pain

Interpretation:

Give 100 mg of Demerol intramuscularly immediately, then give 50 mg of Demerol intramuscularly every 4 hours as needed for pain.

The abbreviation "prn" can often be a source of confusion if not interpreted carefully. In the last example, the medication (Demerol) can be administered if a dosing interval of *at least 4 hours is maintained*. The nurse assesses the patient's need for the Demerol to control pain or the patient requests the medication and it may be administered *only* if it has been *4 hours or more* since the previous injection.

Roman Numerals

Most prescriptions today are written using Arabic numerals, however some prescribers may still use Roman numerals. The use of Roman numerals may make it more difficult to alter the quantity of a written prescription. A list of Roman numerals is shown in **Table 15-2**.

TABLE 15-2 Values of Single Roman Numerals

ROMAN NUMERALS	VALUE
ss or $\overline{ss}$	½
I or i	1
V or v	5
X or x	10
L or l	50
C or c	100
D or d	500
M or m	1,000

All small Roman numerals may be written with a line above them (as is done for "ss" at the top of this table).

Examples of the use of Roman numerals are as follows:

iv	four
xxviii	twenty-eight
LX	sixty
XC	ninety
CXX	one hundred and twenty

Note: Roman numerals may be written in lowercase or uppercase letters.

International System of Units (The Metric System)

The **International System of Units (SI)**, commonly known as the metric system, is the internationally used system of weights and measures. The three basic units of the **metric system** are the meter (length), the gram (weight), and the liter (volume). The technician must be able to convert to and within the units of the metric system.

International System of Units (SI) internationally used system of weights and measures; commonly known as the metric system

metric system a system of weights based on the meter (length), the gram (weight), and the liter (volume)

gram a base unit of weight in the metric system

liter a basic unit of volume in the metric system

Gram

The **gram** is the basic unit of weight in the metric system. The gram is defined as the weight of 1 cubic centimeter of distilled water at 4°C. The abbreviation for grams is **g**. Never use **gr**, which stands for the apothecary unit of grains.

Liter

The **liter** is the basic unit of volume used to measure liquids in the metric system. It is defined as 1,000 cubic centimeters of water. One cubic centimeter is equivalent to 1 milliliter; thus 1 liter (L) equals 1,000 milliliters (mL).

Note: By definition 1 mL of water is equal to 1 g of water.

Meter

meter a basic unit of length in the metric system

The **meter** is the basic unit of length used to measure distances in the metric system. The meter is 1/10,000,000 of the distance from the North Pole to the equator (or a little larger than 1 yard). Multiples or parts of these basic units are named by adding a prefix. Each prefix has a numerical value, as shown in **Table 15-3** and **Table 15-4**.

TABLE 15-3 Metric Prefixes

PREFIX	NUMERICAL VALUE
mega-	1,000,000
kilo-	1,000
deci-	0.1
centi-	0.01
milli-	0.001
micro-	0.000,001

TABLE 15-4 Common Metric Abbreviations Found in Pharmacy

ABBREVIATION	MEASURE
mcg	microgram
mg	milligram
g	gram
kg	kilogram
mL	milliliter
L	liter
mm	millimeter
cm	centimeter
m	meter

Examples of the use of the metric prefixes are as follows:

1 milligram (mg)	1/1,000 gram	0.001 g
1 microgram (mcg)	1/1,000,000 gram	0.000001 g
1 kilogram (kg)	1000 grams	1000 g
1 milliliter (mL)	1/1,000 liter	0.001 L
1 deciliter (dL)	1/10 liter	0.1 L

Conversions

Conversion of units is often required when working with medications. It is extremely important to note that a decimal error of just one space will result in a 10-fold over- or underdose, which can cause severe harm or even death to the patient. Metric conversions are listed in **Table 15-5**.

TABLE 15-5 Metric Conversions

1,000 g	=	1 kg
1,000 mg	=	1 g
1,000 mcg	=	1 mg
1,000 mL	=	1 L
100 mL	=	1 dL

EXAMPLE

Convert 22 grams to milligrams.

Solution by proportion:

1 g is equal to 1000 mg. It is possible to convert between grams and milligrams using proportions. (Proportions are covered in detail in the next section of this chapter.)

$$\frac{1{,}000\ \text{mg}}{1\ \text{g}} = \frac{X\ \text{mg}}{22\ \text{g}}$$

$$X = 22{,}000\ \text{mg}$$

EXAMPLE

Convert 150 milliliters to liters.

Solution by dimensional analysis:

1 L is equal to 1,000 mL. Milliliters can be converted to liters using dimensional unit analysis.

$$150\ \text{mL} \times \frac{1\ \text{L}}{1{,}000\ \text{mL}} = 0.15\ \text{L}$$

Important:

- A 1,000-fold difference results when the decimal point is moved three places to the right or left.
- Approach this logically; milliliters are a smaller unit than liters, therefore more of them are needed to equal a liter.

Ratio and Proportion

Nearly every calculation involving medications can be broken down into a simple ratio and proportion. Developing skill in setting up ratios and proportions will be a valuable aid to the technician in solving medication problems quickly and accurately.

Ratio

ratio the relationship of two quantities (e.g., 1:10 is read as one part in ten parts)

A **ratio** is the relationship between two quantities. It may be expressed in the form 1:10 or 1:2,500, or it may be expressed as a fraction: 1/10 or 1/2,500. The ratio expression 1:10 or fraction 1/10 can be read as one in ten, one-tenth, or one part in ten parts.

Note: When expressing values as a ratio *strength*, it is customary to set the first number equal to one. (This will be discussed later in the chapter.)

EXAMPLE

A handful of twenty jelly beans contains one red jelly bean.

Interpretation:

The ratio of red jelly beans to total jelly beans is expressed as 1 in 20 or 1:20 or as a fraction 1/20.

Proportion

proportion formed using two ratios that are equal (e.g., ½ = 5/10)

A **proportion** is formed when two ratios are equal (or proportional) to one another. For example, 1:2 = 5:10. When two ratios or fractions are equal, their cross product is also equal. The cross product is obtained by multiplying the denominator of one ratio by the numerator of the other, as follows:

$$\frac{1}{2} = \frac{5}{10} \text{ therefore, } 2 \times 5 = 10 \times 1$$

The cross products are equal: 10 = 10. This confirms that the ratio 1:2 is equal (proportional) to the ratio 5:10.

Is 1:3 proportional to 4:12?

$$\frac{1}{3} = \frac{4}{12} \text{ yes, } 3 \times 4 = 1 \times 12$$

The cross products are equal: 12 = 12. Therefore, 1:3 is proportional to 4:12.

This characteristic of proportions is very useful in solving problems that arise in drug administration. If any three of the values of a proportion are known, the fourth value can be determined.

EXAMPLE

The prescriber orders 20 mg of a drug for a patient. The drug is available in a 10-mL vial that contains 50 mg of drug. How many milliliters will be needed to supply the dose of 20 mg?

Solution:

Three things are known from the statement of the problem:

1. The vial contains 10 mL of drug solution.
2. 50 mg of drug are in the 10-mL vial.
3. 20 mg is the desired dose.

A ratio can be written for the drug in the vial:

$$\frac{50 \text{ mg}}{10 \text{ mL}}$$

A ratio can also be written for the required dosage:

$$\frac{20 \text{ mg}}{X \text{ mL}}$$

Thus the proportion is

$$\frac{50 \text{ mg}}{10 \text{ mL}} = \frac{20 \text{ mg}}{X \text{ mL}}$$

Note in the proportion that the units are labeled and like (identical) units are located in the same position in each fraction or ratio (that is, mg is in the numerator on both sides and mL is in the denominator on both sides). It is important to correctly equate the units of the proportion.

(*Continues*)

EXAMPLE *(CONTINUED)*

Important:

These three conditions must be met when using ratio and proportion:

1. The numerators must have the same units.
2. The denominators must have the same units.
3. Three of the four parts must be known.

To solve the last example, equate the cross products and solve for the unknown (X):

$$\frac{50\text{ mg}}{10\text{ mL}} = \frac{20\text{ mg}}{X\text{ mL}}$$

$$50\,(X\text{ mL}) = 10 \times 20$$

$$50\,(X\text{ mL}) = 200$$

$$X = 4\text{ mL}$$

Therefore, 4 mL of the solution will supply the 20-mg dose of drug ordered.

Note that a proportion is similar to the way we think logically: if this is so, then that will follow. Problems can be analyzed with the if-then approach. For example, in the last example, we could say IF 50 mg of drug are contained in 10 mL of drug solution, THEN 20 mg of drug will be contained in X mL of solution. To use the IF-THEN approach, the first ratio of a proportion is always formed from the quantity and strength (concentration) found on the label of the drug on hand.

EXAMPLE

An ampicillin oral suspension contains 250 mg of the drug in each 5 mL. How many milliliters should be measured into a medication syringe to obtain a dose of 75 mg of ampicillin?

Solution:

Step 1. Set up the proportion beginning with the drug on hand:

IF THEN

$$\frac{250\text{ mg}}{5\text{ mL}} = \frac{75\text{ mg}}{X\text{ mL}}$$

Step 2. Then cross multiply:

$$250\,(X\text{ mL}) = 5\,(75)$$

$$250\,(X\text{ mL}) = 375$$

$$X = 1.5\text{ mL}$$

The Apothecary System

apothecary system an early English system of weights and liquid measures

The **apothecary system** was the traditional system used in the practice of pharmacy. Today only components of it may be found on some prescriptions. The fluid dram sign (ʒ or ℨ) is sometimes used by physicians to represent 1 teaspoonful. The apothecary symbol for one ounce is ℥i. Due to confusion and errors, the use of these symbols is discouraged and should eventually result in their elimination. Examples of apothecary notations are shown in **Table 15-6**.

Apothecary System of Volume (Liquid) Measures

The apothecary liquid measures are the same as the avoirdupois (English) measures of ounces, pints, and quarts. The smallest unit of volume in the apothecary system is the minim (♏) which is not in common use today. The minim should

TABLE 15-6 Apothecary Notations

ʒ or ʒ	teaspoonful
ʒ ss or ʒ ss	one-half teaspoonful
ʒ iss or ʒ iss	one and a half teaspoonfuls
ʒ iiss or ʒ iiss	two and a half teaspoonfuls
℥i	one ounce
℥ss	one half-ounce or one tablespoonful
℥iss	one and a half ounces
℥iiss	two and a half ounces

TABLE 15-7 Liquid Measures in the Apothecary System

MEASURE	EQUIVALENT
1 tablespoonful (℥ ss)	3 teaspoonfuls (ʒiii or ʒiii)
1 fluid ounce (℥)	2 tablespoonfuls
1 pint	16 fluid ounces
1 quart	2 pints
1 gallon	4 quarts

not be confused with the drop because they are not equivalent. The size of a drop varies with the properties of the liquid being dispensed or measured. Also, the symbol for minim (♏) is often confused with the symbol for micrograms (μ) and it should not be used to avoid this error as well. **Table 15-7** shows the common units of liquid measure in the apothecary system.

Apothecary System of Weights

grain a base unit of weight in the apothecary system

The apothecary system of weights is based on the **grain** (gr), which is the smallest unit in the system. The origin of the grain is uncertain, but it is believed that at one time solids were measured by using grains of wheat as the standard.

In practice, the technician will rarely see apothecary units of weight with the exception of the grain, which may sometimes be used in ordering medications such as these:

Nitroglycerin (1/100 gr, 1/150 gr, 1/200 gr, 1/400 gr)
Phenobarbital sodium (1/4 gr, 1/2 gr, 1 gr)
Aspirin or acetaminophen (5 gr, 10 gr).

Converting from the Apothecary System to the Metric System

Before reviewing the types of calculations used in determining medication dosages, we need to examine conversions between systems of measurement. It was mentioned previously that nearly all medication orders today are written using the metric system. Occasionally some orders may still be written using the apothecary system. The technician must be able to convert from the apothecary system to the metric system and within both systems. **Table 15-8** provides conversion factors between the apothecary and the metric systems. Many conversions can easily be made using the ratio and proportion method discussed earlier in this chapter.

TABLE 15-8 Conversions between the Apothecary and Metric Systems

APOTHECARY	METRIC EXACT CONVERSION	METRIC APPROXIMATE CONVERSION
1 teaspoonful, ʒ or ʒ	No longer in use	5 mL
1 tablespoonful (℥ ss)	No longer in use	15 mL
1 fluid ounce (℥)	29.6 mL	30 mL
1 pint	473 mL	480 mL
1 quart	946 mL	960 mL
1 gallon	3,784 mL	3,840 mL
1 grain	64.8 mg	65 or 60 mg
1 ounce	28.4 g	30 g
1 pound	454 g compounding 2.2 kg person's weight	No approximate conversion used
1 inch	2.54 cm	No approximate conversion used

EXAMPLE

How many milligrams of nitroglycerin are in one 1/150 gr tablet of the drug?

Solution:

This problem requires conversion from the apothecary system to the metric system. Use the equivalent 1 gr = 60 mg. The proportion is:

$$\overset{\text{IF}}{\frac{1\,\text{gr}}{60\,\text{mg}}} = \overset{\text{THEN}}{\frac{1/150\,\text{gr}}{X\,\text{mg}}}$$

Cross multiplying:

$$1\,(X\,\text{mg}) = 60\,(1/150)$$

$$X\,\text{mg} = 0.4\,\text{mg}$$

Therefore, nitroglycerin ordered as 1/150 gr is the same product as nitroglycerin 0.4 mg.

EXAMPLE

Four fluid ounces are equal to how many milliliters?

Solution:

$$\frac{1\,\text{ounce}}{30\,\text{mL}} = \frac{4\,\text{ounces}}{X\,\text{mL}}$$

Cross multiplying:

$$1\,(X\,\text{mL}) = 4\,(30\,\text{mL})$$

$$X\,\text{mL} = 120\,\text{mL}$$

Calculation of Days' Supply

It is often necessary when entering prescription data to calculate the "days' supply" of a medication, meaning simply how many days will it be until the medication is finished when used as directed by the prescriber. This is important to determine when a prescription needs to, or may, be refilled. Insurance companies as well as state and federal laws set limits on when patients may obtain more medication.

The number of days' supply is calculated using the following steps:

Step 1. Take the total quantity dispensed.

Step 2. Divide that by the quantity to be taken each day.

EXAMPLE

A prescription for 60 tablets of ibuprofen 800 mg states that the patient should take 1 tablet every 6 hours as needed. How many days' supply is provided?

Solution:

The patient may take a maximum of 4 tablets per day (1 tablet every 6 hours in a 24-hour day). Thus:

$$\frac{4 \text{ tablets}}{1 \text{ day}} = \frac{60 \text{ tablets}}{X \text{ days}}$$

$$X = 15 \text{ days}$$

The patient has received a 15-day supply (if he takes all of the doses). The prescription may last longer if he does not need to take the tablets as often as prescribed, but it should not be completed in less than 15 days.

For doses of oral liquids, the number of milliliters per dose will be used to calculate the amount per day. The number of milliliters per dose multiplied by the number of days will equal the total dispensed.

EXAMPLE

A prescription is received to dispense 200 mL of amoxicillin suspension 250 mg/5 mL. The dose is 1 and ½ teaspoonfuls three times a day until gone. How many days should it take for the medication to be finished (i.e., what is the number of days supplied)?

Solution:

Step 1. 1 and ½ teaspoonfuls is 7.5 mL.

Step 2. 3 doses daily × 7.5 mL = 22.5 mL.

Step 3. $$\frac{22.5 \text{ mL}}{1 \text{ day}} = \frac{200 \text{ mL}}{X \text{ days}}$$

$$X = 8.89 \text{ days}$$

The medication will last approximately 9 days.

Calculations must also be made for ear- and eyedrops, inhalers, and topical preparations. These types of calculations can be a little more complicated and involve some estimation because it is not always possible to determine the exact amount used per day (especially with ointments and creams). Assumptions must be made for the number of drops per milliliter that an eyedrop solution contains. Fifteen or 20 drops per milliliter may be seen. A 5-mL bottle would thus contain between 75 and 100 drops. If 4 drops per day are used, then the bottle would last 19 to 25 days. This also assumes that a patient never uses any "extra" drops if she "misses" the eye with the first drop. Days supplied for ointments and creams vary not only with the frequency of use each day but also with the size of the area to be covered (an elbow takes much less than an entire leg) and the directions given (which may include apply sparingly or liberally). Pharmacies and insurance companies may have a number of days allowed based on the size of the package dispensed.

Calculation of Amount to Dispense

A prescriber may write a prescription/medication order that indicates the amount of drug per dose, the number of doses per day, and the number of days to take the medication. It is then left to the pharmacy filling the order to calculate the correct amount to dispense, whether it is dispensed as a certain number of capsules or tablets or as milliliters of liquid.

EXAMPLE

A prescription for erythromycin suspension 200 mg/5 mL is received with the directions: 1 tsp qid for 7 days. How many milliliters of the erythromycin suspension are needed to fill the prescription?

Solution:

1 teaspoonful is equal to 5 mL.

$$5 \text{ mL} \times 4 \text{ doses per day} = 20 \text{ mL each day}$$

$$20 \text{ mL/day} \times 7 \text{ days} = 140 \text{ mL}$$

140 mL of erythromycin suspension must be dispensed to complete the therapy as ordered.

Calculations Related to Solutions

Solutions are formed in two ways:

1. By dissolving a solid (the *solute*) in a liquid (the *solvent*),or
2. By mixing two liquids together to form a solution.

An example of the first method is adding salt to water to make a normal saline solution. Mixing Zephiran chloride solution with water to make an antiseptic wash is an example of the second method.

Percentage Solutions

Many solutions are available in or are prepared to a specified percentage strength. To produce a solution of the desired strength, it is necessary to calculate the exact amount of drug needed to prepare a specified final volume of product. Although most solutions that are not commercially available are prepared by the pharmacist, the pharmacy technician must understand the concept of percentage to interpret medication labels.

percentage a number representing an amount per hundred (e.g.,5% represents 5 parts per 100)

A **percentage** is defined as the number of parts per hundred parts and is expressed as follows:

$$\text{Percentage (\%)} = \frac{\text{No. of parts}}{\text{100 parts}} \times 100$$

Parts is expressed in grams (in the case of solids) and milliliters (in the case of liquids). To calculate the percentage of active ingredient in a product, the amount of active ingredient is divided by the total amount of the product. To convert the result to a percentage, it is multiplied by 100:

$$\frac{\text{Active ingredient}}{\text{Total quantity of product}} \times 100 = \text{Percentage (\%)}$$

Problems in percentage solutions are generally concerned with three types of percentages:

1. Weight to volume (% W/V)
2. Weight to weight (% W/W)
3. Volume to volume (% V/V).

A weight-to-volume percentage is defined as the number of grams of solute (or drug) in 100 mL of solution. Typical % W/V examples include the following:

- 1 L of D5W, which contains 5 g of dextrose in each 100 mL of solution
- 1/4% solution of pilocarpine HCl, which contains 1/4 g (0.25 g) of pilocarpine HCl in each 100 mL of solution.

EXAMPLE

What is the percentage weight to volume (% W/V) of sodium chloride (solid solute) in normal saline solution if 9 g of the salt are dissolved in enough water to make 1,000 mL of solution?

Solution

$$\frac{\text{Amount of salt in grams: } 9\text{ g}}{\text{Total volume of solution: } 1000\text{ mL}} \times 100 = 0.9\%\text{ W/V}$$

A weight-to-weight percentage (% W/W) is defined as the number of grams of solute (or drug) in 100 g of a solid preparation. Typical % W/W examples include the following:

- A 10% ointment of zinc oxide, which contains 10 g of zinc oxide in each 100 g of ointment
- Hydrocortisone cream 1/2%, which has 1/2 g (0.5 g) of hydrocortisone in each 100 g of cream.

The third form of percentage is a volume-to-volume percentage (% V/V), which is defined as the number of milliliters of solute in each 100 mL of solution. Examples of this form include the following:

- Rubbing alcohol 70%, which contains 70 mL of absolute alcohol in each 100 mL of the solution
- A 2% solution of phenol, which contains 2 mL of liquefied phenol in each 100 mL of solution.

When the type of percentage is not stated, assume that for solutions of a solid in a liquid the percentage is % W/V, for solutions of a liquid in a liquid the percentage is % V/V, and for mixtures of two solids the percentage is % W/W.

Note: Concentrated hydrochloric acid and glacial acetic acid are two examples of *solutions* given as a weight-to-weight percentage and should be clearly labeled as a W/W solution.

Ratio Strength Solutions

Concentration expressions for weak solutions (or solids) may also be expressed in terms of ratio strength. A 0.1% solution of drug is interpreted to be 0.1 g of drug in 100 mL of solution. The ratio strength could be expressed as 0.1:100. However, it is customary to give a ratio strength with the first number of the ratio as "1." The correct expression of the 0.1% solution as a ratio strength is 1:1,000. This would be interpreted as 1 g of drug in 1,000 mL of solution. Any concentration can be restated as a ratio strength when converted using proportions.

Important:

1. A ratio strength is written with a colon (1:20) and *not* as a fraction (1/20). Note the first number in the ratio strength is a 1.
2. As with percentages, solids are given in grams and liquids in milliliters.

EXAMPLE

Express the strength of a 2.5% W/V solution as a ratio strength.

Solution:

2.5% W/V means 2.5 g of drug in 100 mL of solution.

$$\frac{2.5\text{ g}}{100\text{ mL}} = \frac{1\text{ g}}{X\text{ mL}}$$

$$X = 40$$

The ratio strength is expressed as 1:40 W/V. (This product contains 1 gram of drug in every 40 mL of solution.)

Dilution and Alligation

A physician may order a commercially prepared dosage form to be diluted to a lower strength for a patient. Liquid dosage forms such as suspensions or solutions, or semisolid dosage forms such as creams or ointments, may all be diluted with a diluent that is compatible with the original product.

These problems can be solved by using:

1. Proportions, as discussed earlier in the chapter
2. The equation (Q1)(C1) = (Q2)(C2) where Q1 is the original quantity, C1 is the original concentration, Q2 is the final quantity, and C2 is the final concentration.
3. Alligation.

(Q1)(C1) = (Q2)(C2)

Important: Three conditions must be met when using (Q1)(C1) = (Q2)(C2):

1. Three of the four parts must be known.
2. Each quantity must have the same units.
3. Each concentration must be expressed in the same format (percentage or ratio).

EXAMPLE

The physician orders 10% coal tar ointment be diluted to 2.5% coal tar ointment. How many grams of petrolatum (Vaseline) must be added to 30 grams of the 10% ointment to correctly dilute this product?

Solution:

(Original Quantity) (Original Concentration) = (Final Quantity) (Final Concentration)

(30 g) × (10%) = (X g) × (2.5%)

X = 120 g (**Note** : 120 g is **not** the correct answer.)

EXAMPLE *(CONTINUED)*

where X is the *total quantity* of 2.5% ointment that can be made when 30 grams of 10% ointment are diluted with petrolatum. Since X is the total weight of the final product, the weight of the original ointment must be subtracted from the diluted ointment to calculate the amount of petrolatum needed:

$$120\,g - 30\,g = 90\,g$$

Therefore, to make this product, 30 grams of 10% coal tar ointment is incorporated (mixed) with 90 grams of petrolatum to make 120 grams of 2.5% coal tar ointment.

EXAMPLE

How many milliliters of 5% acetic acid solution must be used to make 125 mL of 2% acetic acid solution?

Solution:

(Original Quantity) (Original Concentration) = (Final Quantity) (Final Concentration)
(X mL) × (5%) = (125 mL) × (2%)

X = 50 mL of 2% acetic acid solution.

To make this product, measure 50 mL of 5% acetic acid solution and add enough water (75 mL) to make 125 mL of solution, which will have a strength of 2% acetic acid.

alligation the relative amounts of solutions of different percentages from a mixture of a given strength

Alligation is a method generally used to solve problems in which two liquids, solids, or semi-solids of *different strengths* are combined to create a final strength. The final strength must be somewhere between the two strengths of the two components (weaker than the strongest strength and stronger than the weakest strength). Alligation can also be used in place of the (Q1)(C1) = (Q2)(C2) equation.

EXAMPLE

The physician orders 10% coal tar ointment to be diluted to 2.5% coal tar ointment. How many grams of petrolatum (Vaseline) must be added to 30 grams of the 10% ointment to correctly dilute this product? (This is the same question posed in the preceding example, but will be solved using the alligation method.)

Note: The final product has a strength of 2.5%, which is weaker than 10% and stronger than 0% (because petrolatum contains no coal tar).

Solution:

- Put the percent strengths *available* in the first two columns.
- Put the percent strength *ordered* in the next column.
- Subtract on the diagonal to calculate the *parts* of each component needed in the last column:

10%		2.5 parts (of 10% ointment)
	2.5%	
0%		7.5 parts (of petrolatum)

- Then solve by proportion:

$$\frac{2.5\text{ parts}}{7.5\text{ parts}} = \frac{30\,g}{X\,g}$$

$$X = 90\,g$$

EXAMPLE

How many grams of 2.5% hydrocortisone ointment and how many grams of 1% hydrocortisone ointment must be used to make 120 g of 2% hydrocortisone (HC) ointment?

Solution:

2.5%		1 part of 2.5% HC ointment
	2%	
1%		0.5 part of 1% HC ointment
		1.5 parts total

- The parts must be added because the total quantity of the final ointment is given:

$$\frac{1 \text{ part}}{1.5 \text{ parts}} = \frac{X \text{ g}}{120 \text{ g}}$$

$$X = 80 \text{ g of } 2.5\% \text{ HC ointment}$$

$$\frac{0.5 \text{ part}}{1.5 \text{ parts}} = \frac{X \text{ g}}{120 \text{ g}}$$

$$X = 40 \text{ g of } 0.5\% \text{ HC ointment}$$

Double-check: 80 g + 40 g = 120 g, which is the amount of 2% hydrocortisone ointment ordered.

Calculation of Fractional Doses

Health care professionals encounter fractional or partial medication dosages because physicians often order medication for a patient in a strength that differs from the strength of the commercially prepared product.

The ratio and proportion method can be used to solve all problems of fractional dosages. Since the concentration of the medication on hand is known, it forms the "IF" ratio of the proportion. The "THEN" portion allows for calculation of the amount of drug product necessary for the fractional dose.

EXAMPLE

The physician orders 1 million units of penicillin G for a patient. The penicillin G available is prepared as a solution containing 250,000 units/mL.

Solution:

Find the strength of the product available. This expression forms the IF ratio of the proportion:

$$\overset{\text{IF}}{\frac{250{,}000 \text{ units}}{1 \text{ mL}}} = \text{THEN}$$

Place the number of units wanted in the THEN ratio and solve for the unknown X:

$$\overset{\text{IF}}{\frac{250{,}000 \text{ units}}{1 \text{ mL}}} = \overset{\text{THEN}}{\frac{1{,}000{,}000 \text{ units}}{X \text{ mL}}}$$

$$250{,}000\ X = 1{,}000{,}000$$

$$X = 4 \text{ mL}$$

To supply 250,000 units of penicillin G, 4 mL of the solution is required.

Remember to label all parts of the proportion carefully with the appropriate units.

EXAMPLE

The physician orders 250 mcg of cyanocobalamin (vitamin B_{12}) daily. The vitamin B_{12} solution available is labeled 1,000 mcg/mL. How many milliliters should be given to the patient?

Solution:

The concentration of B_{12} available is 1,000 mcg/mL. It forms the IF ratio of the proportion. Place the number of micrograms needed in the THEN ratio and solve for the unknown X:

$$\overset{\text{IF}}{\frac{1000\,\text{mcg}}{1\,\text{mL}}} = \overset{\text{THEN}}{\frac{250\,\text{mcg}}{X\,\text{mL}}}$$

Solving for X yields:

$$X = 0.25\,\text{mL}$$

To supply 250 mcg of vitamin B_{12} requires 0.25 mL of the B_{12} solution available.

EXAMPLE

A patient is to be given 25 mg of diphenhydramine (Benadryl) by mouth. The Benadryl elixir is available in a strength of 12.5 mg/5 mL. How many milliliters should be given to the patient?

Solution:

$$\overset{\text{IF}}{\frac{12.5\,\text{mg}}{5\,\text{mL}}} = \overset{\text{THEN}}{\frac{25\,\text{mg}}{X\,\text{mL}}}$$

$$X = \frac{125}{12.5}$$

$$X = 10\,\text{mL}$$

EXAMPLE

A medication order calls for 750 mg of calcium lactate to be given po tid. On hand are tablets labeled calcium lactate 0.5 g. How many tablets should be given for each dose?

Solution:

Note: Remember when using ratio and proportion the units must be alike. Grams cannot be used in a proportion opposite milligrams. Therefore, in this example 0.5 g must be converted to milligrams or 750 mg converted to grams. Changing the grams to milligrams yields:

$$0.5\,\text{g} = 500\,\text{mg}$$

The IF/THEN proportion would read:

$$\overset{\text{IF}}{\frac{500\,\text{mg}}{1\,\text{tab}}} = \overset{\text{THEN}}{\frac{750\,\text{mg}}{X\,\text{tab}}}$$

$$X = 1.5 \text{ or } 1\tfrac{1}{2} \text{ tablets}$$

Calculation of Dosages Based on Weight

The recommended dosages of drugs are often expressed in the literature as a number of milligrams per unit of body weight per unit of time (refer to package inserts, *Physicians' Desk Reference,* or other standard drug references). Such dosage expressions are commonly used in depicting pediatric doses. For example, the recommended dose for a drug might be 5 mg per kg per day (5 mg/kg/day). The drug may be given all at once or divided into two or more doses for the day. This information can be utilized by the pharmacist to:

- Calculate the dose for a given patient.
- Evaluate that the dose ordered is in the appropriate range for the patient.

EXAMPLE

The physician orders rifampin capsules for a 66-pound child. The recommended dosage for rifampin is 10 mg/kg/dose. How many 150-mg capsules of rifampin should be given to this patient for each dose?

Solution:

Step 1. Because the dose provided is based on a kilogram weight, convert the patient's weight to kilograms by proportion. Since 1 kg = 2.2 lb, then:

$$\frac{1\,\text{kg}}{2.2\,\text{lb}} = \frac{X\,\text{kg}}{66\,\text{lb}}$$

$$X = 30\,\text{kg}$$

Step 2. Calculate the total daily dose using the recommended dosage information: 10 mg/kg. This is interpreted as "Give 10 mg of the drug for each kilogram of body weight."

$$\frac{10\,\text{mg}}{1\,\text{kg}} = \frac{X\,\text{mg}}{30\,\text{kg}}$$

$$X = 300\,\text{mg}$$

Step 3. Calculate the number of capsules needed to supply 300 mg per dose. The strength of the capsules available is 150 mg/capsule.

$$\frac{150\,\text{mg}}{1\,\text{cap}} = \frac{300\,\text{mg}}{X\,\text{cap}}$$

$$X = 2 \text{ capsules per dose}$$

EXAMPLE

The physician orders gentamicin 6 mg/kg/24 hours to be given in divided doses every 8 hours. How many milliliters of gentamicin injection (40 mg/mL) should be administered to a 132-pound patient for one dose?

Solution:

Step 1. Calculate the daily dose for a 132-pound patient. (*Note:* The calculation can be done in one step by inserting the conversion unit 2.2 lb for 1 kg in the ratio.)

$$\frac{6\,\text{mg}}{1\,\text{kg}\,(2.2\,\text{lb})} = \frac{X\,\text{mg}}{132\,\text{lb}}$$

$$X = 360\,\text{mg of Gentamicin per day (24 hours)}$$

Step 2. Calculate the number of milligrams of gentamicin needed for one dose:

$$\frac{360\,\text{mg}}{24\,\text{hours}} = \frac{X\,\text{mg}}{8\,\text{hours}}$$

$$X = 120\,\text{mg per dose}$$

Step 3. Calculate the number of milliliters to be given per dose:

$$\frac{40\,\text{mg}}{1\,\text{mL}} = \frac{120\,\text{mg}}{X\,\text{mL}}$$

$$120 = 40\,(X\,\text{mL})$$

$$X = 3\,\text{mL}$$

Calculation of Dosages Based on Weight and Height

body surface area (BSA) the measurement of the height and weight of a patient to establish an estimate of his or her body surface

nomogram a chart that determines body surface area from height and weight

Some drugs may be dosed based on a patient's **body surface area (BSA)**, which is expressed as square meters (m^2). The BSA is determined by taking the weight and height of a patient for use in a nomogram or in an equation. A **nomogram** is a chart that contains columns with both metric (cm, kg) and avoirdupois (in., lbs) values for height and weight. Thus, the BSA can be determined based on pounds and inches or kilograms and centimeters without making conversions. Once calculated, the body surface area is then placed in a proportion with the dose when it is ordered per square meter.

Figure 15-2 is a body surface area nomogram. (A different nomogram is available for children.) Note the three columns labeled "Height," "Body surface area," and "Weight."

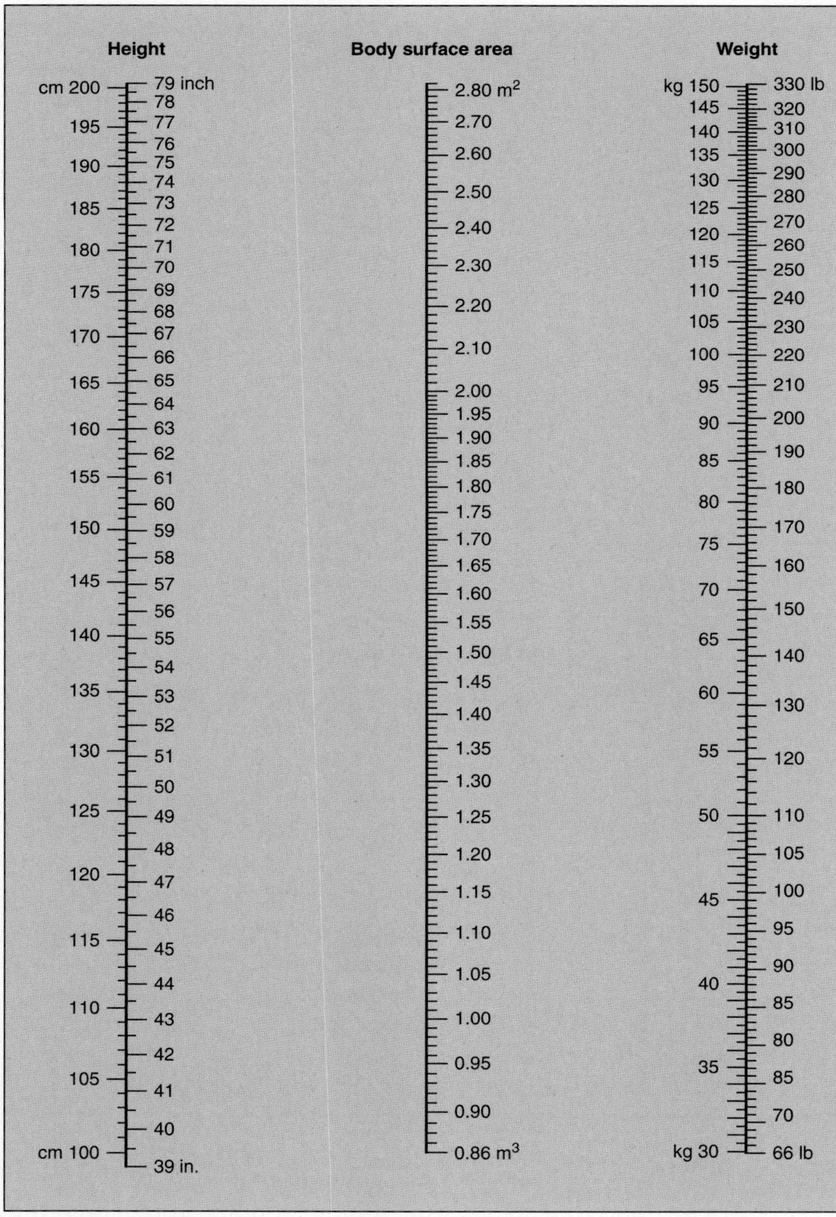

Used with permission from Lentner C. (1981). *Geigy Scientific Tables: Units of Measurement, Body Fluid, Composition of Body, and Nutrition* (8th ed.). Novartis Basel, Switzerland.

FIGURE 15-2 Nomogram from Geigy Scientific Tables.

To determine the patient's body surface area, a ruler or straightedge is needed. The following steps demonstrate the use of the nomogram:

Step 1. Determine the height and weight of the patient. This information may be given in metric values (e.g., height 150 cm, weight 50 kg) or in avoirdupois values (height 59 inches, weight 110 pounds). Mixed values can also be used (height 150 cm, weight 110 pounds).

Important: Be very careful to use the correct side of each column.

Step 2. Place the straightedge on the nomogram connecting the point on the Height column with the point on the Weight column that represent the patient's values. The patient weighs 110 pounds and stands 59 inches tall. The 110 pounds on the Weight column and 59 inches on the Height column are connected using the straightedge.

Step 3. Where the straightedge crosses the center column (Body surface area) a reading is taken. This value is the patient's body surface area in square meters. In our example, BSA = 1.43 m^2.

Important: Use caution when reading the nomogram because the divisions between the numbered sections vary in value along each of the columns.

Step 4. If a dose is ordered as 10 mg/m^2, this gives the proportion:

$$\frac{10\text{ mg}}{1\text{ m}^2} = \frac{X\text{ mg}}{1.43\text{ m}^2}$$

$$X = 14.3\text{ mg}$$

If the dose is not available in square meters, a dose can be estimated for a child by placing the child's BSA into a ratio with the body surface area of an average adult (1.73 m^2).

$$\text{Child's dose} = \frac{\text{Child's body surface area in m}^2}{1.73\text{ m}^2\text{ (BSA of average adult)}} \times \text{Adult dose}$$

EXAMPLE

If the dose of aminophylline is 500 mg for an adult, what is the estimated dose for a child with a calculated BSA of 0.52 m^2?

Solution:

$$\text{Child's dose} = \frac{0.52\text{ m}^2}{1.73\text{ m}^2} \times 500\text{ mg}$$

$$= 0.3 \times 500\text{ mg}$$

$$= 150\text{ mg of aminophylline}$$

With practice, the health care practitioner can become proficient in using the nomogram and will find it a useful tool for calculating dosages.

Calculations Involving Intravenous Administration

Pharmacists may be required to determine the flow rates for intravenous infusions and to calculate the volume of fluids administered over a period of time. Infusion solutions may be a large volume and run continuously at a specified rate, or a

piggyback refers to a small-volume IV solution (25 to 250 mL) that is run into an existing IV line over a brief period of time (e.g., 50 mL over 15 minutes)

smaller volume and run intermittently (for a certain period of time and repeated at intervals throughout the day). Sometimes a second IV solution is connected to and run through the line of a primary solution. These are known as **piggyback** or secondary solutions. The calculations necessary to perform these tasks can all be accomplished by the use of ratios and proportions.

Chapter 18 provides information on the techniques involved in IV administration, the equipment used, and the documentation to be prepared by the nurse administering the IV solutions.

Calculating the Rate of IV Administration

When a physician orders intravenous solutions to run for a specific number of hours, the pharmacist may have to compute the administration rate in milliliters per hour, milliliters per minute, or drops per minute to comply with the order. The rate expression used will be determined by the method of solution delivery; pumps will be calculated in milliliters per hour or milliliters per minute, and gravity feed administration sets calculated in drops per minute.

The flow rate may be calculated through the following steps using the ratio and proportion method:

Step 1. Calculate the number of milliliters the patient will receive per hour.

Step 2. Calculate the number of milliliters the patient will receive per minute.

Step 3. Determine the number of drops per minute that will equal the number of milliliters computed in step 2. The number of drops per milliliter (gtt/mL) given for the specific IV set being used must be considered in this step.

Because it is not possible to obtain a fraction of a drop, always round off the number of drops per minute to the *nearest whole drop*.

EXAMPLE

The physician orders 3,000 mL of dextrose 5% in water (D5W) IV over a 24-hour period. If the IV set is calibrated to deliver 15 drops per milliliter, how many drops must be administered per minute?

Solution:

Step 1. Calculate milliliters per hour:

$$\frac{3{,}000\text{ mL}}{24\text{ hr}} = \frac{X\text{ mL}}{1\text{ hr}}$$

$$X = 125\text{ mL/hr or }125\text{ mL/60 min}$$

Step 2. Calculate milliliters per minute:

$$\frac{125\text{ mL}}{60\text{ min}} = \frac{X\text{ mL}}{1\text{ min}}$$

$$X = 2.1\text{ mL/min}$$

Step 3. Calculate drops per minutes using the specified drops per milliliter of the IV set:

$$\frac{15\text{ gtt}}{1\text{ mL}} = \frac{X\text{ gtt}}{2.1\text{ mL (amt needed/min)}}$$

$$X = 32\text{ gtt/min}$$

EXAMPLE

The physician orders 2 L of lactated Ringer's solution (LR) to be administered over a 12-hour period. The IV set is calibrated to deliver 10 gtt/mL. How many drops per minute should the patient receive?

Solution:

Step 1. Determine the number of milliliters to be administered in 1 hour. Since the answer requested is in milliliters, first convert the liter quantity to milliliters:

$$2\ \text{L} = 2{,}000\ \text{mL}$$

$$\frac{2000\ \text{mL}}{12\ \text{hr}} = \frac{X\ \text{mL}}{1\ \text{hr}}$$

$$X = 167\ \text{mL/hr or}$$

$$= 167\ \text{mL/60 min}$$

Step 2. Calculate the number of milliliters per minute:

$$\frac{167\ \text{mL}}{60\ \text{min}} = \frac{X\ \text{mL}}{1\ \text{min}}$$

$$X = 2.8\ \text{mL/min}$$

Step 3. Calculate the number of drops per minute, knowing that the IV set delivers 10 gtt/mL:

$$\frac{10\ \text{gtt}}{1\ \text{mL}} = \frac{X\ \text{gtt}}{2.8\ \text{mL}}$$

$$X = 28\ \text{gtt/min}$$

Note: One may only need to calculate through step 1 or 2 depending on how the administration rates must be expressed for the method of delivery used.

The following example shows how to calculate the time required to administer an IV solution when the volume and flow rate are known.

EXAMPLE

How many hours will it take to complete an IV infusion of 1.5 L of D5W being administered at the rate of 2.5 mL/min? This problem is a variation of the flow rate problem considered earlier.

Solution:

Step 1. Calculate the number of minutes required to administer the total volume of the solution:

$$\frac{2.5\ \text{mL}}{1\ \text{min}} = \frac{1500\ \text{mL}}{X\ \text{min}}$$

$$X = 600\ \text{min}$$

Step 2. Convert the minutes to hours:

$$\frac{60\ \text{min}}{1\ \text{hour}} = \frac{600\ \text{min}}{X\ \text{hours}}$$

$$X = 10\ \text{hours}$$

EXAMPLE

A physician orders 0.9% sodium chloride solution with 10 mEq potassium chloride per liter at a rate of 125 mL/hr. How many liters of solution must be provided to cover a 24-hour period?

Solution:

$$\frac{125\ \text{mL}}{1\ \text{hr}} = \frac{X\ \text{mL}}{24\ \text{hr}}$$

$$X = 3{,}000\ \text{mL or 3 liters of solution per 24-hour period}$$

Calculations Involving Piggyback IV Infusions

A physician may order medications to be run piggyback with IV electrolyte fluids. The medications are usually dissolved in 50 or 100 mL of an IV solution and run for short periods of time through the open IV line. The flow rate for these piggyback infusions is calculated the same way as the rate for the regular IV solutions.

EXAMPLE

A physician orders an IV piggyback of cefazolin sodium (Ancef, Kefzol) 500 mg in 100 mL to be administered over 1 hour. The piggyback IV set is calibrated to deliver 10 gtt/mL. How many drops per minute should be given?

Solution:

Step 1. The entire 100 mL is to be infused in 1 hour. Calculate the number of milliliters per minute:

$$\frac{100\ \text{mL}}{60\ \text{min}} = \frac{X\ \text{mL}}{1\ \text{min}}$$

$$60X = 100$$

$$X = 1.7\ \text{mL/min}$$

Step 2. Calculate the number of drops per minute:

$$\text{Drop rate} = \frac{10\ \text{gtt}}{1\ \text{min}} = \frac{X\ \text{gtt}}{1.7\ \text{mL}}$$

$$X = 17\ \text{gtt/min}$$

A health care provider may need to account for the volume of the piggyback and the time of its administration when calculating the daily fluid requirements, or fluid intake, of a patient.

When fluids are not restricted, calculating daily fluid intake simply involves adding all of the volumes administered to a patient in a 24-hour period. Daily volumes are determined by each fluid/drug and its ordered infusion rate:

- Cefazolin 100 mL qid = 100 mL × 4 doses per day = 400 mL in 24 hours
- Standard hydration fluid D5W at 75 mL/hr × 24 hours = 1,800 mL in 24 hours
- Add to determine total intake = 1,800 mL + 400 mL = 2,200 mL in 24 hours if the piggyback is run in concurrently.

OR if the standard fluid is stopped when giving the piggyback, the:

- 75 mL/hr × 20 hours = 1,500 mL
- Plus 400 mL from piggyback cefazolin
- Total = 1900 mL in 24 hours.

Prevention of Medication Errors

Medication errors may fall into several categories including omitting the dose, administering the wrong dose, administering an extra dose, administering an unordered drug, administering by the wrong route, and administering at the wrong time. The focus here is on considering the errors that occur when a drug order is misinterpreted. How amounts are expressed in the original order (weights, volumes, and units) may cause interpretational errors. The pharmacist and all personnel assisting them (technicians and interns) are vital to catching, preventing, and correcting this type of error.

For example, writing ".5" instead of "0.5" can result in a 10-fold error if the decimal point is missed. In general, the following rules should be followed when transcribing orders to reduce the possibility of errors. These are important for all health care professionals (physicians, nurses, pharmacists, interns, technicians, etc.) to follow:

- Never leave a decimal point "naked"; that is, always place a zero *before* a decimal expression of less than 1. Example: 0.25 is correct, whereas .25 is incorrect.
- A whole number should be shown with no decimal point or "trailing" 0. The decimal may not be seen and result in a 10-fold overdose. Example: 2.0 mg is incorrect because it may be read as 20 mg. The correct way to write this is simply 2 mg.
- Avoid using decimals when a whole number can be used as an alternative. Example: 0.5 g should be expressed as 500 mg and 0.4 mg should be expressed as 400 mcg.
- A space should be left between a number and the units for clarity in reading the number.
- Use the metric system, converting when necessary.
- Always spell out the word *units*. The abbreviation "U" for unit can be mistaken for a zero. Example: 10 U may be interpreted as 100 if the U is unclear. The safer way is to write 10 *units*.

Summary

Accuracy in pharmaceutical calculations is one of the most critical and important functions in the profession of pharmacy. *A pharmacy technician should have every calculation regarding drugs or compounding checked by a pharmacist before preparing or dispensing any medication order.* Pharmacists frequently double-check each other in this important matter because life and death can hinge on a proper or improper dose being administered. Emergency situations or other life-threatening situations are never an excuse for undue haste and lack of sufficient double-checks. Care and vigilance are required whenever drug doses or formulations are calculated.

TEST YOUR KNOWLEDGE

Calculations

Convert the following to Arabic numbers:

1. viii
2. xxiv
3. XLV
4. CXXV
5. DCCL

Convert the following:

6. 2,500 mg = ______________ g
7. 7.5 g = ______________ mg
8. 0.3 L = ______________ mL
9. 250 mcg = ______________ mg
10. 1.5 kg = ______________ g
11. 0.05 g = ______________ mcg
12. 1.5 dL = ______________ mL

Solve the following problems by setting up the proportion and finding the unknown quantity:

13. Digoxin elixir contains 50 mcg of digoxin in each milliliter. How many micrograms of the drug are in 0.3 mL of the elixir?
14. A solution of gentamicin contains 3 mg of gentamicin per milliliter. How many micrograms of gentamicin are in 0.2 mL of the solution?
15. Benadryl elixir contains 12.5 mg per 5 mL (teaspoonful). How many milliliters are needed to provide 30 mg of the drug?
16. A physician orders 24 mg of theophylline to be administered orally to a pediatric patient. If theophylline solution contains 80 mg of theophylline per 15 mL (tablespoonful), how many milliliters of the solution should be administered?
17. A bottle of erythromycin suspension contains 250 mg of erythromycin in every 5 mL of suspension. How many grams of erythromycin are in a 200-mL bottle?

Convert the following:

18. 2 fluid ounces (℥ii) to teaspoonfuls
19. 24 pints to gallons
20. 1.5 quarts to fluid ounces
21. 138 pounds to kg

22. 2.5 pounds of ointment to grams
23. ℥ iiss to mL
24. 2 quarts to liters
25. 5 gr to mg

Calculate the following doses/amounts:

26. If a physician orders ʒ ii three times a day for 10 days, how many milliliters of solution must be dispensed to fill the prescription?
27. Sixty tablets of lorazepam 0.5 mg are ordered for a patient with these directions given: 1–2 tablets every 8 hours as needed for nausea. What is the minimum number of days this order should last?
28. Loratadine syrup 5 mg/5 mL is dispensed to a patient in a 4-oz bottle. How many days will this last if a dose of 5 mg is taken twice a day?
29. An antacid is prescribed to be taken 1 ounce four times a day. How many 12-oz bottles will the patient need for a month (30 days) of therapy?
30. Calculate the percentage strength of a solution made from 102 g of sucrose and enough water to make 120 mL of solution.
31. How many grams of hydrocortisone are present in 40 g of a 2.5% hydrocortisone ointment?
32. How many milliliters of alcohol are in 30 mL of a mouthwash made with 18% V/V alcohol?
33. How many grams of dextrose does a patient receive from 3 L of 5% dextrose in water?

Calculate the following using the (Q1)(C1) = (Q2)(C2) equation:

34. How many grams of petrolatum must be added to 15 grams of 20% ichthammol ointment to dilute it to a 12% ichthammol ointment?
35. To make 240 mL of a solution that contains 20% alcohol, how many milliliters of 70% alcohol must be used?
36. How many grams of 1.5% Bactroban ointment can be made from 30 grams of 2% Bactroban ointment?
37. How many milliliters of 17% benzalkonium chloride solution must be diluted to make 480 mL of 2% benzalkonium chloride solution?

Using alligations, recalculate Questions 34 through 37 and then calculate the following:

38. How many milliliters of 70% dextrose solution must be diluted to make 2 liters of 20% dextrose solution?
39. To make 120 g of 1.5% hydrocortisone ointment, how many grams of the following must be weighed?
    a. 5% hydrocortisone ointment
    b. petrolatum

40. How many grams of 3% coal tar ointment can be compounded by adding petrolatum to 1 pound of 5% coal tar ointment?

41. How many milliliters of water must be added to 120 mL of 95% alcohol to dilute it to 75% alcohol?

42. A patient is to receive a 120-mg dose of gentamicin. The drug is available in a vial containing 80 mg/2 mL of drug. How many milliliters should be given to the patient to obtain the correct dose?

43. After reconstitution, a multiple-dose vial of a penicillin G potassium solution contains 100,000 units per milliliter. How many milliliters of this solution must be administered to a patient who requires a 450,000-unit dose?

44. A physician orders 40 mg of Demerol for a patient. How many milliliters of a Demerol solution with a strength of 100 mg/mL should the patient receive?

45. The nurse is asked to administer an intramuscular dose of 0.45 mg of an investigational drug. How many milliliters must be withdrawn from a vial containing 200 mcg/mL of the drug?

46. An elderly patient is to be given a 120-mg dose of phenytoin by administering an oral suspension containing 50 mg/5 mL of phenytoin. How many milliliters of the suspension should be administered for each dose?

47. The recommended dose of cefuroxime (Ceftin) for a pediatric patient is 20 mg/kg/day. How many milligrams must be given daily to a 80-pound child?

48. Acyclovir (Zovirax) is administered in a dose of 15 mg/kg/day. How many milligrams of the drug must be administered for each dose to a 175-pound adult if the drug is to be given three times a day?

49. The recommended dose for methotrexate is 2.5 mg/kg once every 14 days. How many milligrams of this drug must be administered to a 125-pound adult for each dose?

50. Chlorpromazine HCl is to be administered in a dose of 0.25 mg/lb. How many 25-mg tablets of chlorpromazine HCl should be administered for each dose to a 91-kg patient?

51. A new drug is to be dosed at 40 mg/kg/dose. Calculate the number of milligrams a 48-kg adult should receive for each dose.

Solve the following problems using the nomogram of Figure 15-2.

52. Find the BSA for the following patients:
a. 114 pounds, 57 inches
b. 88 kg, 185 cm
c. 45.5 kg, 42 inches

53. If the adult dose of amoxicillin is 500 mg, estimate the dose for a child whose BSA is 0.27 m^2.

54. If the adult dose of furosemide (Lasix) is 40 mg, estimate the dose for a child whose BSA is 0.62 m^2.

55. If a dose of drug is ordered at 5 mg/m^2, what is the dose for a child who weighs 55 pounds with a height of 41 inches?

56. If a dose of drug is ordered at 25 mg /m^2, what is the dose for a child who weighs 8 kg with a height of 68 cm?

57. The physician orders 1,500 mL of D5W solution to be administered over a 12-hour period. The IV set is calibrated to deliver 20 gtt/mL. Calculate the number of drops per minute the patient must receive.

58. An IV infusion containing 500 mL is to be administered at a drip rate of 40 gtt/min.

The IV set is calibrated to deliver 20 gtt/mL. Calculate the number of minutes it will take to administer the entire infusion solution.

59. A physician orders a solution to be run continuously at 75 mL/hr.
   a. How many 500-mL bags must be prepared for the patient to cover a 24-hour period?
   b. Using an IV set that is calibrated to deliver 15 gtt/mL, how many drops per minute must it be set at to infuse the solutions?

60. An IV piggyback of cefazolin containing 1 g of drug in 100 mL is to be infused over 1 hour. The IV set to be used is calibrated to deliver 15 gtt/mL. How many drops per minute should be administered?

61. A piggyback infusion solution of heparin sodium containing 25,000 in 500 mL is to be infused at a rate of 1,000 units per hour. The IV set is calibrated to deliver 30 gtt/mL. How many drops per minute should be administered?

62. What should the rate be (in drops per minute) to infuse a piggyback solution of 300 mg of cimetidine in 50 mL of normal saline (0.9% sodium chloride solution) over 45 minutes? The set to be used delivers 25 drops/mL.

Suggested Readings

Ansel, H.C. (2010). *Pharmaceutical calculations* (13th ed.). Philadelphia, PA: Lippincott Williams & Wilkins.

Capriotti, T. (2004). Basic concepts to prevent medication calculation errors. *MEDSURG Nursing 04, 13*(1), 62–65.

Cohen, M.R. (2007). *Medication errors* (2nd ed.). Washington, D.C.: American Pharmacists Association.

Kelly, L.E., & Colby, N. (2003). Teaching medication calculation for conceptual understanding. *Journal of Nursing Education 03, 42*(10), 468–471.

Preston, R.M. (2004). Drug errors and patient safety: The need for a change in practice. *British Journal of Nursing 04, 13*(2), 72–78.

Richardson, L.I., & Richardson, J. (2004). *The mathematics of drugs and solutions with clinical applications* (6th ed.). New York, NY: Pearson Publishing Co.

Trim, J. (2004). Clinical skills: A practical guide to working out drug calculations. *British Journal of Nursing 04, 13*(10), 602–606.

CHAPTER

16

Extemporaneous Compounding

Competencies

Upon completion of this chapter, the reader should be able to:

1. Define a Class A prescription balance, a counter balance, and a solution balance.
2. Describe what is meant by *extemporaneous compounding*.
3. Explain the circumstances that may require the extemporaneous compounding of a drug dosage form.
4. Outline the steps required to accurately weigh a pharmaceutical ingredient.
5. Describe the meaning of the term *geometric dilution*.
6. Explain the difference between a solution and a suspension; an ointment and a cream.
7. Describe the process of levigation.
8. List some of the steps involved in the process of compounding suppositories.
9. Give an example of the ingredients found in an enteral solution.
10. List the essential equipment used in the compounding process.

Key Terms

chemical sterilization
Class A prescription balance
counter balance
electronic balance
extemporaneous compounding
filtration
geometric dilution
graduate
levigation
meniscus
radiation
suspending agent
tare
taring
thermal sterilization
triple beam balance
triturate

Introduction

This chapter familiarizes students with the terminology, equipment, and principles of extemporaneous compounding and their roles in providing this service. The student should understand this to be an introduction to compounding; experience is needed to develop this valuable skill. While it is beyond the scope of this chapter to review all types of compounding, the most common and relevant practices are reviewed. The student is referred to compounding textbooks for more detailed knowledge.

Extemporaneous compounding is a true pharmaceutical service, not simply the redistribution of a commercially available commodity, but rather the preparation of drugs not readily available from manufacturers. This service requires specialized knowledge of the physical and chemical properties of drugs and their vehicles. This knowledge is based on sound scientific principles; however, the practice is closer to an art.

Extemporaneous Compounding

extemporaneous compounding the act of preparing a drug product at the time it is required with materials on hand

Extemporaneous compounding may be defined as the timely preparation of a drug product according to a physician's prescription, a drug formula, or a recipe in which the amounts of the ingredients are calculated to meet the needs of a particular patient or group of patients.

Extemporaneous pharmaceutical compounding is among the most exciting, challenging, and rapidly expanding areas in pharmacy today. Practically every medical discipline incorporates pharmaceutical dosage forms in their everyday practice. Many pharmaceutical products are either no longer produced or become temporarily unavailable due to lack of sales, shortage in raw supplies, or plant closures. Many commercially available products are in dosage forms that may not be convenient for dosing a specific patient. These are some of the challenges that are overcome with modern compounding techniques. Veterinary medicine, sports medicine, ophthalmology, hormone replacement therapy, and pain management have opened up vast new areas for the compounder. The compounding of sterile products such as ophthalmics, injectables, and intravenous prescriptions, when done following proper procedure, is both very challenging and professionally rewarding. With the development of modern equipment and devices, the properly equipped compounding pharmacy is capable of delivering the highest quality specialty dosage forms.

Traditional Equipment

Class A prescription balance balance scale that has a sensitive balance range of 6 mg with a maximum capacity of 120 g

The tools of pharmaceutical practice are those used to measure, transfer, transform, and handle medications in any way desired. Those involved in nonsterile compounding are classic, and every pharmacy technician should be familiar with their proper handling.

Every pharmacy is required to have a **Class A prescription balance** (**Figure 16-1A**). Class A balances have a sensitivity requirement of 6 mg and maximum capacity of 120 g. A scale's sensitivity is the smallest weight required to move the indicator at least one degree.

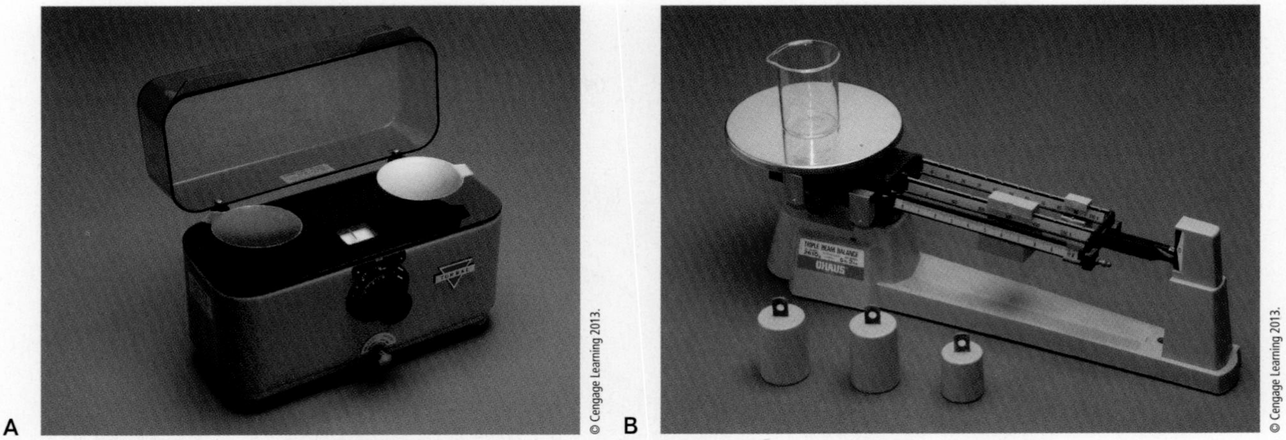

FIGURE 16-1 **A.** The Class A prescription balance. **B.** A triple beam balance.

triple beam balance a single-pan unequal arm balance used for weighing large amounts

counter balance a double-pan balance capable of weighing relatively large quantities; they have a sensitivity of 100 mg and a weight limit of about 5 kg

A **triple beam balance** is a single-pan instrument with an unequal arm that acts as a compound lever (**Figure 16-1B**). These balances are less accurate than Class A balances, but because of their weighing capacity of about 20 kg, they are useful for measuring large masses.

Counter balances are double-pan balances that, like triple beam balances, are not intended for measuring small weights, but are capable of weighing large quantities. They have a sensitivity of 100 mg and a limit of about 5 kg.

Weights used with the balances should be of good quality and stored correctly. Weights made of corrosion-resistant metals such as brass are preferred (**Figure 16-2**). Metric weight sets are commonly available in a range from less than 1 g to 50 g. Always use forceps to transfer the weights, and take care not to drop them. Keep the weights covered in their original case when not in use.

Spatulas (**Figure 16-3**) are used to transfer solid ingredients to weighing pans. They are the preferred mixing instruments with semisolid dosage forms such as ointments and creams. These are available in stainless steel and hard rubber or plastic. Care must be used with materials that corrode metals, such as iodine, salts of mercury, or tannins. Use rubber spatulas for these agents. Check that spatulas

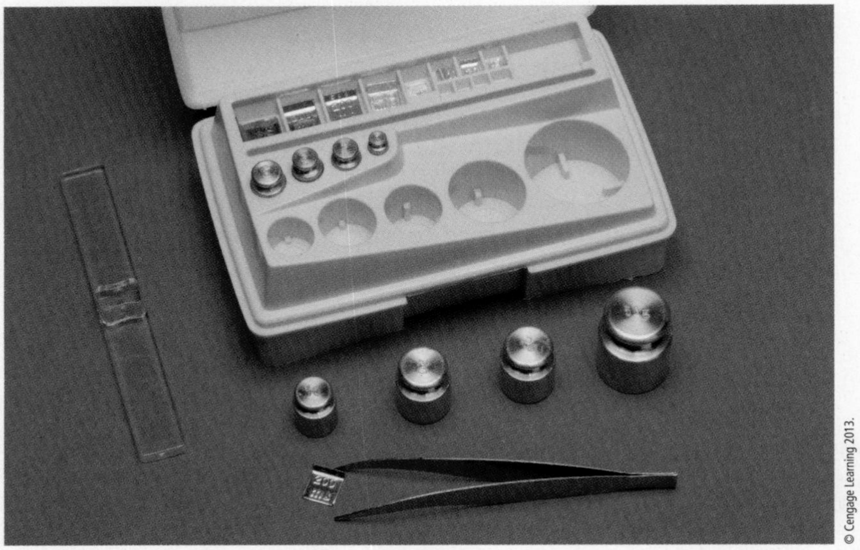

FIGURE 16-2 Pharmaceutical weights should be corrosion resistant and handled with forceps.

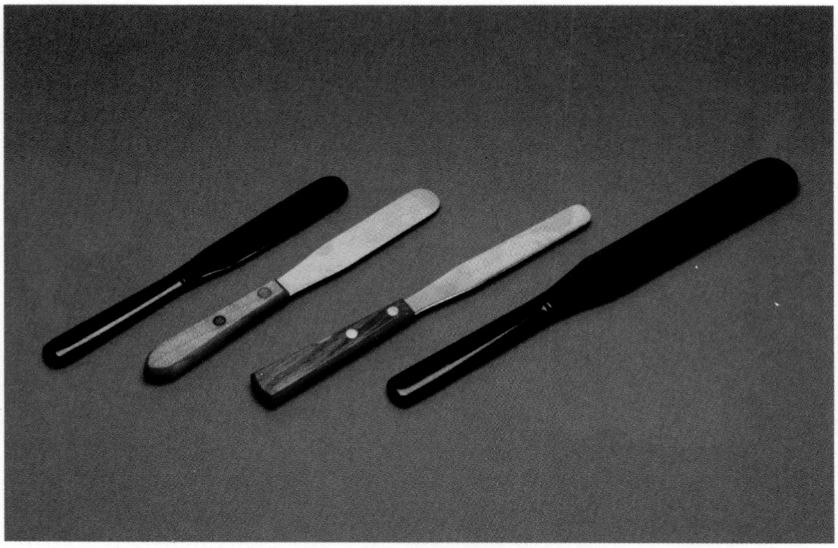

FIGURE 16-3 Spatulas, available in stainless steel and hard rubber or plastic, are used to transfer solid ingredients to weighing pans.

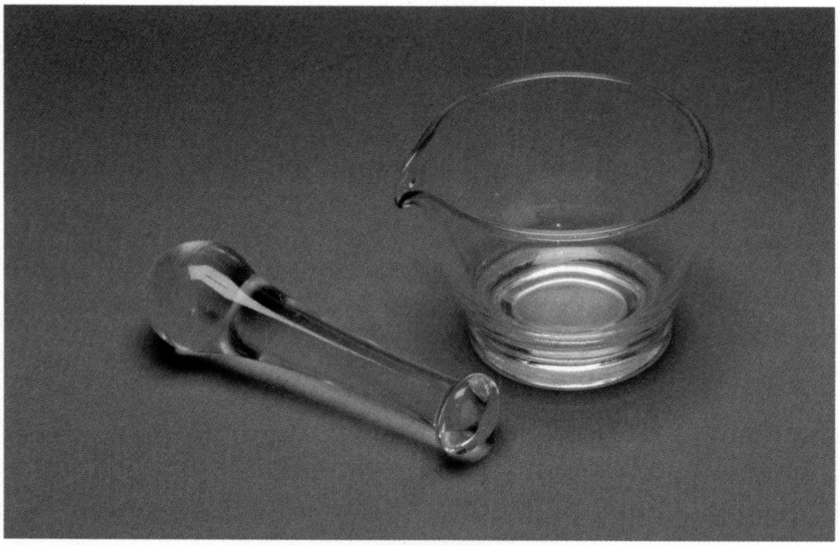

FIGURE 16-4 A glass mortar and pestle is preferable for mixing liquids and semisoft dosage forms.

are clean. Common practice in many universities and compounding labs is to use rubber spatulas when in doubt about corrosion.

Weighing papers, preferably nonabsorbable paraffinic glassine paper, should always be used to weigh powders and other solid and semisolid pharmaceuticals to prevent contamination or damage to the weighing pans. For small amounts of powders, the paper should be creased diagonally from each corner and then flattened and placed on the pans. This ensures a collection trough in the paper. Discard the paper after each product has been mixed to prevent contamination.

Essential equipment that technicians must be familiar with include the mortar and pestle, commonly available in three types: glass (**Figure 16-4**), Wedgwood (**Figure 16-5**), and porcelain (**Figure 16-6**), which is quite similar to the Wedgwood mortar in use and appearance. Wedgwood and porcelain mortars are relatively coarse and are used to grind and/or **triturate** crystals and large particles into fine powders. Both are earthenware, are somewhat porous, and are easily stained.

triturate to reduce particle size and mix one powder with another

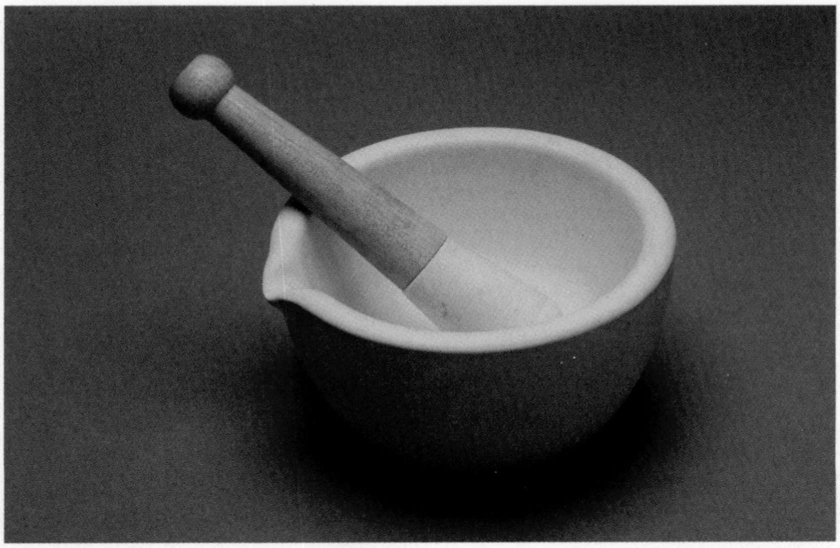

FIGURE 16-5 A Wedgwood mortar is very similar to a porcelain mortar and is used for the same purposes.

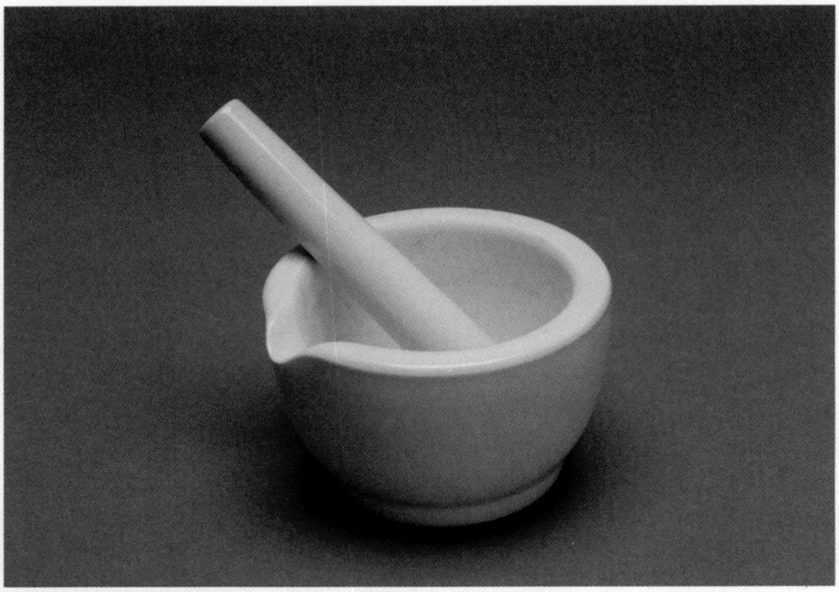

FIGURE 16-6 A porcelain mortar and pestle is used for trituration of crystals and large particles.

Glass mortars are preferable for mixing liquids, semisoft dosage forms, and colored substances with a propensity to stain.

When mixing ingredients, always place the most potent or active ingredient into the mortar first. Then add an equal amount of the next most potent ingredient and mix thoroughly. Once this amount has been mixed until uniform, continue by mixing the first combination with the next ingredient in equal quantities. This process is repeated until all ingredients have been added. Because each addition is approximately equal to the amount in the mortar, the process is called **geometric dilution**. Here is an example of geometric dilution:

geometric dilution the addition of approximately equal amounts of prescribed drugs when mixing in a mortar

Ingredients: 5 g of salicylic acid, 10 g of ibuprofen, in 60 g of petrolatum. To geometrically dilute, we mix 5 g of salicylic acid with 5 g of ibuprofen with a spatula

Next, we take the remaining 5 g of ibuprofen and mix it together with the initial salicylic acid/ibuprofen combination until uniform. We now have 15 g of a total mixture.

We mix the 15-g combination with 15 g of petrolatum and combine until uniform as well.

We then continue until all of the petrolatum has been incorporated.

Ointment slabs are composed of ground glass plates or a large plate of plastic, often square or rectangular, that provides a hard, nonabsorbable surface for mixing compounds. When combining creams and ointments, spatulas are used to spread the material, using a shearing force to mix ingredients. Some pharmacists use disposable, nonabsorbent parchment paper to cover the work area, which is not as durable as the ointment slabs, but saves time in cleaning.

graduate a marked (or graduated) conical or cylindrical vessel used for measuring liquids

Accurately measuring liquids is an essential skill technicians must master. Equipment consists of conical **graduates** (containers marked with calibrated measurements; **Figure 16-7**), cylindrical graduates (**Figure 16-8**), and syringes. Beakers are generally not accurate enough for prescription work and, hence, are used only for fluid transfer.

Conical graduates are the easiest to use, with wide mouths and narrow bases, and are the easiest to clean. Liquids may be stirred in them with the aid of a stirring rod. As the diameter of the graduate increases, the accuracy of the measurement decreases. This design makes the narrow-diameter cylindrical graduates preferable when greater accuracy is desired.

Graduates are available in sizes ranging from 10 to 4,000 mL. When selecting a graduate, always choose the smallest graduate capable of containing the volume to be measured. Avoid measurements of volumes that are below 20% of the capacity of the graduate, because the accuracy is unacceptable. For example, a 100-mL graduate cannot accurately measure volumes below 20 mL. When measuring small volumes, such as 30 mL and less, it is often preferable to use a syringe. Disposable plastic injectable and oral syringes are readily available in all pharmacies and have essentially replaced the use of smaller-sized graduates.

When measuring liquids in a graduate, it is important for the reading to be done at eye level (**Figure 16-9**). The surface of a liquid has a concave or crescent

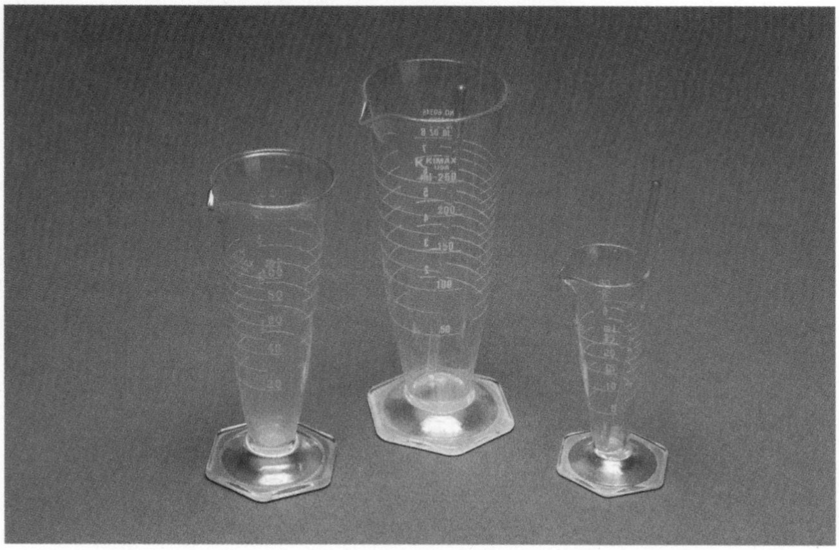

FIGURE 16-7 Conical graduates have a wide mouth and a narrow base.

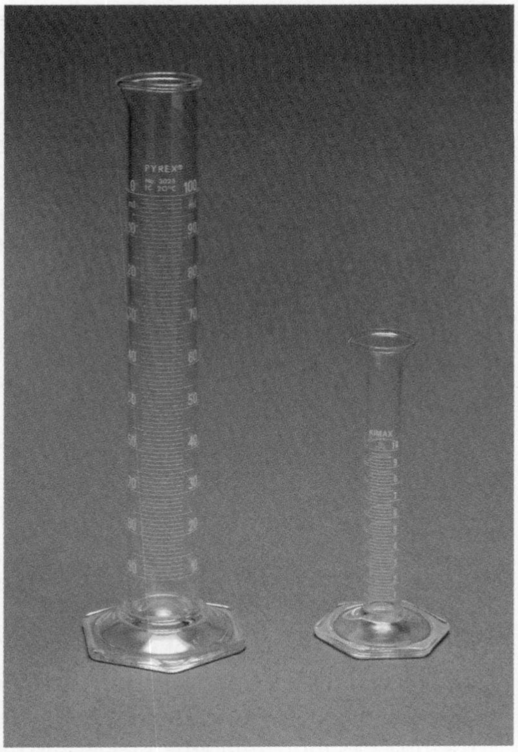

FIGURE 16-8 Cylindrical graduates provide greater accuracy than do conical graduates.

meniscus the shape of the outer surface of a liquid; it can be a concave or crescent shape, which is caused by surface tension

shape that bulges downward, called the **meniscus**. When measuring liquids, the correct reading is the mark at the bottom of the meniscus.

Most graduates are marked "TD" (to deliver). They are calibrated to compensate for the excess of fluid that adheres to the surface after emptying the graduate. Caution must be used to differentiate this from older glassware marked "TC" (to contain), or errors in accuracy will result. Keep in mind that even TD glassware will retain excessive amounts of viscous liquids if not drained completely. Essentially, no liquid should remain in the graduate after emptying.

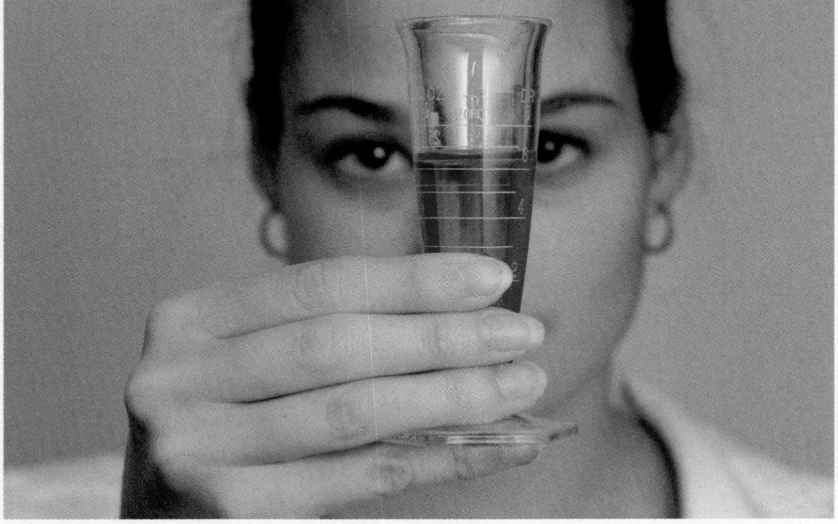

FIGURE 16-9 When reading liquids, they must be viewed at eye level.

Modern Equipment

electronic balance a digital weighing balance scale that varies based on its purpose; can be used to weigh bulk quantities greater than 1 g. Standard prescription balances are accurate up to 1 mg or smaller quantities down to 0.001 mg

Modern pharmacy compounding labs are equipped with digital **electronic balances**. These balances greatly increase the ease and accuracy of the weighing process. These balances do away entirely with the need for the counterweights that were used with the earlier torsion balances. Because they are self-leveling and self-calibrating, they remove a great deal of potential error and stress from the weighing process. They allow for greater accuracy and improved record keeping, due to their ability to be interfaced with printers and computer software programs that enable the retention of a record of weights and calibrations. The more sophisticated software programs will actually enable the weights to be applied directly to log the formula being prepared.

Electronic balances (**Figure 16-10**) will vary based on their purpose. Bulk balances are used to weigh quantities greater than 1 g. Standard prescription balances are accurate to 1 mg, whereas analytical balances are accurate to 0.001 mg.

Because chemicals are never weighed directly onto the table of the balance, different receptacles are used to contain the chemicals being weighed. The most common receptacles used to be glassine weigh papers; however, most compounders now use different types of weigh boats. Weigh boats come in several shapes, sizes, and materials, depending on their use. Some have an octagonal shape, allowing several chemicals to be weighed into the same weigh boat in separate corners, making the process more efficient. Electronic balances allow this process because they can be reset to a zero reading, which is known as **taring**, for each chemical added.

taring the process of resetting an electronic balance to a zero reading

A formula with six chemicals can be weighed into one weigh boat by taring the balance after each chemical has been weighed. Weigh boats also allow more efficient transportation of chemicals from the balance to the processing area.

The recent development of the *mini-ointment mill* has added a whole new dimension to semisolid compounding. An ointment mill allows the incorporation of solid ingredients into cream, gel, and ointment bases by milling the active ingredients to minute particle size and efficiently incorporating and dispersing the active ingredient throughout the base. This process is similar to methods used in the commercial manufacture of creams, gels, and ointments and enhances the

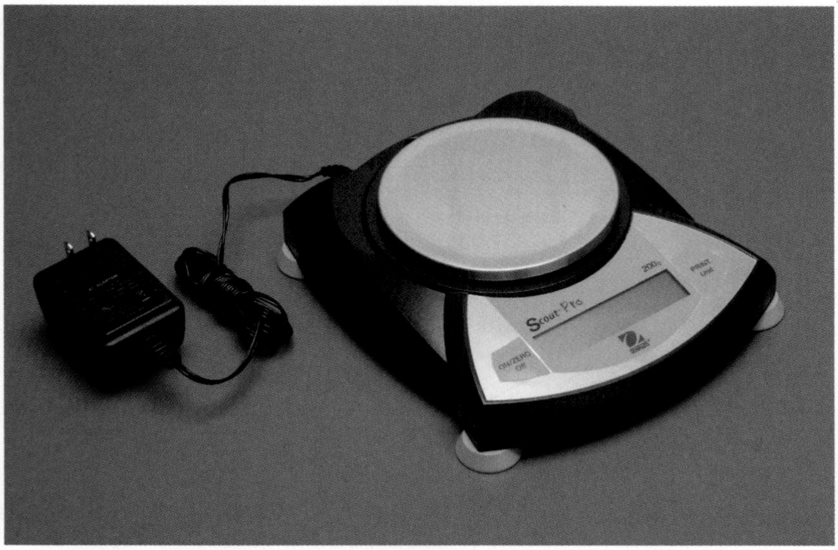

FIGURE 16-10 An electronic balance.

effect of the active ingredients in the base. The old method of using the ointment tile or pad along with geometric dilution, although effective, could not result in the same particle size and distribution of active ingredient. The ointment mill also allows a greater concentration of active ingredient to be incorporated into the base. When making an ointment or cream using the mill, the active ingredient is usually combined with a small amount of the base in the weigh boat. This combination is milled while increasing amounts of the base are added. The final product is evenly dispersed and smooth to the touch.

The electronic mortar and pestle (EMP) is a modern, motorized piece of equipment used to combine multiple ingredients into ointment, gel, and cream bases. It is far more efficient than using a hand-operated mortar and pestle for many reasons. Its rapid rotation allows for greater dispersion of ingredients. The more elaborate EMPs have computer controls. The EMP saves processing time because not only can it be set to operate by itself, but it is able to produce a large quantity of product in one single operation. Many finished products are both mixed and blended in their final dispensing container, thus reducing handling and preserving the purity of the final product. The newest of the EMPs allows the mixing of up to 500 g of finished product. Although the EMP allows for faster blending of the product, the compounder must be aware of the grittiness of an EMP-produced cream before it is dispensed. The pharmacist must check visually and physically for particle size and smoothness of application as discussed below.

Today, basic compounding equipment commonly includes a combination thermostatically controlled hot plate and magnetic spinner. This combination allows semisolids and liquids to be heated and stirred at the same time. It also allows viscous liquids to be heated without burning them. A magnetic stirring rod is placed in the bottom of the holding vessel, and it is spun by a magnet within the hot plate. The speed of the stirring rod is controlled by a rheostat.

New pressure-driven tube heat sealers and tube-filling devices allow the compounder to package creams, gels, and ointments in collapsible plastic tubes and seal them in much the same way a manufacturer would. The final product is elegantly presented. In instances where products must be packaged in metal tubes, modern crimping devices allow the application of a professional-looking seal. The most popular tube sizes range from 3 to 120 g. Tubes can also be filled from the large-size electronic mortar and pestle jar or by using special tube-filling devices.

Homogenizers are used both to reduce the particle size of active ingredients and to disperse and emulsify them into suspensions, emulsions, and low-viscosity lotions. Homogenizers are necessary in the compounding of sterile suspensions in ophthalmics and sterile injectables where particle size and dispersion are critical to the efficacy of the dosage at the site of use.

Traditional Weighing Techniques

The critical first step in any pharmaceutical dispensing is the selection of the proper drug and dose. Qualitative and quantitative accuracy are hallmarks of our profession. Technicians given the responsibilities of compounding must learn the skills and work carefully under the supervision of a pharmacist.

Prior to weighing with a Class A balance, the technician should gather and organize all materials in a level, well-lit, draft-free area. The balance should be leveled by adjusting the thumbscrew at the base of the legs until the pointer rests at zero. Place weighing papers on each pan and adjust the balance again if necessary. The beam weight should be all the way to the left and set at zero. When equilibrium is reached, the balance is arrested (locked) in place by a lock screw. The desired weights are placed in the right pan using forceps. The desired material is placed on the left pan using a spatula. When weighing less than 1 gram, one may wish to shift the weight beam to the appropriate weight. The balance is carefully unlocked to observe the movement of the pointer, which will shift to the side with the greater weight. Relock the balance and use a spatula to subtract or add material being weighed. This process is repeated until equilibrium is reached and the indicator is at the zero point. The balance is then locked, the lid closed, and the lock released one final time to verify the equilibrium. The weight should be checked by a pharmacist. If it is correct, the material can be removed from the balance in the cradle of the folded weighing paper. Weights should be checked three times: when selected, when resting on the pan, and when returned to the kit.

When weighing, the sensitivities and limitations of the balance used must be kept in mind.

Compounding Liquids

Liquids are probably the most common form of compounded medications. Extemporaneous, nonsterile compounds most often involve solutions and suspensions, whereas emulsions and lotions are less popular. Solutions are clear liquids in which the drug is completely dissolved. The simplest compound solution involves the addition of a drug in liquid form to a vehicle such as water or syrup. This involves careful liquid measurement of the drug, using graduates or syringes, and then dilution to the final volume desired. Gentle shaking effects thorough dispersion of additives.

Compounding Solids

When solids are required in solution, they must be carefully weighed, using a prescription balance. Most solids dissolve readily in a solvent, but others require intervention. Some solids may be reduced in size by grinding in a mortar to increase dissolution rates. Other times, the vehicle is heated to enhance dissolution, but care must be used since some drugs decompose at higher temperatures. Dissolution of a solute may require vigorous shaking or stirring.

Compounding Suspensions

Suspensions are liquid preparations of drugs containing finely divided drug particles distributed uniformly throughout the vehicle. Suspensions appear cloudy in nature, and shaking is often required to resuspend drug particles that have settled. Depending on particle size, some suspensions settle so rapidly that a uniform dispersion cannot be maintained long enough for an accurate dose to be withdrawn. Such preparations require a **suspending agent**, a thickening agent that gives some structure to a suspension. Typical agents are carboxymethylcellulose, methylcellulose, bentonite, tragacanth, and others. Some suspending agents may bind the drug, limiting availability, so these agents should be carefully selected.

> **suspending agent** a chemical additive used in suspensions to "thicken" the liquid and retard settling particles

Some solid drugs may be added directly to a suspending vehicle; others, however, need to be "wetted" first. That is, the powder to be added is first mixed with a wetting agent, such as alcohol or glycerin, in a mortar with a pestle. This displaces the air from the particles of the solid and allows them to mix more readily with a suspending vehicle. Compounders must take care to use as little wetting agent as possible because if too much is used, the solid drug may crystallize out of the vehicle, thus preventing a uniform group of finely defined particles. Next, the vehicle is added in portions and mixed with mortar and pestle until a uniform mixture results. This mixture is then blended into the remaining vehicle. The mortar and pestle can be rinsed with small portions of the vehicle and added until the final volume is reached. Suspensions should be dispensed in tight, light-resistant containers that contain enough air space for adequate shaking. The bottle should contain the auxiliary label "Shake well." Refrigeration may be used to slow separation.

Compounding Ointments and Creams

These two semisolid external dosage forms are still popular choices for extemporaneous compounds and share common preparation techniques. Ointments are oil based in nature, whereas creams are water based. Given the commercial availability of unmedicated cream and ointment bases, their preparation is more of historic interest, but we will focus on the addition of drugs to these bases. In the simplest cases, physicians often desire the combined effects of two or more ointments or creams in a specified proportion. This usually involves the thorough mechanical mixing of the weighed bases on an ointment slab using a spatula until a uniform preparation has been obtained. Using the spatula, transfer the material into an ointment jar big enough for the final volume (**Figure 16-11**). When filling the ointment jar, use the spatula to bleed out air pockets. Tapping the jar on the countertop will settle the contents. Wipe any excess material from the outside of the jar, including the screw threads on the cap. Cover the jar and label it appropriately.

Drugs in powder or crystal form, such as salicylic acid, precipitated sulfur, or hydrocortisone, are often prescribed to be mixed into cream or ointment bases. Large particles should be reduced to fine powder with a mortar and pestle. The

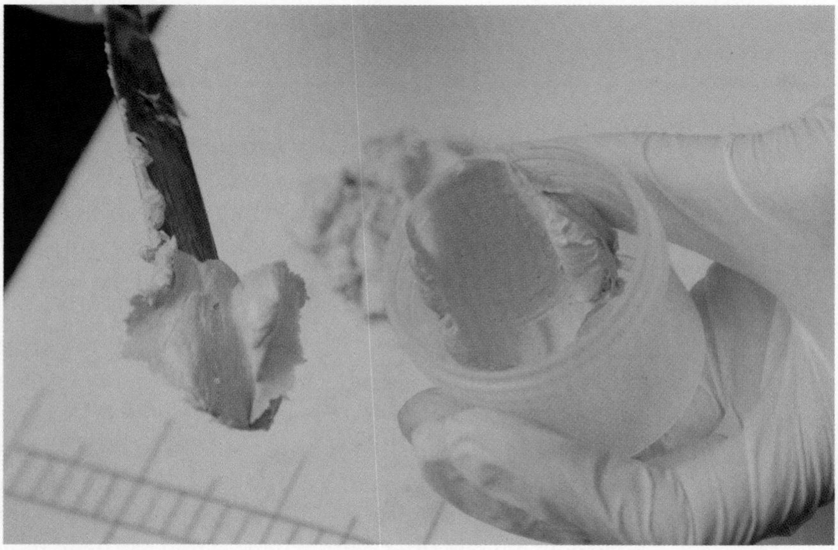

FIGURE 16-11 When creating an ointment or cream, use the spatula to transfer the compound into the jar.

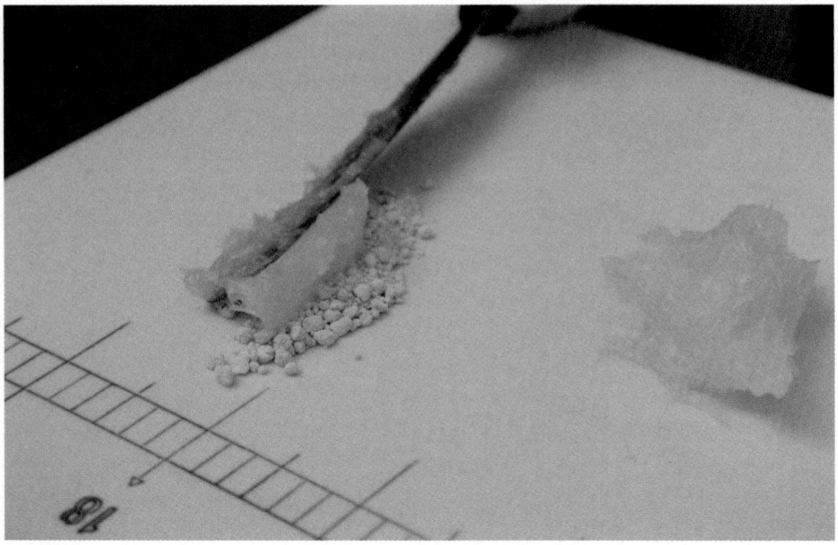

FIGURE 16-12 Gradually mix the medication and base until the substance is uniform.

ointment base may be placed on one side of the working area, with the powders to be incorporated on the other. Using a spatula, mix a small portion of powder with a portion of the base on an ointment slab (**Figure 16-12**). Geometric dilution may be used when mixing the powders with the base. Repeat this until all powder is incorporated into the base and a uniform product is produced.

Occasionally, the direct mixture method results in a gritty product with poorly dispensed clumps of powder that fail to blend in despite vigorous mixing. The solution is to first reduce the particle size of the powder by levigating it. **Levigation** is the mixing of a powder with a vehicle in which it is insoluble to produce a smooth dispersion of the drug. The dispersion is then mixed with the base. When using ointments, mineral oil is a good levigating agent. When working with creams, glycerin or water can often be used. Care must be used to not use too much levigating agent because this may cause the solids to crystallize and come out of the vehicle, causing grittiness.

levigation the mixing of particles with a base vehicle, in which they are insoluble, to produce a smooth dispersion of the drug by rubbing with a spatula on a tile

Compounding Transdermal Gels

Ointments and creams are used to introduce and maintain the presence of drugs in the body topically. Their effectiveness is usually limited to the drug's ability to pass through the skin barrier. Transdermal gels are able to disrupt the lipid layers of the stratum corneum of the skin without damaging it the way harsher agents can. The most popular form of transdermal gel is the pluronic lecithin organogel, or PLO gel.

PLO allows the medication to slip through the stratum corneum into systemic circulation via dermal-epidermal blood flow. PLO gels are used in all disciplines of compounding. These gels are extremely effective for the delivery of pain management drugs to local sites with excellent results and decreased liver absorption. Combinations of localized pain trigger receptor agonists (i.e., drugs that block pain) can be incorporated into a single gel and applied with excellent results. These gels have many positive uses. They are used in veterinary medicine to allow ease in dosing. Cats, which can be difficult to medicate, will respond extremely well to PLO gels administered to the pinna or inner flap of the ear. They can also be used to deliver drugs to pediatric patients who might otherwise be difficult to dose. A good example of this is the dosing of the drug secretin to treat autism. It replaces the need for daily injections and the absorption is equivalent.

These gels are easily compounded using the electronic mortar and pestle and run through an ointment mill. The active ingredient is dissolved in a solvent and combined with isopropyl palmitate and Pluronic F-127. They are then blended and mixed to allow the formation of small emulsion units called *micelles*, which transport the drug across the skin barrier.

There are many other new forms of gels, such as aqueous gels, that are water miscible and easily washable and act as effective carriers for drugs across the skin barrier. Although not every drug can be introduced in gel form and the expiration dating of gels is usually less than 6 months, they have proven to be a valuable tool for compounding.

Compounding Troches, Lollipops, and Gummy Bears

Pharmacists used to compound pastilles and troches by using a hand-rolling technique. They incorporated certain types of drugs into a candy base and were able to produce a hard disk or barrel-shaped troche or pastille that could be placed in the cheek and allowed to dissolve. Modern compounders are able to produce troches that can contain a much wider array of active ingredients and can be sugar free and elegantly colored and flavored. The advent of the troche mold allows the active ingredient to be calculated and combined into a premeasured amount of base to make a much more uniform product.

The various types of troche bases, such as soft, chewy, and hard, allow for greater flexibility in dosing. The different bases are used to adjust the time that the drug takes to be absorbed, along with adapting to the personal preference of the patient. The recent development of lollipop molds now allows medication to be incorporated in this very attractive and fun dosage form (see Figure 5-3). Actiq, which is a commercial pain medication with the active ingredient fentanyl, started out as a custom-compounded product. It was designed to allow the pleasant dosing of a narcotic analgesic to both children and hospice patients. Lollipops are a good dosage form for ease of compliance. As with troches, they can be made sugar free and in literally 101 flavor combinations.

Gummy bears are another dosage form used to deliver medication to children. The same base is used in their formulation as is used for soft troches. The base is melted and the active ingredient, suspending agents, sweetener, and choice of flavors are combined and introduced into a precalibrated mold. Children particularly like this dosage form.

Flavoring

The development of modern flavoring techniques, along with a multitude of different flavors, sweeteners, and flavoring vehicles, has added a great deal of flexibility to modern compounding. Flavors can be either oil soluble or water soluble. Powdered flavorings can be added to dry bulk powders for veterinary use, such as an apple flavoring for horses. Specific flavors have been developed for either level of pH balance. There are flavors to enhance most dosage forms.

The development of more sweetening products now allows the compounder to make a greater assortment of sugar-free products. Flavoring is very important in medication dosing compliance because it allows very bitter drugs to be made more palatable. Dosage forms can be changed; for example, tablets can be pulverized, suspended, and flavored, creating a different dosage form of the same drug. This is especially useful in dosing children and also those patients who have difficulty swallowing. Commercially available liquid products can be flavor-enhanced to make them taste better. Prescriptions can be flavored for animals based on preference. Cats like tuna fish, whereas dogs like liver flavors. Small birds like tutti-frutti flavors. Hundreds of bases, flavors, and flavor combinations are now available.

Compounding Suppositories

Suppositories are solid dosage forms intended for insertion into body orifices, predominantly rectal or vaginal, where they melt or dissolve to release their active ingredients. Extemporaneous manufacture of suppositories remains a vital art today for several reasons. Industrial manufacturers market relatively few products in suppository form in this country, in part because rectal administration is not socially popular. So, although the products are limited, there is a subgroup of patients who cannot tolerate oral medications, but who also are not candidates for parenteral drug therapy.

Suppositories must be manufactured so that they remain solid at room or refrigerated temperatures, yet melt readily at body temperature—a fine line indeed. This process is accomplished by using special bases, such as cocoa butter or polyethylene glycol. Polyethylene glycols are available in various molecular weight ranges. Those of 200, 400, or 600 are liquids; those over 1,000 are solid and wax-like. Often, combinations of liquid (low molecular weight) and solid polyethylene glycol are used to achieve a suppository that melts as desired. By increasing the waxy portion of the blend, we gain a suppository that melts more slowly and provides more sustained action.

To prepare suppositories, the base material is melted and the active ingredients are added. The material is poured into molds and chilled until congealed. Then they are removed from the mold. **Figure 16-13** illustrates suppository molds.

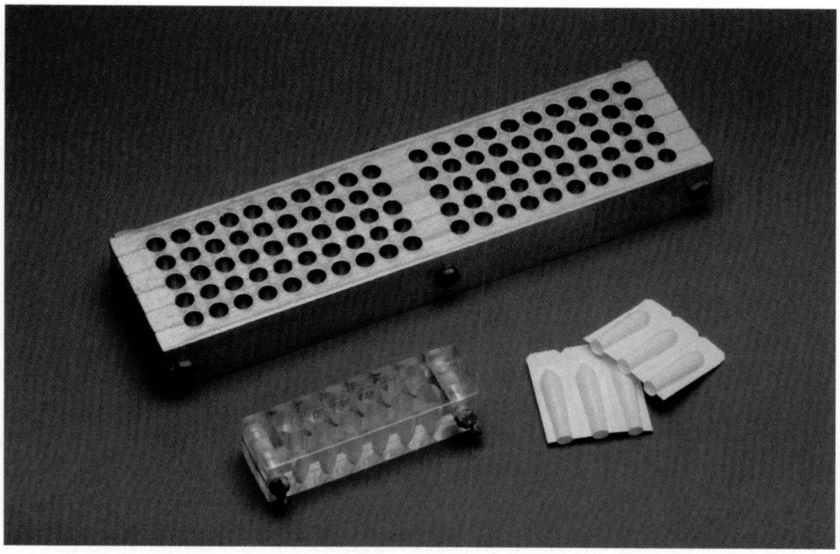

FIGURE 16-13 Suppository molds.

Most modern compounding labs tend to use disposable suppository strip molds. These are precalibrated to the specific bases, are easier to fill and dispense, and can be heat-sealed to present an elegant and professional-looking product. Modern compounders melt the base by placing it in a beaker with a magnetic stirrer at the bottom, then heating it on an electric hot plate with a stirrer. The mixture must be allowed to cool almost to the point of congealing, so as not to melt the plastic molds and also to properly fill the mold cavity.

Suppositories (both commercial and extemporaneous sources) are still commonly used to deliver analgesics, hormones, antiemetics, laxatives, and vaginal anti-infectives.

Compounding Capsules

Extemporaneous capsule manufacturing remains a popular means of providing unusual (and often low) doses of oral medication. You may recall that commercially available capsules cannot be divided. Tablets can only be reliably broken in quarters at best and usually only halves depending on shape. A typical situation that might require capsule compounding is when a drug is only available in 50-mg tablets or capsules, but the physician has prescribed 12.5-mg doses, or what would amount to a one-quarter dose. If crushed, the resulting powder would be too small to handle accurately.

To facilitate measuring, first dilute the crushed tablet (or emptied capsule) with inactive filler and measure a portion containing the desired amount. Select empty, hard gelatin capsules (available in eight sizes, with 000 being the largest and 5 the smallest). In general, the smallest capsule capable of containing the final volume is used because patients often have difficulty swallowing large capsules. To fill each capsule, place the powder on a tile or paper and press the body of the capsule repeatedly into the powder until it is filled (**Figure 16-14**). Be careful not to touch the powder with your fingers. This is called the *punch method* of capsule filling. Place the cap onto the body and weigh the result, using an empty capsule the same size as the **tare**. Adjust the weight, if needed, by adding or removing powder.

tare a weight used to counterbalance the container holding the substance being weighed

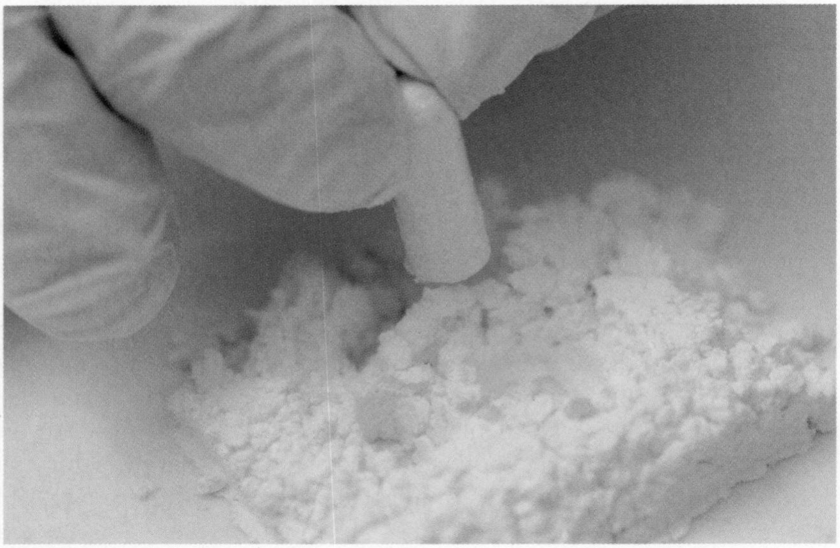

FIGURE 16-14 The punch method is used to fill the capsule with the prepared medication.

To keep the capsule clean during the process, the compounder may wear rubber gloves or finger cots. Because some material is lost in the process, always calculate a little extra material to compensate for this loss.

For the earlier example in which a 12.5-mg dose is required, select a #3 capsule and set the final weight at 200 mg. To make 10 capsules, three 50-mg tablets are needed, which would produce 12 doses, in theory. Twelve doses of 200 mg require 2,400 mg of final powder. Three tablets might weigh 700 mg, to which we would add 1,700 mg of diluent, such as lactose powder, by trituration. We would pack 200 mg of this powder into each capsule to yield the 12.5-mg dose.

The use of capsule-filling machines can greatly facilitate the capsule-filling process. These machines vary from a strictly manual to a highly automated process. The use of a machine requires the prior development of a formulation that will deliver a given dose of a drug in a precalculated volume of powder. As such, machines are useful for manufacturing batches of a standard formula.

The machines require the loading of capsules into a molded plate. The capsule bodies may be separated by hand or by an automated process, leaving the capsule openings aligned with the surface of the plate. The formulated powder is poured over the plate, and spreaders are used to fill the capsules. The capsules are then closed by hand or by an automated process. The machine is inverted to release the filled capsules. The machines are useful for filling many capsules in a timely manner, because they are designed to fill from 50 to 300 capsules with each operation.

Compounding Lotions

Lotions are liquid preparations intended for external application. The most common lotions are "shake" lotions, in which insoluble substances are dispersed by agitation. Often, gums or other agents are used as suspending agents to prevent rapid settling of suspended particles. To prepare shake lotions, place the measured powders of the formula into a mortar and triturate until well blended. Slowly add a liquid levigating agent and triturate to form a smooth paste, free of gritty particles. Add the vehicle in small portions with continued trituration. After roughly two-thirds of the vehicle has been added, transfer the solution to a graduated vessel and rinse the mortar with remaining vehicle to bring the lotion to its final volume. Transfer this to a well-sealed bottle and label "Shake well."

Compounding Enteral Preparations

Pharmacy departments may also prepare enteral nutrition products. Although enteral literally means "in the intestine," the term is commonly used to mean a refined liquid diet, often administered by nasogastric tube to patients unable to eat solid foods.

Preparation of enteral products usually involves simple dissolution of powdered material in a blender, following package directions. At times, however, varied dilutions of feedings are needed to match a patient's clinical state. We use pharmaceutical calculations to prepare a two-thirds- or three-fourths-strength formula. For example, suppose a package of powdered dietary supplement is normally diluted to 500 mL. To prepare a two-thirds-strength enteral formula, we divide 500 mL by two-thirds to yield 750 mL. Each packet should be dissolved to 750 mL to yield the more diluted two-thirds mixture required.

At times, these oral feedings are supplemented with additional electrolytes, such as sodium chloride or potassium chloride. The pharmacy technician may be required to convert weight in milligrams to milliequivalents (mEq).

The use of clean equipment, precise measurement, and proper packaging, labeling, and storage of enteral nutrition products is important. They often require refrigeration after preparation, and each product has a recommended expiration period.

Sterile Compounding, On-Site Sterility, and Pyrogen Testing

Many compounding labs are equipped to prepare sterile compounds, including ophthalmic drops and ointments, injectable solutions and suspensions, and intravenous drugs. This is an area of practice where many drugs must be prepared near the time of actual use due to the instability of the final products. Great care must be taken to ensure the integrity of these compounds. The products must be prepared in a sterile environment. Special equipment is required to prepare these compounds. The creation of new on-site testing for selective impurities and sterility allows for the proper compounding of the products.

Pyrogens, dead cell particles that can cause fevers if allowed to exist in the sterile product, are easily prevented by proper techniques. Their presence in a product can now be tested on-site prior to the release of the drug to the patient. One such test is *Pyro Test*, which can give a final result within 1 hour of preparation. Sterility can also be verified by the use of similar on-site tests, such as *Q-Test*. These tests are designed to use only minute volumes of the finished product. There are also products that test the accuracy of the person performing these procedures. Periodic testing of personnel is necessary to maintain the standard of the compounding facility. Most responsible compounders will send a specified percentage of their products for outside testing to ensure the integrity of their procedures.

Sterilization

When talking about sterilization, understanding the concept of maintaining the integrity of the pharmaceutical product to be dispensed is vital. Proper sterilization techniques start with using iodine scrub to wash the hands and nails thoroughly under the sink for several minutes before applying gloves, arm sleeves, hairnets, and lab coats to ensure aseptic procedure is intact. Technicians can spread microorganisms into the laminar hood by wearing jewelry, coughing, sneezing (and not wearing a mask), or having loose facial hair. No food, beverages, or gum should be allowed in the sterile area. The hood should always be cleaned properly with alcohol after each compounded prescription is completed. We discuss four methods of sterilization in this chapter: thermal, chemical, filtration, and radiation.

thermal sterilization sterilization using heat; moist heat and dry heat are methods of thermal sterilization

There are two types of **thermal sterilization**: moist heat and dry heat. Moist heat is used to coagulate the protein contained in microorganisms. Dry heat causes death by oxidation. Microorganisms need protein to survive and thermal sterilization prevents this organism from surviving. Moist heat sterilization is performed in an autoclave, which uses steam under pressure for a specified period of time. Dry sterilization is performed in an oven between 140° and 260°C to kill spores and other microorganisms. This method of sterilization is preferred for products such as mineral oil, paraffin, and zinc oxide.

>>> **ALERT! >>>**

The recent unfortunate nationally publicized incident involving infractions in proper compounding procedures of a compounding pharmacy, and the resultant patient injury and death, necessitates the need to stress the following basic understanding about pharmacy compounding: Foolproof, proven formulation information is required; the compounding facility must have a well-trained and competent compounding staff and must follow comprehensive standard operating procedures that are fully compliant with USP/NF Chapters <795>/<797>; and of greatest importance is that those individuals involved in extemporaneous compounding, for both nonsterile and sterile preparations, must have a full understanding and appreciation of their professional and ethical responsibilities to ensure safe patient outcomes for anyone using the preparations they compound.

chemical sterilization the process of completely removing or destroying all microorganisms by exposure to a chemical

filtration the process of passing a liquid through a porous substance that arrests suspended solid particles

radiation the use of x-rays, ultraviolet rays, or short radio waves to sterilize, for example, hospital supplies, vitamins, antibiotics, steroids, plastic syringes, and needles

Chemical sterilization uses chemical agents to prevent microorganism proliferation. The most common chemical agent used in this process is ethylene oxide. This chemical only requires a temperature of 54°C for approximately 4 to 16 hours, and can be used for rubber and plastic items. This type of sterilization can never be used in IV solutions due to possible chemical reactions.

Filtration, aside from being the easiest, is the most often-used form of sterilization in most pharmacies. In order for a filter to prevent passage of all bacteria, it must be no more than 0.22 micron in size. Filters are used for IV, IM, and ophthalmic preparations, since heat and chemicals often damage these solutions. The smallest bacteria can be eliminated using a 0.22-micron filter. This filter is widely used as a standard in a majority of compounding procedures.

Radiation is a form of sterilization normally used in hospitals, laboratories, and large institutions. This method, which uses x-rays, ultraviolet rays, or short radio waves, is largely used to sterilize hospital supplies, vitamins, antibiotics, steroids, plastic syringes, and needles.

Most pharmacies will prepare sterile products in either a horizontal or vertical airflow hood; each provides a Class 100 clean environment. The horizontal laminar flow hood consists of three major components: a prefilter, a high-efficiency particulate air (HEPA) filter, and a work surface. The horizontal hood blows clean air from the back of the hood to the front, maintaining a clean area within 3 inches from the back of the hood and 6 inches from the front edge of the hood. The constant airflow through the HEPA filter prevents all particles greater than 0.3 micron in size from entering the sterile area.

The vertical airflow hood sends the sterile filtered air from the top of the cabinet to the base and recirculates it within the cabinet. It is a closed system that better protects the person performing operations within the clean barrier. Vertical flow hoods can be used for those products toxic to humans and the environment, such as chemotherapeutic drugs.

Both types of hoods must be cleaned with the proper chemical compounds before each operation. A more detailed and thorough discussion of laminar airflow hoods is presented in Chapter 21.

Labeling of Finished Products and Record Keeping

Extemporaneous products should be labeled with neat, well-designed labels, in accordance with hospital policy. Outpatient prescription labels must contain all information required by state and local laws. Auxiliary labels should be affixed if applicable. The label should contain the ingredients and proportions of the compounded prescription. If a master compounding form was used, the internally assigned lot number should appear on the label.

EXTEMPORANEOUS PREPARATION
GENTIAN VIOLET 10%

MATERIALS
- 1 glass flask 600ml
- Absolute alcohol 300ml
- Gentian Violet 30gm
- Stirring rod
- 1 oz. amber dropper bottle

LABEL
- Gentian violet solution
- 10% W/V
- In 95% absolute alcohol
- Volume: 300 ml
- Control # _____
- Tech/R.Ph. _____ Exp. date _____

Procedure
1. Clean all materials to be used and rinse with absolute alcohol.
2. Weigh out 30 gram gentian violet and have pharmacist check it.
3. Measure out 300ml absolute alcohol and have pharmacist check it.
4. In glass flask, dissolve the gentian violet in the absolute alcohol. Stir well until in solution.
5. Measure out 30ml and put in 1 oz. glass amber dropper bottle.
6. Have pharmacist check label.
7. Put label on product.
8. Have pharmacist check final product.

Date Prepared	Control #	Ingredients	Mft. & Lot #	Amt. Used	Check by R.Ph	Expiration Date of Prod. Made	Quant. Prep.	Sample Label	Tech.

FIGURE 16-15 Master formula record.

In general, no specific expiration date can be assigned to an extemporaneous compound unless the institution has a policy for assigning reasonable expiration dates. Even with such a policy, some judgment is needed on the part of the supervising pharmacist. It may suffice to list the date of preparation on the label.

Accurate record keeping is essential in extemporaneous compounding. Master formula records (**Figure 16-15**) are excellent sources for both directions for compounding and uniform record keeping. When using a master form, record all lot number information on the form, and use the internal lot number on the prescription label. These master records also contain the amount of ingredients used and the initials of the pharmacy technician or preparer and the pharmacist who checked all measurements in the finished product. All worksheets should be filed as permanent records.

For single extemporaneous compounds without master records, such as those involving outpatient prescriptions, the lot numbers and manufacturers of the ingredients can be recorded on the prescription.

Cleaning Equipment

Cleaning the compounding equipment is as important as the preparation and labeling of the product—this part of the process should not be overlooked. Improperly cleaned equipment can contaminate the next preparation and be dangerous to the patient. Cleaning is sometimes not as simple as washing dishes because oily residues, such as ointments, often must be dissolved. Proper cleaning may require a rinse with organic solvents, such as alcohols or acetate, to facilitate removal. When working with these volatile solvents, the student must be aware of their flammable nature as well as the risk of inhaling fumes. Although these fumes are generally safe for limited exposure, care must be taken to wash solvents down the drain with cold water to limit exposure. Occupational safety data sheets should be available in every pharmacy, outlining the hazards of each substance.

Summary

Bulk compounding by pharmacy technicians should be viewed as a challenge and a rewarding skill. The student can readily appreciate the necessity of competence in other aspects of pharmacy, such as calculation, dose forms, and pharmaceutical terminology. The responsibility of bulk compounding should not and will not be required of technicians who are not trained or not competent with these skills. Any bulk compounding must be done only under the close supervision of a licensed pharmacist, and in some states, must be done only via master manufacturing records.

Bulk compounding is a difficult art to master, but it is one of the most rewarding. It remains one service no other health care profession can provide.

TEST YOUR KNOWLEDGE

Multiple Choice

1. The concave surface of a liquid in a graduate is called the
  a. sight line.
  b. metric point.
  c. meniscus.
  d. tare.

2. Clear liquids in which drugs are completely dissolved are called
  a. suspensions.
  b. emulsions.
  c. lotions.
  d. solutions.

3. The hazards of using organic solvents are
  a. their flammability.
  b. their lack of odor.
  c. their explosive nature.
  d. their acidity.

4. A packet of external nutrition supplement diluted to what strength would yield the greatest volume?
a. full strength
b. three-fourths strength
c. two-thirds strength
d. none of the above

5. A master formula record should contain
a. directions for compounding.
b. a record of lot numbers.
c. the initials of the preparer and checking pharmacist.
d. all of the above.

6. What type of balance can weigh large quantities?
a. Class A prescription balance
b. solution balance
c. counter balance
d. electronic balance

7. A thickening agent that gives some structure to a suspension is called
a. a gel agent.
b. a cream agent.
c. a suspending agent.
d. a soluting agent.

8. The punch method is used to compound
a. capsules.
b. suppositories.
c. solids.
d. ointments.

9. What piece of equipment is used to transfer solid ingredients to weighing pans?
a. graduate
b. syringe
c. spatula
d. beaker

10. The device used to reduce the particle size of active ingredients is
a. a homogenizer.
b. an electronic mortar and pestle.
c. a hot plate.
d. an ointment mill.

Matching

Match the piece of equipment to its use.

1.	______ Class A prescription balance	a. used to measure liquids
2.	______ mortar and pestle	b. used to grind large particles
3.	______ spatula	c. used to mix and transfer ingredients
4.	______ graduate	d. used to weigh small quantities
5.	______ ointment slab	e. used to mix ointments

Fill in the Blank

1. The timely preparation of a drug product according to a prescribed recipe is called ____________.
2. The correct reading of a liquid is at the bottom of the ____________.
3. The mixing of a powder into a vehicle in which it is insoluble to produce a smooth dispersion is called ____________.
4. The resetting of a balance to a zero reading is known as ____________.
5. ____________ are dead cell particles that can cause a fever.

Suggested Readings

Parrot, E. L. (1970). *Pharmaceutical technology*. Minneapolis, MN: Burgess Publishing.

Shrewsburg, R. (2001). *Applied pharmaceutics in contemporary compounding*. Englewood, CO: Morton Publishing.

University of the Sciences in Philadelphia (2005). *Remington: The Science and Practice of Pharmacy* (21st ed.). Easton, PA: Lippincott, Williams, and Wilkins.

CHAPTER

17

Sterile Preparation Compounding

Competencies

Upon completion of this chapter, the reader should be able to:

1. List three routes of administration and give an example.
2. List several advantages of administering a drug by the parenteral route.
3. Define an ISO Class 5 area.
4. Define a buffer area.
5. Define an ante-area.
6. Understand and explain the difference between a vertical flow hood and a horizontal flow hood.
7. Describe the proper order for garbing and entering a clean room.
8. Understand and describe the concept of unidirectional airflow and "first air."
9. Understand and explain the difference between compounding a low-risk versus a medium-risk versus a high-risk level preparation.
10. Understand and describe the appropriate steps in compounding sterile preparations.

Key Terms

compounded sterile preparation (CSP)
intermittent infusion
intra-arterial
intra-articular
intracardia
intradermal (ID)
intramuscular (IM)
intraperitoneal
intrapleural
intrathecal
intravenous (IV)
intraventricular
intravesicular
intravitreal
parenteral
sterile
subcutaneous (SC)

Introduction

parenteral a sterile, injectable medication; introduction of a drug or nutrient into a vein, muscle, subcutaneous tissue, artery, or spinal column; often refers to intravenous infusions of nutritional solutions

sterile free from living microorganisms

compounded sterile preparation (CSP) relates to the compounding of preparations, such as intravenous admixtures, ophthalmics, and intrathecals, prepared in a controlled sterile environment

A **parenteral** (*para* + *enteron*) product is an example of a sterile preparation. Parenteral products are products that bypass the gastrointestinal (GI) tract. They are administered by injection through some other route, thereby bypassing the gastric mucosa, the skin, and other membranes. Hence, parenteral products must be **sterile** (free from living microorganisms), free from particulate matter, and free from bacterial endotoxins. *Bacterial endotoxins* are a type of pyrogen. A *pyrogen* is any fever-causing substance.

Administration of a sterile preparation by injection might be necessary because the drug is destroyed when taken orally, inactivated in the GI tract, or poorly absorbed. An injection may also be used when the patient is unable to swallow or take anything by mouth, is unconscious, or is uncooperative. Administering a drug by the parenteral route is also used when rapid drug absorption is essential, such as in emergency situations.

According to the U.S. Pharmacopeia (USP), **compounded sterile preparations (CSPs)** are parenteral products and include compounded biologics, diagnostic agents, drugs, nutrients, radiopharmaceuticals, aqueous bronchial and nasal inhalations, baths and soaks for live organs and tissues, irrigations for wounds and body cavities, ophthalmic drops and ointments, and tissue implants.

Parenteral Routes of Administration

The route of administration chosen depends on the drug characteristic, the effect desired, and the required site of action.

Intravenous Route

intravenous (IV) within a vein; administering drugs or fluids directly into the vein to obtain a rapid or complete effect from the drug

intermittent infusion the administration of an IV infusion over a period of time followed by a period of no administration. The same cycle is usually repeated at scheduled times, hence the name *intermittent*

An **intravenous (IV)** injection is administered directly into the vein. Because the medication is rapidly diluted with blood, a rapid effect of the drug, along with a predictable response, is seen. Drugs may be given by IV bolus, a continuous infusion, or an intermittent infusion. A *bolus* is used to deliver a relatively small volume of drug over a short time and is often written as "IV push." This is useful in emergency situations where a rapid therapeutic effect is desired. For some drugs that cannot be given quickly without causing adverse effects to the patient, **intermittent infusions** are sometimes used. Intermittent infusion is also used for drugs that need to be given at defined intervals over a specific amount of time in order to be most effective. They are used to deliver a relatively small volume of solution. When the patient has an established IV administration set, the intermittent infusion is piggybacked through the established primary IV administration set. A *piggyback* is a second medication that is infused through the primary IV administration set and is usually 250 mL or less. This eliminates the need for another needlestick and also dilutes the medication to reduce irritation of the vein (see **Figure 17-1**).

Intramuscular Route

intramuscular (IM) within the muscle

An **intramuscular (IM)** medication is injected deep into a large muscle mass, such as the upper arm, thigh, or buttocks. Typically, no more than 2.5 mL (but up to 5 mL depending on muscle mass) of medication may be administered IM as a solution or suspension. Sterile preparations given by the IM route act more quickly than when given by the oral route, but not as quickly as if the drug was

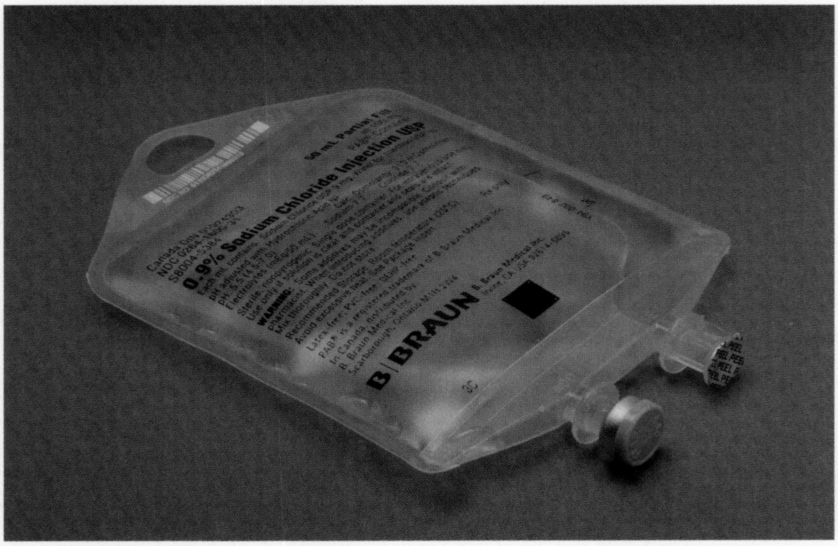

FIGURE 17-1 A continuous infusion allows for the introduction of large volumes of solution, usually run at a constant rate and given over an extended period of time.

given by the IV route. Depending on the solubility of the drug and the vehicle it is in, a sustained-release action can be achieved as the drug is released from muscle tissue at a prolonged rate. IM injections are often painful, and if an adverse effect occurs from the sterile preparation, reversing the effect can be difficult.

Subcutaneous Route

subcutaneous (SC) under the skin

Sterile preparations given by the **subcutaneous (SC)** route can be solutions or suspensions. They are given beneath the surface of the skin. The volume of medications administered by this route must be not more than 2 mL. SC injections are not absorbed as well and have a slower onset of action than injections given by the IV or IM route.

Intradermal Route

intradermal (ID) situated or applied within the skin

Sterile preparations given by the **intradermal (ID)** route are injected into the top layer of the skin. The injection is not as deep as a SC injection. Preparations used for diagnostic purposes, such as an allergy test or a tuberculin test, are often given by the ID route. The volume of solution is limited to 0.1 mL, and the onset of action and rate of absorption from this route are slow.

Intra-Arterial Route

intra-arterial into an artery

The **intra-arterial** route of administration occurs when the sterile preparation is injected into the artery and thus delivers the medication directly to the desired location. A preparation used for diagnostic purposes, such as radio-opaque materials for an arteriogram, is one example. Another example of this route of administration is for the delivery of cancer chemotherapy directly to the desired site of action.

Other Parenteral Routes of Administration

intra-articular into a joint, such as the elbow or knee

intracardia into the heart

Other parenteral routes of administration are as follows:

- An **intra-articular** preparation is injected into a joint such as the elbow or knee.
- An **intracardia** preparation is injected directly into the heart muscle.

intraperitoneal into the peritoneal or abdominal cavity

intrapleural into the sac surrounding the lungs

intraventricular into a ventricle of the brain or heart

intravesicular into the urinary bladder

intravitreal into the vitreous chamber of the eyeball behind the lens

- An **intraperitoneal** preparation is injected into the peritoneal or abdominal cavity.
- An **intrapleural** preparation is injected into the sac surrounding the lungs.
- An **intraventricular** preparation is injected directly into a ventricle of the brain.
- An **intravesicular** preparation is instilled into the urinary bladder.
- An **intravitreal** preparation is injected into the vitreous humor of the eye.
- An **intrathecal** preparation is injected into the space around the spinal cord. Preservative-free drugs must be used for this route of injection, because a preservative may damage the nervous system.

Definitions for Compounding Sterile Preparations

intrathecal within the subdural space of the spinal cord

The following are definitions you will need to know for compounding sterile preparations:

- *Admixture*—parenteral dosage forms are combined for administration as a single entity.
- *Ante-area*—an ISO Class 8 or better area where personnel perform hand hygiene and garbing procedures, staging of components, order entry, CSP labeling, and other high-particulate generating activities. Such an area is maintained under positive pressure in comparison to the rest of the pharmacy, but negative to the buffer area. The ante-area is supplied with high-efficiency particulate air (HEPA) filters.
- *Aseptic processing*—process in which product components, containers, closures, and the product itself are sterilized separately and then brought together and assembled in an aseptic environment, under at least ISO Class 5 conditions; the primary objective of aseptic processing is to create a sterile product.
- *Aseptic technique*—a means of manipulating sterile products without contaminating them.
- *Beyond-use date (BUD)*—USP Chapter <797>, definitions, states that the BUD is the date or time after which a CSP shall not be stored or transported. The date is determined from the date or time the preparation is compounded.
- *Buffer area*—usually an ISO Class 7 area where the laminar flow hood is located. It has positive pressure to the rest of the pharmacy and is supplied with HEPA-filtered air. Activities that occur in this area include the preparation and staging of components and supplies used when CSPs.
- *Critical area*—an ISO Class 5 environment/area.
- *Critical site*—any opening or surface that can provide a pathway between the sterile product and the environment (e.g., the hub of the needle, the tip of the syringe, the open neck of the ampoule, the top of the vial closure, the ribs of the plunger on a syringe).
- *Direct compounding area (DCA)*—a critical area within the ISO Class 5 primary engineering control (PEC) where critical sites are exposed to unidirectional HEPA-filtered air, also known as "first air."
- *First air*—the air exiting the HEPA filter in a unidirectional air stream that is essentially particle free.

- *Hypertonic*—a solution containing a higher concentration of dissolved substances (hyperosmotic) than the red blood cell, which causes the red blood cell to shrink.
- *Hypotonic*—a solution containing a lower concentration of dissolved substances (hypoosmotic) than the red blood cell, causing the red blood cell to swell and possibly burst.
- *ISO Class 5 area*—the air in this type of area has no more than 3,520 particles per cubic meter of air 0.5 micron and larger. This is equivalent to the air in a Class 100 area, which is the number of particles per cubic foot of air 0.5 micron and larger.
- *ISO Class 7 area*—the air in this type of area has no more than 352,000 particles per cubic meter of air 0.5 micron and larger. This is equivalent to a Class 10,000 area.
- *ISO Class 8 area*—the air in this type of area has no more than 3,520,000 particles per cubic meter of air 0.5 micron and larger. This is equivalent to a Class 100,000 area.
- *Isotonic*—a solution with an osmotic pressure close to that of body fluids. Use of an isotonic solution minimizes patient discomfort and damage to red blood cells. Dextrose 5% in water and sodium chloride 0.9% solutions are approximately isotonic.
- *Preparation*—a compounded sterile preparation (CSP), that is a sterile drug or nutrient compounded in a licensed pharmacy or other health care–related facility pursuant to the order of a licensed prescriber; the article may or may not contain sterile products.
- *Primary engineering control (PEC)*—a device such as a laminar airflow workbench (LAFW), biological safety cabinet (BSC), or compounding aseptic isolator (CAI) that provides an ISO Class 5 environment for the exposure of critical sites when compounding sterile preparations.
- *Product*—a commercially manufactured sterile drug or nutrient that has been evaluated for safety and efficacy by the Food and Drug Administration (FDA). Products are accompanied by full prescribing information, which is commonly known as the FDA-approved manufacturer's labeling or product package insert.
- *Sterilizing filter*—a filter that, when challenged with the microorganisms *Brevundimonas (Pseudomonas) diminuta*, at a minimum concentration of 10^7 organisms per square centimeter of filter surface, will produce a sterile effluent; a sterilizing filter has a pore size rating of 0.2 or 0.22 micron.
- *Unidirectional flow*—airflow moving in a single direction, in a robust and uniform manner, and at sufficient speed to reproducibly sweep particles away from the critical processing area.
- *Validation/verification*—establishing documented evidence that provides a high degree of assurance that a specific process will consistently produce a product meeting predetermined specifications and quality attributes.

United States Pharmacopoeia 35/National Formulary 30

The new Chapter <797>, Pharmaceutical Compounding—Sterile Preparations, became official on May 1, 2012. The chapter has four specific categories of CSPs: low-risk level, medium-risk level, high-risk level, and immediate-use.

Low-Risk Level CSPs

Compounding is classified as *low risk* under these prevailing conditions:

1. CSPs are compounded using only sterile ingredients, product, components, and devices entirely within an ISO Class 5 environment or better.
2. Compounding involves simple aseptic manipulations with not more than three commercially manufactured sterile products, including an infusion or diluent solution, and not more than two entries into any one sterile container or package of sterile product or administration container/device to prepare the CSP.
3. Manipulations are limited to penetrating stoppers on vials with sterile needles and syringes, opening ampoules, and transferring sterile liquids in sterile syringes.
4. In the absence of passing a sterility test, the storage periods cannot exceed the following time periods before administration:
   a. stored for not more than 48 hours at controlled room temperature.
   b. stored for not more than 14 days at a cold temperature of 2° to 8°C.
   c. stored for not more than 45 days in a solid frozen state between −25° and −10°C.

Medium-Risk Level CSPs

Medium-risk level CSPs are compounded under low-risk conditions, and one or more of the following exists:

1. Compounding requires pooling of sterile products that will be administered to either multiple patients or to one patient on multiple occasions.
2. Compounding involves complex aseptic manipulations other than the single-volume transfer.
3. The compounding process requires unusually long duration, such as that required to complete dissolution or homogeneous mixing.
4. In the absence of passing a sterility test, the storage periods cannot exceed the following time periods before administration:
   a. stored for not more than 30 hours at controlled room temperature.
   b. stored for not more than 9 days at a cold temperature of 2° to 8°C.
   c. stored for not more than 45 days in a solid frozen state between −25° and −10°C.

Compounding a total parenteral nutrition solution or filling reservoirs of injection and infusion devices with more than three sterile drug products are examples of medium-risk level compounding.

High-Risk Level CSPs

The following compounding conditions may result in contamination or leaves the products at high risk to become contaminated:

1. Compounding with nonsterile ingredients or a nonsterile device before sterilization.
2. Sterile ingredients or components are exposed to air quality inferior to ISO Class 5; this includes storage in environments inferior to ISO Class 5 of opened or partially used packages of commercially manufactured sterile products with no antimicrobial preservative system.
3. Nonsterile preparations containing water that are stored for more than 6 hours before being sterilized.

4. Compounding personnel are observed to be improperly garbed and gloved.
5. No examination of labeling and documentation from suppliers or direct determination that the chemical purity and content strength of the ingredients meet their original or compendia specification.
6. In the absence of passing a sterility test, the storage periods cannot exceed the following time periods before administration:
   a. stored for not more than 24 hours at controlled room temperature.
   b. stored for not more than 3 days at a cold temperature of 2° to 8°C.
   c. stored for not more than 45 days in a solid frozen state between –25° and –10°C.

An example of high-risk level compounding is preparing a CSP from nonsterile ingredients.

Immediate-Use CSPs

The immediate-use CSP category is intended only for emergency situations or when immediate patient administration of a CSP is needed. It may be used for only low-risk level CSPs and may not be used for any hazardous drugs. Immediate-use CSPs are exempt from the requirements of low-risk level CSPs only if:

1. Unless required for the preparation, the compounding process is continuous and does not exceed 1 hour.
2. The finished product is compounded with good aseptic technique and is under continuous supervision until administered.
3. Administration begins not later than 1 hour after the start of preparation.
4. Unless administered immediately by the person who prepared it, the CSP bears a label listing patient identification information, ingredients and amounts, the name or initial of the person who prepared it, and the exact 1 hour beyond-use time and date.

Sterile Product Preparation Area

The horizontal laminar flow workbench draws air in through a prefilter (**Figure 17-2**). The prefiltered air is pressurized in the plenum for even distribution of air to the HEPA filter. Prefilters should be checked regularly and changed as needed. A record of these checks and changes of the prefilter should be kept. The *plenum* of the hood is the space between the prefilter and the HEPA filter. The air is blown across the work surface toward the operator. The air from the HEPA filter is unidirectional (laminar flow) and should have uniform velocity. Federal Standard 209E recommends airflow from the filter have a velocity of 90 feet per minute, plus or minus 20%. USP 35/NF30 Chapter <797> states that the airflow must be sufficient to sweep particles away and provide an ISO Class 5 environment. The prefilter in the laminar flow workbench protects the HEPA filter from premature clogging. The HEPA filter consists of banks of filters, separated by corrugated aluminum pleats. The HEPA filter is 99.97% efficient at removing particles 0.3 micron and larger. To put this in perspective, the smallest particles visible to the human eye are about 40 to 50 microns in size. When working in horizontal flow, the compounding personnel must be careful to never put their hand behind an object. In other words, nothing must come between the critical site and the HEPA filter.

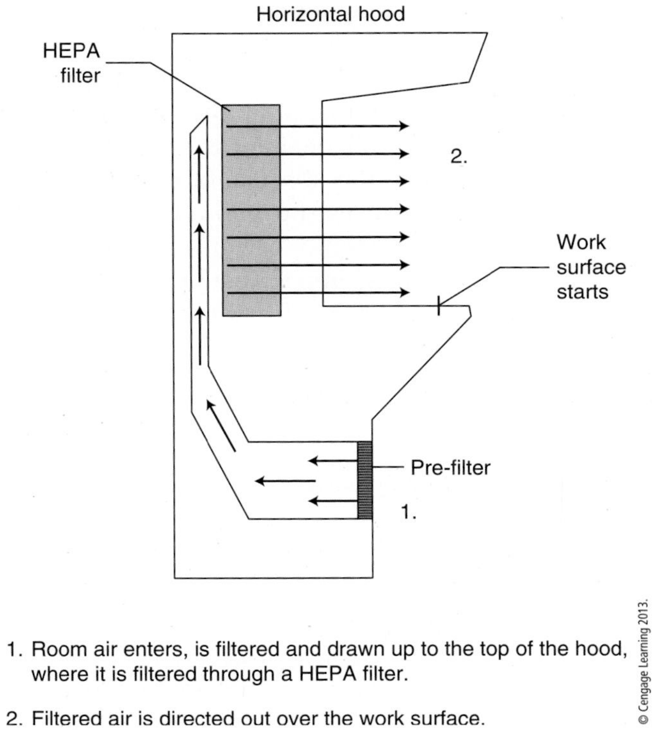
Horizontal hood
HEPA filter
2.
Work surface starts
Pre-filter
1.
1. Room air enters, is filtered and drawn up to the top of the hood, where it is filtered through a HEPA filter.
2. Filtered air is directed out over the work surface.

FIGURE 17-2 Horizontal laminar flow workbench.

A vertical laminar flow workbench works like the horizontal flow hood in that air is drawn in through the prefilter and pressurized in the plenum (**Figure 17-3**). The main difference is that the air is blown down onto the work surface instead of at the operator. This means the operator, when working in a vertical flow hood, will modify his or her aseptic technique so that his or her hands and any objects are never above an object in the hood. Nothing should come between the HEPA filter and the critical site.

The biological safety cabinet (BSC) is a type of vertical laminar flow workbench that provides protection to the product by having vertical HEPA-filtered air, protection to the operator by having the air intake at the open front of the hood, and protection to the environment by having the exhausted air pass through a HEPA filter (**Figure 17-4**). Ideally all of the exhaust should be directed outside to the roof.

Buffer Area

Primary engineering controls (PECs) must maintain an ISO Class 5 environment while compounding of the sterile preparation occurs (e.g., under dynamic conditions). It usually must be kept in the buffer area, located away from excess traffic, doors, air vents, or anything that could produce air currents greater than the velocity of the airflow from the HEPA filter. The buffer area should be an ISO Class 7 area with positive pressure of 0.02 to 0.05 inch of water between this area and the ante-area. ISO Class 7 areas must be supplied with HEPA-filtered air and achieve not less than 30 air changes per hour. A recirculating PEC may supply 15 of those 30 air changes per hour.

Certification of all ISO-classified areas needs to be done no less than every 6 months. This includes testing the integrity of the HEPA filter, determination of air changes per hour in the classified rooms, and the total particle counts of the ISO 5, 7, and 8 areas.

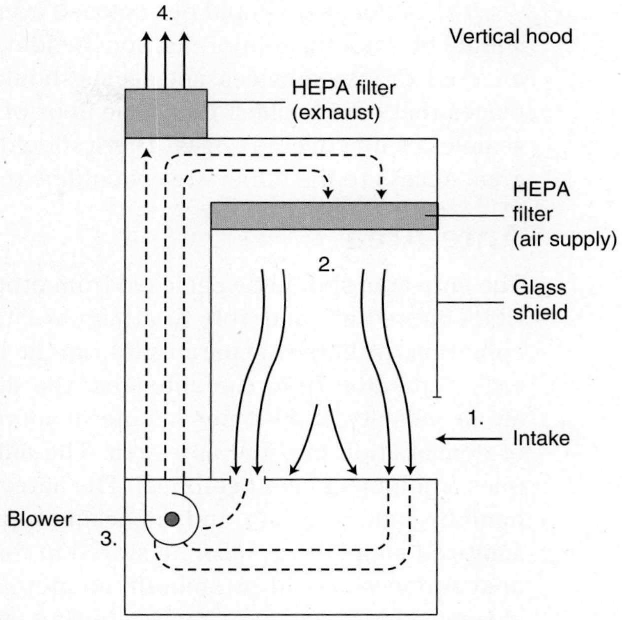

1. Room air enters the laminar airflow. This makes up about 30% of the air in the hood.
2. HEPA-filtered air enters and makes up 70% of the air in the hood.
3. Air from the work area is drawn down into the base and pulled back through the unit.
4. Air is exhausted after being filtered through carbon or HEPA filters.

FIGURE 17-3 Vertical laminar flow workbench.

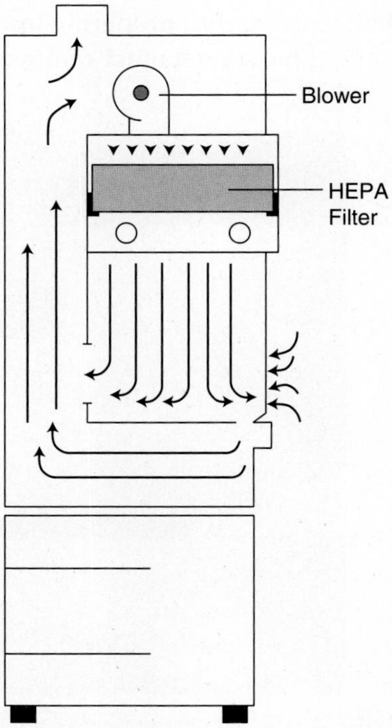

FIGURE 17-4 Biological safety cabinet.

The buffer area should be enclosed from other pharmacy operations. Surfaces should be smooth, nonporous, nonshedding, and able to be easily cleaned and disinfected. Cracks, crevices, and seams should be avoided, as should ledges or other places that could collect dust. The floor of the buffer area should be smooth and seamless with covered edges. There should be no sink or floor drains in the buffer area. Access to the buffer area should be restricted to only qualified personnel.

Ante-Area

The ante-area should be enclosed from other pharmacy operations, supplied with HEPA-filtered air, and able to attain an ISO Class 8 environment under dynamic conditions. A barrier separates it from the buffer area. For a buffer area not physically separated from the ante-area, the displacement airflow typically requires an air velocity of 40 ft per minute or more from the buffer area across the line of demarcation into the ante-area. The ante-area is used to decontaminate supplies, equipment, and personnel. The ante-area is the support area for performing hand hygiene, gowning, and unpacking supplies from cardboard boxes. Clean and sanitized supplies can also be stored in this area. As in the buffer area, the ante-area surfaces should be smooth, nonporous, nonshedding, and able to be easily cleaned and disinfected. Cracks, crevices, and seams should be avoided, as should ledges or other places that could collect dust. The floors should be smooth and seamless with covered edges. There should be a line of demarcation in the ante-area that separates the clean side from the dirty side.

Personnel Cleansing and Garbing

Careful cleansing of hands and arms and correct donning of garb (personal protective equipment; **Figure 17-5**) is critical in the prevention of microbial contamination in CSPs. Personnel entering the ante-area shall don attire as described below.

Before entering the buffer area or segregated compounding area (a designated space, restricted to preparing low-risk level CSPs with 12-hour or less BUD), compounding personnel must remove personal outer garments, all cosmetics, and all

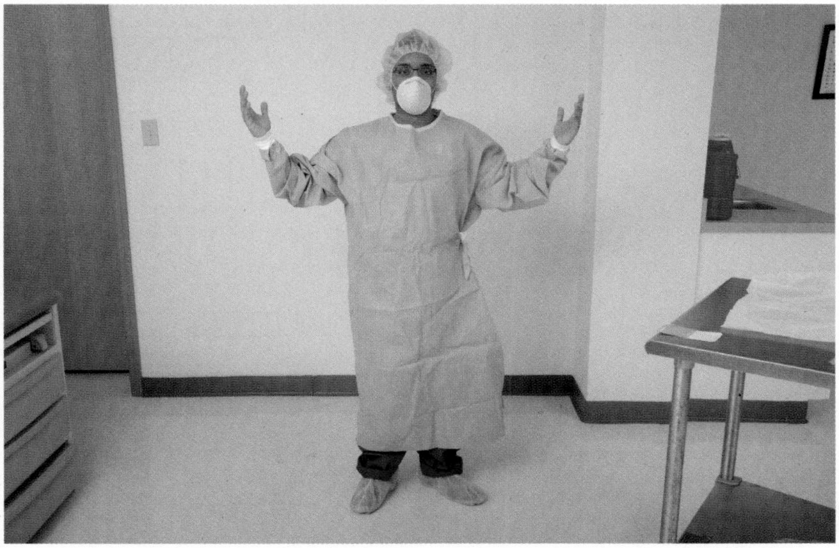

FIGURE 17-5 Personal protective equipment (PPE) with gown, shoe covers, rubber gloves, face mask, and hair cover.

hand, wrist, and other visible jewelry or piercings (e.g., earrings, lip or eyebrow piercings), because they can interfere with the effectiveness of the garb. Artificial nails or extenders may not be worn while working in the sterile compounding area. Natural nails must also be kept neat and trimmed.

Garb must be donned in an order that proceeds from those considered dirtiest to cleanest, as shown in the following figures:

1. Don shoe covers (**Figure 17-6A**).
2. Don hair covers and beard covers (if necessary) (**Figure 17-6B**).
3. Don face mask (**Figure 17-6C**).
4. Perform a hand-cleansing procedure by removing debris from underneath fingernails (**Figure 17-6D**).
5. Wash hands and forearms to the elbows with soap (either nonantimicrobial or antimicrobial) and water for at least 30 seconds while in the ante-area (**Figure 17-6E** and **Figure 17-6F**). (Use of antimicrobial scrub brushes is not recommended.)
6. Rinse all soap from arms (**Figure 17-6G**). Completely dry hands and forearms, using either lint-free disposable towels or an electronic hand dryer (**Figure 17-6H**).

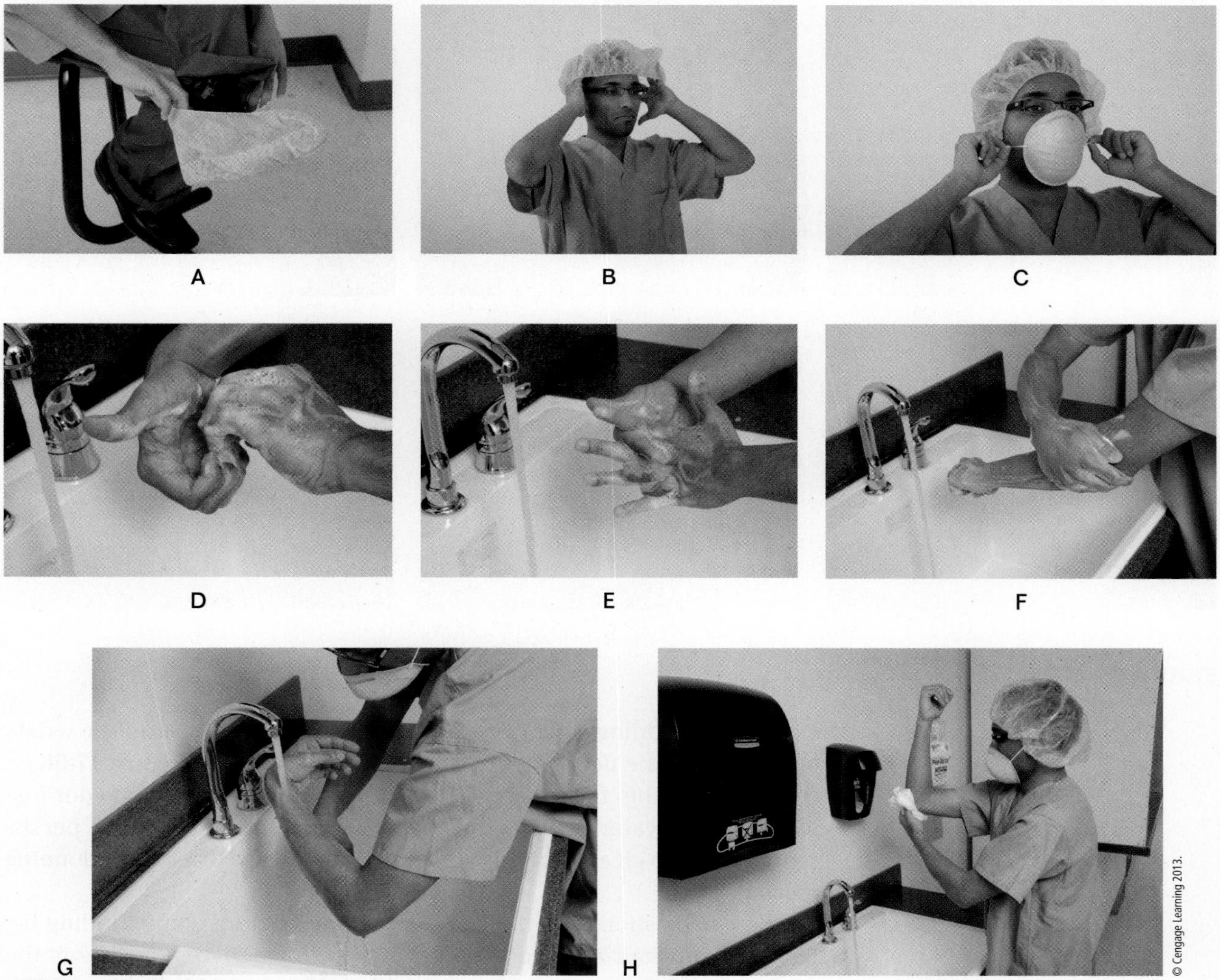

FIGURE 17-6A–H Procedure for donning PPE for sterile compounding.

(Continued)

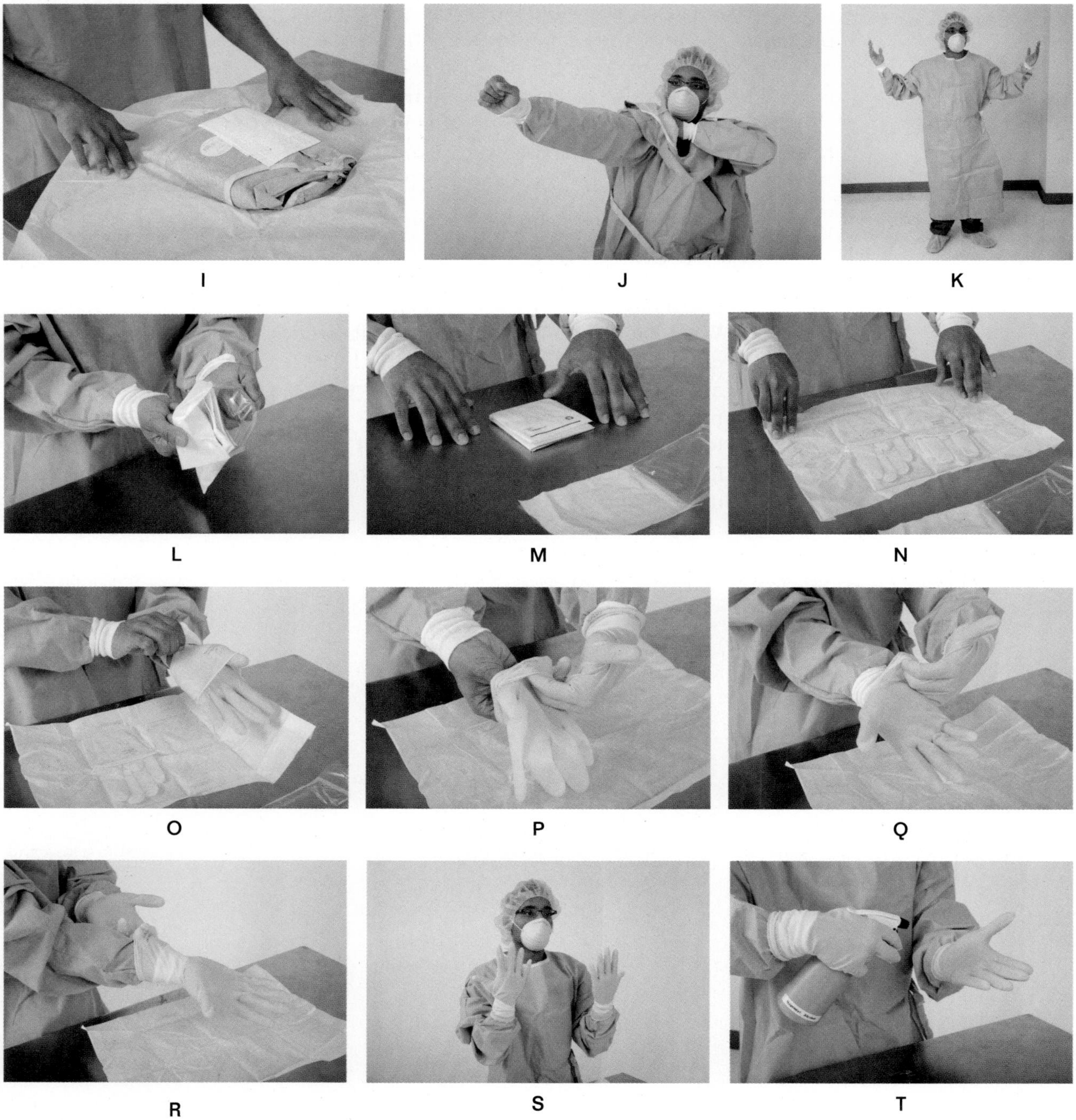

FIGURE 17-6I–T (Continued)

7. Don a nonshedding gown with sleeves that fit snugly around the wrists and closes at the neck (**Figure 17-6I**, **Figure 17-6J**, and **Figure 17-6K**).
8. Once inside the buffer area, prior to donning sterile, powder-free gloves, use a waterless, alcohol-based surgical hand scrub with persistent activity to cleanse hands again. Allow hands to dry before donning sterile gloves.
9. Sterile gloves should be the last item donned before compounding begins. The appropriate size gloves should be opened, removed from the package, and the inner package unfolded (**Figure 17-6L**, **Figure 17-6M**, and **Figure 17-6N**).

10. The first glove should be picked up by the folded-down cuff of the gloves. The hand should be now touching the inside of the glove (**Figure 17-6O**).
11. The ungloved hand should never touch the outside of the glove. The cuff of the glove should not be fully pulled up at this time.
12. Next, two fingers of the gloved hand should be inserted into the cuff of the other glove such that the gloved hand is now touching the outside of the glove (**Figure 17-6P**).
13. The glove should be pulled on and the cuff pulled up over the sleeve of the gown. The cuff of the second glove should be pulled over the coat (**Figure 17-6Q**, **Figure 17-6R**, and **Figure 17-6S**).
14. Routine application of sterile 70% isopropyl alcohol (IPA) throughout the compounding process and whenever nonsterile surfaces are touched is essential (**Figure 17-6T**).

Introduction of Supplies into the Ante-Area

All supplies and equipment must be removed from their outer cardboard packing and sprayed with sterile 70% IPA and wiped down as they are transferred into the ante-area for storage. Nothing should cross the line of demarcation in the ante-area without being sanitized.

Training of Compounding Personnel

All personnel who prepare CSPs must be thoroughly trained by expert personnel in the principles and practical skill of garbing procedures, aseptic work practices, achieving and maintaining ISO Class 5 environmental conditions, and cleaning and disinfecting procedures. This training should be completed and documented before any compounding personnel begin to prepare CSPs. Compounding personnel must complete didactic training, pass written competence assessments, and undergo skill assessment using observational audit tools, such as a checklist and media fill testing.

Compounding personnel must also demonstrate proficiency of proper hand hygiene, garbing, and cleaning procedures. The personnel should be observed during the process of performing hand hygiene and garbing procures. This should be documented using a checklist format, allowing for the maintenance of a permanent record of training. After completion of garbing, a gloved fingertip sample should be taken, using sterile contact agar plates. The evaluator will collect a gloved fingertip and thumb sample from both hands of the compounding personnel onto trypticase soy agar (TSA) with lecithin and polysorbate 80, which will be incubated at 30° to 35°C for 48 to 72 hours. This evaluation process must be successfully completed three times before the compounding personnel are allowed to perform the initial media fill. Reevaluation of all compounding personnel for this competency must occur at least annually for low- and medium-risk levels and semiannually for high-risk levels, using one or more sample collections during the media-fill test procedure, before being allowed to continue compounding CSPs for human use.

The risk of contamination of a CSP is highly dependent on proper hand hygiene and garbing practices, compounding personnel's aseptic technique, and the presence of surface contamination, assuming that all work is performed in a certified and properly functioning ISO Class 5 PEC with secondary engineering controls, an

ISO Class 7 buffer area, and an ISO Class 8 ante-area. Sampling of compounding personnel glove fingertips is performed for all CSP risk level compounding, because direct touch contamination is the most likely source of introduction of microorganisms into CSPs prepared by humans. This sampling is used to evaluate the competency of personnel in performing hand hygiene and garbing procedures, in addition to educating compounding personnel on proper work practices, which includes frequent and repeated glove disinfection using sterile 70% IPA during actual compounding of CSPs. However, disinfecting gloves immediately before sampling will provide false-negative results and is not allowed.

Media fill testing to evaluate aseptic work skills should be performed initially before beginning to prepare CSPs and at least annually thereafter for low- and medium-risk level compounding, and semiannually for high-risk level compounding. The media test is done by using a growth-promoting media, such as soybean casein digest, in place of the drug product. The test should mimic as closely as possible the most complicated procedure the compounding personnel perform, and should be done under worst-case conditions. Sterile media may be purchased for use in low- and medium-risk level media fills. For high-risk level compounding, the media used is commercially available, nonsterile soybean casein digest medium, made up to a 3% solution. Normal processing steps should then be mimicked. The purpose of any media fill is to evaluate the compounding personnel's aseptic technique, the compounding process used, and the environment of the facility.

>>> ALERT! >>>

The objective of USP Chapter <797>is to describe the conditions and practices in CSPs to ensure safety in their preparation to prevent harm to patients that could result from (1) microbial contamination, (2) excessive bacterial endotoxins, (3) variability in the intended strength of correct ingredients, (4) unintended chemical and physical contaminants, and (5) ingredients of inappropriate quality. Contaminated or inappropriately prepared CSPs are potentially hazardous to patients once administered.

Recent adverse events relating to CSPs resulting in patient harm and death have focused extensive attention on the need for pharmacy compounding personnel to be meticulously conscientious in precluding contamination of CSPs. This chapter describes the appropriate steps in compounding sterile preparations.

Surface Cleaning and Disinfection

A major source of contamination can be the clean-room environment. Therefore, careful attention to cleaning and disinfecting is required. Compounding personnel are responsible for ensuring that the frequency of cleaning is in accordance with what is stated in USP Chapter <797>. All cleaning and disinfection procedures must be written as standard operating procedures and followed by all compounding personnel. The ISO Class 5 environment must be cleaned and disinfected frequently, at a minimum at the beginning of each shift, before each batch is prepared, every 30 minutes during continuous compounding of CSPs, when there are spills, or when surface contamination is known or suspected. Work surfaces in the ISO Class 7 buffer area and in the ISO Class 8 ante-area should be cleaned and disinfected at least daily, and dust and debris must be removed when necessary from storage sites for compounding supplies. Floors in the buffer area and ante-area must be cleaned and disinfected daily when no compounding activities are occurring. The walls, ceiling, and shelving of the buffer area and ante-area must be cleaned and disinfected on at least a monthly basis. All cleaning materials, such as mops, sponges, and wipes, must be nonshedding and used in the clean room only.

Visual observations of cleaning and disinfection competency should occur during initial training and at the end of any media fill test. This should be documented by using a checklist format and the documentation maintained in personnel training files.

Surface sampling using contact plates is useful for evaluating the cleaning and disinfection procedures, personnel work practices as far as component/vial disinfection, and the overall state of the facility. Surface sampling using a contact plate filled with TSA, which has polysorbate 80 and lethicin added as neutralizing agents, should be done periodically in all ISO classified areas. Sampling should only be done at the conclusion of compounding.

Working in the Primary Engineering Control

One must always use good aseptic technique when compounding sterile preparations. Compounding personnel must be careful not to get a false sense of security concerning the sterility of the products just because they were prepared in the primary engineering control (PEC). The ISO Class 5 environment does not remove particulates or microbial contamination from the surfaces of the containers or other items being placed in the PEC. The laminar flow workbench is not a sterilization device; it must be properly used and maintained to provide the ISO Class 5 environment.

Products and supplies not in an overwrap are first wiped with a nonshedding wipe soaked with sterile 70% IPA before being placed in the PEC. Items should be checked for cracks, tears, and particles before use in compounding sterile preparations. If items are in a protective overwrap, the overwrap may be removed at the edge of the hood and the item placed in the hood in uninterrupted unidirectional airflow. One exception to this practice is the needle. It should not be opened until immediately before use. Needles in the wraps are placed within the first 6 inches of the hood.

Compounding materials in a horizontal flow workbench are placed to the right or left of the direct contiguous work area (DCA). Critical sites must be in uninterrupted airflow at all times. The operator must work without placing a hand or object behind a critical site. The operator must work at least 6 inches inside the horizontal flow workbench. As the unidirectional airflow hits the operator, it must split and go around him or her. This can create turbulence, allowing an ingress of air from the buffer area into the PEC. Remember that the PEC is not a means of sterilization. It can only provide an ISO Class 5 environment when properly maintained, cleaned and disinfected, and used by the operator with good aseptic technique. A PEC will not compensate for bad technique. The most common method of contamination of a CSP is for it to be touched by the operator.

When an item is in a horizontal laminar flow workbench, it disturbs the unidirectional flow of the air behind the object, approximately three times the diameter of the object. If the vial or bottle is placed next to the side wall of the hood, it disturbs the airflow behind it, approximately six times the diameter of the object. Therefore, any nonsterile item has the potential to contaminate articles downstream with particles or microorganisms. Once again, it is very important for first air to be maintained.

When working in a vertical laminar flow workbench, supplies must be placed so the compounding personnel may work without putting their hands or an item over the top of a critical site. Movements in and out of the VLFW should be minimized. Articles to be thrown away can be dropped over the edge into the trash or left in the first 6 inches of the hood until the manipulations are completed.

Needles

Sterile and pyrogen-free needles are wrapped in plastic with a twist-off top or wrapped in paper. Whatever the type of wrap, it should be inspected before using, because tears or pinholes in the wrapping materials will compromise the sterility of the needle. Needles come in various sizes—the larger the gauge of the needle, the smaller the bore of the needle. Many facilities use an 18- to 21-gauge needle. The needle length is measured in inches, with the most common lengths for pharmacy being 1 to 1.5 inches.

The basic parts of the needle are the bevel tip, the bevel, bevel heel, shaft, and hub. The needle shaft is encased in a rigid plastic sheath to cover the needle and allow for ease in handling. This sheath is left on until the needle is ready to be used. The entire needle is considered a critical site (**Figure 17-7**).

Syringes

Sterile and pyrogen-free disposable plastic syringes are packed in either paper or rigid plastic. Before using, the wrap should be inspected carefully for holes or tears to ensure the syringe is intact and sterile. The basic parts of the syringe are the barrel, piston, top collar, plunger, flange, and tip—either a slip tip where the needle is held on the friction, or a Luer-Lock tip, where the needle is screwed into place (**Figure 17-8**). The critical sites on the syringe include the tip of the syringe and the ribs of the plunger. Syringes have calibration marks that allow the

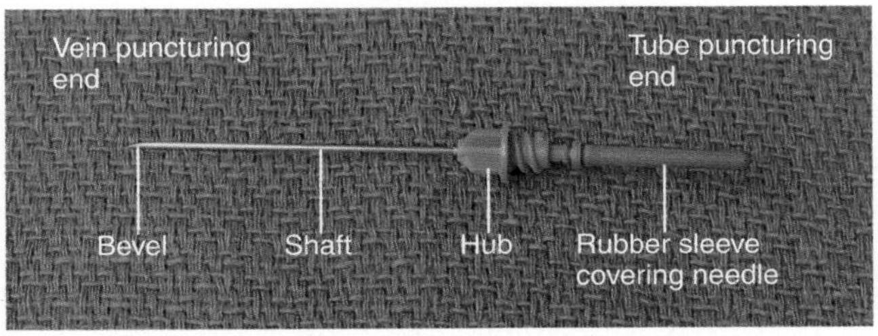

FIGURE 17-7 Parts of a needle.

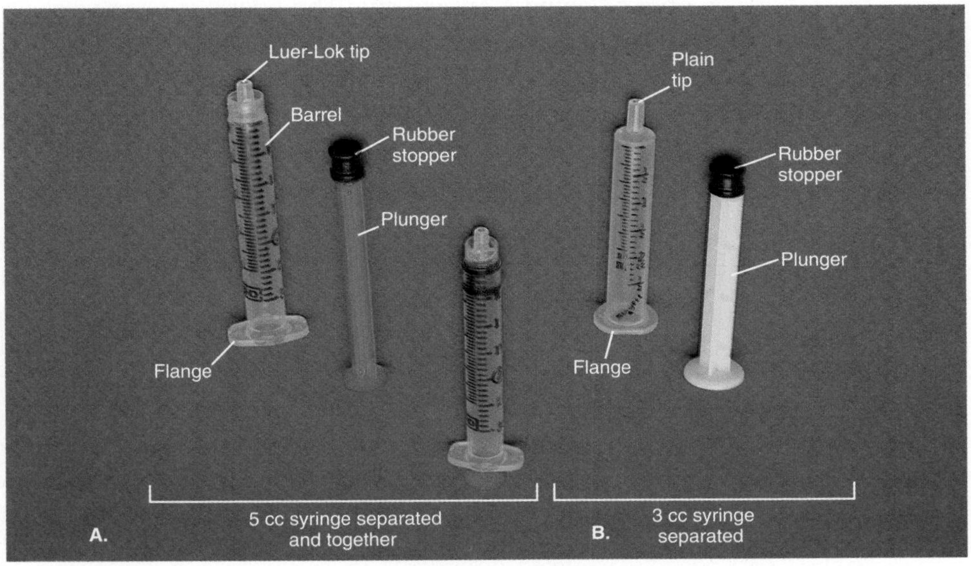

FIGURE 17-8 Parts of a syringe: **A.** A 5-mL syringe separated and together with a Luer-Lock tip. **B.** A 3-mL syringe separated with a plain tip.

technician to estimate accurately to one-half of the interval marked. The larger the syringe, the larger the intervals marked on the syringe area. The final edge of the rubber tip of the plunger that comes in contact with the syringe side wall is lined up with the calibration mark that corresponds to the volume of solution desired.

Preparing the Horizontal Laminar Flow Workbench (HLFW)

The hood (**Figure 17-9**) of the HLFW is disinfected with sterile 70% IPA. The sterile IPA is poured onto the surface of the workbench. This allows for better wetting of the surfaces than using a spray bottle (**Figure 17-10A**). Wet nonshedding wipes with 70% sterile IPA (**Figure 17-10B**). Wipe the light cover and then the side walls (**Figure 17-10C** and **Figure 17-10D**). The technique is to wipe up and down, working out from the HEPA filter. Do not go from the edge of the hood back in over wiped surfaces (**Figure 17-10E**). Wipe the workbench in the same manner. Start at the

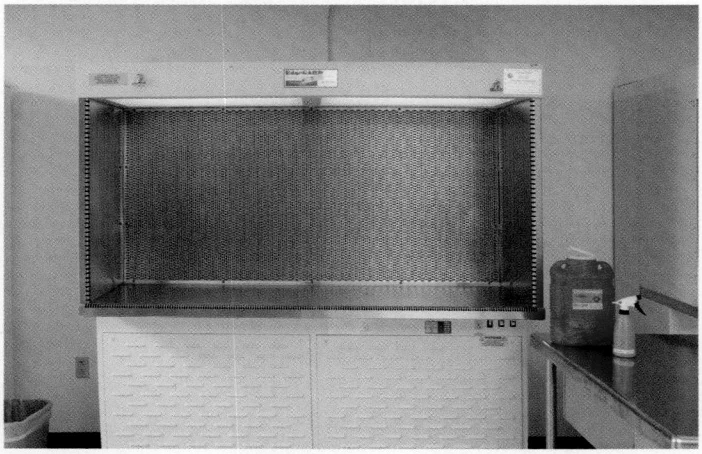

FIGURE 17-9 Horizontal laminar flow workbench.

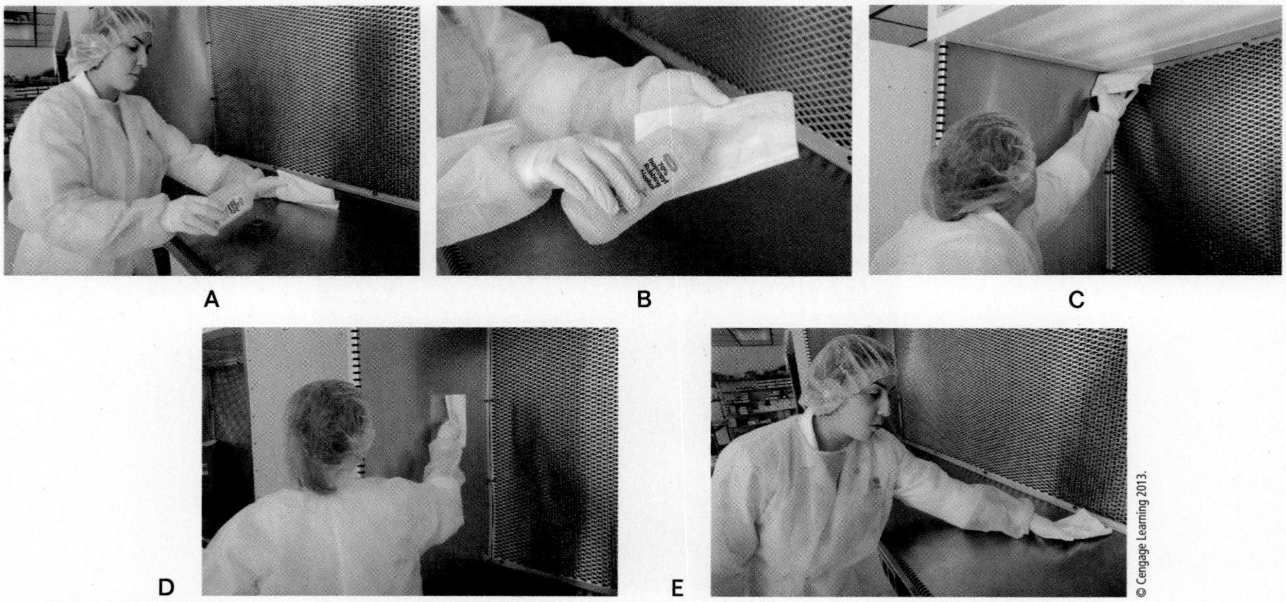

FIGURE 17-10A–E Preparation of a horizontal laminar flow workbench.

back on one side by the HEPA filter, and wipe from side to side, moving the wipe forward the width of your hand each time. The last place to be wiped is the front edge. Discard the wipes in the trash, being careful not to touch the trash container.

Aseptic Technique: Using a Needle and Syringe

(The following instructions are given for a right-handed person. If the operator is left-handed, the directions should be reversed.)

1. Select an appropriately sized syringe, one large enough to contain the volume of solution desired.
2. Inspect the integrity of the outer wrap for defects such as pinholes, tears, or breaks in the wrap.
3. At the edge of the hood (in the 6-inch supply staging area) peel back the paper on the syringe or remove the syringe from a plastic container (**Figure 17-11A**).
4. Place the syringe in the hood. Do not push the syringe through the paper wrap.
5. Select a wrapped needle and peel back the paper tabs while not touching the needle hub. Keep the hub in uninterrupted HEPA-filtered air (**Figure 17-11B**).
6. Holding back the paper, hold the needle in a vertical position in the unidirectional airflow.
7. Hold the syringe in a horizontal position, roll the left hand containing the needle to the right, and connect the needle hub to the syringe (**Figure 17-11C**).

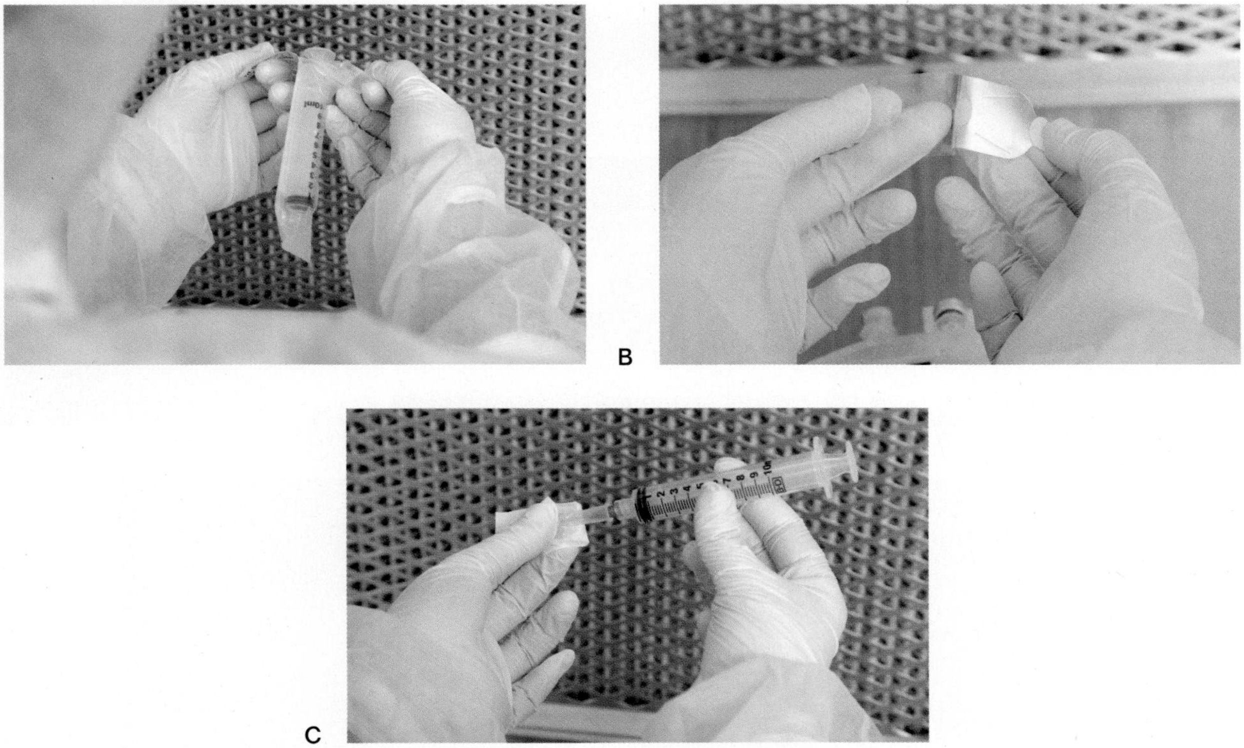

A B C

FIGURE 17-11A–C Aseptic technique using a needle and syringe.

8. Turn the syringe counterclockwise to lock the needle on the syringe.
9. Hold the syringe by the barrel (a noncritical site) firmly with four fingers. Push the plunger in to seat and loosen the plunger.

Using Ampoules, Filter Needles, and an Intravenous Solution

Ampoules are single-dose containers (**Figure 17-12**). Once the tip is broken, you have an open system with a large critical site. The contents of the ampoule should be used immediately and not stored for any length of time.

The ampoule should be wiped with a nonshedding wipe soaked in 70% IPA before being placed in the PEC.

The neck of the ampoule should be wiped with a sterile alcohol wipe in the event glass particles fall into the solution when the ampoule is broken (**Figure 17-13**). The ampoule must be dry so the hands do not slip while attempting to break it open.

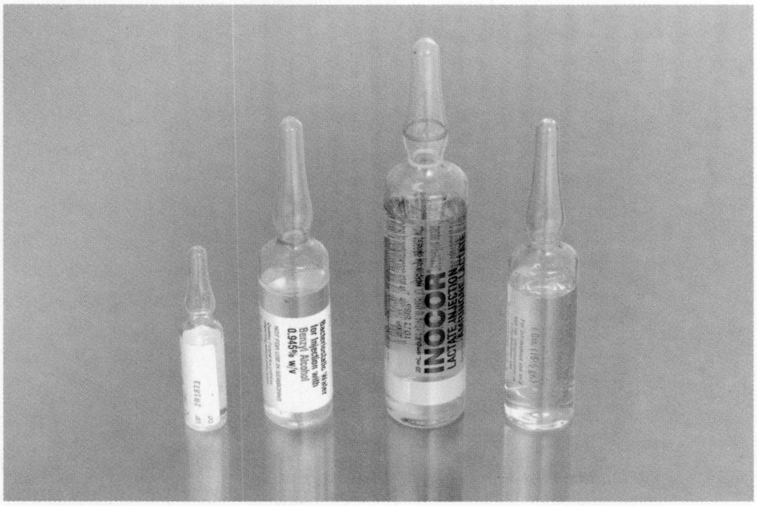

FIGURE 17-12 Single-dose ampoule containers.

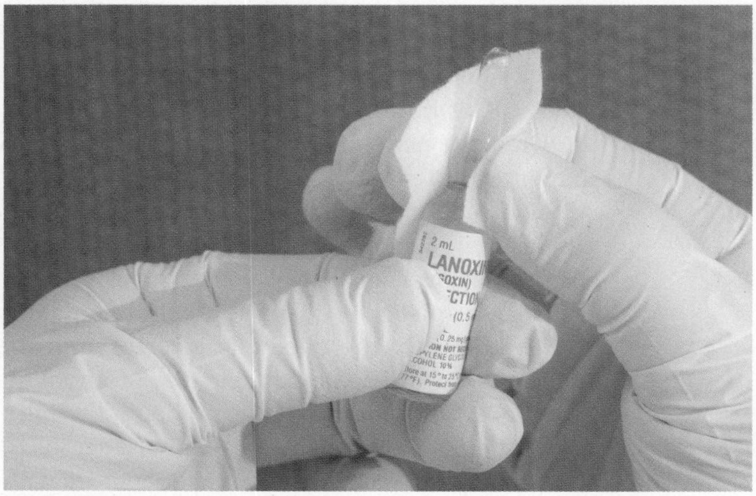

FIGURE 17-13 Wipe the neck of the ampoule with a sterile alcohol wipe and then dry before breaking.

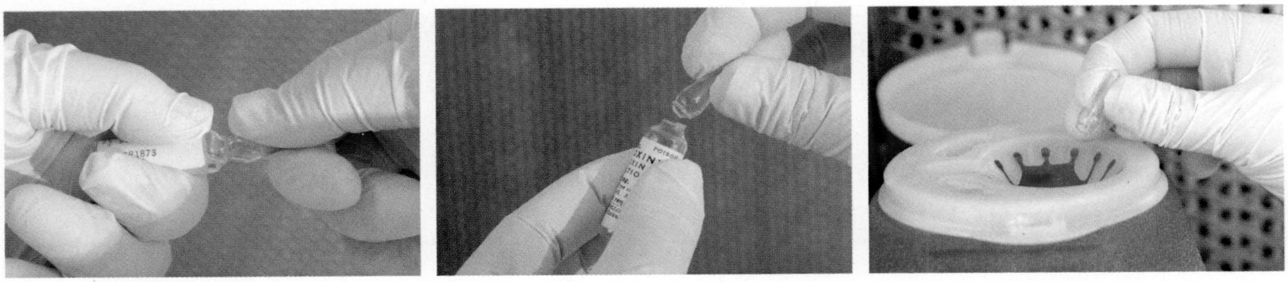

A B C

FIGURE 17-14 **A.** Apply pressure with the fingers on either side of the ampoule for, **B.** an even break. **C.** Place the top to the side or in a sharps container.

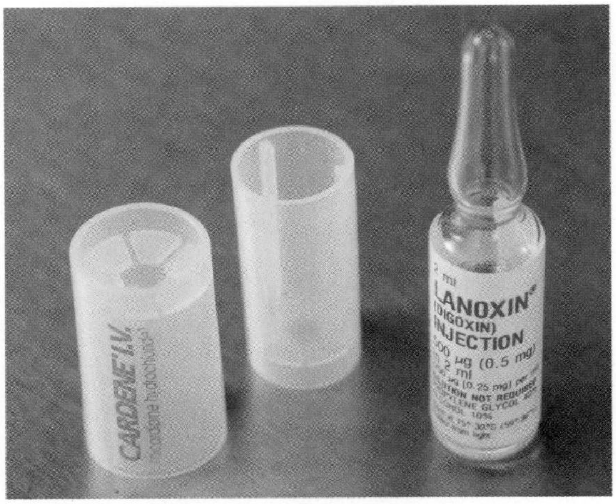

FIGURE 17-15 An ampoule breaker is shown on the left.

Open the ampoule toward the side wall of the laminar flow hood, because glass particles and small amounts of fluid are dispersed when the ampoule is broken. Do not wrap the ampoule in gauze to open it, because this could allow particles to fall into the ampoule. (For this reason, ampoule solutions are always filtered before use; see discussion below.) Position the thumbs about a half inch apart on either side of the constricted neck of the ampoule to apply pressure with the fingers, as if breaking a pencil in half (**Figure 17-14A**, **Figure 17-14B**, and **Figure 17-14C**). You may use an ampoule breaker if you prefer (**Figure 17-15**). If the ampoule does not break easily, rotate it a quarter of a turn before trying again.

Once the ampoule is broken, place the top to the side, and place the ampoule in uninterrupted unidirectional airflow.

The needle cover (a noncritical site) is removed by grasping the needle cover between two fingers of the left hand and pulling the needle cover off. Do not twist the needle cover, as this will unscrew the needle from the syringe. The needle cover may also be placed on a sterile alcohol prep pad pointing toward the HEPA filter.

The bevel of the needle is inserted into the shoulder of the ampoule, with the bevel down. The ampoule is tilted to pool the drug solution into the shoulder of the ampoule (**Figure 17-16**). When inserting the needle into the ampoule, the needle should not touch the outside edge of the ampoule. If this does happen, the contaminated needle should be replaced with a new needle on the syringe. The opening of the ampoule and the needle are critical sites, so care must be taken to keep them in uninterrupted unidirectional airflow.

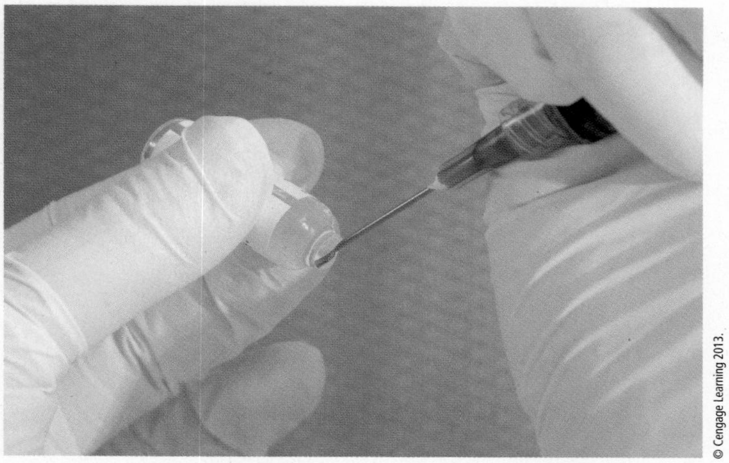

FIGURE 17-16 Tilt the ampoule to pool the solution and insert the bevel of the needle in the shoulder of the ampoule.

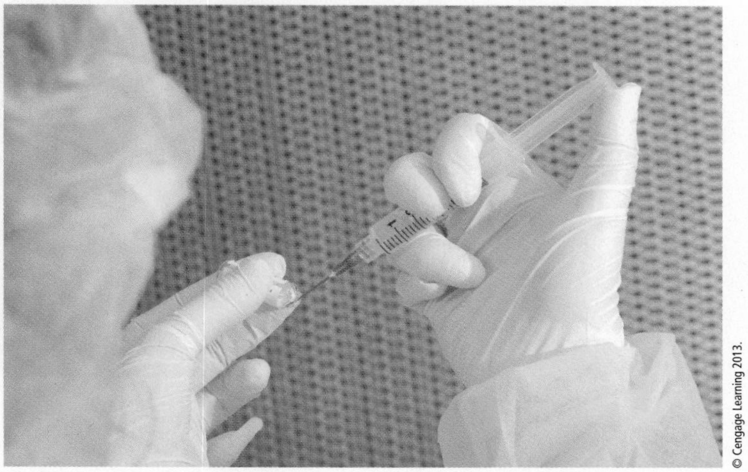

FIGURE 17-17 Withdraw the solution by using the thumb (or forefinger if necessary).

The solution is withdrawn, using the thumb on the plunger end plate and withdrawing the plunger. If the thumb is not long enough to withdraw the solution into the syringe, the first finger can be used to extend the length of the plunger withdrawal (**Figure 17-17**).

Any unused solution in the ampoule should be discarded.

If air is in the syringe, it must be removed to obtain an accurate measurement of the volume of solution. Turn the syringe to a vertical position with the needle pointing up, and tap the syringe firmly with the fingertips to loosen air bubbles from the plunger and side walls (**Figure 17-18**).

The plunger is drawn back to pull any solution in the needle shaft back into the barrel of the syringe. The plunger is then pushed in slowly to expel the air until the first drop of solution appears on the bevel of the needle. Do not spray drug solution into the hood. Any excess solution is put back into the ampoule.

Open the outer wrap for the intravenous solution bag and place it in the PEC. Position the bag so the injection port is facing the unidirectional air from the HEPA filter.

Wipe the injection port with a sterile alcohol prep pad in one direction to remove particles and disinfect the injection port.

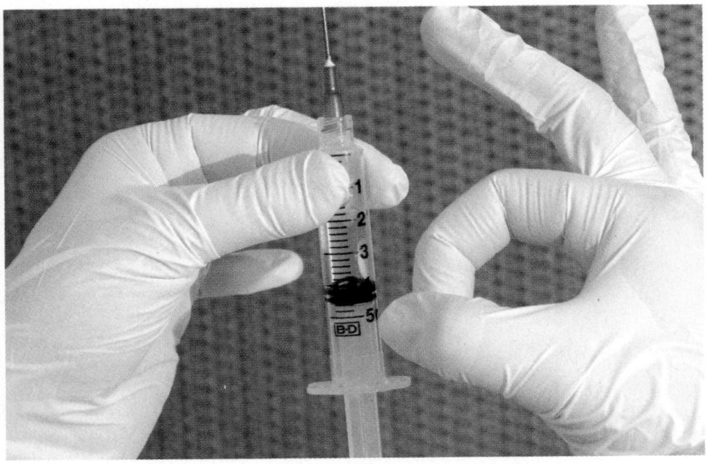

FIGURE 17-18 Tap or flick the syringe to loosen any air bubbles.

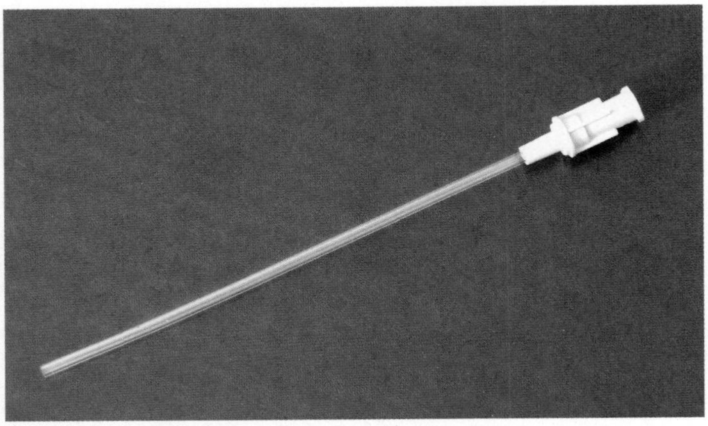

FIGURE 17-19 A filter needle.

Any solution taken from an ampoule must be filtered with a 5-micron filter, because glass particles can fall into the ampoule when it breaks open. Most often, a filter needle is used (**Figure 17-19**). A filter needle is a sterile needle that contains a 5-micron filter to remove glass particles. The filter needle may be used for withdrawing the solution from the ampoule. This filters the solution as it enters the syringe. A regular needle must then be put on the syringe before the solution can be injected into the IV bag. Another filtering method is to withdraw the solution with a regular needle and then put on a filter needle before injecting the solution into the IV bag. This method is described next.

To filter the solution in the syringe as it is injected into the IV bag, the filter needle is attached to the syringe after the regular needle is removed. Holding the filter needle, the regular needle is removed by unscrewing the syringe from the needle (**Figure 17-20A**).

The left hand is rolled 90 degrees to the right, the filter needle is aligned with the syringe tip, and the syringe is screwed onto the filter needle (**Figure 17-20B**).

The cover of the filter needle is removed. The filter needle is inserted into the center of the injection port of the IV bag. Care must be taken so the needle does not penetrate the side of the injection port of the IV bag itself (**Figure 17-21**).

The IV solution is mixed by kneading the bag. The compounded IV solution must be checked for precipitates, particulates, undesirable color changes, and gas evolution before release to the nurse or patient (**Figure 17-22**).

A B
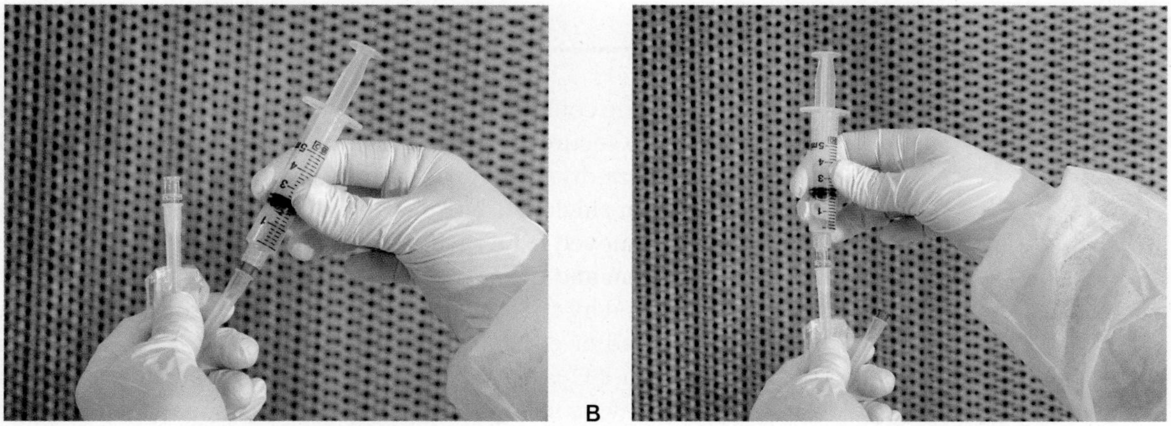

FIGURE 17-20 **A.** The regular needle is removed from the syringe and is, **B,** screwed onto the filter needle.

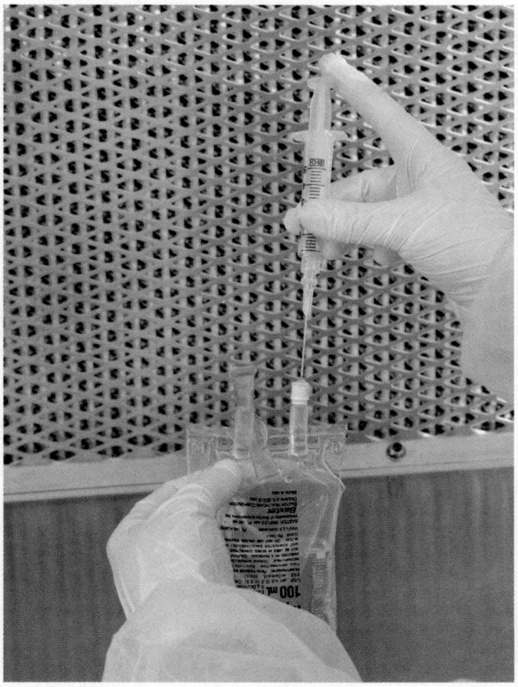

FIGURE 17-21 The filter needle is inserted into the injection port of the IV bag and added to the IV solution.

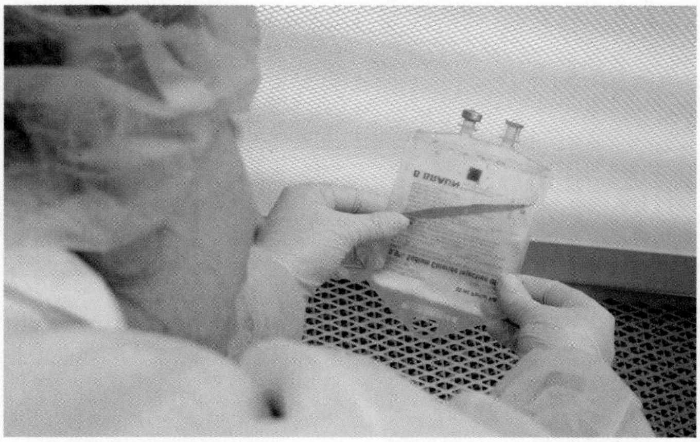

FIGURE 17-22 After the IV solution has been kneaded, it should be checked for particulates, color changes, and other possible problems.

Vials

Vials can be glass or plastic containers with rubber closures and aluminum or flip-top seals crimped in place to secure the closure. They can be filled with sterile solution, lyophilized powder (freeze-dried), or dry powders or they may be empty, evacuated containers. Vials come in single-dose or multiple-dose sizes. Multiple-dose containers can have product removed from them on multiple occasions. They usually contain a preservative system and the BUD is 28 days after the initial entry or opening, unless otherwise specified by the manufacturer. Single-dose containers can be used for up to 1 hour if opened or entered in worse than an ISO Class 5 environment. If entered or opened in an ISO Class 5 or cleaner environment, the contents of the single-dose container may be used for 6 hours. However, opened ampoules cannot be stored for any length of time. The first person using a vial or other container must label the container with the date, time of the initial entry, and his or her initials.

Withdrawing Solution from a Vial

The vial must be wiped with a nonshedding wipe wet with sterile 70% IPA before being placed in the hood. Once placed in the hood, the flip-top plastic cap is removed to reveal the rubber closure (stopper) (**Figure 17-23A**).

The top of the closure is wiped in one direction with a sterile alcohol wipe (**Figure 17-23B**). Wiping in one direction helps to remove particles, and the alcohol disinfects the closure. This minimizes the chance of contaminating the drug when the needle is pushed through the rubber closure. While the alcohol is drying, the needle and syringe should be put together as described in the ampoule section above,

Remove the needle cover placed between the ring finger and the little finger, or on a sterile alcohol pad with the opening pointing toward the HEPA filter (**Figure 17-24A**). Draw in a volume of air equivalent to the amount of drug solution that will be withdrawn from the vial. Since the vial is a closed system, to get solution out you must put air in (**Figure 17-24B**).

While holding the base of the vial with one hand, the needle is placed in the center of the rubber closure, bevel up, at approximately 45 degrees (**Figure 17-25**). This is to help prevent coring of the stopper when the needle is inserted through the closure. Do not touch the aluminum seal with the needle. As the closure is penetrated, the needle is elevated to a vertical position while exerting pressure laterally on the needle. Make sure the critical sites stay in uninterrupted unidirectional air

Invert the syringe and needle. Do not place a gloved hand between first air and the critical sites (**Figure 17-26**).

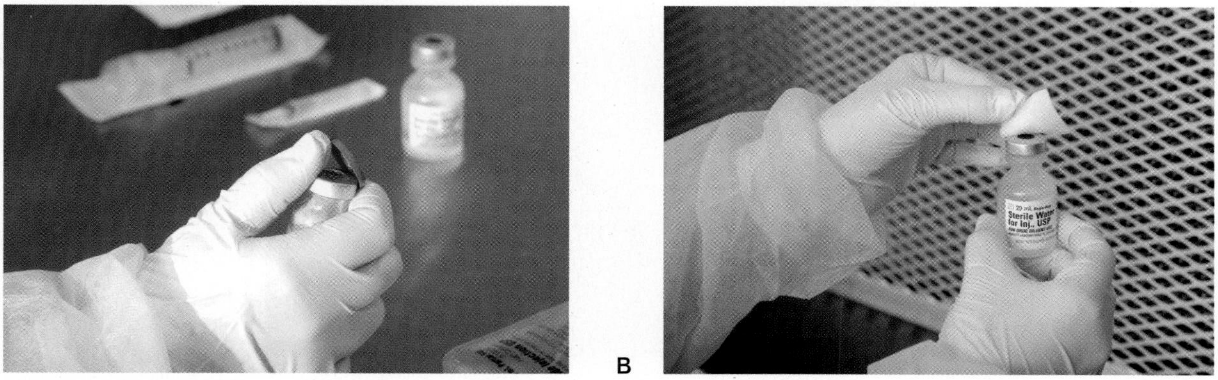

A B

FIGURE 17-23 **A.** Flip the plastic top of the vial and then, **B**, wipe the top with a sterile alcohol wipe.

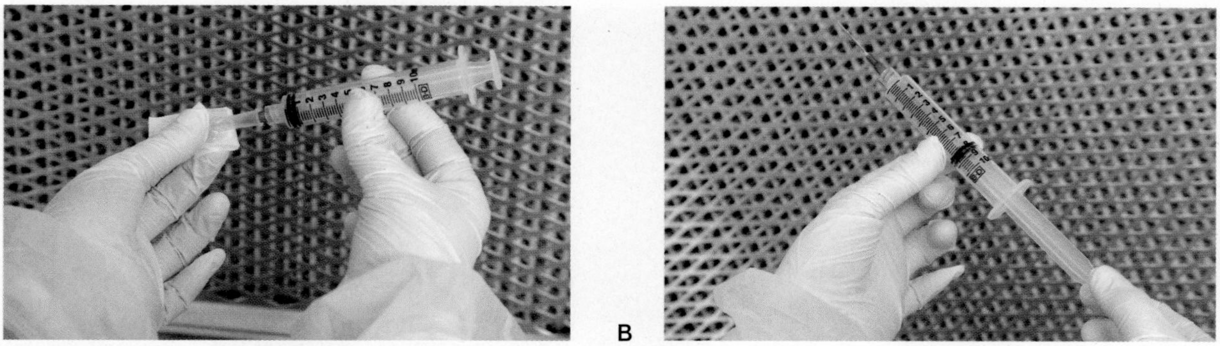

A B

FIGURE 17-24 One method for removing the needle cover is to use a sterile alcohol pad, **A,** after which, **B,** air is drawn into the syringe in the amount of the drug solution.

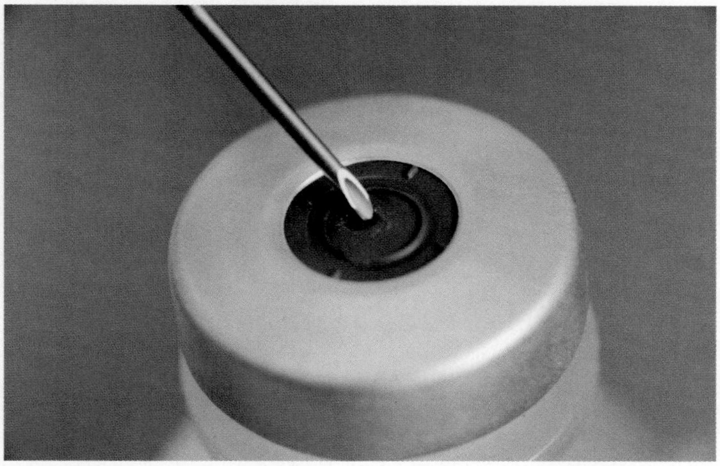

FIGURE 17-25 With bevel up, the needle should be placed at a 45-degree angle to the rubber closure on the vial.

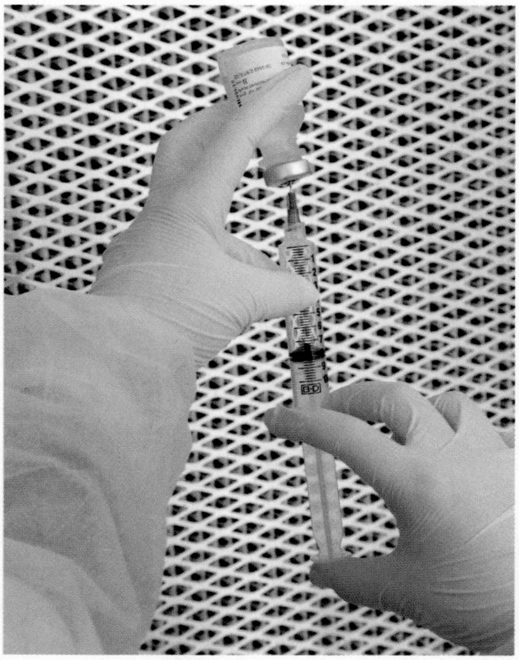

FIGURE 17-26 Invert the syringe and needle and create positive pressure in the vial by injecting the air from the syringe.

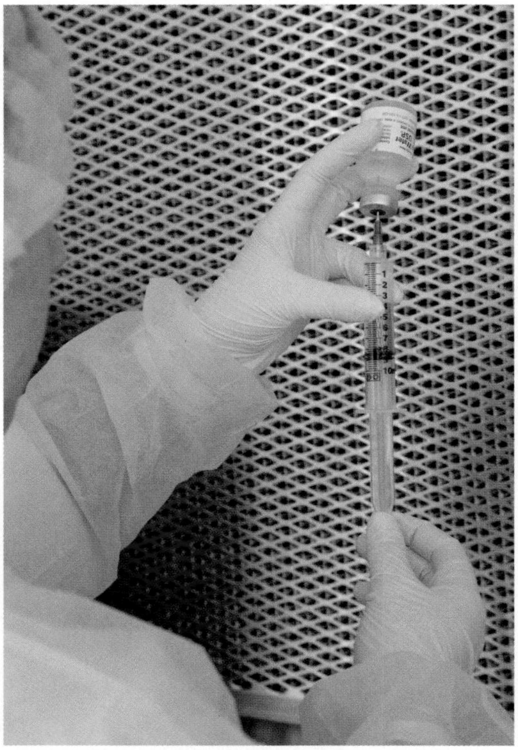

FIGURE 17-27 Pull the plunger back using the flat top of the plunger, making sure not to touch the critical site of the ribs of the plunger.

Inject the air into the syringe, creating positive pressure in the vial. This will help push the drug solution back into the syringe when the pressure on the plunger is released (see Figure 17-26).

Withdraw the needle tip to just above the inside of the rubber closure to keep the tip of the needle in solution. Allow the positive pressure inside the vial to push the liquid back into the syringe. If more solution is needed, pull back on the plunger slowly. Place the middle finger and thumb on the flat top of the plunger and push against the collar of the syringe with the index finger to pull back on the plunger. The plunger should be pulled back to an amount slightly larger than desired. Take care not to touch the ribs of the plunger, because this is a critical site (**Figure 17-27**).

Invert the vial and syringe. Tap on the syringe with the fingertips to dislodge any air bubbles from the plunger and side walls. Push up the plunger to inject the air back into the vial, and adjust the plunger until the appropriate amount of solution is in the syringe (**Figure 17-28**).

While holding the inverted vials with one hand, hold the syringe barrel with the other and turn the vial and syringe over, taking care to protect the critical sites. The needles and syringe are then withdrawn from the vial.

Reconstitution

Vials containing lyophilized drugs or sterile drug powder must first be reconstituted with a diluent to put the drug into solution. When the drug product is lyophilized or in a powder form, it is usually because the drug has limited stability in solution. Sometimes the drug will come with a special diluent for reconstitution,

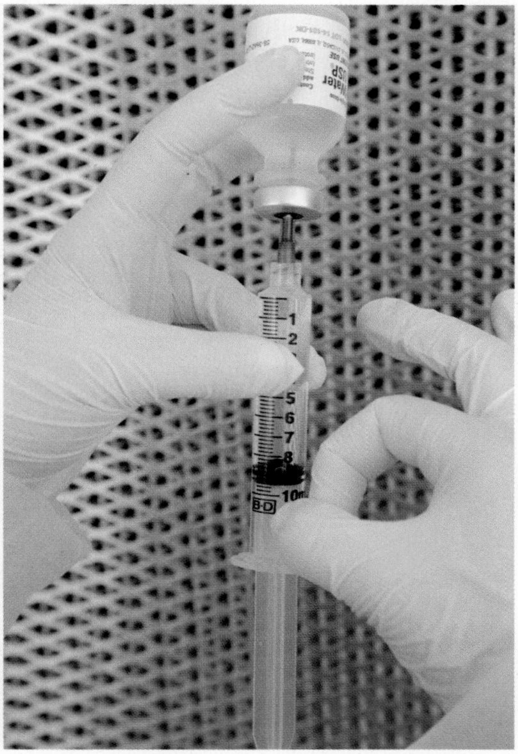

FIGURE 17-28 Tap on the syringe to release any air bubbles back into the vial.

and the diluent is specified on the label or in the product information. The label of the vial should be read to determine the proper diluent and the volume needed before reconstituting. In this example, sterile water for injection is used as the diluent.

Air is injected into the sterile water for the injection vial, and the correct volume needed for reconstitution is withdrawn.

The water is then injected into the vial, reconstituting the lyophilized drug. The excess air should be allowed to go back into the syringe so the vial will not contain positive pressure. If this is not done, some of the drug may be forced out of the vial when the needle is removed (**Figure 17-29**).

The vial should be shaken and checked for clarity, particulates, unexpected color changes, extra-long dissolution time, and gas evolution before withdrawing the necessary amount of drug solution. The reconstituted solution does not need filtering unless a particle or a rubber core is found floating in solution upon inspection of the vial.

Visual Inspection of Parenteral Solutions

Each completed sterile preparation must be inspected and verified by the pharmacist. The operator also must check the completed sterile preparation immediately after compounding it. It must be checked for:

- Correct labeling
- Correct intravenous solutions, including strength and quantity
- Correct drug additives, including strength and quantity
- Particulate matter, crystals, and precipitates.

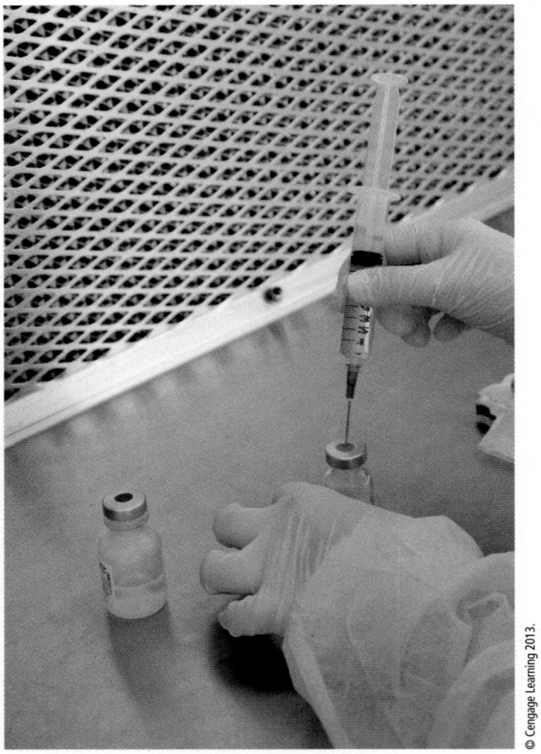

FIGURE 17-29 Sterile water is injected into the vial to reconstitute the drug. Any excess air should be allowed to go back into the syringe.

Sterilization Methods

The pharmacist is responsible for choosing the appropriate sterilization method for high-risk level CSPs and the necessary equipment. Three methods are commonly used: filtration, moist-heat (steam) sterilization, and dry-heat sterilization.

Filtration

Filtration is the most common method of sterilization of CSPs in the pharmacy. Care must be taken to choose the correct filter. One must take into consideration the volume that is to be filtered and the temperature and pressure at which filtration will occur. Filters used to sterilize CSPs must be sterile, pyrogen-free, and have a nominal porosity of 0.2 or 0.22 micron. Filtration occurs by a combination of mechanisms: sieving, adsorption, and entrapment. Filter manufacturers have compatibility data on their membrane and housing types with various solvent systems. They are a great source of information when selecting a filter.

Hydrophilic filter membranes wet spontaneously with water and are used to filter aqueous solutions, and aqueous solutions contain water-miscible solvents.

Hydrophobic filter membranes do not wet spontaneously with water and are used to filter gases and solvents.

Filter Integrity Test

All sterilizing membranes must undergo a filter integrity test after filtration has occurred (bubble point test). This test is a simple, nondestructive test that checks the integrity of the filter membrane and of the housing. It is based on the fact that liquid is held in the capillary structure of the membrane by surface tension. The minimum pressure required to push the liquid from the largest pores in the membrane is the *bubble point*.

The test is performed by wetting the filter with water and applying pressure on the upstream side. The pressure is increased until bubbles are seen coming out the downstream side of the filter. The typical water bubble point for a pore size rating of 0.2 micron is >50 psig (pounds per square inch gauge). If the bubble point of the filter is 50 psig as stated on the certificate of quality, to pass the integrity test you cannot exceed the bubble point at a pressure less than 50 psig.

Heat Sterilization

Moist-heat (steam) sterilization is a common method of terminally sterilizing the product in its final container. However, it can only be used to sterilize products that are aqueous. Steam (at 121°C and 15 psig), when it comes in contact with a cooler object, condenses and loses heat to the object, which releases about 524 kcal/g. This kills the microorganisms. In order for steam sterilization to work, the steam must contact the object or be made inside the closed vial or ampoule from the water that is in the CSP. This is why items like oils or powders that do not wet cannot be sterilized by steam. Steam sterilization also does not destroy bacterial endotoxins.

Dry-heat sterilization requires higher temperatures and longer exposure times than moist-heat sterilization. Dry-heat sterilization can be used to sterilize oils and powders. It should be used only on products that cannot be sterilized by steam. The commonly used temperature for dry heat is 170°C.

Dry-heat depyrogenation is used to sterilize and destroy bacterial endotoxins on equipment. A cycle of 30 minutes at 250°C is usually adequate.

Summary

The pharmacy technicians who prepare CSPs must be highly motivated and very conscientious. They must be thoroughly trained and follow written procedures at all times. Due to the possibility of microbial contamination or errors in compounding, all personnel must pay attention to every detail and thoroughly document the compounding process they followed. The pharmacist is responsible for double-checking and supervising all compounding activities. Quality must never be compromised. The pharmacy technician fulfills an important role in compounding sterile preparations.

TEST YOUR KNOWLEDGE

Multiple Choice

1. When working in a horizontal laminar flow hood, you must work at least ________ in from the outside edge of the work surface.

a. 2 inches
b. 4 inches
c. 6 inches
d. 8 inches

2. Which of the ISO classifications listed below is equivalent to a Class 100 area?
   a. ISO Class 3
   b. ISO Class 5
   c. ISO Class 6
   d. ISO Class 7

3. When working in a laminar flow hood
   a. you must protect all critical sites by never putting your hand or an object between a critical site and the HEPA-filtered air.
   b. you must never put your hand behind an object in a vertical flow hood.
   c. you must always spray your vials thoroughly with 70% IPA before placing them in the hood.
   d. you should always unwrap your needles and lay them down in the hood before attaching them to the syringe.

4. In the definition of Class 100, Class 10,000, and Class 100,000 rooms, we are always talking about total particles ________ micron(s) in size and larger.
   a. 0.3
   b. 0.5
   c. 1.2
   d. 5

5. A tuberculin skin test is given by which route of administration?
   a. intravenous
   b. intrapleural
   c. intradermal
   d. intramuscular

6. The compounding of a total parenteral nutrition solution would be an example of
   a. low-risk level compounding.
   b. medium-risk level compounding.
   c. high-risk level compounding.
   d. immediate-use CSPs.

7. When choosing a sterilizing filter, which of the following items must be considered?
   a. the volume of product to be filtered
   b. the compatibility of the membrane with the product to be filtered
   c. whether the solution to be filtered is hydrophobic or hydrophilic
   d. all of the above

8. Concerning the placement of items in the laminar flow workbench and working in the laminar flow workbench, choose the correct answer.
   a. Items should be placed in a horizontal flow hood to the right or left of the work area.
   b. Items in a vertical laminar flow hood should be placed so that when working in the hood, your hand never goes over the top of a critical site.
   c. An object placed in a horizontal flow hood disturbs the airflow three times the diameter of the object downstream of the object.
   d. All of the above.

9. The pore size of a sterilizing filter is
   a. 0.2 micron.
   b. 0.45 micron.
   c. 0.12 micron.
   d. 5.0 microns.

10. A sterile product is one that is
   a. free from all pyrogens.
   b. free from all viruses.
   c. free from all living microorganisms.
   d. free from all endotoxins.

11. Please choose the correct statement concerning USP media transfers.
   a. An operator must successfully complete one media fill before compounding any sterile products.
   b. An operator who passes a written exam may compound sterile products until the chief pharmacist gets time to watch his or her aseptic technique.
   c. An operator who has successfully completed a media fill must requalify semiannually if the operator is preparing low-risk level products.
   d. Once an operator successfully completes one media fill for high-risk compounding, the operator needs to revalidate quarterly by completing one media fill.

12. Choose the *most correct* answer about transferring products into the ante-area.
   a. Bottles, bags, and syringes must be removed from brown cardboard boxes before being brought into the ante-area.
   b. Vials stored in laminated cardboard may not be brought into the ante-area.
   c. Stainless steel carts may be used to transfer items into the ante-area directly from the storage area.
   d. Large-volume parenteral bags of IV solution must be removed from their protective overwrap before being brought into the ante-area.

13. Please choose the *most correct* conclusion to this statement. The plenum in a laminar flow workbench is
   a. where the air is prefiltered.
   b. the area where air is pressurized for distribution over the HEPA filter.
   c. the area where compounding takes place.
   d. an area that serves no purpose.

Suggested Readings

Buchanan, E.C., & Schneider, P.J. (2005). *Compounding sterile preparations*. Bethesda, MD: American Society of Health-System Pharmacists.

Controlled Environment Testing Association (CETA). (2005, November 8). *CETA applications guide for the use of compounding isolators in compounding sterile preparations in healthcare facilities* (CAG-001-2005). Raleigh, NC: Author.

International Organization for Standardization. (1999, May 1). *Cleanrooms and associated controlled environments—Part 1: Classification of air cleanliness* (ISO 14644-1:1999). Geneva, Switzerland: Author.

U.S. Food and Drug Administration, Guidance for Industry. (2004, September). *Sterile drug products produced by aseptic processing: Current good manufacturing practice*. Silver Spring, MD: Author.

U.S. Pharmacopeial Convention. (2007). Chapter <797>: Pharmaceutical compounding—Sterile preparations. In *U.S. pharmacopeia, 31st ed./National formulary, 26th rev., second supplement*. Rockville, MD: Author. Retrieved from http://www.usp.org/USPNF/pf/generalChapter797.html

Other Recommended Readings

Agalloco, J., & Akers, J.E. (2005). Aseptic processing: A vision of the future. *Pharmaceutical Technology*. Aseptic Processing supplement, s16.

Centers for Disease Control and Prevention, National Institute for Occupational Safety and Health. (2004). *NIOSH alert: Preventing occupational exposures to antineoplastic and other hazardous drugs in health care settings* (DHHS/NIOSH publication 2004–2165). Atlanta, GA: Author.

Eaton, T. (2005). Microbial risk assessment for aseptically prepared products. *American Pharmaceutical Review, 8*(5), 46–51.

Guideline for hand hygiene in health care settings. (2002). *MMWR, 51*(RR-16). Retrieved from http://www.c.c.gov/handhygiene

Power, L., & Jorgenson, J. (2006). *Safe handling of hazardous drugs*. Bethesda, MD: American Society of Health-System Pharmacists.

Trissel, L.A. (2005). *Handbook on injectable drugs* (13th ed.). Bethesda, MD: American Society of Health-System Pharmacists.

CHAPTER

18

dministration of Medications

npetencies

n completion of this chapter, the reader should be able to:

- Specify the drug information that should be reviewed by the health care practitioner prior to administering a drug to a patient.
- Describe the clinical and technical concerns required for administering medications by the following routes: oral, topical, rectal, vaginal, intraocular, intranasal, and into the ear.
- dentify five methods by which the person administering medications can reduce medication errors.
- Discuss the characteristics and professional concerns of a drug administrator or drug technician.
- Differentiate the directions that should be given to a patient receiving a buccal tablet and a gelatin capsule.
- Differentiate between labeling requirements for internal and external drug preparations.
- List five situations in which a drug is discontinued or drug administration is interrupted.
- Describe the procedure to be followed if a patient states, "I cannot swallow that large tablet."
- Discuss some causes of medication errors. Explain the universal policy to be observed if a medication error is detected.
- List the requirements for each health care practitioner who accepts the responsibility for the administration of medications.

Terms

dosage schedule
hypoglycemic
hospital-acquired infection
medication administrator
PRN (*pro re nata*) order
STAT order
systemic action
verbal order

Introduction

This chapter focuses on the clinical, professional, and technical aspects of medication administration. Although policies and procedures vary from institution to institution (and the institution's policy takes precedence over what is written here), the person who administers medications must always respect the dignity, privacy, safety, and autonomy of the patient. Patient cooperation is essential to the administration of most forms of medications. Even those patients who appear comatose, confused, or otherwise compromised should have the proposed procedure explained to them. Each health care practitioner who accepts the responsibility for the administration of medications must become familiar with the patient population, the institution's policies concerning medications, the approved methods of medication administration, the formulary and other resources that are available for reference and information, and the institution's expectations of the person who administers medications. All are very serious responsibilities.

Medication Orders

Drug administration is initiated with the physician's (prescriber's) *medication order*. No drug is given to a patient without physician authorization. Numerous kinds of medication orders exist. Orders written in the chart at the time of admission, which may be subsequently increased, decreased, or deleted, are the most common type of medication orders. Another type of drug order is a **verbal order**, which may be given by the physician to a nurse or pharmacist, usually via the phone, when an emergency or unusual circumstance arises. Prior to initiation, verbal orders should be repeated to the prescriber. Verbal orders are always transcribed in the patient's chart, signed by the order taker, and cosigned by the physician on the next visit to the hospital. Verbal orders should be cosigned by the physician within 24 hours or as specified by hospital policy. Medication orders are also written upon transfer and discharge of patients and upon changes in the patient's condition or required medical therapy.

verbal order
an order for a drug or other treatment that is given verbally to an authorized receiver by an authorized prescriber

Orders for drugs that should be administered immediately are called **STAT orders**. The immediacy relates to the patient's condition, such as the need for pain relief, when the patient is experiencing clinical distress, or when the patient has a drug or allergic reaction. The person administering drugs always gives top priority to making sure the patient receives a STAT drug in timely fashion. Orders written by the physician that are to be given to the patient only if required by the patient's condition are **PRN (*pro re nata*) orders**. One-time orders are written for specific circumstances, such as patient sedation for a test or procedure. Standing orders sometimes accompany a patient on admission to the hospital, or may be the printed drug regimens prescribed by the physician or a physician group to treat particular conditions (e.g., women who are admitted to the obstetrical unit preceding childbirth). These orders may be prewritten and signed by the physician or stamped on the chart with the physician's signature. Medication orders may also be included in physician-, unit-, or patient-specific protocols, pathways, and standards of care.

STAT order
statim; order for drugs to be given immediately

PRN (*pro re nata*) order order for drugs to be given as needed when a clinical situation arises

Institutional policy may permit drug orders to be written by persons other than physicians, including doctors of osteopathic medicine, physician's assistants, clinical nurse practitioners, dentists, podiatrists, and, in some states, pharmacists. These policies must be known and observed.

Information Needed on Drug Orders

To properly administer a drug, the following information is needed for each drug order:

- Patient's full name.
- Room number, bed number, and other identifiers required by hospital policy (e.g., medical record numbers, ID bar codes).
- Name of drug (clearly written). Several medications that need to be written in full with no abbreviations include morphine, morphine sulfate, magnesium sulfate.
- Dosage strength (e.g., 10 mg). Some abbreviations and conventions are no longer acceptable:
  - Do not use a trailing zero after a whole number. For example, "2.0 mg" is not acceptable; use "2 mg" instead.
  - Do not use a decimal point without a leading zero. For example, ".2 mg" is not acceptable; use "0.2 mg" instead.
  - Do not use apothecary symbols. For example, do not use drams and grains; use metric system abbreviations instead (mg, g, etc.).
  - Do not use "µg"; use "micrograms" or "mcg" instead.
  - Do not use U or IU; use "units" or "International Units," respectively, instead.
  - Do not use BIW and TIW; instead, write out "twice a week" or "three times a week," respectively, and state the days.
  - Do not use OD, Q.D., q.d.; instead, write out "once daily" and the time of day when the drug should be given would help as well.
  - Do not use QOD, Q.O.D., q.o.d., qod; instead, write "out every other day." (See Chapter 30.)
- Dosage schedule (e.g., STAT, tid).
- Route of administration (e.g., sublingual, subcutaneous, instill in left eye).
- Length of time drug is to be given (e.g., for 24 hours, 1 week, length of hospital stay, as needed).
- Prescriber's signature. Must be legible. Date and timed order is required.

For additional information related to the use of abbreviations, please refer to the Chapter 30 on preventing and managing medication errors.

The drug order is entered into the patient's medication order forms, which is done by hand or as part of a computerized physician order entry (CPOE) system. The order is then transmitted to the pharmacy to be filled. Illegibility of handwritten physician orders has been identified as a key contributor to medication errors, which is leading to the development and implementation of CPOE systems. The person who administers the drug verifies the label on the drug by comparing it with the order on the patient's medication record.

Computerized medication systems are being used more to provide additional levels of automated checking—from the time of drug order, to delivery to the patient, to the drug being administered. One rule of thumb is to never administer a medication without checking it three times against the order or medication administration record (MAR). Leave all medications fully labeled in their unit-dose packages until they are at the bedside. The last check just prior to administration is the most important, because it is the last chance to pick up an error.

The Medication Administrator

medication administrator a person who administers or gives medications to patients

The **medication administrator** (nurse or other authorized health care practitioner) should appreciate the responsibility inherent in her or his role. This person should be knowledgeable about the responsibilities of the other members of the health team regarding drug administration and communicate effectively with them. The medication administrator should always give priority to patient care, treating each patient with dignity and professional concern regardless of physical or mental impairment, lifestyle orientation, religious beliefs, or cultural background.

The medication administrator must be totally familiar with the policies and procedures that prevail in a particular hospital and always know the physician, nurse, or pharmacist to whom he or she directly reports. Any unusual physical or emotional change noted by the medication administrator during medication rounds should be immediately reported to the charge nurse. Professional confidentiality regarding any patient is of prime importance. Patients have, at all times, a right to have personal matters respected and held in confidence. Pharmacy technicians should report to work dressed in appropriate hospital attire, with a name identification badge, in keeping with the dignity of the position and the respect they should expect from others.

hospital-acquired infection an infection or illness that occurs as a result of a patient's stay in a hospital or health facility

The individual administering medications should be in good health, free of communicable infections (e.g., a head cold, a sore throat, an open lesion). This is of importance for both the patient and the drug administrator. Patients are susceptible to **hospital-acquired infections** (infections incurred in the hospital). Often the patient is weak, has had surgery or radiation therapy, and the immune system may be compromised for these or other reasons (e.g., aging process, malnutrition). The drug administrator who is at a low physical ebb due to exhaustion or poor health is more likely to make a drug administration error than a person who is well, alert, and fully attentive. In addition, a drug administrator (e.g., nurse) who is in poor health is more apt to pick up an infection from a patient.

Any person who gives direct patient care must ensure and maintain good health through proper nutrition, exercise, and healthy living habits. In the case of an upper respiratory infection or other indisposition, the drug administrator should inform the supervisor for a change of assignment away from direct patient care for the duration of the illness. Personal protective devices to ensure standard precautions are in place for bloodborne disease transmission must be used during medication delivery as required. If the patient is in isolation due to an infectious, transmittable disease, the drug administrator should follow hospital policy regarding protection.

In all events, persons who are about to administer drugs should thoroughly wash their hands before handling any drugs and rewash their hands between patients when hospital policy or aseptic technique requires it. Hand hygiene is the single most effective infection control measure.

Administration of the Drug

Prior to drug administration, the medication administrator should become familiar with the following information regarding the drug:

- General and special uses or indications
- Usual dose or dosage range
- Special precautions (e.g., do not give with food, observe patient for rash)

- Side effects that may occur
- Foods or other drugs that should not be given with the drug
- Time when onset of action is expected.

By reviewing this information before administering the drug, mistakes and errors can be avoided and the patient's well-being better ensured. Hospital policy will indicate how involved the medication administrator becomes in providing this information to the patient. Generally, the registered nurse or the pharmacist has the responsibility to answer drug information questions and to counsel the patient on proper drug use.

Patient Rights

Nearly every patient in the hospital will receive drugs during their stay. Each patient is entitled to the "five rights" of safe, appropriate drug administration. Drug rights of the patient include the right drug, right dose, right route (or right dosage form), right time, and right patient. These rights should be memorized and checked prior to each drug administration.

The Right Drug

The right drug is verified by checking the physician's (prescriber's) order sheet and the nurse's (or pharmacist's) drug administration form, drug Kardex, or drug summary on the patient's computer profile. Thousands of drugs are available and many sound alike, are spelled alike, and look alike. The use of abbreviations for drug names has become a risky practice, and many hospitals are limiting or eliminating the use of medication abbreviations entirely as a risk reduction strategy. One or two letters in a name can mean an entirely different drug (e.g., Zantac or Zyrtec, Lasix or Luvox). Capital letters (called *tall man lettering*) are now used to differentiate between look-alike and sound-alike drugs (e.g., vinCRISTINE, vinBLASTINE). The prescriber must be contacted if there are any questions or doubts concerning the order. Most drugs used in hospitals today are in unit-dose packages. The name is clearly visible on each drug dosage form.

Labels should be checked *three times* before the drug is administered. The expiration date should also be checked. The Institute for Safe Medication Practices (ISMP) has identified top high-risk drugs. These are medications that have been involved frequently in serious errors. Examples include insulin and chemotherapy drugs. It is important to follow the hospital's special safety precautions when administering these high-alert drugs.

The Right Dose

Accurate dosage strength is critical to beneficial drug administration. Giving the wrong strength, particularly to children or infants, can be and has been fatal. The right dose is further checked with special care given to decimal points. A zero before the decimal, called a *leading decimal* (e.g., 0.1 mg), should be noted. Care should be taken if there is a zero after the decimal, called a *trailing zero*, which can be misleading and can be misread, leading to a 10 times greater dosage error (e.g., 1.0 is one, not ten). Orders for units must always be written out. The abbreviation U for units can be misread as a 0 and lead to a 10 times greater dosage error.

Proper dosage strength should never be presumed by anyone in the prescribing, dispensing, or administering process. Physicians must clearly indicate the desired strength on the medication order, pharmacists are expected to further verify the dosage to be sure it is within appropriate therapeutic limits, and nurses are expected to further check that the dosage strength ordered by the physician was accurately dispensed by the pharmacist. After the drug and dosage strength has gone through these three checkpoints, the last checkpoint resides with the person who administers the drug to the patient. If any dosage changes have been made along the way, the change should be clearly indicated on the patient's chart and other medication records. Children, the elderly, and patients with impaired liver and kidney function are at the greatest risk of adverse drug events related to medication dosage.

The Right Route/Dosage Form

In addition to ensuring that the right drug in the right strength has been selected, it is important to check and be sure that the drug is given by the right route in the right dosage form. Drugs come in many different dosage forms. Liquids come as solutions, tinctures, suspensions, syrups, and elixirs. Oral solid dosage forms come as tablets, gelatin capsules, caplets, enteric-coated tablets, extended-release capsules, sublingual tablets, and buccal tablets. External preparations include creams, ointments, and lotions. Some medications in ointment form contain potent active ingredients. The length of the ointment strip must be carefully measured by the drug administrator. Injectable medications must be carefully checked to determine whether the injection should be administered by an intramuscular route, intravenous route, subcutaneous route, or other route of administration. Drop-type drugs must be checked and used only as indicated for the eye, ear, or nose. There are many suppository dosage forms, such as rectal, vaginal, and urethral.

Dosage forms are *not* interchangeable, so it is important that the right drug is administered in the right dosage form. It is also important to note when a drug dosage form has been changed by the prescriber (e.g., an injectable drug [IM] is changed to an oral dosage [PO]). Every drug order should include the route of administration. If a question arises, the proper dosage form should be confirmed before the drug is administered.

The Right Time

dosage schedule the frequency, interval, and length of time a medicine is to be given

hypoglycemic a drug that lowers the level of glucose in the blood; used primarily by people with diabetes

Time of drug administration (i.e., **dosage schedule** or frequency) is an important factor in pharmacotherapy. Drugs should be given at the time ordered, allowing for an ordinary deviation of a half hour, unless timing is critical. Patients with diabetes may receive their **hypoglycemic** drugs a half hour before meals, unless otherwise specified. Patients on therapeutic drug monitoring are involved in pharmacokinetic laboratory studies. Dosage time is related to drug half-life and the time the phlebotomist will draw blood for the serum analysis. Time of drug administration can be a critical factor in pharmacokinetic laboratory results. Time of drug administration can also be of great concern to the patient who is waiting. A patient who has been ordered an analgesic for pain relief to be given every 4 hours for the first 24 hours after an operation should receive this drug on time. Delays for this patient increase the pain and anxiety and slow the recovery process.

Many drugs are now administered "per parameters." An example is a cardiac medication that is administered if the heart rate and blood pressure are within a certain range and held if outside the range. Knowledge of when the physician wants the medication administered, any hospital-, unit-, or physician-specific applicable per-parameters policy, and the actual monitoring required prior to administration are required. It is less confusing for the patient if, when possible, drug administration times in the hospital are kept close to when the patient would normally take them at home, being considerate of the patient's individual waking and sleeping times. This also facilitates an accurate assessment of therapeutic effects.

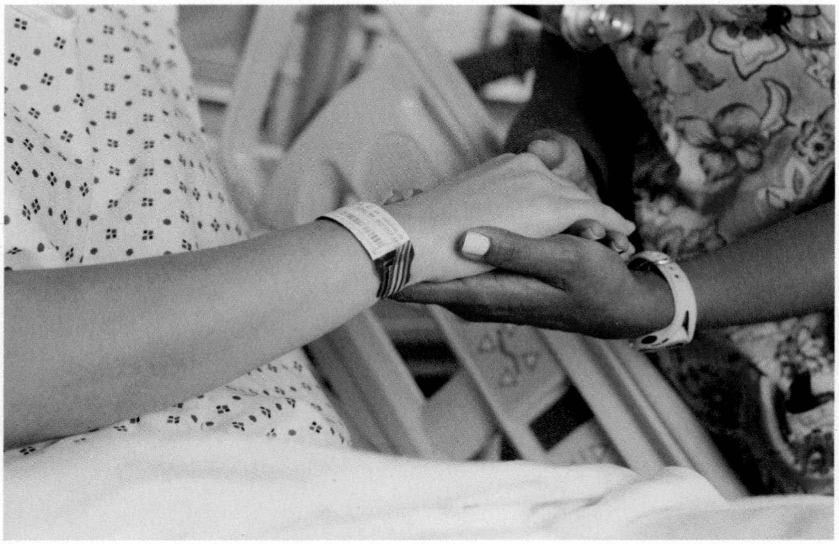

FIGURE 18-1 It is critical to be certain that medications are being delivered to the correct patient. The medication administrator must always verify the patient's identity.

The Right Patient

The last requirement is to verify that the right patient is the one to receive the drug. The patient should be asked, "Please tell me your name and date of birth"; this is checked against the patient's identification band (**Figure 18-1**). Just addressing the person by name is not sufficient. People may respond positively even if they have not clearly heard their name, due to distractions, deafness, or language barriers. Beds are often shifted to different positions in the room, so identifying a person as the patient in room 120, bed 3, is insufficient and may be misleading. Hospitals are implementing computerized medication systems that utilize bar coding or other methods of patient verification; this information can then be compared to the actual medication order or medication profile.

Oral Drug Administration

After the patient has been properly identified, the patient is either given the medication to swallow, to place under the tongue (sublingual tablets), or to place between the cheek and the gum (buccal tablets). If the patient is to self-administer an oral tablet, the nurse or medication administrator should remain with the patient until the drug has been swallowed. Drugs are never left at the patient's bedside without a physician's order. Drugs left at the bedside may be forgotten, discarded, or hoarded for future use. The patient should be instructed to place a sublingual tablet under the tongue and leave it there until it dissolves (**Figure 18-2**). A patient ordered a buccal tablet should be told to place the tablet between the gum and the cheek and allow it to dissolve (**Figure 18-3**). Throat and mouth troches or lozenges should not be swallowed or chewed but allowed to remain in the oral cavity until dissolved. In the case of a medicated mouthwash used for oral and throat infections, the patient should be told to swish the liquid around in the mouth and then either swallow or expectorate (spit out) according to the nature of the substance and the dosage directions.

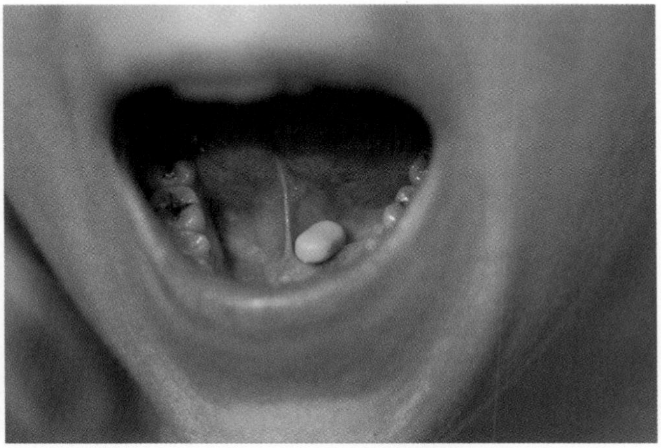

FIGURE 18-2 A sublingual tablet is placed under the patient's tongue to dissolve.

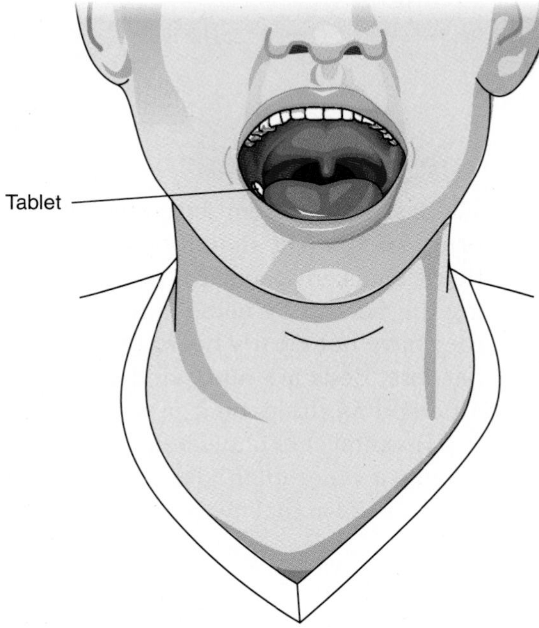

FIGURE 18-3 A buccal tablet is placed between the patient's cheek and gums to dissolve.

If a medication is to be swallowed, the patient usually should be given an adequate amount of water (at least 4 ounces or a full 8-ounce glass of water if possible) to allow for easy swallowing, dissolution of the tablet or capsule, and prevention of esophageal erosion. Esophageal erosion can occur when an oral medication lodges and remains in the esophagus and does not move into the stomach. Particular care must be given to tablets with a corrosive potential, such as a compressed potassium chloride tablet.

The exceptions to the rule for administering sufficient water with an oral dosage form are in the cases of cough syrups intended to soothe and work in the throat area, medicated mouthwashes intended to be swallowed or expectorated, and after administering either a buccal or sublingual tablet. There are times when a liquid other than water may be indicated. If there is no contraindication, the patient may prefer to follow the drug with a drink of milk or fruit juice. However, some drugs have definite contraindications. The person administering the drug should know which liquids should not be administered with particular medications (e.g., fruit juices and sodas, such as cola beverages, should never be given with penicillin tablets; milk or milk products should not be given with certain categories of antibiotics or certain laxatives, such as Dulcolax™).

Before leaving the patient, the person administering the drug should make sure the patient has taken the drug and has had no difficulty in swallowing the medication or following other instructions. If the patient asks questions about the drugs, an adequate answer should be given. If the person administering the drug is limited either on time or knowledge when the question is asked, a follow-up visit should be made. Such answers as "that is what the physician ordered" or "this is given to you to make you feel better" are not adequate. This is in fact dismissing the patient's questions and need for information. The patient is entitled to information regarding the drugs he or she is ordered. In most cases the medication administrator will refer these questions to the physician, nurse, or pharmacist responsible for the care of the patient, who will further discuss the question.

Medication administration must be documented immediately *after* the drug is taken. Documentation should never be done prior to administration, because the person administering the drug could be called away from the bedside unexpectedly.

Topical Drug Administration

A topical drug is one applied to the skin or mucous membranes. Topical medications are intended to either produce local effects or provide a sustained release (e.g., transdermal patches). The person applying an ointment should wear disposable gloves and explain the procedure to the patient. The area should be cleaned and any ointment remaining from a previous administration removed. Ointments should be applied in thin layers using cotton swabs or a tongue depressor.

Liquid medications, such as lotions and suspensions, should first be shaken well and then applied as directed with quick sprays. Both the patient and the drug administrator should be careful not to inhale the aerosol spray. In some cases, directions may require that the area be covered with sterile gauze after application. Special care should be given to patients with burn injuries because they are most susceptible to infections. Generally, absorption of topically applied medications is less predictable than other routes of administration.

Eyedrop and Eye Ointment Application

Always aseptically clean hands by scrubbing well or wearing disposable gloves before instilling eyedrops. To preserve the cleanliness of the delivery orifice, do not touch the tip of the dropper or container to the patient's eye or an external surface. Position the patient with his or her head tilted back. The lower eyelid can be gently pulled forward to create a well into which the drop or drops can be inserted (**Figure 18-4**). Be careful not to touch the eye or conjunctival sac with the medication dispenser.

Accurately apply the drop or number of drops as directed. Many eyedrops have systemic effects; therefore, additional drops should not be given. Before the drops are administered, check the label for the drug name, strength, and directions for use, including which eye (or, if directed, both eyes) should be treated. Check labels for an expiration date. Never use any expired drug. If an ointment is

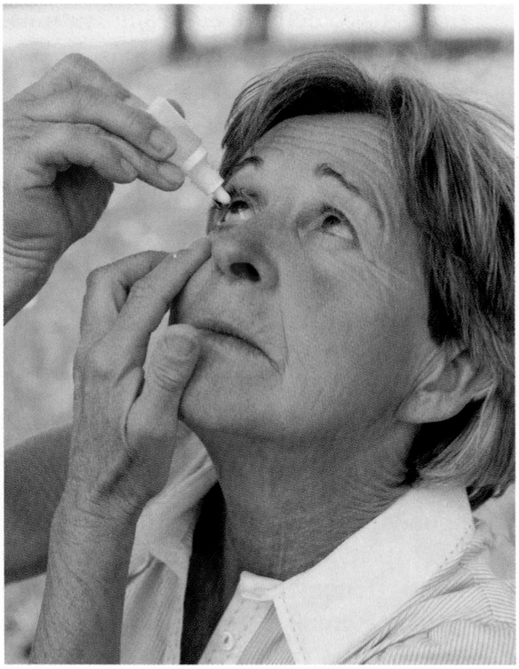

FIGURE 18-4 Make sure you are using proper technique when instilling eyedrops to avoid causing infection or damage to the eye.

used, discard the first bead (because it is considered contaminated), instruct the patient to look up, and then apply a thin line of ointment to the slightly retracted lower eyelid without allowing the tip of the tube to touch the eye.

After instillation of either eyedrops or ointment, instruct the patient to close the eye for a few minutes to permit the dispersal of the drug through the eye. If a tear appears, wipe it away with sterile gauze. If there is any noticeable change in the eye (e.g., increased redness, discharge, signs of irritation), report it right away to the supervising nurse or pharmacist.

Administration of Ear and Nose Preparations

To instill eardrops, the patient should be sitting with the unaffected ear resting on the shoulder or lying down with the affected ear facing up. It will be more comfortable for the patient if the solution to be instilled is warmed slightly with your hand or by placing the solution under warm water for a few minutes prior to instillation. For an adult or a child older than age 3, the ear should be gently pulled up and back (**Figure 18-5**). For a child younger than age 3, the ear should be gently pulled down and back to make the ear canal more accessible.

Drops are inserted directly into the canal without touching the tip of the dropper or nozzle to the ear. The patient should remain positioned for a few minutes to keep the drops from running out of the ear. If a cotton plug is ordered, it should be sterile and gently placed just at the opening of the canal. Administer only the prescribed number of drops after carefully reading the label.

Nose drops should be applied with the patient's head resting on the back of the neck. The patient should be instructed to breathe through the mouth. Instill the required number of drops, and instruct the patient to keep the head back for a few minutes and not to blow the nose for a few minutes. Nose sprays are used

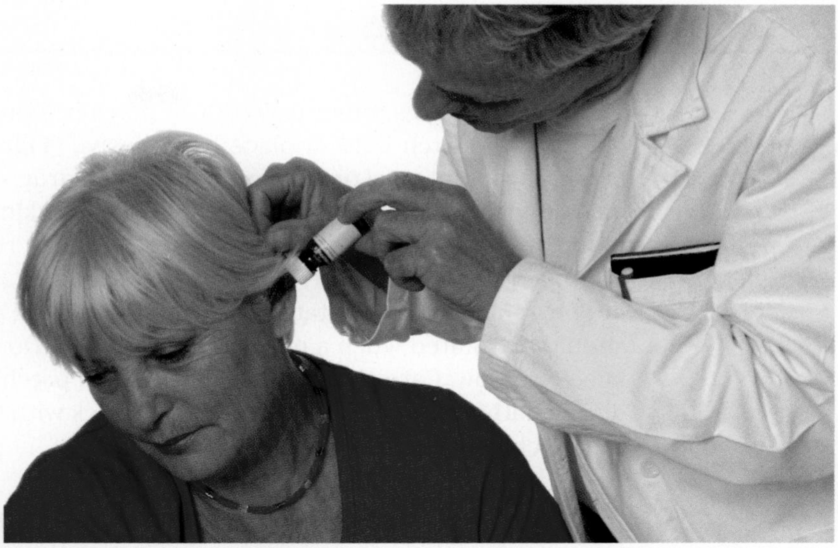

FIGURE 18-5 Instillation of eardrops requires proper positioning of the patient. The ear should be pulled up and back for adults for proper medication administration.

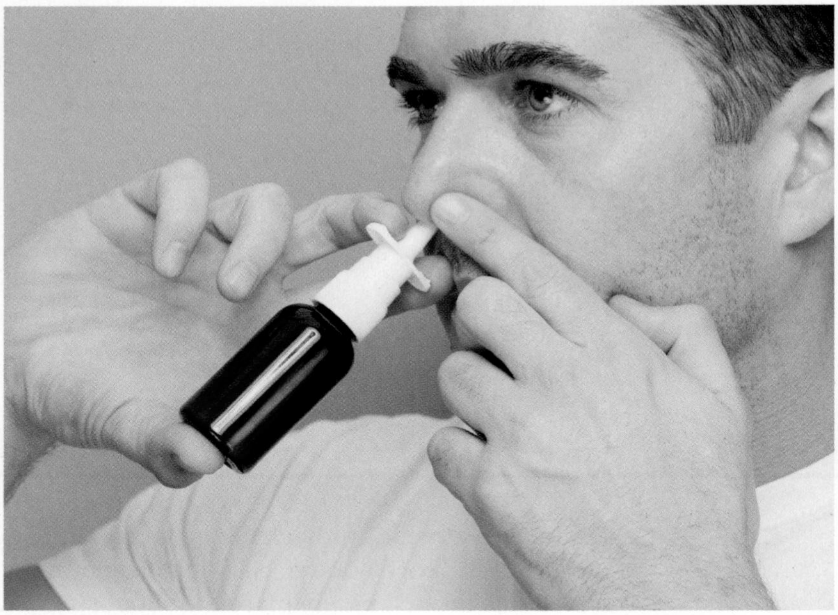

FIGURE 18-6 Nasal sprays can be self-administered by placing the applicator in the tip of the nostril and giving it a quick squeeze.

with the patient's head in an upright position. The spray is applied by squeezing the applicator bottle quickly and firmly while it is placed in the tip of the nostril (**Figure 18-6**). Repeat the process with the other nostril. Use only as directed, because active ingredients in the spray enter directly into the circulatory system and may have untoward systemic effects. Other drugs in nebulizer form come with specific instructions in the package insert. These should be carefully followed to properly administer the drugs.

Application of Transdermal Drugs

systemic action affects the body as a whole

Transdermal drugs, often called drug patches, consist of an active drug ingredient inside a patch held in place by adhesive (**Figure 18-7**). The drug is applied externally for internal or **systemic action**. A drug such as nitroglycerin (for chest pain) is placed in a transdermal patch on the skin where it is picked up by the bloodstream for action over a sustained period of time. The area where the patch is applied should be clearly dry and free of hair (e.g., upper arm). The patch should not be applied to any irritated, callused, or scarred area. The location of the patch should be rotated when a new patch is applied. Do not place the patch below the knee or elbow. Care should be taken that the patch does not come off at night or during bathing. If the patch does fall off, check with the supervisor. The location of the patch needs to be documented.

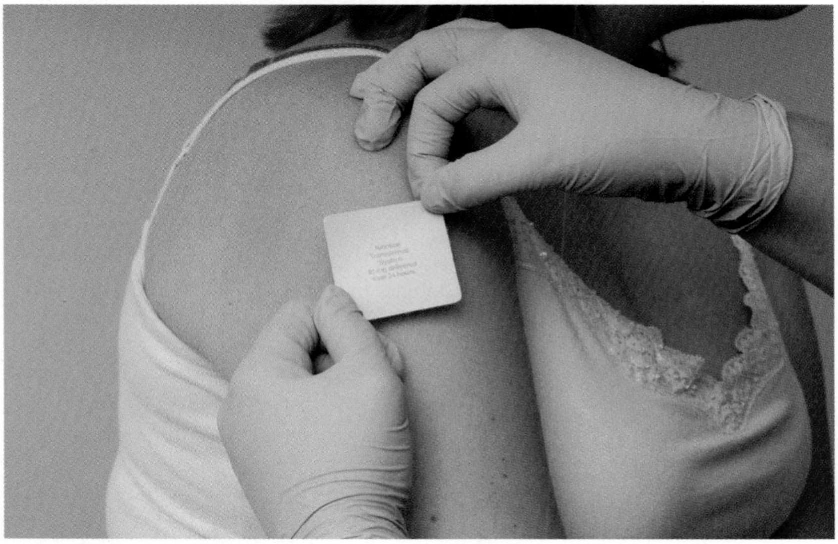

FIGURE 18-7 Transdermal patch.

Insertion of Suppositories

Prepare a treatment by checking the label on the box. Make sure the suppository feels firm. The cocoa-butter base may begin to soften or melt at warm temperatures. If this occurs, briefly place the suppository, with foil wrapper intact, in cold water to increase firmness. Have a tube of lubricating ointment available, and use a pair of disposable gloves. Inform the patient concerning the drug administration procedure, and position the patient as instructed. Drape the patient and provide for privacy. For rectal insertion, the patient should be on one side (generally the left side unless contraindicated) with one leg extended and other leg flexed at the knee. Don gloves, unwrap the suppository and lubricate the rounded end (or follow more specific manufacturer's instructions), and lubricate your gloved index finger. Instruct the patient to take slow, deep breaths to aid relaxation. Insert the suppository into the rectum beyond the anal sphincter (approximately the length of your index finger for an adult, less for a child), and encourage the patient to retain it for at least 30 to 40 minutes. For vaginal insertion, encourage the patient to void, then position her on her back with knees flexed and legs spread apart. The drug administrator should put on gloves and remove the suppository foil wrapper. Rectal ointment and vaginal suppositories and ointments are inserted using an applicator that accompanies the suppository or cream. Further directions for use are found in the package insert.

Injectable Drug Administration

Many techniques and various routes exist for the use of injectable medications. Injectable drugs can be given directly into a blood vessel (intravascular), into a vein (intravenous), into an artery (intra-arterial), into select muscles (intramuscular), under the skin (hypodermic or subcutaneous), or into the skin (intradermal) by medication administrators, and into the spinal cord (intrathecal) or the heart (intrapericardiac) by practitioners specially trained in these techniques.

Many of these injection techniques require special manipulative skill. They are considered invasive procedures, frequently using very potent drugs. Information and competency development are beyond the scope of this book.

Discontinuance of Drug Administration

Persons involved in drug administration need to be very alert to the times when drug discontinuance, interruption of dosage schedules, or modification of scheduled dosage patterns are prescribed or indicated.

Drug administration should be withheld if the patient gives evidence of experiencing an adverse drug reaction (e.g., hives; a rash occurring on the body, face, neck, arms, or legs; difficulty in breathing; double vision or seeing various colors that are not objectively present). If the drug administrator observes any of these conditions or the patient speaks about them, the supervising nurse should be contacted before the next dose is given. In other clinical situations, hospital policy or physician orders may direct stoppage of a drug due to certain indicators (i.e., drugs given "per parameters"). For example, do not give digoxin if the apical pulse rate falls below 60 beats per minute.

Surgeons and anesthesiologists usually give specific orders for medication immediately before and after surgery. Many times, physicians or hospital policy will instruct that all or certain drugs be given with a sip of water prior to surgery even if the patient is NPO ("nothing by mouth"). An example would be to continue blood pressure medication even though the patient is NPO for surgery to ensure the blood pressure remains within normal limits pre- and intraoperatively. Some physicians or hospital policies may discontinue all standing medication orders prior to the patient going to surgery. At that time, drugs needed prior to, during, and immediately after surgery are reordered. All health professionals involved in medication dispensing and administration must carefully scrutinize the preoperative and postoperative drug orders for the surgical patient. Mistakes in this area could jeopardize the surgical outcome.

The patient may be scheduled for physical therapy, x-rays, or other activities that take the patient off the floor during the scheduled times of medication administrations. If this occurs, the supervising nurse should be contacted as to the appropriate action to take regarding giving the medication when the patient returns.

Other interruptions of drug administration can occur when the patient's orders read "nothing by mouth," and the patient is on oral drug therapy. In some situations, for various reasons, the patient may refuse to take the drug. In each case, the supervising nurse, the pharmacist, or the prescribing physician must be contacted to clarify the appropriate action to be taken regarding drug administration.

If a patient is in a program for therapeutic drug monitoring, the drug dosage schedule or laboratory phlebotomy schedule may have to be modified according to the half-life of the drug to obtain the accurate drug blood serum levels that are required for optimum drug therapy dosing. These patients may require an individualized drug dosage administration schedule to be planned by the physician, pharmacist, and medical technologist. Information regarding interrupted drug administration, refusal of the patient to take a drug, and modified drug schedules should always be charted in the medication records and reported to the supervising nurse.

Unit-Dose Drug Administration

A unit-dose drug comes individually packaged and labeled and requires no further packaging or labeling. This system cuts down on the problem of medication errors and preserves the integrity and safety of the product. In a unit-dose drug delivery system, a pharmacist checks every drug order prior to the administration of the drug. The unit-dose system provides each patient with a storage bin, usually in a medication cart, in which no more than a 24-hour supply of drugs is available for the individual patient. The package is opened at the patient's bedside, and the name, label, strength, and patient are checked against the medication administration record. Currently, unit doses frequently include drug-specific bar codes to facilitate automation of the medication system.

Crushing Medications

Crushing medications to assist patients who have difficulty swallowing pills or capsules is recommended only after serious consideration and consultation between the physician and the pharmacist. Medications are designed in tablet or capsule form to ensure their absorption in the correct area of the gastrointestinal tract and to eliminate or minimize digestive problems. Crushing may seriously interfere with these safety measures. Crushing cannot be used for enteric-coated or sustained-action medications (e.g., Pronestyl-SR). Notify the pharmacy about the need to crush specific medications, and follow the pharmacist's advice regarding the safety of this action. The ISMP publishes a list of drugs that should not be crushed.

If crushing is necessary and approved by institutional policy, each medication must be crushed individually, mixed with a palatable food (e.g., applesauce, Jell-O), and given to the patient separately. Attempt to give the patient as much of the drug in the first spoonful so that very little is wasted if the patient refuses the remainder. Never mix all of the patient's medications in one cup.

Internal and External Medications

Any caregiver who has been in practice for an extended period of time can cite examples of inaccuracies that they read about, heard about, or were involved in. One that comes to mind is that of an elderly monk admitted to the hospital for a severe scalp burn. Someone attempting to dry a wet lesion dropped a sunlamp on his head. The burn became infected, and he was admitted to the hospital. His first morning in the hospital, his caregiver poured out and left at the bedside 2 ounces of mouthwash in a small waxed paper cup, the same cup as the one the patient had received a liquid medication in the previous evening. When the caregiver returned to assist him with oral hygiene, she asked what happened to the mouthwash. She got the simple answer, "I swallowed it." The aide reported the incident; the patient was carefully monitored, and outside of excessive urination, was fortunately discharged with no other apparent side effects. This story illustrates the fact that one cannot be too careful in providing medications for hospitalized people.

Internal medications (to be swallowed, ingested, or injected) and external medications (to be applied to the outside of the body or an adjoining orifice) should always be stored separately. These drugs are labeled differently. External preparations require a red external use label. Black or another color is used for internal medications. Drugs labeled for topical use are also external preparations and usually carry a red-lettered label.

Ancillary directions (e.g., "Shake well before using," "Refrigerate," "Do not refrigerate," "For external use only") should be carefully read and followed.

Medication Teaching

Patients and families knowledgeable about their drug regimens can be important links in ensuring safe medication administration, understanding the individual therapeutic medication effect, attaining the intended medication effect, and limiting untoward effects. As part of the medication team, the pharmacist or medication administrator should consistently involve the patient and family in the medication process and provide them as much information as appropriate. Active participation and an individualized approach based on patient needs are the standard (**Figure 18-8**). Remember that patients will be administering their own medications upon discharge. Listen carefully to patients and families during medication administration. If they question a medication or a dose, double-check it with a

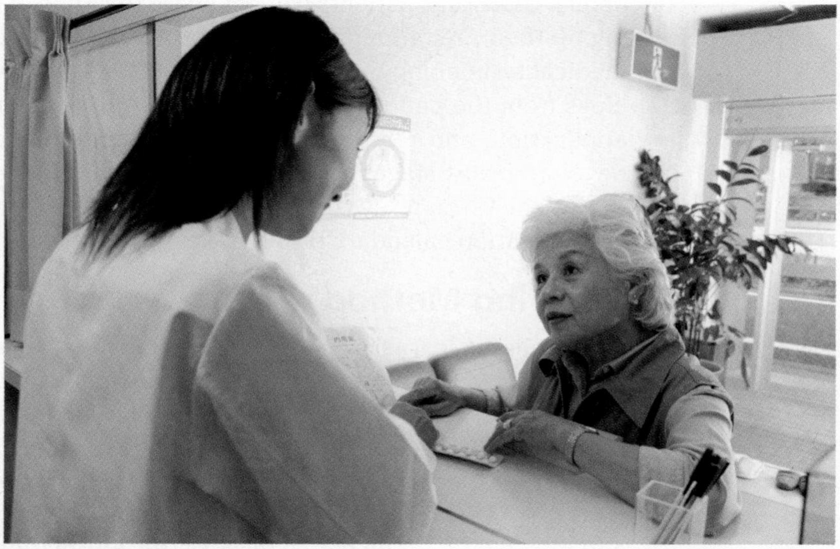

FIGURE 18-8 It is vital that pharmacists and other members of the medical team communicate and educate patients about their medications, effects, and proper administration.

supervisor. Many errors have been prevented by an astute patient or family member, and anyone has the potential to make a mistake.

The provision of medication information to patients and their families takes some preparation and planning. The patient's physician, pharmacist, and nurse are responsible for establishing the teaching need and priorities, developing the teaching plan, and evaluating learning outcomes. The medication administrator's role is to participate in this process as requested and as appropriate. As the medication administrator, he or she will learn helpful information that will be important to communicate to the patient care team. This individual will also have a unique opportunity to participate in the teaching process. Information on the patient's readiness to learn, education level, best learning method (e.g., verbal, written, demonstration), and time available for teaching (i.e., expected discharge date) is needed to prepare to teach. It is always best to start with finding out what the patient knows and what the patient would like to know about the medications. Many excellent sources of medication teaching materials are available, and every hospital has access to many resources.

Readiness to Learn

With today's shorter lengths of stay, the best time for patient teaching may be a narrow window. Signs of readiness to learn include stable physical condition, pain control, patient alertness, the ability to concentrate for at least short periods of time, and patient interest in learning about medication. When the time frame available for teaching is particularly short, the teaching plan may include instruction done by others along the patient's "continuum of care," including long-term care facility staff, a home care or visiting nurse, the outpatient pharmacy, and family.

Age and Education Level

Age, developmental level, and educational level must all be considered as a teaching plan is formulated by the nurse or pharmacist. Age and years of schooling alone may not be the only guides to how to deliver information, but they do provide a starting point. When the patient's education has been of a basic level, it is best to address the teaching at an eighth-grade level. In many parts of the country, significant numbers of patients cannot read at all or have a very limited reading ability. Generally, patients will not share this type of information and do well covering up their limitations. It is a good rule of thumb to avoid the use of scientific or medical terminology, and to give examples to support and reinforce learning. Take clues from the patient; this is ultimately the best guide on patient understanding, application, and retention. Examples of different teaching approaches based on developmental stages are asking adolescents if they want their parents present during the teaching session and providing elderly patients with memory aids such as medication calendars or pill boxes.

Learning Method

How a person learns is a complex and individual process, but learning is facilitated when a number of methods and senses are involved. A good plan includes the methods of instruction. These may include a combination of the following: written materials, verbal instruction, demonstration, providing examples, video- or audiotapes, and a question-and-answer session. Information is best absorbed when given over a period of time (e.g., give written material to the patient to read in the morning, and return later in the day to discuss the information and answer questions). Many patients now have access to the Internet at home, and they can be given hospital or general website addresses that include patient educational materials on medication. Clear discharge instructions, medication information leaflets, and providing a number for the patient to call with questions after discharge are all standard ways to reinforce valuable information given to the patient under the stressful circumstances of illness, hospital discharge, or transfer to another facility.

Teaching Plan

The patient's nurse and/or pharmacist in collaboration with the physician will develop the teaching plan. Formation of a teaching plan focuses on the needs of the patient and the information to be taught. The plan will include learning objectives stated as outcome objectives (i.e., what the patient will learn by the completion of instruction). Objectives should be practical, achievable, and measurable. Include the patient's objectives in the plan when possible. Examples of teaching and learning objectives are as follows:

- The patient will be able to list three signs of digitalis toxicity that require physician notification.
- The patient will describe rotation of sites for insulin injection.
- The patient's son will demonstrate correct insulin injection technique.

Objectives provide a basis for evaluating the effectiveness for teaching. The ultimate objective is that the patient has the information and skills necessary for safe medication administration.

Teaching Process

Try to select the most suitable and comfortable location to provide instruction. A comfortable location with limited distractions will allow the patient to concentrate on the information and ask questions. Prior to initiating teaching, the teaching plan and the objectives should be reviewed. It is then important to communicate what will be covered with the patient to the other team members and ensure it is documented. At least two methods of instruction are recommended to improve understanding and retention.

When possible, provide the patient with written material from a patient teaching text, from a computerized program, or from the instructor. When a preprinted text is used, it needs to be reviewed for content, education level, size of type, and so forth, prior to giving it to the patient. Teaching of complex information is generally done by the physician, nurse, or pharmacist, and should be given in more than one session. The definition of "complex" information will vary according to the patient, but any learning that requires cognitive and psychomotor capabilities is considered "complex." Examples of complex learning include self-injection, taking a radial pulse reading prior to cardiac medication, and taking a child's temperature. In each of these situations, the patient or family members need to have information on the reason for the procedure, how to perform the skill or procedure, and what action they are to take based on the results. When participating in teaching complex information, a second or third teaching session should be scheduled to provide the patient with an opportunity to absorb the information, formulate questions, and give a return demonstration as indicated.

Reinforcement

Provide patients with praise and encouragement during their learning process. Describe their progress in terms of readiness for discharge, self-independence, accomplishment of a skill, or being knowledgeable about their medication.

Evaluation of Learning

Since the ultimate goal of the teaching process is to effect learning and change behavior, the evaluation of learning is the final stage of the teaching/learning process. According to the nature of the information, an evaluation method may include requesting the patient to speak back the instructions or to give a return demonstration (e.g., taking a pulse).

Professional Responsibility for Drug Administration

Drug administration is the shared privilege and responsibility of different health disciplines, each one with carefully delineated functional activities. Medication administration is just one part of the medication process, which includes prescribing, dispensing, administering, monitoring, and systems and management control. Physician's delegates, such as physician's assistants and nurse practitioners, have the responsibility to prescribe rational and selective drug therapy that is dependent on the patient's medical profile and the drug's therapeutic characteristics.

Pharmacists are responsible for screening medication orders for rational drug therapy and appropriateness in particular, individualized cases. In some instances, the pharmacist is invited to participate in the multidisciplinary planning of a particular patient's drug regimen. The pharmacist evaluates the choice of a drug for a particular pathology, and if doubt arises, the physician is contacted. Further consideration is given to the drug dose, the time intervals between doses, and the patient's past drug history regarding allergies, drug sensitivities, and past untoward drug reactions. The pharmacist further considers the drug benefit/risk ratio regarding the possibility of a drug-drug interaction, a drug-food interaction, or a drug-laboratory test interaction. If there is apparent serious drug risk involvement, the pharmacist further consults with the physician regarding appropriate drug administration.

If the pharmacist evaluates the regimen to be within the bounds of sound therapy, the drug is dispensed, for an inpatient, through the nursing service in most situations. If the pharmacy completely controls the drug use process, a medication administrator (technician) may then assume the final responsibility for proper drug administration. However, in most institutions, the nursing department in collaboration with the pharmacy department is responsible for the final step in the drug use process (i.e., administration of the drug and observation of the patient regarding the therapeutic outcome of the drug action).

According to hospital policy, the task of actually giving the medication to a patient may be delegated to a trained medication technician. Yet the responsibility for the drug's outcome remains with the licensed health professionals involved. Basically, the right drug, for the right reason, must be given to the right patient at the right time in the right dosage strength and in the right drug dosage form. This is the core responsibility of the drug administration process. Responsibility for the outcome is shared by the professionals of medicine, nursing, and pharmacy.

Legal Responsibilities in Drug Administration

Many states and many health care institutions have very specific policies and procedures that must be carried out exactly as written. Currently, many states require a registered nurse to administer all medications. At the same time, other states and health institutions, due to fiscal, technical, personnel, and patient loads, are changing or modifying existing regulations. Basic requirements do not change, even if the assigned or designated personnel change.

Every hospital is required to have a policy and procedural manual to ensure patient safety and patient care. The persons involved in drug administration activities must know and observe these policies and procedures. When medication errors are made, they are usually related to the patient's five rights. To prove negligence, it must be established that drug administration policy was not followed, careless shortcuts were taken, or the medication order and administration procedure were not adequately checked by the responsible licensed professional.

For many years, health care has assumed a myth of infallibility. Errors have been underreported and covered up. Given the dramatic increase in prescription drug use, the toxicity of many medications, and the fact that health care professionals are human and do make mistakes, errors are a reality. The current thinking is that much will be gained in error reduction by refocusing from a culture of blame to one of systems improvement. The systems improvement approach recognizes that humans are more likely to err under certain conditions and environments and that those conditions can be modified to reduce error. By having more errors and near-misses reported, and by conducting studies to improve those environments, medication systems can be rewired for error prevention. Where do you fit in medication error prevention?

- Be aware of the risk and reality of medication errors. It is unrealistic to believe you will never be involved in an error.
- Report all errors and near-misses consistently based on your hospital's policies and procedures.
- Utilize medication resources, and attend in-service education programs. Recognize that it is no longer possible to be knowledgeable on every medication—there are just too many new drugs and too much new information constantly available.
- Know your patient's allergies.
- Be alert to high-risk medications, safe medication practices, and specific safety protocols.
- Recognize the role certain practices have in errors: illegible handwriting, trailing zeros, leading decimal points, abbreviations, use of the abbreviation U for units, and so forth.
- Practice meticulous medication administration practices, such as identification of every patient every time, stating the drug-dose-reason for every drug every time, and always listening to patients and families.
- Provide information to patients and families, and facilitate their active involvement in care.
- Participate in performance improvement activities, the implementation of computerized medication systems, and other medication safety improvements.

Refer to Chapter 30 on preventing and managing medication errors for a thorough discussion of this topic.

Adequate patient drug use control, drug use evaluation, and drug use surveillance must be top priorities to ensure patient safety. Detected errors must be reported immediately to the licensed supervisor. The goal of the performance improvement process is to identify individual and system problems that, if corrected, will help to avoid future errors.

Trends in Drug Administration

Drug administration methods are frequently called *drug delivery systems*. Drug firms have made large investments in researching and developing new methods to target drug administration dosage forms to maximize effectiveness and to limit unwanted systemic effects. The future may see pharmacy technicians specializing in the maintenance, utilization, and monitoring of these new and often unique devices and drug administration delivery systems.

If contemporary trends, particularly the working definition for pharmaceutical care, continue to prevail, pharmacy technicians of the future may require specific knowledge, judgment, techniques, and skills to participate in the health care team as competent pharmacy medication technicians. The current trend for hospitalized patients is to complete a drug reconciliation of their home medications and new hospital medications. Reconciliation may be necessary for surgical patients because all patient medications are cancelled preoperatively and subsequently reordered postoperatively, and in many instances the preoperative drug regimen changes postoperatively. Additional reconciliation may be necessary when patient medications are stopped and reordered as the patient moves from one level of care to another in the hospital environment (e.g., moving from the intensive care unit to an intermediate care unit).

Summary

The administration of medication is a serious responsibility, requiring the possession of clinical information and skills. It includes not only information about the drugs being given, but also the proper procedures for safe administration, communication with team members, and documentation. Skills in administration ensure that the patient receives medication in the safest and most therapeutic manner with the least chance of mistakes, untoward reactions, or spread of infection.

TEST YOUR KNOWLEDGE

Multiple Choice

1. The drug administration process begins with
   a. the physician's prescription.
   b. the pharmacist dispensing the drug.
   c. the nurse evaluating the patient.
   d. the request for a drug.

2. Medication orders include
   a. drugs ordered by the physician after medical rounds.
   b. telephone drug orders in emergencies.
   c. standing drug orders for particular patient categories.
   d. all of the above.

3. A PRN drug is administered
   a. routinely.
   b. at night before sleep.
   c. before meals.
   d. when the patient asks for the medication or when the patient's condition requires it.

4. Patient rights include the
   a. right drug.
   b. right time.
   c. right route.
   d. right dose.
   e. right patient.
   f. all of the above.

5. Prior to administering a drug, the medication administrator should
   a. check the patient's correct identification using two identifiers.
   b. check the drug against the order three times.
   c. leave the medication in the unit-dose package and check the expiration date.
   d. all of the above.

6. A drug may be left at the patient's bedside if
   a. the patient requests that the drug be left.
   b. the patient is asleep.
   c. the patient wants to discuss the drug with the pharmacist.
   d. none of the above.

7. At least 4 ounces of water should be given following the drug administration of
   a. a buccal tablet.
   b. a medicated mouthwash.
   c. an aspirin tablet.
   d. a sublingual tablet.

8. Sufficient water given after administration of a solid oral dosage form
   a. assists the patient in swallowing.
   b. prevents esophageal irritation.
   c. aids drug solubility.
   d. all of the above.

9. After administration of eyedrops, the patient should be advised to
   a. not move the head.
   b. not sneeze.
   c. close the eye(s) for a few moments
   d. immediately wipe away any tears.

10. Transdermal drug patches are placed
    a. on the upper arm or inside the forearm.
    b. below the knee.
    c. directly above the wrists.
    d. on the most accessible spot.

11. Outcomes of the performance improvement process for medication errors include
    a. identifying problems in the medication administration process.
    b. determining the need for staff education.
    c. reducing the possibility of future errors.
    d. all of the above.

12. When administering an enteric-coated medication to a child or geriatric patient, the administrator may take which of the following actions?
    a. Give the medication crushed in applesauce.
    b. Dissolve the medication in water.
    c. Give the medication with sufficient juice.
    d. None of the above.

Matching

Determine if the following dosage forms are internal or external. Answers are used more than once.

1. ______ ointment		a. internal drug
2. ______ topical preparation		b. external drug
3. ______ tablet		
4. ______ elixir		
5. ______ intramuscular injection		

Fill in the Blank

1. An order for a drug that must be administered immediately is called a __________ order.
2. Never administer a medication without checking it __________ times against the MAR.
3. An infection incurred in the hospital is called a __________ infection.
4. A __________ medication is one that is given under the tongue.
5. A __________ focuses on the needs of the patient and the information to be presented to the patient.

Suggested Reading

Gourley, D. R., Wedemweyer, H. F., & Norvell, M. (2006). Administration of medications. In T. R. Brown & M. C. Smith (Eds.), *Handbook of institutional pharmacy practice* (4th ed.). Baltimore, MD: Lippincott Williams & Wilkins.

CHAPTER

19

Drug Information

Competencies

Upon completion of this chapter, the reader should be able to:

1. Describe and participate in the steps of the systematic approach to answering a drug information question.
2. Describe the characteristics of tertiary, secondary, and primary resources.
3. Differentiate between reputable and questionable websites.
4. Identify useful tertiary resources and websites.
5. Devise a system to keep current in pharmacy practice.

Key Terms

drug information
drug information center (DIC)
evidence-based medicine (EBM)
medical information
primary resources
secondary resources
tertiary resources

Introduction

Over the centuries, pharmacy practice has evolved from a more product-oriented profession to a more patient-oriented profession. Traditionally, pharmacists focused primarily on compounding and dispensing medications. This changed as mass manufacturers of drug products reduced the need for pharmacists to compound drugs. More recently, technological advancements and the addition of pharmacy technicians have allowed pharmacists to focus more time on improving patient outcomes through the provision of pharmaceutical care.

To meet the demands of their profession, pharmacists have developed and maintained effective drug information skills. The public and health care professionals turn to pharmacists for accurate and unbiased drug information. Pharmacists use their drug information skills on a daily basis to ensure that patients receive safe and appropriate drug therapy. Today, the management of vast amounts of information and the provision of evidence-based drug information continues to be the most essential responsibility of all pharmacists.

Pharmacy technicians need to have effective drug information skills for many reasons. Pharmacy technicians can assist the pharmacist in improving patient outcomes in a variety of practice settings. In a community pharmacy, technicians can assist in researching questions asked by the customers who walk into the pharmacy or by the physicians who call into the pharmacy. In a hospital setting, a technician can assist in researching acute care questions that originate from the many health care professionals working within the hospital.

Regardless of practice setting, pharmacy technicians can play a significant role in triaging inquiries as they come into the pharmacy. After completing proper training, the experienced technician can determine which questions need the attention of the pharmacist and which can be answered by the technician. Proper handling of routine and repeat questions by the technician can help save the pharmacist's time. Technicians must have strong verbal communication skills and an effective knowledge base of medications and medical conditions in order to handle these inquires in an accurate and appropriate manner. It is also beneficial to the technician if he or she has an extensive knowledge base of where to find reliable drug information and how to interpret this information. The technician can verify prescriptions, check dosages, and learn more about medications by using the appropriate drug information resource. Last but not least, pharmacy technicians also need effective drug information skills to keep current with the profession. Effective knowledge of drug information can ultimately prevent the occurrence of medication errors and lead to optimal patient care.

drug information information about drugs and the effects of drugs on people, the provision of which is part of each pharmacist's practice

medical information information pertaining to health

This chapter introduces the pharmacy technician to evidence-based drug information practice and will outline the possible roles of the pharmacy technician. The content of this chapter may or may not be in compliance with all states' laws and regulations. The pharmacy technician is strongly encouraged to review the laws that govern the state in which he or she practices to determine what activities can be delegated by the pharmacist to the pharmacy technician.

Definition of Drug Information

The term **drug information** simply means information pertaining to drugs. The more contemporary term **medical information** is often used alternatively to also encompass information pertaining to health, but not directly related to

evidence-based medicine (EBM) the use of information about health practices and drugs that has been validated as useful and accurate by appropriate reference sources

medications. Alternatively, the term **evidence-based medicine (EBM)** is being used more and more frequently because it emphasizes that health information should be validated by appropriate sources. Health care professionals need to practice according to the best evidence gained from the strongest research available and disregard all other information that is generated by poorly conducted research. EBM requires advanced knowledge of drug information and research evaluation and is most likely beyond the scope of the responsibilities of the pharmacy technician. Inquiries requiring knowledge of EBM should be directed to the pharmacist.

For the purposes of this chapter, the more traditional term *drug information* will be used, although one should realize that the knowledge and expertise of pharmacists extends beyond medications. For example, pharmacists are often consulted about dietary supplements, nonpharmacological methods of managing illness, dietary modifications, and disease prevention.

The provision of drug information can be grouped into two categories: patient specific or population based. Pharmacists and pharmacy technicians most often receive patient-specific drug information requests. For example, a woman suffering from postpartum depression needs an antidepressant medication that would allow her to continue to safely breastfeed her infant. In this specific situation, patient-specific information is needed, such as the woman's medical history including information on her recent pregnancy, her medication history, and any allergies she may have. The patient's values and beliefs regarding the importance of breastfeeding her infant should also be taken into consideration. Information about the infant will also be required. Once all of this information has been collected, an extensive search for drug information is needed to subsequently provide an individualized, evidence-based recommendation.

On the other hand, population-based drug information involves researching and evaluating drug information as it relates to a group of patients in general. When providing population-based information, the pharmacist focuses on the general use of a drug in a group of patients and not in an individual patient. For example, a physician requests that the pharmacy department consider adding a particular drug to the hospital formulary. A pharmacist in turn would retrieve and evaluate all of the research that has been performed on the drug and subsequently compare this drug to other similar drugs that are already in the formulary. The pharmacist would then develop an evidence-based decision about whether the drug would potentially benefit future patients admitted to the hospital.

The drug information activities and responsibilities of a pharmacist are outlined in the American Society of Health-System Pharmacists (ASHP) guidelines in the "Provision of Medication Information by Pharmacists" section. The pharmacy technician should become familiar with this document before aiding pharmacists in answering drug information requests. One can find these guidelines (as well as many other important ASHP policy positions, statements, and guidelines) on the ASHP's website (www.ashp.org).

Drug Information Specialists

Although all pharmacists are responsible for providing drug information, some pharmacists have chosen to undergo extensive training and specialization in the field of drug information practice. These pharmacists are referred to as *drug information specialists or medical information specialists*. Drug information specialists have extensive knowledge of drug information resources, strong literature evaluation skills, problem-solving skills, and expertise in information technology, and they are effective communicators of verbal and written drug information. For more detailed information on drug information specialists, please see the article by Brand and Kraus listed in the Suggested Readings section at the end of this chapter.

Drug Information Centers

drug information center (DIC) a center directed by a drug information specialist, most commonly funded by or located in a hospital, academic institution, or pharmaceutical company; it provides information and education on drugs, develops policies or guidelines for appropriate use of medications, and coordinates medication error programs

A **drug information center (DIC)** is usually directed by drug information specialists. The first DIC was established in 1962 at the University of Kentucky Medical Center. According to a 2009 publication by Rosenberg et al., the United States has at least 75 active drug information centers.

The purposes of a DIC vary and depend on the practice setting in which the drug information center is located. A DIC is most commonly funded by or located in a hospital or an academic institution. Some drug information centers provide free drug information services, while others provide drug information for a fee (fee for service). A client could pay an annual fee to contract with a particular drug information center regardless of the number of times the client uses the DIC. Alternatively, the client may pay for each individual question answered or every project (i.e., formulary monograph) completed by DIC personnel. Also, pharmaceutical companies usually have a medical information department that employs health care professionals (usually drug information specialists) to answer questions regarding a company's medical products. These departments also function in a similar manner to drug information centers. Health care professionals and the public often phone the medical information department for help with locating drug information.

A function common to all drug information centers is the handling of drug information requests. Requests can be received via the telephone, e-mail, regular mail, or in person. Requestors of information can be physicians, nurses, pharmacists, pharmacy technicians, and patients. Other functions of a DIC include, but are not limited to, the provision of education through lectures and newsletters, development of policies or guidelines for appropriate use of medications, management of formularies and quality assurance activities, and coordination of adverse drug reaction and medication error programs. If the opportunity arises, pharmacy technicians can support the drug information specialist in performing all of these activities. Specifically, the pharmacy technician may be expected to collect statistics on the number of drug information requests received, the profession of the requestor using the drug information center, the types of questions asked, and the time spent answering questions on a monthly basis. The technician may assist in maintaining a filing system of old requests and a filing system of important information collected on medications or medical topics of interest to allow for rapid and easy access.

In certain drug information centers where computerized databases are used to document and store drug information questions for subsequent easy retrieval, the technician can assist in maintaining and updating the database. The pharmacy technician can help compile information to be published in a newsletter. A pharmacy technician with effective technological skills can help edit the newsletter to give it a consistent appearance. The technician can also assist in the collection of data for research projects, adverse drug reactions, medication errors, quality assurance projects, and formulary management activities. If a pharmacy technician would like to consult with a drug information center, a directory of drug information centers has been published by Koumis and Rosenberg in the *American Journal of Health-System Pharmacy* (see references at the back of this chapter).

The Systematic Approach to Answering a Drug Information Question

The pharmacy technician should have an understanding of the systematic approach to answering a drug information question, originated by Watanabe and colleagues in 1975. The pharmacy technician should use this systematic approach in most communications with health care professionals and patients to ensure that all communications are handled appropriately and minimize the risk of error. The systematic approach was later modified to involve a total of seven steps:

1. Determine the demographics of the requestor.
2. Obtain background information.
3. Determine and categorize the ultimate question.
4. Develop a search strategy and conduct search.
5. Evaluate, analyze, and summarize the information obtained.
6. Formulate and provide a response.
7. Conduct a follow-up, and document the question from beginning to end.

Requestor Demographics

Usually, requestors of information approach or call the pharmacist or drug information center and immediately provide an initial question. One should proceed by quickly writing down the initial question and then asking for the requestor's full name (first names alone are not sufficient), profession, specialty (if speaking with a medical professional), address, phone numbers, fax numbers, e-mail, and any other contact information thought necessary.

Understanding the requestor's profession or specialty is important in determining the depth and complexity of information needed. For example, a physician's question would most often require extensive research and a detailed scientific response, whereas a patient's inquiry could usually be answered rapidly without as much extensive research. In addition, when communicating with a patient, it is necessary to use lay terms to ensure that the patient understands the information provided.

A pharmacy technician may perform this first step of the systematic approach and then triage the inquiry. If the inquiry is beyond basic, the technician should triage the request to the most appropriate individual. All inquiries should be documented. An example of a drug information request documentation form is shown in **Figure 19-1**. This form can be altered to best fit the practice setting. A pharmacist or drug information specialist should usually perform the next step of obtaining background information, especially if the question appears to be of an urgent nature or of high complexity.

Background Information

Obtaining background information is the most important step in the systematic approach and requires effective communication and listening skills. To perform this step well, an extensive knowledge base is needed of different medical conditions and medications. This step generally should be performed by the pharmacist or drug information specialist. If this step is not performed appropriately, serious consequences may occur in that inaccurate or irrelevant information may be provided and valuable time may be wasted.

Date: ____________________ Time: ________________ Received by: ____________________

Requestor's Demographics

Name: ______________________________________ Hospital Location: _______________

Affiliation: ___________________________________

Address: ___________________________
Street address
____
City State Zip

Profession:
MD RPh PharmD RN PhD
Consumer/Patient

Specialty ____________________
Other ____________________

Phone Number: ( ) - Fax Number: ( ) -

Pager Number: ( ) - E-mail Address:

Background Information:

Patient Specific? Yes No If Yes, fill out below:
MR#____________ **Location:** ___________ **Gender:** Female Male **Age:**_______
Height: _______ **Weight:** _______ **Allergies:** _____________________________________
Relevant PMH / HPI / Diagnosis (including organ fxn):

Medications:

Initial Question:

Ultimate Question:

Classification of Request:

Product Availability	Compatibility/Stability	Reference Material
Pharmacokinetics	Dosage/Administration	Drug Interactions
Adverse Reactions/Toxicity	CAM/Dietary Supplements	Product Identification
Pregnancy/Lactation/Repro	Therapeutic Use	Compounding

Other ____

Urgency of Response: STAT Other ___________________
Method of Request: Phone In Person E-mail 3rd Person Other

FIGURE 19-1 Drug information request form.

Actual Response Provided (attach continuation of response and support materials if necessary):

All References Used (indicate whether information found or not):

Response Information

Date: ______________ Time: ______________ ❒ Verbal ❒ Written

Answered by: ____________________ Approved by: ______________

Response given via: ❒ Phone ❒ Letter ❒ In Person ❒ Fax ❒ E-mail ❒ Other

Total time needed to complete request: ________________________

FIGURE 19-1 (Continued)

During this step, the pharmacist or drug information specialist will determine if the request is patient specific or population based and will proceed to ask important relevant questions to determine the true drug information need. Pharmacy technicians should observe the pharmacist as he or she interviews the requestor to obtain more detailed information. Pharmacy technicians with extensive experience may also perform this step if the question is deemed not urgent or is easily understood by the technician. An experienced technician will be able to use judgment to determine whether the question needs the attention of the pharmacist or drug information specialist. The experienced technician must demonstrate effective listening, communication, and interviewing skills to perform this step. The technician must also have an extensive knowledge base of drugs and diseases.

Determination and Categorization of the Ultimate Question

Determining the ultimate question (true drug information need) is accomplished easily once sufficient background information has been obtained. Often, the initial question differs significantly from the ultimate or final question. Once the ultimate question is identified and clear, the pharmacy technician or the drug information specialist can then quickly categorize the request and the next step can begin. The question should be categorized by type. For example, the question can be categorized as a drug interaction question or a drug identification question. For a list of possible categories of drug information questions, see the drug information request documentation form in Figure 19-1. Categorization of the request is important in that it helps direct the researcher to the resources that would best answer the question (e.g., a drug interaction textbook).

Search Strategy and Information Collection

The experienced pharmacy technician can contribute significantly to the development of a search strategy and collection of pertinent information. The technician must first develop a search strategy starting with general resources (**tertiary resources**) and work toward more specific resources (**primary resources**) through use of indexing and abstracting services (**secondary resources**). These three different types of resources are described later in this chapter.

The experienced technician should be able to identify when a search through secondary and primary resources is needed for a given question (e.g., physician inquiry, detailed or complex question) and when tertiary resources would be sufficient to answer the question (e.g., patient or nurse inquiry, general question). The pharmacy technician must have good knowledge of all the resources available to answer drug information questions in the drug information center, pharmacy, affiliated medical library (if applicable), and on the Internet.

The technician must also be proficient in conducting literature searches and using computerized databases and print resources. Once the necessary resources have been consulted and the information collected, the technician should then promptly provide this information to the pharmacist or drug information specialist for evaluation. The pharmacy technician must also remember to anticipate other questions that must be answered to provide a complete response. For example, if a requestor of information needs the drug of choice to treat a patient's community-acquired pneumonia, the drug name will most likely not be sufficient to completely answer the request. The drug dosing regimen, route of administration, duration of therapy, monitoring parameters, common side effects, and potential drug interactions would be additional information needed by the requestor, although the requestor did not specifically ask for it.

tertiary resources general research resources, including package inserts, textbooks, compendia, computer databases, and review articles; commonly consulted when initiating a search strategy; usually used to educate oneself about a medical condition or medication

primary resources specific research resources and most current sources of information, including original research articles published in professional journals; also include descriptive patient case reports, observational studies, and experimental studies

secondary resources research resources such as indexing and abstracting services; usually available electronically and quickly link the reader to the primary literature

Evaluation, Analysis, and Synthesis of Information

This step requires strong literature evaluation skills and, therefore, should be left to the pharmacist or drug information specialist. Knowledge of EBM, study design, research, and statistical concepts is essential to be able to evaluate the medical literature and apply the information to clinical practice and patient-specific situations. The pharmacy technician's involvement in this step would depend on the training and experience of the technician.

Formulation and Provision of a Response

After careful analysis and synthesis of information, the pharmacist or drug information specialist formulates a response and then accurately conveys the response back to the requestor of information. This requires strong verbal and written communication skills. If a written response is required, the pharmacy technician may assist in drafting and referencing the response. However, ultimately the pharmacist or drug information specialist must review the written response for accuracy and completeness. If specific drug therapy recommendations are made, it is important to have the requestor repeat back the information provided to ensure that he or she has the correct information.

Follow-Up and Documentation

The pharmacy technician can assist in following up on all completed requests to determine whether the information provided was appropriate, recommendations provided were actually followed, and if the response was adequate to meet the requestor's needs. This process ensures and documents the quality of services provided by the pharmacy, pharmacy department, or drug information center. The pharmacy technician is also responsible for assisting in the appropriate documentation of all requests from beginning to end, and should make sure all references used were properly documented on the drug information request documentation form or computerized database.

Drug Information Resources

One of the technician's possible responsibilities in a pharmacy or drug information center is managing the inventory of all resources. Resources should be stored in an organized fashion and kept up to date. The technician may be responsible for ordering references, keeping track of subscription expiration dates, and ensuring that ordered resources are actually received by the pharmacy or drug information center. The technician may also assist in maintaining a filing system of important information for easy and rapid access by all pharmacy or drug information center personnel.

The pharmacy technician should also have knowledge of all of the available resources in the pharmacy, drug information center, nearby medical libraries (if applicable), and on the Internet. The technician must be proficient in the retrieval of drug information, whether it comes from the shelves of a library or a computerized database. The technician may also assist in the printing and photocopying of necessary information.

The experienced technician should also be able to differentiate between reputable resources and those of questionable quality. As mentioned earlier, the three different types of drug information resources are tertiary, secondary, and primary resources. Each type has advantages and disadvantages that the pharmacy technician should be able to describe and keep in mind when researching drug information requests.

Tertiary Resources

A list of tertiary resources (i.e., general resources) is provided in **Table 19-1**. Tertiary resources are package inserts, textbooks, compendia, computer databases, and review articles. These resources are best if peer reviewed, authored by an expert in the field to which the resource pertains, and easy to navigate. Tertiary resources can allow for rapid comprehensive access to information, are commonly consulted when initiating a search strategy, and are usually used to educate oneself about a medical condition or medication.

One of the significant disadvantages of tertiary resources is that they are usually somewhat out of date by the time they are published. This is due to the

TABLE 19-1 Tertiary Resources Listed by Information Provided

Adverse Drug Reactions
Anne Lee's *Adverse Drug Reactions*
Aronson's *Side Effects of Drugs Annual*
Davies's *Textbook of Adverse Drug Reactions*
Meyler's *Side Effects of Drugs*
Compatibility and Stability
ASHP's Interactive Handbook on Injectable Drugs: IV Decision Support by Lawrence A. Trissel
Bing's *Extended Stability for Parenteral Drugs*
Gahart's *Intravenous Medications*
King's *Guide to Parenteral Admixtures*
Trissel's *Handbook of Injectable Drugs*
Trissel's *Stability of Compounded Formulations*
White's *Handbook of Drug Administration via Enteral Feeding Tubes*
Complementary and Alternative Medicine
AltMedDEX System, published by Micromedex (www.thomsonhc.com—subscription required)
The Complete German Commission E Monographs
Natural Standard Herb & Supplement Guide: An Evidenced-Based Reference
PDR for Herbal Medicines
Rakel's *Integrative Medicine*
The Review of Natural Products
Tyler's *Herbs of Choice*
Tyler's *Honest Herbal*
Compounding
Allen's *The Art, Science, and Technology of Pharmaceutical Compounding*
Allen's *Compounded Formulations: The Complete U.S. Pharmacist Collection*
Jew's *Extemporaneous Formulations for Pediatric, Geriatric, and Special Needs Patients*
Trissel's *Stability of Compounded Formulations*
Cultural Competence
Halbur's *Essentials in Cultural Competence in Pharmacy Practice*

TABLE 19-1 (Continued)

Drug Availability

American Drug Index

Drug Facts and Comparisons

Drug Topics Red Book

Thomson's *Red Book*

Drug Identification

Ident-A-Drug Reference

IDENTIDEX System, published by Micromedex (www.thomsonhc.com—subscription required)

Drug Information and Literature Evaluation

Ascione's *Principles of Scientific Literature Evaluation: Critiquing Clinical Drug Trials*

Dawson's *Basic and Clinical Biostatistics*

De Muth's *Basic Statistics and Pharmaceutical Statistical Applications*

Malone's *Drug Information: A Guide for Pharmacists*

Riegelman's *Studying a Study and Testing a Test: How to Read the Medical Evidence*

Snow's *Drug Information: A Guide to Current Resources*

Drug Interaction Resources

Drug Interaction Facts

DRUG-REAX System, published by Micromedex (www.thomsonhc.com—subscription required)

Hansten and Horn's *Drug Interaction Analysis and Management*

Foreign Drugs

European Drug Index

Index Nominum: International Drug Directory

Martindale's *The Complete Drug Reference*

USP Dictionary of United States Adopted Names (USAN) and International Drug Names

General Drug Information References

American Hospital Formulary Service (AHFS) Drug Information

APhA's *Peripheral Brain for the Pharmacist*

Drug Facts and Comparisons

Drug Information Handbook, by Lexi-Comp Inc. (also available electronically at www.lexi.com—subscription required)

DRUGDEX System, published by Micromedex (www.thomsonhc.com—subscription required)

Mosby's GenRx

Physician's Desk Reference (PDR)

Remington's *The Science and Practice of Pharmacy*

Thomson's *Red Book*

USP DI Volume I (health care professional), *Volume II* (patient), and *Volume III* (legal requirements)

(*Continued*)

TABLE 19-1 (Continued)

Geriatric Resources

Brocklehurst's *Textbook of Geriatric Medicine and Gerontology*

Cassel's *Geriatric Medicine: An Evidence-Based Approach*

Geriatric Dosage Handbook, by Lexi-Comp Inc. (also available electronically at www.lexi.com—subscription required)

The Merck Manual of Geriatrics

Immunology

Concepts in Immunology and Immunotherapeutics

ImmunoFacts

Infectious Disease

Mandell, Douglas, and Bennett's *Principles and Practice of Infectious Diseases*

Internal Medicine

Cecil's *Textbook of Medicine*

Conn's *Current Therapy*

Harrison's *Principles of Internal Medicine*

The Merck Manual of Diagnosis and Therapeutics

Laboratory Data Interpretation

Laboratory Test Handbook

Traub's *Basic Skills in Interpreting Laboratory Data*

Medical Dictionaries

Davies's *Medical Abbreviations*

Dorland's *Illustrated Medical Dictionary*

Stedman's *Medical Dictionary*

Nephrology

Drug Prescribing in Renal Failure: Dosing Guidelines for Adults

Nonprescription Products

Facts and Comparisons' *Nonprescription Drug Therapy Guiding Patient Self-Care*

Handbook of Nonprescription Drugs

PDR for Nonprescription Drugs and Dietary Supplements

Pray's *Nonprescription Product Therapeutics*

Oncology/Hematology

DeVita's *Cancer: Principles and Practice of Oncology*

Dorr's *Cancer Chemotherapy Handbook*

Hoffman's *Hematology: Basic Principles and Practices*

Patient Safety

Cohen's *Medication Errors*

Pediatric Resources

AAP Red Book: Report of the Committee on Infectious Diseases

Nelson's *Textbook of Pediatrics*

TABLE 19-1 (Continued)

Pediatric Resources (continued)

Neofax

Pediatric & Neonatal Dosage Handbook, by Lexi-Comp Inc. (also available electronically on www.lexi.com—subscription required)

Teddy Bear Book: Pediatric Injectable Drugs

Pharmaceutical Calculations

Ansel's *Pharmaceutical Calculations*

Zatz's *Pharmaceutical Calculations*

Pharmacogenomics

Zdanowicz's *Concepts in Pharmacogenomics*

Pharmacokinetics

Applied Pharmacokinetics: Principles of Therapeutic Drug Monitoring

DiPiro's*Concepts of Clinical Pharmacokinetics*

Winter's *Basic Clinical Pharmacokinetics*

Pharmacology and Therapeutics

DePiro's *Pharmacotherapy: A Pathophysiologic Approach*

Goodman and Gilman's *The Pharmacological Basis of Therapeutics*

Katzung's *Basic and Clinical Pharmacology*

Koda Kimble's *Applied Therapeutics: The Clinical Use of Drugs*

Melmon and Morrelli's *Clinical Pharmacology*

Pharmacy Law

Abood's Pharmacy Practice and the Law

Darvey's Legal Handbook for Pharmacy Technicians

Pharmacy Law Digest

Reiss and Hall's Guide to Federal Pharmacy Law

Reproduction, Pregnancy, and Lactation

Briggs's *Drugs in Pregnancy and Lactation*

Chemically Induced Birth Defects

REPRORISK System, published by Micromedex (www.thomsonhc.com—subscription required)

Shepard's *Catalog of Teratogenic Agents*

Toxicology

Casarett and Doull's *Toxicology: The Basic Science of Poisons*

Clinical Toxicology of Commercial Products

Ellenhorn's *Medical Toxicology: Diagnosis and Treatment of Human Poisoning*

Goldfrank's *Toxicologic Emergencies*

Material Safety Data Sheets (MSDS) from the USP

POISONDEX System, published by Micromedex (www.thomsonhc.com—subscription required)

TOMES System, published by Micromedex (www.thomsonhc.com—subscription required)

Veterinary Medicine

Merck Veterinary Manual

significant amount of time that elapses between when the resource is written and when it is actually published (i.e., long lag time). Therefore, one must always take into account the resource's date of publication when using it for drug information. Review articles published in journals and certain references published in updatable binder format (e.g., *Drug Facts and Comparisons*) do not have as significant a lag time. Also, one must keep in mind that the information provided in a tertiary resource is subject to the author's interpretation of the primary literature (i.e., original research) on the topic. Sometimes the author's opinion may not necessarily be accurate or complete. Since tertiary resources are general resources, they usually lack specific details, forcing the reader to conduct further research of the primary literature for more information.

A discussion on tertiary resources would not be complete without discussing package inserts. Before a medication can be made available to the public for use, the medication must be evaluated for efficacy and safety in animal and human studies. If the medication is reasonably effective and safe, the Food and Drug Administration will grant approval for the manufacturer to market the drug. In this process, the manufacturer compiles a package insert, which is a document that provides prescribing information and other data derived from premarketing studies. The package insert (i.e., drug labeling, product information, prescribing information, etc.) is usually the first comprehensive source of information one can obtain on a drug as it is first marketed. The package inserts provide the following information on the drug: pharmacology, pharmacokinetics, summary clinical studies, indications for use, contraindications, warnings, precautions, adverse effects, dosage and administration, overdosage, how supplied, preparation instructions, patient information, and so forth. For more information on new prescription drug labeling by the Food and Drug Administration, please see the reference by Lal and Kremzner.

The pharmacy technician should know how to access the most up-to-date package insert of all drugs. The best method is to obtain a package insert from the manufacturer's website (e.g., www.pfizer.com). The prescribing information available from the manufacturer's website will be the most recently revised. Usually, one may obtain the prescribing information by simply typing "www.brandname.com" (e.g., www.zyvox.com). A package insert can also be found attached to the drug product itself at the point of dispensing. The *Physician's Desk Reference* may also be used to obtain a package insert; however, the information may not be as current as that obtained from the manufacturer's website or on the product package itself. Package inserts for older or generic drugs can be obtained by calling the manufacturer.

Secondary Resources

Secondary resources are indexing and abstracting services such as MEDLINE (www.pubmed.gov), International Pharmaceutical Abstracts (IPA), Iowa Drug Information Service (IDIS), EMBASE (European Medline), and Journal Watch. Secondary resources are usually available electronically and quickly link the reader to the primary literature. The pharmacy technician must undergo training in properly searching secondary resources such as MEDLINE and IPA. This training will allow the technician to perform appropriate literature searches and identify useful information. The pharmacist or drug information specialist may either train the pharmacy technician on the proper use of secondary resources or inform the pharmacy technician of available educational programs.

Pharmacy technicians should be aware that each secondary resource indexes different journals and meeting abstracts; therefore, it is often necessary to search more than one secondary resource to perform a thorough literature search. Some secondary resources can be expensive to subscribe to (e.g., IPA, IDIS), while others are free (e.g., MEDLINE).

Primary Resources

Primary resources are the original research articles, published in journals such as the *Annals of Pharmacotherapy, American Journal of Hospital Pharmacy,* and the *Journal of the American Medical Association*. The primary literature also includes descriptive patient case reports, observational studies (i.e., cohort, case-control, cross-sectional studies), and experimental studies (i.e., clinical trials, crossover trials).

The primary literature is the most current source of information and provides a very detailed description of a study (i.e., objective, methods, statistics, results, and conclusion). This allows the reader to make his or her own evaluation and interpretation of the study, compare it to the results of other studies, and apply the study results to patients encountered in practice. Excellent literature evaluation skills are necessary to critically evaluate each study and to be able to apply it to clinical practice. The pharmacy technician should be familiar with all components of an original research article to facilitate communication between the technician and other health care professionals. When answering a drug information request, a significant amount of time is often required to collect pertinent primary literature and evaluate all of the primary literature to locate the best evidence on a particular topic.

The Internet

A discussion on drug information practice would not be complete without a discussion of the Internet and how it has changed the provision of drug information. Tertiary (e.g., most websites), secondary (e.g., MEDLINE, Internet subscriptions to computerized databases), and primary literature (i.e., electronic full-text articles) may be found on the Internet. Medication package inserts can be downloaded easily off the Internet (e.g., a package insert for metformin may be easily found at www.glucophage.com). The Internet allows for rapid and easy access to a wealth of information. It may help save space in the practice by allowing for electronic subscriptions and electronic storage of documents. It also allows for rapid dissemination of important information to others through e-mail.

Pharmacy technicians must, however, be cautious when using the Internet for drug information. Anyone can create a website, and many websites may provide false or misleading information. Each site providing drug or medical information must be carefully evaluated for reliability and accuracy. Reliable websites provide balanced information (benefits and risks of medications), author's qualifications and expertise, protection of patient confidentiality, references, the date information provided was last revised, and contact information for the site's creator. The funding sources of the website should be clearly stated so one can identify any possible conflicts of interest. In general, websites that sell products or advertise products are more likely to provide biased information.

Even if a site provides all the above stated information, professional judgment and knowledge must always be used to determine whether information provided on the site is accurate and reliable. A list of reputable websites including government sites is provided in **Table 19-2**. Pharmacy technicians should always encourage patients to consult a pharmacist or health care professional before following any medical advice obtained from a website.

TABLE 19-2 Useful Websites

Adverse Reaction Reporting

Food and Drug Administration MedWatch Program (www.fda.gov/medwatch)

Dietary Supplements

Center for Food Safety and Applied Nutrition (www.fda.gov/food)

ConsumerLab.com—subscription required for full information (www.consumerlab.com)

National Center for Complementary and Alternative Medicine (www.nccam.nih.gov)

Natural Medicines Comprehensive Database—subscription required (www.naturaldatabase.com)

Office of Dietary Supplements (http://ods.od.nih.gov)

USP-verified dietary supplements (www.usp.org/USPVerified)

Health-Related News and Updates

Centers for Disease Control and Prevention (www.cdc.gov)

CNN Health (www.cnn.com/health)

Medscape—free registration (www.medscape.com)

New York Times—Health (www.nytimes.com/pages/health/index.html)

NPR (www.npr.org/sections/health)

The Pharmacist's Letter—subscription required (www.pharmacistsletter.com)

Reuters Health—subscription required (www.reutershealth.com)

Yahoo! Health News (health.yahoo.com/news)

Interpreting Medical Abbreviations/Acronyms

Medi-Lexicon (www.medilexicon.com)

Medical Dictionaries

Medi-Lexicon (www.medilexicon.com)

PubMed MeSH Database (www.ncbi.nlm.nih.gov/mesh)

Select Medical Websites

American Academy of Geriatric Psychiatry (www.aagponline.org)

American Academy of Ophthalmology (www.aao.org)

American Academy of Pediatrics (www.aap.org)

American Cancer Society (www.cancer.org)

American College of Allergy, Asthma and Immunology (ACAAI) (www.acaai.org)

American College of Emergency Physicians (www.acep.org)

American College of Obstetricians and Gynecology (www.acog.org)

American College of Physicians (www.acponline.org)

American College of Surgeons (www.facs.org)

American Dental Association (www.ada.org)

American Diabetes Association (www.diabetes.org)

American Gastroenterological Association (www.gastro.org)

American Geriatrics Society (www.americangeriatrics.org)

American Heart Association (www.americanheart.org)

American Hospital Association (www.aha.org)

American Lung Association (www.lungusa.org)

American Medical Association (www.ama-assn.org)

American Medical Informatics Association (www.amia.org)

TABLE 19-2 (Continued)

Select Medical Websites (continued)

American Neurological Association (www.aneuroa.org)
American Psychiatric Association (www.psych.org)
American Psychological Association (www.apa.org)
American Urological Association (www.auanet.org)
Association of American Medical Colleges (www.aamc.org)
Institute for Healthcare Improvement (www.ihi.org)
Joint Commission (www.jointcommission.org)
World Health Organization (WHO) (www.who.int)

Medication Error Reporting

Institute for Safe Medication Practices (ISMP) (www.ismp.org)
National Coordinating Council for Medication Error Reporting and Prevention (NCCMERP) (www.nccmerp.org)

Patient Health Information Websites

ASHP's Safe Medication (www.safemedication.com)
MedlinePlus (www.medlineplus.gov)

Pharmacy Technician Websites

American Association of Pharmacy Technicians (www.pharmacytechnician.com)
National Pharmacy Technician Association (NPTA) (www.pharmacytechnician.org)
Pharmacy Technician Certification Board (www.ptcb.org)

Pharmacy Websites

American Association of Colleges of Pharmacy (www.aacp.org)
American College of Clinical Pharmacy (www.accp.com)
American Council on Pharmaceutical Education (www.acpe-accredit.org)
American Pharmacists Association (www.aphanet.org)
American Society of Consultant Pharmacists (www.ascp.com)
American Society of Health-System Pharmacists (www.ashp.org)
American Society for Pharmacy Law (www.aspl.org)
National Association of Boards of Pharmacy (www.nabp.net)
National Association of Chain Drug Stores (www.nacds.org)

Reproduction, Pregnancy, and Lactation

Agency for Toxic Substances and Disease Registry (www.atsdr.cdc.gov)
Clinical Teratology (http://depts.washington.edu/terisweb)
Drugs and Lactation Database (LactMed) (http://toxnet.nlm.nih.gov/cgi-bin/sis/htmlgen?lact)
FDA Pregnancy Exposure Registries (www.fda.gov)
March of Dimes (www.marchofdimes.com)
MOTHERISK (www.motherisk.org)
National Center on Birth Defects and Developmental Disabilities (NCBDDD) (www.cdc.gov/ncbddd)
Office of Health Assessment and Translation (OHAT) (http://ntp.niehs.nih.gov)
Organization of Teratology Information Specialists (OTIS) (www.otispregnancy.org)
REPROTOX—subscription required (www.reprotox.org)
The Teratology Society (www.teratology.org)

(Continued)

TABLE 19-2 (Continued)

Secondary Resources (Indexing and Abstracting Services)
EMBASE—subscription required (www.embase.com)
Google Scholar (www.scholar.google.com)
International Pharmaceutical Abstracts (IPA)—subscription required (http://science.thomsonreuters.com)
Iowa Drug Information Service—subscription required (www.uiowa.edu/~idis)
National Library of Medicine (http://nlm.nih.gov)
PubMed (www.pubmed.gov)
TOXNET: Toxicology Data Network (http://toxnet.nlm.nih.gov/index.html)
Additional Governmental Websites
Agency for Healthcare Research and Quality (AHRQ) (www.ahrq.gov)
Center for Food Safety and Applied Nutrition (CFSAN) (www.fda.gov/food)
Centers for Disease Control and Prevention (CDC) (www.cdc.gov)
Centers for Medicare and Medicaid Services (www.cms.gov)
ClinicalTrials.gov (www.clinicaltrials.gov)
Directory of Health Organizations Online (DIRLINE) (http://dirline.nlm.nih.gov)
Food and Drug Administration (FDA) (www.fda.gov)
National Cancer Institute (NCI) (www.nci.nih.gov)
National Center for Complementary and Alternative Medicine (nccam.nih.gov)
National Guidelines Clearinghouse (www.guidelines.gov)
National Institute for Occupational Safety and Health (NIOSH) (www.cdc.gov/niosh)
National Institutes of Health (NIH) (www.nih.gov)
National Library of Medicine (NLM) (www.nlm.nih.gov)
Occupational Safety and Health Administration (OSHA) (www.osha.gov)
Surgeon General Reports (www.surgeongeneral.gov/library/reports.htm)
U.S. Department of Health and Human Services (DHHS) (www.dhhs.gov)
U.S. Pharmacopeia (USP) (www.usp.org)
Website Evaluation Tool
Health on the Net Foundation (HON) (www.hon.ch)

Necessary Drug Information Skills for the Pharmacy Technician

In summary, the pharmacy technician must have effective drug information skills, which require strong communication and listening skills. The technician must have a strong knowledge base of medical conditions, medications, resources, and strong research and technological capabilities. The technician must follow all ethical principles and always behave in a courteous, professional, and caring manner.

The pharmacy technician is also expected to stay current with advances in pharmacy practice. The technician should participate in the pharmacy or drug information center's methods for staying current (e.g., journal clubs, educational conferences, continuing education, journal circulation). It is recommended that the technician subscribe to *Pharmacist's Letter®* (www.pharmacistsletter.com) and the Pharmacy Technician's Letter (www.pharmacytechniciansletter.com)

to keep current. The technician should review newsletters published by the Institute for Safe Medication Practices (www.ismp.org) and frequently consult its website to help prevent medication errors. The technician should also subscribe to receive MedWatch Safety Alerts from the U.S. Food and Drug Administration (www.fda.gov/medwatch). This is imperative to staying informed about new medication safety information and product recalls. This service is free and the technician can choose to receive these alerts through e-mail or text messages or one can follow MedWatch on Twitter.

Summary

Pharmacy technicians who possess effective drug information skills are an asset to any pharmacy practice setting. Pharmacy technicians can triage drug information inquiries, retrieve drug information from the most appropriate resources, and assist in researching and documenting these questions. They can assist in ordering and maintaining drug information resources. If proficient in the correct use of resources, the technician can also verify prescriptions, dosages, etc. All of these skills are crucial to ensuring safe medication practices and remaining current in the ever-changing field of medicine.

TEST YOUR KNOWLEDGE

Multiple Choice

1. Place the following steps of the systematic approach to answering a drug information question in the order in which they should be performed.
   i. Develop a search strategy and conduct search.
   ii. Secure the demographics of the requestor.
   iii. Document and conduct follow-up.
   iv. Obtain background information.
   v. Formulate and provide a response.
   vi. Perform evaluation, analysis, and synthesis of information.
   vii. Determine and categorize the ultimate question.
      a. ii, iv, vii, i, vi, v, and iii
      b. ii, iv, vii, vi, i, v, and iii
      c. ii, iv, vi, vii, v, i, and iii
      d. ii, vii, iv, i, vi, v, and iii

2. Although all the steps of the systematic approach are important, which of the following steps is the most important?
   a. Secure the demographics of the requestor.
   b. Obtain background information.
   c. Formulate and provide a response.
   d. Perform evaluation, analysis, and synthesis of information.

3. Which of the following resources provides you with a general overview of a topic?
   a. tertiary resources
   b. secondary resources
   c. primary resources
   d. none of the above

4. Which of the following resources suffers the most from a long lag time (i.e., is somewhat outdated by the time it is published)?
   a. tertiary resources
   b. secondary resources
   c. primary resources
   d. none of the above

5. Which of the following statements regarding the use of the Internet for drug information are true?
   i. Websites that sell or advertise products are more likely to provide biased or misleading information.
   ii. Government websites are reputable and can be used for drug information with confidence.
   iii. Patients should be encouraged to follow any medical advice obtained from a website without the need to consult with a health care professional.
   iv. The Internet allows for rapid and easy access to a wealth of information and allows for rapid dissemination of information through e-mail.
   v. You may find tertiary, secondary, and primary resources on the Internet.
      a. i, ii, iii, iv, and v
      b. ii and iii
      c. i, ii, iv, and v
      d. iii and v

6. More reputable websites should
   a. provide balanced information.
   b. provide references.
   c. provide the author's qualifications and expertise.
   d. all of the above.

7. A useful tertiary resource to answer a drug information question on the safety of a certain medication during pregnancy is
   a. *American Drug Index.*
   b. *Index Nominum.*
   c. *Ident-A-Drug.*
   d. Brigg's *Drugs in Pregnancy and Lactation.*

8. A useful tertiary resource to identify a medication is
   a. *Index Nominum.*
   b. *Ident-A-Drug.*
   c. Brigg's *Drugs in Pregnancy and Lactation.*
   d. *Geriatric Dosage Handbook.*

9. Which of the following is/are possible drug information responsibilities of the pharmacy technician?
   a. triaging drug information requests to the most appropriate individual
   b. documenting drug information requests
   c. retrieving drug information from the most appropriate resources
   d. all of the above

10. Which of the following is/are necessary drug information skills for the pharmacy technician?
    a. effective communication and listening skills
    b. strong knowledge base of available drug information resources
    c. ability to maintain oneself current in a systematic manner
    d. all of the above

Fill in the Blank

1. Package inserts and textbooks are examples of ______________ resources.
2. Indexing and abstracting services provide ______________ resources.
3. Original research articles published in journals are examples of ______________.
4. Drug information can be grouped into two categories: ______________ information and ______________ information.

Suggested Readings

American Society of Health-System Pharmacists. (1996). ASHP guidelines on the provision of medication information by pharmacists. *American Journal of Hospital Pharmacy, 53*, 1843–1845.

Brand, K.A., & Kraus, M.L. (2006). Drug information specialists. *American Journal of Health-System Pharmacy, 63*, 712–714.

Koumis, T., Cicero, L.A., Nathan, J.P., & Rosenberg, J.M. (2004). Directory of pharmacist-operated drug information centers in the United States—2003. *American Journal of Health-System Pharmacy, 61*, 2033–2042.

Koumis, T., & Rosenberg, J.M. (2005). Update of directory of drug information centers. *American Journal of Health-System Pharmacy, 62*, 1348.

Lal, R., & Kremzner, M. (2007). Introduction to the new prescription drug labeling by the Food and Drug Administration. *American Journal of Health-System Pharmacy, 64*, 2488–2494.

Malone, P.M., Kier, K.L., & Stanovich, J. E. (2001). *Drug information: A guide for pharmacists* (4th ed.). New York, NY: McGraw-Hill.

Rosenberg, J.M., Koumis, T., Nathan, J.P., Cicero, L.A., & McGuire, H. (2004). Current status of pharmacist-operated drug information centers in the United States. *American Journal of Health-System Pharmacy, 61*, 2023–2032.

Rosenberg, J. M., Schilit, S., Nathan, J. P., Zerilli, T., & McGuire, H. (2009). Update on the status of drug information centers in the United States. *American Journal of Health-System Pharmacy, 66*, 1718–1722.

Watanabe, A.S., & Conner, C.S. (1978). *Principles of drug information services: A syllabus of systematic concepts*. Hamilton, IL: Drug Intelligence Publications.

Watanabe, A.S., McGart, G., Shimomura, S., & Kayser, S. (1975). Systematic approach to drug information requests. *American Journal of Hospital Pharmacy, 32*(12), 1282–1285.

CHAPTER

20

Drug Distribution Systems

Competencies

Upon completion of this chapter, the reader should be able to:

1. Outline the major activities in the overall drug distribution process.
2. Briefly explain the methods by which a prescriber's original orders are transmitted to the pharmacy.
3. Explain why the pharmacist must review a direct prescriber's order entry for a medication.
4. Describe the roles of the pharmacist and the current and possible future role of the pharmacy technician in the drug distribution process.
5. Indicate the differences between the four major drug distribution systems.
6. State the purpose, functions, and advantages of the unit-dose drug distribution system.
7. List the important points to consider in labeling medications.
8. Describe the purpose, functions, and advantages of the profile-enabled automated dispensing cabinet drug distribution system.
9. List the drug distribution activities that can be generated through computer technology.
10. Explain how automation can affect the incidences of medication errors.
11. Describe various ways in which the pharmacy technician is directly involved in the computerization process.

Key Terms

bar code medication administration (BCMA)
computerized prescriber order entry (CPOE)
dumbwaiters
floor stock system
individual prescription system
medication administration record (MAR)
no carbon required (NCR) form
Pharmacy and Therapeutics Committee (P&T)
pneumatic tube system
radio-frequency identification device (RFID)
robotics
turnaround time
unit-dose distribution system
unit-of-use

Introduction

Controlling drugs, monitoring utilization, and assisting in the distribution of medications to patients are among the pharmacist's most important contributions to health care. New regulations and the constantly changing health care environment require the methods of distributing and controlling drugs to undergo continuous reevaluation and review. Advancing technologies permit the pharmacist to move from the traditional product-focused dispensing role to the role of therapeutic adviser for both patients and prescribers. This shift in roles enables the pharmacist to become more active in improving therapeutic outcomes in disease management. An improvement in outcomes generally translates to reduced costs of care while improving the overall quality of care.

The pharmacy technician's role in the area of drug dispensing and distribution has expanded dramatically in recent years consistent with the changes in technology and pharmacy law. These changes have allowed the technician to better assist the pharmacist, which translates into their greater value as a member of the health care team. Pharmacy state boards are exploring numerous methods of integrating technicians into processes traditionally performed by pharmacists to allow time for the pharmacist to be more involved in the management of a patient's therapy. An important proposal under review by a number of pharmacy boards is a process called "tech–check–tech" (TCT). For example, in the area of medication cart filling, preliminary studies have shown that the process of having technicians check other technicians scores better than having a pharmacist check a technician's work. This appears to be the result of a technician having fewer interruptions than a pharmacist, thus improving the focus on the job of checking. Some pharmacy boards have approved the use of the TCT process.

After reviewing this chapter, the student should have an understanding of the overall drug distribution process and how the various drug distribution systems integrate into the delivery of patient care. The technician should be able to distinguish between the different types of distribution systems and clearly define the technician's role in the overall drug distribution process. The information provided is designed to support the technician in actively participating in both pharmacy system planning and development.

Drug Distribution

The drug distribution system begins to operate when a prescriber requests a medication to treat some diagnosed condition of a specific patient. The flowchart in **Figure 20-1** diagrams the generic process. Various methods are used to complete each step in the process, but we will focus on those more commonly used today.

Prescriber Ordering

Prescribers who order medications in a hospital must be certified by the appropriate hospital medical staff committee to practice within the hospital. A prescriber is defined as a licensed physician, a licensed physician's assistant, a licensed nurse practitioner, a licensed dentist, or any other professional category defined by the state's pharmacy board as eligible to prescribe a medication.

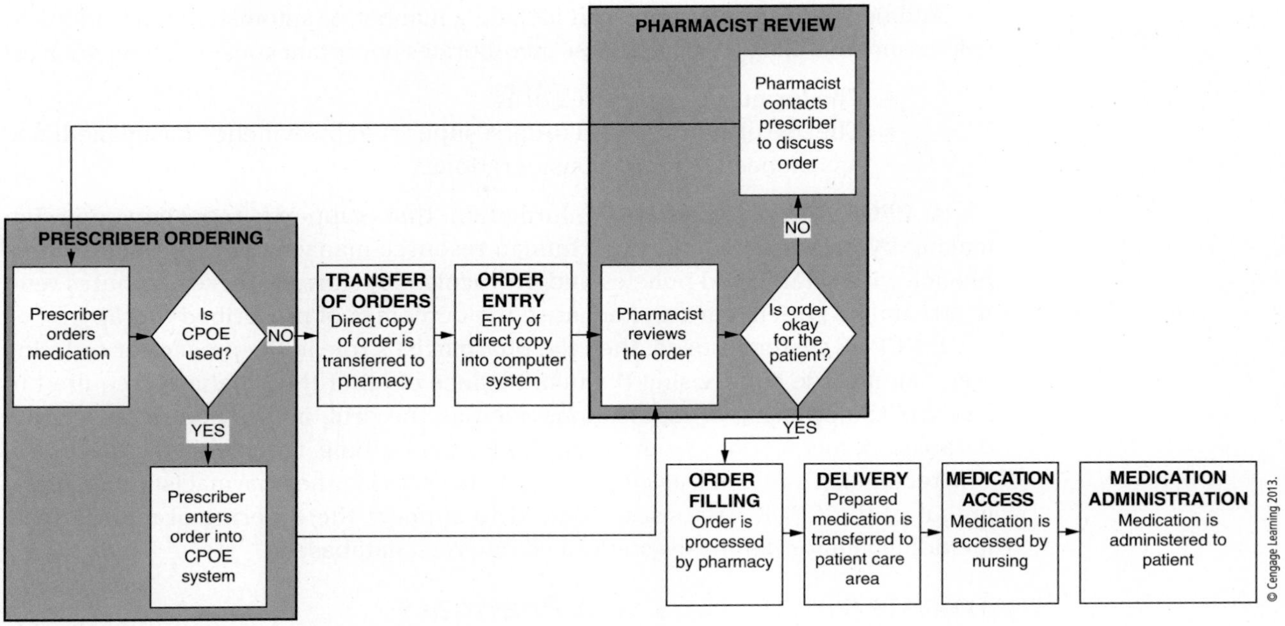

FIGURE 20-1 Drug distribution process.

All medication orders must appear in the patient's medical record. They can be written on a specific form by the prescriber, provided verbally to a nurse by a prescriber, or entered directly into a computer by the prescriber. Most hospitals have policies that require a prescriber to verify and sign any orders written by a caregiver in a patient's medical record within 24 hours if the order was provided verbally by the prescriber to the caregiver. A pharmacy technician cannot take a verbal medication order from a prescriber. A multiple-copy order form known as a **no carbon required (NCR) form** is commonly used when an order is written into a patient's medical record to aid in the distribution of the order to the appropriate caregivers.

no carbon required (NCR) form carbonless copy paper, non-carbon copy paper, or NCR paper is an alternative to carbon paper, used to make a copy of an original, handwritten (or mechanically typed) document without the use of any electronics

computerized prescriber order entry (CPOE) a drug order entered into a hospital-wide computer system and transmitted to a pharmacy

If the hospital has a **computerized prescriber order entry (CPOE)** system, then the prescriber enters the patient-specific medication order directly into that system. The medication order is queued electronically in the computer system for the pharmacist to review prior to production. If CPOE has been implemented by a hospital, then all work associated with the two steps discussed next, transferring orders to a pharmacy and order entry, is eliminated.

Numerous studies have shown that when a medication order is entered directly by a prescriber into a CPOE system the result is a significant reduction of errors due to:

- The elimination transcription errors
- Instant access to complete and accurate patient information
- The use of automatic dose calculation prompts specific to the requested medication
- The integration of clinical decision support software to prompt the prescriber for drug interactions, possible deviation from approved protocols, conflict with patient-known allergies, etc., in the order entry process
- The timely transfer of a medication order to a pharmacy for processing.

Additionally, CPOE systems can include a number of automated applications to help ensure that the ordering process incorporates important considerations such as:

- The formulary status of a drug
- The use of standardized orders, supported by evidence-based medicine
- Assistance with cost considerations.

A CPOE system generates information that supports reporting, decision making by prescribers, improved human resource management, and better compliance with established policies and protocols. Collectively, these attributes tend to streamline patient care and enhance the outcomes of prescribed therapy.

If a CPOE system is used, then the pharmacist's role in the prescriber ordering step can include supervising the maintenance of all of the databases required to support the ordering of medications such as the drug interaction database, the database of medications from pharmacy for prescribing, the allergy database, etc. The technician's role in this step can include assisting the pharmacist in maintaining all of the CPOE databases required to support the ordering of medications, including vendor databases such as commercial databases.

Transferring Orders to a Pharmacy

If the hospital's medication ordering is 100% CPOE, then the transfer of the prescriber's medication order to a pharmacy is a by-product of the prescriber's entry. However, even when a CPOE system has been installed and used, very few hospitals require all orders to be entered by a prescriber. Thus a manual process must be available to supplement CPOE, and in the case of a CPOE system failure, the manual process will function as a backup process so patient care is not disrupted.

Transmitting the prescriber's written medication order to the pharmacy is achieved in a variety of ways depending on the technology available in the hospital. The Joint Commission and most state boards of pharmacy require that a pharmacy receive, at a minimum, a direct copy of the prescriber's original prescription when filling medication orders. A "direct copy" has been defined to include either an NCR copy or a faxed copy of the original written order. The direct copy eliminates errors caused by attempting to manually transcribe a written order from one form to another.

The prescriber's written medication order must be transcribed into the appropriate computer system by someone other than the prescriber. However, if anyone other than a pharmacist transcribes the order, then state boards of pharmacy require that a pharmacist verify the transcribed order using a direct copy of the original written order. Generally the NCR direct copy is removed from the patient's medical record by nursing and placed in a pick-up tray for pharmacy. Nursing may also send the order to pharmacy via fax or a **pneumatic tube system**.

pneumatic tube system a method for sending a medication order from various locations in a hospital to its pharmacy by placing the order in a "tube" and sending it to a dispatcher, who then forwards it to a specific location

Recent advances in the management of faxed images allow faxed copies of medication orders to be stored electronically for recall by a pharmacy on a computer without the need to print a copy. These advances eliminate the need to store printed copies of medication orders and the need for the manual storage and retrieval of faxed orders that have been processed. However, when faxed orders are stored electronically, the pharmacy must have a backup and retrieval process in place for those electronic files.

The pharmacy technician's role in the step of transferring an order to a pharmacy may include the following tasks:

- Retrieve direct copies of orders from the patient care areas.
- Remove and stage direct copies of orders from a pneumatic tube system for order entry at the pharmacy.

- Maintain backup processes if faxes are stored electronically.
- Maintain any manual storage and retrieval system for direct or faxed copies of medications orders.

Order Entry

The entry of all medication orders into a patient-specific record is the norm for all hospitals regardless of the hospital's size. The method of entry varies significantly. It ranges from transcribing the medication order to a manual patient profile that is maintained with pen and paper and is accessible only by the pharmacy, to an enterprise-wide computerized patient care management system that all caregivers can access. The pen-and-paper manual patient profile is updated by a pharmacist. Generally this document functions as the record of all medications prescribed, dispensed by the pharmacy, and charged to the patient. Manual demographic information is added to the profile to aid the pharmacist in reviewing the patient's medications to identify any therapeutic issues. A completely manual patient profile may be used in small hospitals that do not have the financial resources to computerize the process. The processes used to maintain a manual profile compared to a computerized profile are similar; however, in the computerized version much of the actual work has been automated.

Computerization of patients' medication profiles has revolutionized medication order management. Computerization ranges from stand-alone pharmacy computer systems to fully integrated clinical care enterprise-wide systems serving all patients regardless of the care venue. Many different brands of computerized information management systems are available, each with its own advantages and disadvantages in how it manages a patient's medication orders. Each brand generally is present in health care in different versions. Each version can function much differently than prior versions of the same software. Technicians must devote time to learning the unique attributes of each system encountered to be effective and efficient in its use. Stand-alone pharmacy computer systems are generally interfaced (connected) to several other hospital departments' computerized systems, for example, accounting for charges, admitting for patient demographics, and the laboratory to obtain lab results.

Each computerized system offers the pharmacy a systematic method of medication order entry, patient profile development, label production, fill list generation, and report generation. Most systems provide some form of clinical cross-checking for allergy and sensitivity detection, dosage verification, drug-drug interactions, and food-drug interactions to aid in order entry when the order is keyed into the system. Most computerized information systems will support the common drug distribution systems.

Order entry into automation can be accomplished in several different ways:

- The nurse can enter the initial order into the computer system prior to supplying the pharmacy with a direct copy of the written order. The pharmacist then uses the direct copy to review the order entry for accuracy and then for appropriateness.
- The pharmacy technician can enter the medication order into the computer system and the order is suspended until the pharmacist has verified the entry and conducted her review.
- The pharmacist can enter the order into the computer system and conduct the review simultaneously (most common).
- The prescriber can enter his order directly into the computer system (CPOE) as described earlier in the order entry discussion (preferred).

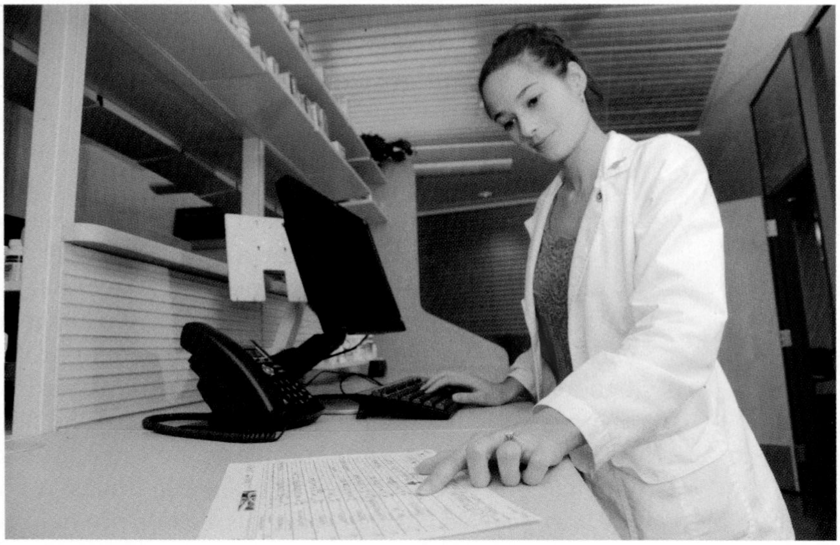

FIGURE 20-2 The pharmacy technician may be responsible for creating and maintaining the patient profile as well as entering the initial order entry for pharmacist review.

The pharmacist and the technician have differing roles when it comes to entering medication orders. The responsibilities are being evaluated by some state boards of pharmacy to determine whether some of the routine functions that pharmacists have performed in the past can be shifted to specially trained technicians.

The pharmacy technician's role in the order entry step may include the following tasks:

- Confirm that all necessary information pertaining to the patient's identification is available in the computer or on the patient profile (e.g., patient name, age, room number or location, hospital identification number, patient weight, allergies and sensitivities, the name of the prescriber).
- If a nurse has received a verbal or telephone order, confirm that the nurse's name follows the name of the ordering prescriber.
- Perform the initial order entry into the computerized profile (**Figure 20-2**) or transcribe it to a hand-generated profile if such a system is in use.
- Enter special patient charges or credits, request reports, maintain supporting databases, etc.

Pharmacist Review

A pharmacist's review of medications requested for use with a patient goes beyond the accurate entry of that order into a patient care computer system. The pharmacist must assess the appropriateness of the medication and its dosage in relation to the age, weight, known allergies or sensitivities, and general health of the patient. The pharmacist's assessment of the effect of combining this new medication with all of the other medications currently used in the patient's treatment to screen out possible drug–drug interactions and unwarranted therapy duplications is vitally important. Additionally, the pharmacist must consider the effect of the medication on the combined conditions currently being treated, because some medications can affect the amount or type of medication used to treat other conditions.

A complete listing of a patient's current medications, medication history, conditions under treatment, and pertinent patient demographic information is critical to the pharmacist's review process. These elements are generally available in the computer-based patient profile:

- Patient's full name, age, weight, gender, hospital identification number, bed location, and admitting prescriber's name
- Provisional diagnosis, secondary diagnosis, and confirmed diagnosis if available
- Allergies (e.g., food, drug, latex), sensitivities, and idiosyncrasies
- Drug history from patient interview
- Names of medications dispensed, dosage, directions for use, quantity dispensed, date, and initials of pharmacist
- IV therapy (e.g., large- and small-volume intravenous solutions) with or without additives, TPN fluids, chemotherapy, and so forth
- Laboratory data if known (e.g., electrolytes, creatinine, cultures, sensitivities)
- Diet (e.g., low-sodium diet)
- Selected diagnostic data related to coronary disease, diabetes, hypertension, and the like.

Depending on the hospital, some profiles contain clinical data such as laboratory results, antimicrobial culture results, and sensitivity reports. Previously used but discontinued drugs may also be visible.

During his order review process, the pharmacist may use any one of the many databases available locally or on the Internet that provides comprehensive drug information. These databases enable the pharmacist to confirm the appropriateness of drug use and dosage while checking for side effects, contraindications, laboratory test interferences, and so forth. If appropriate, much of this information can be copied and pasted into e-mails or other communication methods for discussion with prescribers or other professionals relative to a patient's treatment.

Enterprise-wide computerized patient care systems can generate patient medication profiles for a pharmacist, a caregiver, or a prescriber to use in evaluating a patient's treatment. These profiles generally include all information necessary for adequately supervising appropriate drug usage within the hospital. These profiles generally include complete patient demographics, all scheduled and unscheduled (e.g., PRN [as needed]) drugs, administration frequency, administration route, and appropriate cautionary statements.

If a medication order appears to be appropriate to the pharmacist, then the order is approved for production. However, when the pharmacist has a question about the use of a medication with a particular patient, she will contact the prescriber directly to resolve the question. The pharmacist may conduct either a voice-to-voice or electronic conversation with the prescriber depending on the available technology. The affected medication order is suspended until resolution is obtained.

Although the pharmacy technician does not currently have a role in the pharmacist review step, the future could include various types of prescreening of orders to ensure that all appropriate information is present for the pharmacist review.

Order Filling Process

Approved medication orders are queued by the computerized system for the order filling process. A written patient medication profile is used in lieu of a computerized

Pharmacy and Therapeutics Committee (P&T) the liaison between the department of pharmacy and the medical staff, consisting of physicians who represent the various clinical aspects; this committee selects the drugs to be used in the hospital. The pharmacy director is the secretary and a voting member of this committee

turnaround time the time required from order entry to delivery of medication to the patient care area

system. The hospital's **Pharmacy and Therapeutics Committee (P&T)** is responsible for the development and approval of broad policies and procedures governing the medication distribution system. One such requirement is turnaround time. **Turnaround time** is an important element in the delivery of the initial dose(s) of a new medication order. Generally, most hospitals require medications to be available in the patient care area for the nurse to administer to a patient within no more than 2 hours from the time the order is written by a prescriber. The time requirement for administration of a STAT (immediate) medication order ranges from 20 to 30 minutes from the time the order is written by the prescriber. Thus, each new medication order sent to production has its own clock, and the pharmacy must make every attempt to meet the turnaround time requirements. The order filling process step continues to undergo substantial change due to advances in technology and is the heart of the drug distribution process for the pharmacy technician.

Delivery Step

Many methods are used to move medications from where they are packaged to where they are needed. Almost all of them require the assistance of a technician to be effective. The more common methods in use are:

- Pneumatic tube
- Transportation courier
- Robotic delivery
- Dumbwaiter.

A transportation staging area is generally identified in the pharmacy where finished products are placed in some organized manner for delivery to the patient care area. The type of drug distribution system in use at the hospital will affect the type and frequency of deliveries.

Some hospitals have a centralized transportation courier system that delivers and transports medications, laboratory specimens, and supplies. In other hospitals and institutions, pharmacy technicians transport medications by providing order pickup and delivery. In a unit-dose exchange system, a technician uses a mobile cart to deliver medications in cassettes to the patient care area. Technicians will exchange full cassettes for those used during the previous 24-hour period and return the used cassettes to the pharmacy for crediting unused medications and refilling.

dumbwaiter an in-house elevator used to transport medications and supplies

Mechanical delivery systems like pneumatic tubes and dumbwaiter systems are part of the building's infrastructure. They are generally installed when the building is built or remodeled. The older the systems are, the less intelligent and dependable they are. Newer pneumatic tube systems have built-in intelligence that allows the user to track the delivery to the end user. **Dumbwaiter** systems are simply small elevators. Neither device informs the sender who received the target product. Unless you have some proof that the item arrived at its destination and who received it, then the delivery system can become an issue with missing or lost medications.

The pneumatic tube system utilizes carrier cartridges that are sent from the pharmacy department to terminals in designated patient care areas. This system is similar to that used by banks to handle drive-through transactions. A vacuum is created to pull the carrier to its destination. Any department may be served by such a system if it has a terminal. Each receiver of a pharmacy tube is responsible for returning the tube to the pharmacy. In the event of mechanical problems, a backup system must be available to ensure rapid transfer of needed medications to the area or patient. Delays in drug delivery have been a major source of irritation for nurses and may result in medication errors when the delivery time is excessive. A *significant drawback* to this system is the limitation on sending fluids because of weight and breakage issues.

The elevators and dumbwaiters used to transport medications move in only a vertical direction and may not be convenient to the patient care area; hence, health care personnel must move the materials from the elevator or dumbwaiter's lobby to the patient care area. Elevators and dumbwaiters are also subject to mechanical failures and may impose the need for technicians to use stairways to deliver medications to the nursing staff.

Robots are utilized in some hospitals. These mobile, computerized mechanical devices are programmed to move throughout the facility and deliver medications. They are able to detect and move around obstacles. The robot can call elevators in order to deliver medications to all floors of the hospital. Other hospitals have found small, track-mounted carts that move to and from patient care areas to be useful. The big advantage of this type of transport system is that it can handle bigger and heavier loads than virtually any other system; however, such systems are very expensive to install.

As mentioned earlier, all mechanical systems are subject to failures, and provisions must be made for alternate delivery methods when breakdowns occur. Drug security and control during transfer is a major concern that must always be considered in the selection and use of any transportation method. Pilferage, loss, and waste may create significant legal and financial problems.

The pharmacy technician's role in the delivery of medication may include the following tasks:

- Hand carrying finished medication orders to the appropriate patient care area
- Using a pneumatic tube system, a dumbwaiter system, or a robotic system to deliver finished medication orders to the appropriate patient care area.

Medication Access

The patient's caregiver must access the patient's medication prior to administration. The computerized patient medication profile is generally used to generate the **medication administration record (MAR)** for the caregiver. This tool can be generated on paper or provided electronically as a by-product of computerized order entry. It informs the caregiver as to what, when, how much, and what route to administer a drug. The computerized MAR can even prompt the caregiver electronically when it is time to administer a medication to a patient. The MAR is an essential tool for the accurate administration of medication to patients. If the MAR is manual, then daily updating of the MAR by nursing or pharmacy is essential to ensure all changes on the patient's profile within the past 24 hours are reflected. The goal of a paperless online MAR (e-MAR), along with an automated patient profile, is to provide ready access for the review of a pharmacist, nurse, or prescriber.

medication administration record (MAR) a record maintained by the nursing staff containing information about the patient's medication and its frequency of administration

The type of drug distribution system in use at a hospital affects how a medication is accessed by a caregiver:

- For an individual prescription system, the caregiver begins his search for the medication in the patient's storage bin on the patient care unit. If the medication is not found, then the other storage areas (e.g., the refrigerator, bulk storage areas, patient room) are searched until the medication is found.

- For the unit-dose drug distribution system (discussed in the next section), the caregiver begins his search for the medication in the patient bin or drawer in the medication cart. If the medication is not present in the patient's bin, then the caregiver must review other medication storage sites in the patient care unit to obtain the dose required.
- For the profile-enabled automated dispensing cabinet (ADC) system (discussed in the next section), the caregiver begins his search by accessing the patient's medication profile on the ADC computer. If the medication is present, the device opens the appropriate drawer from which the caregiver can remove the appropriate amount. If the medication is not in the cabinet or its attached devices, then the profile will generally direct the nurse to the storage location.

In all cases if the medication cannot be found, the caregiver contacts the pharmacy. Once the medication has been accessed, the caregiver prepares it for administration. This might require drawing the injectable up in a syringe or other actions that ready the medication for administration. If bar code medication administration (discussed in a later section) has been implemented at the hospital, then the caregiver should make every attempt to ensure that the medication remains in the package with the bar code until it arrives at the patient's bedside. This action allows the medication to be verified by scan to the patient and to his or her medication profile just prior to administration.

The pharmacy technician's role in the medication access can include the following task:

- If a printed MAR is provided by the pharmacy, then the technician may be responsible for generating and distributing updated MARs to the patient care areas every day.

Medication Administration

The administration of medications is generally accomplished by a nurse or other caregiver in the patient care area. The use of a properly implemented bar code medication administration program will significantly reduce the opportunity for errors. Just prior to administration the caregiver must scan his or her identification, the patient's identification, and the medication's identification. If the medication is still appropriate for this patient at this time, then the caregiver is given the okay to administer the medication. This process ensures that medications that might have been discontinued by the prescriber who uses a CPOE system as late as a few seconds prior to administration can be appropriately stopped by the caregiver. The administration of medications is covered in depth in Chapter 18.

Drug Distribution Systems

The overall drug distribution system used by the hospital must be approved by the P&T Committee. Four common drug distribution systems are used in hospital settings:

- Floor stock system
- Individual patient prescription system
- Unit-dose cassette exchange system
- Profile-enabled automated dispensing cabinet system.

Most hospitals use some combination of these approaches for drug distribution. These four approaches will be discussed from the most primitive to the most advanced. Additional components of the drug distribution system are covered in other chapters of this manual and include but are not limited to intravenous admixtures, controlled drug distribution, and interdepartmental requisitions.

Floor Stock System (Non-Patient-Specific Distribution)

floor stock system system in which medications are provided to the nursing unit for administration to the patient by a nurse, who is responsible for preparation and administration

The **floor stock system** of distribution is the most primitive approach to drug distribution. It is not used by itself in hospitals or long-term care facilities anymore; however, it may be used in some limited form to supplement another distribution approach. In a floor stock system of distribution, medications are stocked in the patient care unit *without regard to any individual patient.* As a medication is used, the caregiver records its usage on a patient-specific record, often a card with selected patient demographic information embossed at the top. The information may be written on the card for that patient or a sticker containing the product information could be attached to the card. The patient-specific cards are retrieved daily by pharmacy and entered into the hospital's billing system. In some cases this information is entered on the patient's medication profile as one-time doses. Floor-stocked medications are supposed to be replenished as pharmacy receives confirmation of their use with a patient. Each floor-stocked medication in the patient care areas should be inventoried periodically and unaccounted-for discrepancies reconciled with the nursing staff.

The traditional floor stock system relied heavily on the notion that individuals would record the use of medications. The system also relied on the fact that individuals other than pharmacists were capable of determining the appropriateness of a medication for a specific patient without input from a pharmacist. Full use of this approach to drug distribution is dangerous for patients and error prone. It is important to note that the traditional floor stock system was only connected back to the patient after the medication was used with the patient. Even then, the omission of documentation often failed to record any connection between the floor stock item and the patient. The traditional floor stock system removes important safeguards from the overall system and is relegated to a minor role in today's drug distribution systems.

The Joint Commission and other regulatory bodies are opposed to the use of the floor stock drug distribution approach with very few exceptions (i.e., emergency carts, items generally needed STAT in the patient care areas, or items deemed appropriate by the medical staff's P&T Committee). Medications that require an expanded level of professional supervision and control such as antineoplastic agents and antibiotics are excluded from floor stock supplies. Additional medications identified by *National Patient Safety Goals* as safety hazards are prohibited from floor stock (e.g., injectable potassium chloride).

The caregiver assumes total responsibility for the selection, preparation, and administration of floor stock medications independent of pharmacist oversight. This is **not** the preferred drug distribution system for either hospitals or long-term care facilities and should be strongly discouraged because of the following disadvantages:

- The increased potential for medication errors due to a lack of review by a pharmacist prior to patient administration
- The potential for selection of the wrong medication
- The potential for selection of the wrong dosage
- Use of an expired, contaminated, or deteriorated medication
- Economic loss due to theft or diversion of medication by hospital personnel
- Economic loss due to lack of documentation of use with patients.

The pharmacy technician's role in the floor stock system approach to drug distribution may include the following tasks:

- Routinely conduct floor stock inventories and report discrepancies to the pharmacist.
- Routinely replenish floor stock supplies to appropriate par levels.
- Routinely enter floor stock usage in the appropriate systems to record charges and patient-specific stock usage.

Individual Prescription System (Patient-Specific Distribution)

individual prescription system a system in which a multiple-day supply of each medication is dispensed for a patient upon receipt of prescriptions or medication orders

The **individual prescription system** of drug distribution has been used primarily in long-term care (LTC) facilities. In rare instances it has been used in hospitals, but its use in hospitals is not viewed favorably by most regulatory agencies. A routine medication order for a patient in a long-term care facility may be dispensed as a week's supply up to a month's supply. One-time-use medications are generally dispensed for the course of therapy. Generally, individual prescriptions dispensed for patients in long-term care facilities are not returnable or creditable to the patient once they have left the dispensing pharmacy and been received by the facility for the patient. Pharmacy's involvement is limited in the LTC facility drug distribution system. Pharmacy will conduct an on-site monthly review of the patient's medication therapies and advise the prescriber of any needed changes.

Usually an individual prescription system within a hospital will dispense a multiple-day supply of each medication ordered for a patient. Commonly, a 3- to 5-day supply is provided by the pharmacy. When the original supply is exhausted, the nurse prepares a refill request, and the whole process is repeated. An enormous amount of time and manpower is required. Maintenance of drug containers by the nursing staff in an organized, easily accessible method wastes valuable nursing time. The pharmacy is usually responsible for charges and credits, which are individually entered into the patient's account or forwarded to the business office for processing. Overall this system requires a lot of effort for all participants. In both hospitals and long-term care facilities limited floor stock may be added to provide for rapid access to selected medications (e.g., aspirin, acetaminophen, laxatives, or vitamins). Although this system is an improvement over the floor stock system because it uses patient-specific dispensing, it is not an efficient or practical method of drug distribution.

The pharmacy technician's role in the individual prescription system approach to drug distribution may include the following tasks:

- Pick and package medication for patient-specific medication orders.
- Stage processed orders for delivery to the appropriate location.
- Generate and manage any documents needed to support transportation of medications.

Unit-Dose Distribution System (Patient-Specific Distribution)

unit-dose distribution system a system in which medication is distributed in a single-dose or unit dose form from the pharmacy for use by the individual administering the drug

The **unit-dose distribution system** represents a significant refinement over the individual prescription system. It has been considered the safest, most economical method of distributing drugs in hospitals for a number of years. All unit-dose drug distribution systems provide patient-specific medications individually packaged for each prescribed dose. Medications dispensed to support this model are packaged as close as possible to the actual prescribed dose of the medication.

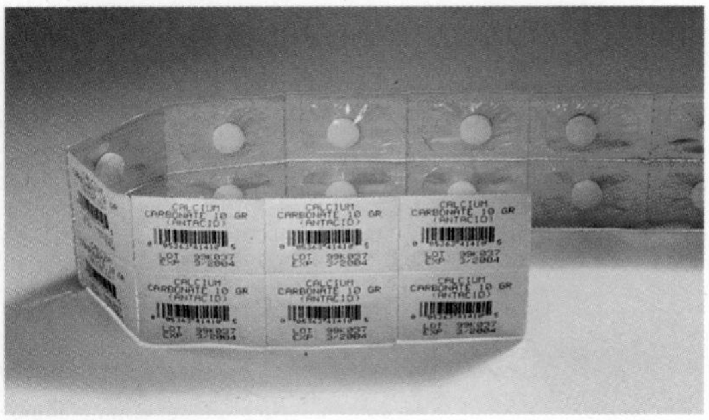

Courtesy of Capsa Solutions.

FIGURE 20-3 Example of unit-dose packaging.

unit-of-use
prescription medication that contains a quantity designed and intended to be dispensed directly to a patient for a specific use without modification

An example of an oral tablet in a **unit-of-use** package is shown in **Figure 20-3**. This type of drug distribution system is considered a hospital system, not simply a pharmacy system, because it involves many departments and disciplines in its planning, development, and operation.

The unit-dose drug distribution system has been the preferred drug distribution model of the federal government, The Joint Commission, the Institute for Safe Medication Practices, the Centers for Medicare and Medicaid Services, and state and local regulatory agencies for a number of years. It has been proven to be an effective drug distribution system with the following advantages:

- Fewer medication errors
- Improved drug control
- Decrease in the overall cost of medication distribution
- More precise medication billing
- Reduced drug inventories throughout the hospital.

A unit-dose drug distribution system can be implemented in various ways; however, the following are some common characteristics of all such systems:

1. The term *unit-dose* refers to the amount of a medication that a prescriber has ordered for a specific patient at a specific frequency by a specific route of administration. Unfortunately, the term *unit-dose* is often used to refer to the type of commercial packaging used to support a unit-dose drug distribution system. This chapter refers to the commercial packaging as *unit-of-use* instead of *unit-dose*.
2. The majority of medications are provided in a patient-specific storage bin or drawer in a “ready-to-use” form. The pharmacy replenishes the medications in the storage bin automatically at least once each day until the order is discontinued (**Figure 20-4**).
3. Hospital policy may affect how multiple-dose medications such as insulin, inhalers, ointments, or creams are handled. Generally, these items are patient specific and stored in the patient-specific bin or drawer. These items are replenished by the pharmacy when they have been fully consumed.
4. A large- or small-volume injection may be considered a “unit-dose,” but it is not normally included in the unit-dose drug distribution system.

Considerations of Unit-Dose Delivery

Virtually all medications can be dispensed as a *unit-dose*, which is defined as containing the individual dose of the drug ordered for a patient. For example, a unit-dose liquid may contain from a fraction of a milliliter to 60 or more milliliters, but *it is the exact amount ordered by the prescriber.* A unit-dose of a solid oral medication

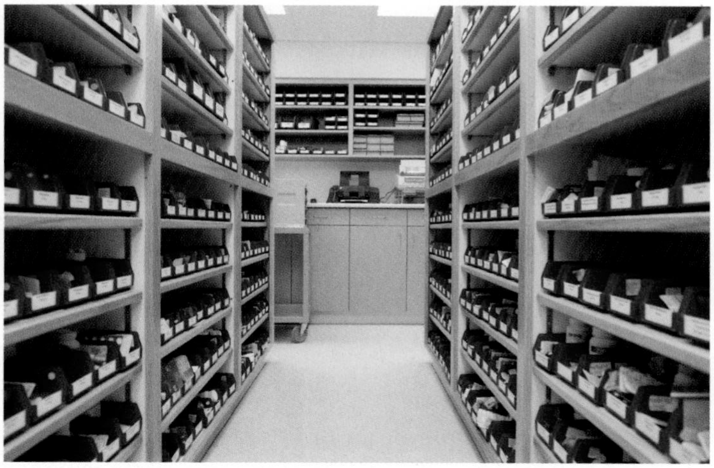

FIGURE 20-4 In a unit-dose drug distribution system, pharmacy technicians replenish the medications provided in patient-specific storage bins.

(tablets, capsules) may contain a fraction of one or more of the particular drugs, but it is the amount to be administered.

The term *single-dose* or *unit-of-use* package contains one discrete dosage unit, such as one tablet, 5 mL of a liquid, or a prefilled syringe containing a standard strength per milliliter. In the event that the dose prescribed and the dose sent vary, an auxiliary label "Note Dosage Strength" should be applied to the package to alert the nursing staff of the difference.

Cassette Exchange System

A common form of the unit-dose drug distribution system is the *cassette exchange system*. This system uses a cassette of individual bins as the storage area for medications. Each bin is labeled for a specific patient and is generally designed to contain a 24-hour supply of the patient's medications. In some long-term care facilities, a 48-hour or longer supply might be appropriate. Generally, each patient care area has two identical sets of cassettes. One set is kept in the patient care area to support the nurse's access to a patient's medication. The other set is kept in the pharmacy where it is replenished each day in anticipation of the daily cassette exchange process. The management of these cassettes is the single largest consumer of a pharmacy technician's time in the hospital environment.

The duplicate cassette maintained in the patient care area might be stored in a cabinet in the nursing station or located on a rolling cart that can be moved by the nurse to each patient's room. Numerous manufacturers supply these carts, which are of various design. Some manufacturers have incorporated mobile computer terminals on the carts to support the decentralized nursing management of medication administration. Regardless of what type of cart is used or where it is stored, it must be kept locked at all times when the caregiver is not actively accessing medications for patients. The storage of patient-specific medications is the primary objective for these carts; however, nursing will also store supplies on the cart to support the administration of medications.

Medication carts can be single sided or double sided and can contain as many as 60 patient-identified drawers for medications. The drawers may vary in length, width, and depth to accommodate the different needs of specific patient care areas. The bins or drawers may have dividers to separate the patient's medications into administration times or administration characteristics; for example, "as-needed" meds may be separated from "routine" meds. Drugs prescribed to be given early in the morning are located in the front of the drawer; those in the middle are given during the day; and those in the rear are scheduled for late evening or at bedtime. A final section might contain PRN (as-needed) drugs. Dividers of different colors may also be used to further distinguish administration periods.

If the cart has a computer terminal, it may limit access to the drawers depending on the vendor's software. The computer terminal is often used to inform the nurse regarding which medications should be administered to the patient at what time. It also can be used to document the administration of the medications, which can then transmit information to the billing system to record charges.

Proper maintenance of the patient bins is an important responsibility of the technician. Each drawer or bin must be properly labeled with a computer-generated, typed, or machine-printed label showing the patient's name, room number, and the prescriber's name. Due to patient confidentiality, care must be taken to prevent a patient's identity from being observed during transport through hospital corridors. Carts and bins should be cleaned frequently. When possible, bins should be taken at regular intervals, or when conditions indicate, to a location where they can be thoroughly washed and sanitized.

New medication orders are filled by a technician and checked by a pharmacist. The technician will fill the medication order with a sufficient supply to last through the next cassette exchange period. This supply of medication is labeled for the specific patient and delivered to the patient care area either by hand or through a pneumatic tube system. If it is delivered by hand, the medications are generally placed in the appropriate patient bin in the patient care area's cassette. If the supply is delivered by pneumatic tube (**Figure 20-5**), then the nursing personnel are responsible for placing the supply in the appropriate patient bin.

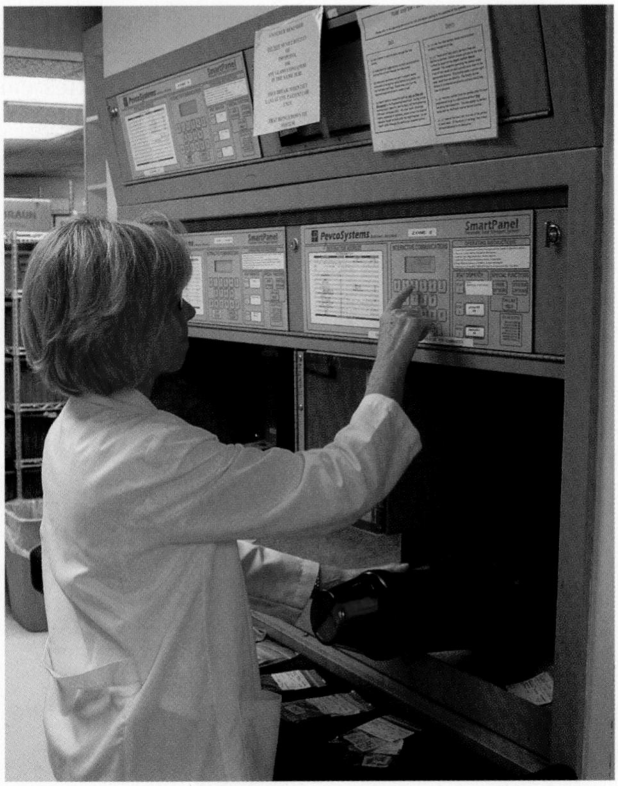

FIGURE 20-5 A pneumatic tube system may be used to transport medication from the hospital pharmacy to the nurses' station.

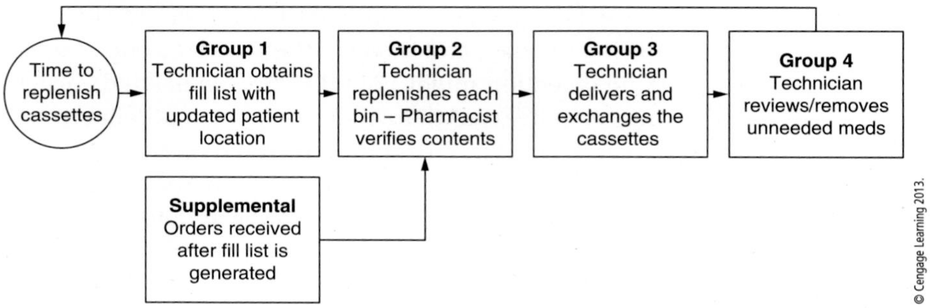

FIGURE 20-6 Flowchart of the replenishment activities for a cassette exchange system.

A small number of drugs, such as antineoplastics, might be prepared and hand delivered directly to the patient care area just prior to administration due to their stability, high cost, or hazardous nature.

A computerized unit-dose drug distribution system can generate automated reports that support the production activities required for day-to-day maintenance of the patient's medication needs. The same computerized information can support the transfer of charges to the patient's account by means of a direct interface to the hospital's financial system. Credits for drugs that are returned would be applied through the same interface. Inventory control can be managed by debiting inventory when dispensing occurs and crediting inventory when returns occur.

Generally the replenishment activities for the cassette exchange system are divided into four primary groups of activities as illustrated in the flowchart shown in **Figure 20-6**.

The cassette replenishment activities generally start at the same time each day, 7 days a week. The time is often set to ensure that most order changes made by prescribers have been entered into the computer system prior to running the "fill lists." The replenishment activities can be accomplished either in the central pharmacy or in a decentralized satellite.

Cassette Replenishment: Obtain Fill List

Group 1 activities are performed by the pharmacy technician as shown by the flowchart in **Figure 20-7**. If the pharmacy is computerized, then one or more computer terminals and printers need to be located in the picking area to permit technicians to generate fill lists, post charges, issue credits, and review patient profiles. A telephone is essential. A small compounding area and packaging area with a sink and running water should be immediately adjacent to the picking area.

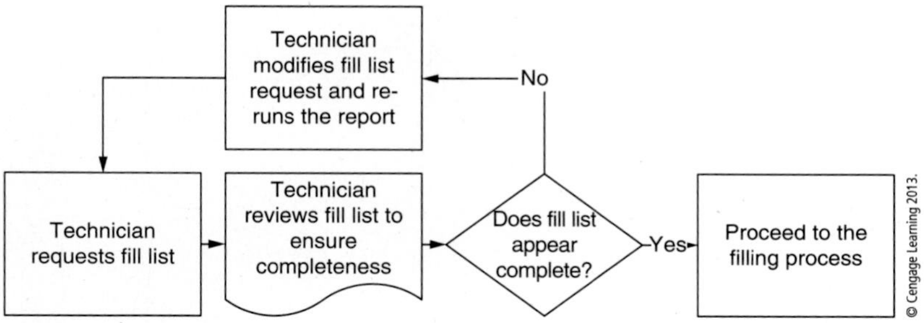

FIGURE 20-7 Flowchart of a pharmacy technician's responsibilities for Group 1 activities (see Figure 20-6).

If the pharmacy is not computerized, then there will not be a fill list. The technician would use the manual patient's profile maintained by the pharmacist to determine what will be needed in the cassettes. A computerized fill list will provide a listing of all medications required for the patient with their dosing frequencies, and it may suggest a quantity. The technician must review the computerized fill list to ensure that it appears to be complete.

The pharmacy technician role in obtaining the fill list for cassette replenishment may include the following tasks:

- Request and evaluate the completeness of the fill list from the computer system.
- Separate the fill list into the patient care areas.

Cassette Replenishment: Filling Process

Once the fill list has been confirmed, the technician will begin the activities associated with Group 2: replenishment of the cassettes as described in the flowchart in **Figure 20-8**. Group 2 activities begin with the technician would remove the bins or drawers of patients who have been transferred since the last exchange of cassettes. The technician then updates the patient bin labels.

The technician begins the review of the bins one at a time to determine what drugs remain in the bin from the previous day. Medications not on the fill list are removed from the bin. In some hospitals, this medication and its quantity would be noted on the fill list for future crediting before restocking. In other hospitals, the removed medications are just evaluated for restocking. If scheduled medications are found in the bin then in some hospitals the technician would be required to notify the pharmacist. The patient-specific bin's medication is replenished to the appropriate quantities identified on the fill list. The exact process used to replenish the bin depends on the policies in the specific hospital. Some hospitals empty the bins and replenish everything. Other hospitals bring the quantity of medications up to the number identified on the fill list.

The area in the pharmacy where unit-dose carts are processed generally consists of cabinets with slanted shelves. Plastic or cardboard bins are arranged to permit easy access by the technician to select the doses needed (**Figure 20-9**). These plastic or cardboard bins should be labeled in large letters showing the drug name (if possible, both the generic and brand names are posted) and strength. Circular cabinets with slanted shelves tend to be more efficient and can permit multiple technicians to work with minimum movement. Shelves should be within

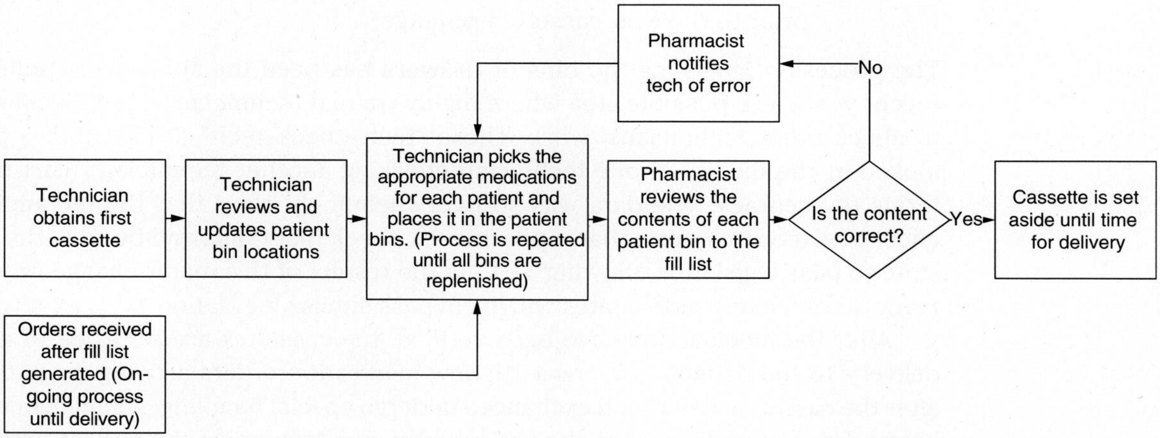

FIGURE 20-8 Flowchart of a pharmacy technician's responsibilities for Group 2 activities (see Figure 20-6).

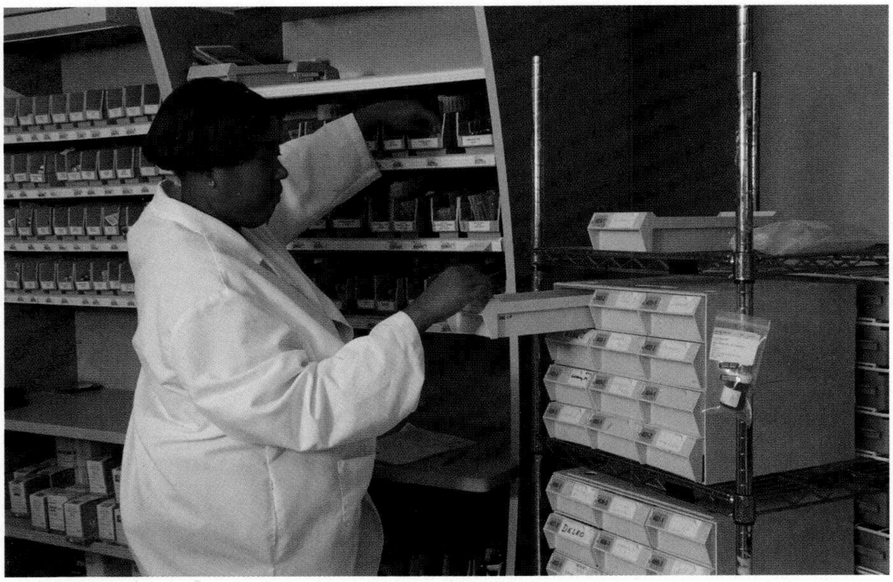

FIGURE 20-9 A vital responsibility of the pharmacy technician is to replenish and stock the medication carts.

easy reach and should require minimal stooping or stretching. Adequate lighting is essential, along with rubber mats on the floor to reduce the strain and fatigue of standing too long in one place. Sufficient space should be available outside the immediate picking area for storage of the transfer carts. This will allow the pharmacist to conduct the checking process with little distraction.

The number and variety of drug bins needed in the picking area change constantly due to the addition of new medications, changes in the fast movers, etc. The technician must ensure that the most frequently needed drugs are the most readily retrievable. Infrequently used items should be relegated to the general stock area. The area should be kept free of clutter and trash. Maintaining a clean and orderly picking area is absolutely necessary for optimum efficiency. Food or beverages should never be consumed in the picking area.

Once all of the bins in a cassette have been replenished, they are set aside for a pharmacist to:

- Check the bin labels to ensure that all patients are represented.
- Verify that each patient bin or drawer has been accurately replenished and that the drugs used to replenish the bin or drawer will not expire prior to the next cassette exchange.

The process of checking the bins or drawers has been the subject of studies in recent years as a possible area where highly trained technicians could be allowed to check other technicians' work. These "tech–check–tech" (TCT) studies have looked at the quality of one technician checking another technician's cart fill in terms of accuracy. The data was so overwhelmingly clear that the technician's check was more accurate than a pharmacist check that California became the first state to pass legislation allowing TCT. As the results of this major change in pharmacy unfold, many more states will likely pass similar legislation.

After the medications have been verified, the cassettes are set aside to await delivery to the patient care areas. All new medication orders arriving for patients after the cassettes have been exchanged undergo special handling. A sufficient number of doses must be sent to the patient care area to support the patient until the next cassette exchange occurs. Additionally, medication for the new order must be added to the patient's exchange bin in the pharmacy if the fill list has already been generated. Failure to do this will result in missed doses and significant rework.

robotics technology based on a mechanical device, programmed by remote control to accomplish manual activities, such as picking medications according to a patient's computerized profile

Robotics and Technology Many types of **robotics** devices are currently available to support the unit-dose drug distribution system. The number of mundane, repetitive tasks can be significantly reduced by the use of technology. A major advantage of automation is a significant decrease in the opportunity for errors through the automation of many repetitive tasks. However, technicians must remember that restocking one of these machines with the wrong medication can cause multiple errors before they are detected and corrected. Undivided attention must be maintained when restocking any automated device. Checking and double-checking is a must to ensure that this type of error is not committed. Some of the devices use bar codes to verify that the right product has been loaded.

One such device, the FastPak™ 330/520 by AmerisourceBergen, can manage up to 520 of the most common oral drugs used in a facility. The machine is interfaced with the main pharmacy computer system. Bulk drugs are repackaged into unit-dose drugs consistent with the patient's profile medication orders. For example, drug A is to be given at 0800, 1400, and 2000; drug B is to be given at 1200; and drug C is to be given at 0700 and 1900. The drugs are packaged in a strip with all of the patient's information. The packaged strip would be sequenced as follows: drug C, drug A, drug B, drug A, drug C, drug A. The use of this type of machine assists the health care provider with the proper sequencing for drug administration and virtually eliminates cart fill errors for oral solids. Additionally, this machine uses lower cost bulk medications to create the unit-doses so that unopened doses maybe reissued. However, if charges are generated at the time of filling, crediting for unused medications must be done manually. All medications other than oral solids must be hand-picked and incorporated into the bin or drawer manually.

Another device, the McKesson ROBOT-Rx® (shown in **Figure 20-10**), can select items other than oral medications for filling the patient's bin or drawer. The device is a three-axis robot that moves horizontally and vertically along rows of bar-coded prepackaged solid oral medications or small-volume vials or ampoules. The device hosts an electronic copy of the patient's medication profile obtained electronically from the main pharmacy computer system. This electronic copy of the patient's medication profile controls what is selected and how much is selected for the patient's bin or drawer.

A disadvantage of the ROBOT-Rx is the need for specialty packaging for all items managed by the robot. The robot can also issue credits for unused doses for items in robot-ready packaging. Restocking the robot is automatic. Items not

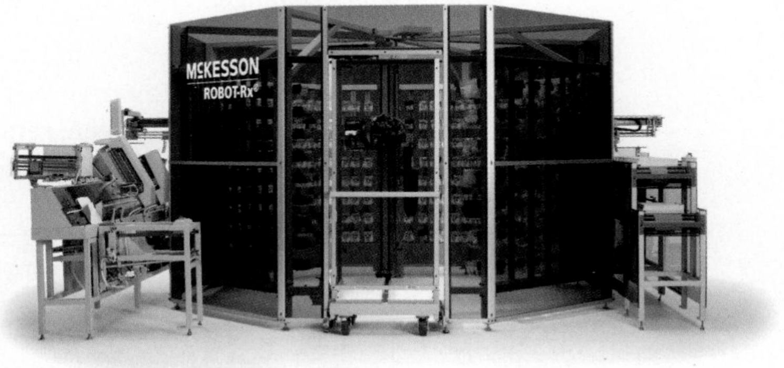

FIGURE 20-10 McKesson ROBOT-Rx® is another advancement in automated technology used in pharmaceutical drug delivery systems.

available to the robot must be hand-picked and incorporated into the patient's bin or drawer manually.

The pharmacy technician's role in replenishing the cassettes may include the following tasks:

- Prepare the cassettes for processing by evaluating and processing any medication returned from the previous day's cassette according to facility policy.
- Ensure that the bins or drawers are clean and ready for processing.
- Verify and update patient identification information on the patient bins or drawers in each cassette.
- If a robot is used, ensure that the robot has sufficient medication to process the cart fill operation.
- Hand-pick all medications present on the fill list that are not supplied by a robotic device and place them in the appropriate patient bin or drawer.
- Hand-pick medications for new orders received after the cassettes have been exchanged and place them in the appropriate patient bin or drawer.
- Hand-pick medications for new orders received after the fill list has been generated and place them in the appropriate bin.
- Place completed cassettes with their fill lists and fill list updates in the holding area until time for delivery.

Cassette Replenishment: Delivery and Exchange Process

At the appropriate time, the replenished cassettes are transported to the patient care area, and the activities listed in **Figure 20-11** are performed by the pharmacy technician. The cassettes are transported to the patient care areas by a pharmacy technician. The technician reviews the cassettes already in the patient care area to identify any medication that should be transferred to the replenished cassettes (e.g., creams, ointments, inhalers). In many hospitals these items are only replaced in the patient care area when nursing service notifies pharmacy that a replacement is needed. If mobile carts are used, the technician exchanges the cassettes and relocks the mobile cart. The old cassette is returned to pharmacy to restart the filling process for the next day.

The pharmacy technician's role in transporting the filled cassettes may include the following tasks:

- Physically transport the replenished cassettes to the patient care area.
- Review each patient bin or drawer for medications that must be transferred to the replenished cassette.
- Physically exchange the cassettes in a mobile cart or other storage area in the patient care area.
- Return all exchanged cassettes to the pharmacy to restart the process for the following day.

Cassette Replenishment: Reviews/Removes Medication

Sometime after the cassettes have been returned to the pharmacy, they are reviewed by the pharmacy technician as shown in **Figure 20-12**. This group of

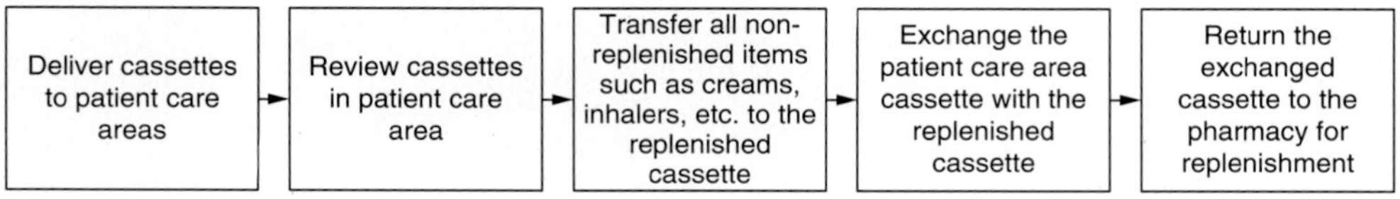

FIGURE 20-11 Flowchart of a pharmacy technician's responsibilities in delivery and transportation of cassettes.

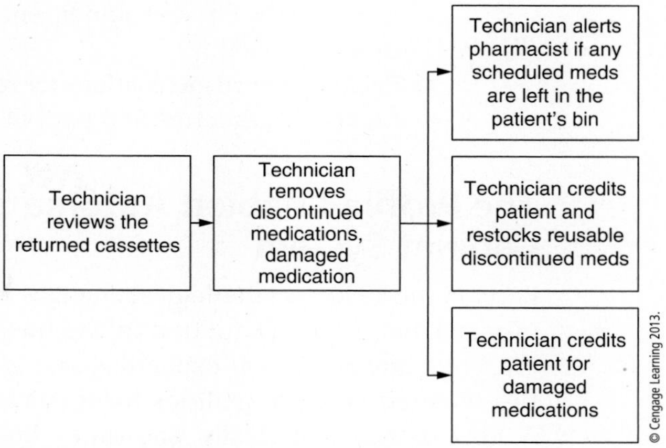

FIGURE 20-12 Flowchart of a pharmacy technician's responsibilities in reviewing the returned cassettes.

activities is an important component of the unit-dose drug distribution system. Medication remaining in the patient's bin generally represents medication that was not given to the patient. You would expect to find discontinued medications and medications given PRN (as needed) in the bin or drawer. However, doses of either damaged medications or any other medication may indicate a failure to administer unless that patient was discharged during the period. If this patient is still active, then the discrepancy should be reported to the pharmacist for follow-up.

Any of the medications returned in the bins or drawers that hospital policy says can be returned to stock should be evaluated for their expiration date and condition of the packaging. If the product has not expired and the packaging appears to be in good condition, then the medication should be restocked in the picking bins used to support replenishment. The technician should be extremely cautious when restocking these items to prevent placing the medication into the wrong bin. Incorrect restocking could lead to a filling error during the replenishment process.

Patient transfers in hospitals are very common due to the changing condition of the patient. The organization of hospital beds is built around the type of care the patient needs. As the patient's health care needs change, so does their location. For example, a patient may be admitted to an internal medicine bed then transferred to surgery. After surgery the patient goes to the postanesthesia recovery unit, followed by transfer to an intensive care bed. Finally the patient may be moved to a different internal medicine bed and then discharged.

It is not uncommon for a patient to be moved three or more times during a single admission. Medications are supposed to be moved with the patient but that often fails to happen, leaving all of that patient's medications in the original location. Generally these misplaced medications are credited and restocked during this group of activities. The impact of transfers and discontinued medication orders can generate a return rate of 25% or more for all medications dispensed for use with patients. The rework associated with this situation is substantial and has encouraged the development of new ways of managing the drug distribution needs within hospitals.

The pharmacy technician's role in reviewing or removing medications may include the following tasks:

- Evaluate the contents of the returned cassette's bins or drawers to identify remaining scheduled medications for reporting to the pharmacist.
- Evaluate the contents of the returned cassette's bins or drawers to remove discontinued items, damaged items, misplaced items, etc.

- If hospital policy requires, enter the appropriate credits for medications returned.
- Evaluate return medications for reuse. Restock medications deemed usable.
- Clean the cassettes and patient bins or drawers if needed.

The Profile-Enabled Automated Dispensing Cabinet System

Early in the 1990s, technological changes set the stage for a radically different way of managing drug distribution in the hospital. The processing speed of computers, combined with their expanding storage capacity and communication capabilities, created new possibilities for medication management device development. A new device generically known as an automated dispensing cabinet (ADC) emerged in the early 1990s. These cabinets were electromechanical devices controlled by computer software applications. The cabinets were built to store many different types of medications and limit access to those medications to only authorized individuals. Those devices have since evolved into intelligent medication storage sites with a sophisticated security system that limits access.

Today's devices can be connected to the electronic version of the patient's medication profile enabling them to be the primary source of medications in the patient care area. The software can limit access to the stored medications based on what has been ordered and approved for use by an individual patient. Some devices will only allow the caregiver to remove the exact dose required for a patient. Security identification is often accomplished through the use of a fingerprint or a login with a password. Up to 95% of all doses needed by patients can be made available through a profile-enabled automated dispensing cabinet.

Pyxis, Omnicell, and McKesson are three of the leading vendors of this type of patient profile-enabled ADCs to hospitals and other facilities. Medstation® 3500 by Pyxis, OmniRx® by Omnicell, and AcuDose-Rx® by McKesson are similar in that medications are securely stored in the patient care areas throughout a hospital. Each system has unique attributes that the vendors use to market their ADCs. These vendors are constantly upgrading and expanding their system offerings.

The ADC is easy to use. Once the caregiver has gained access to the ADC, she identifies the patient needing medications. The computer terminal on the ADC may bring up all of the patient's medications or only those that are currently due to be administered. The caregiver selects the appropriate medication, and the ADC releases a drawer or dispenses the appropriate dose like a vending machine. The caregiver removes the medication and continues with the process of administration. In some machines, the ADC records who removed the medication, how much medication was removed, and the time-date stamp of when the medication was removed.

The advantages for caregivers are significant. The caregiver has only one place to start collecting medications for administration to a patient. The ADC can even direct the caregiver to alternate locations if the requested product is not located in the cabinet. Controlled substances are managed through the ADC, eliminating the traditional controlled substance management systems, which previously were independent from all other drug distribution systems. The majority of medications are always available in the patient care area rather than having to be moved from the pharmacy to the care delivery area. The single most often heard complaint by nursing is the wait they may experience caused by too many caregivers trying to obtain medications at the same time. This can be solved by staggering administration schedules.

The use of profile-enabled ADCs has dramatically changed how pharmacy approaches the drug distribution system challenges. Turnaround time issues can be

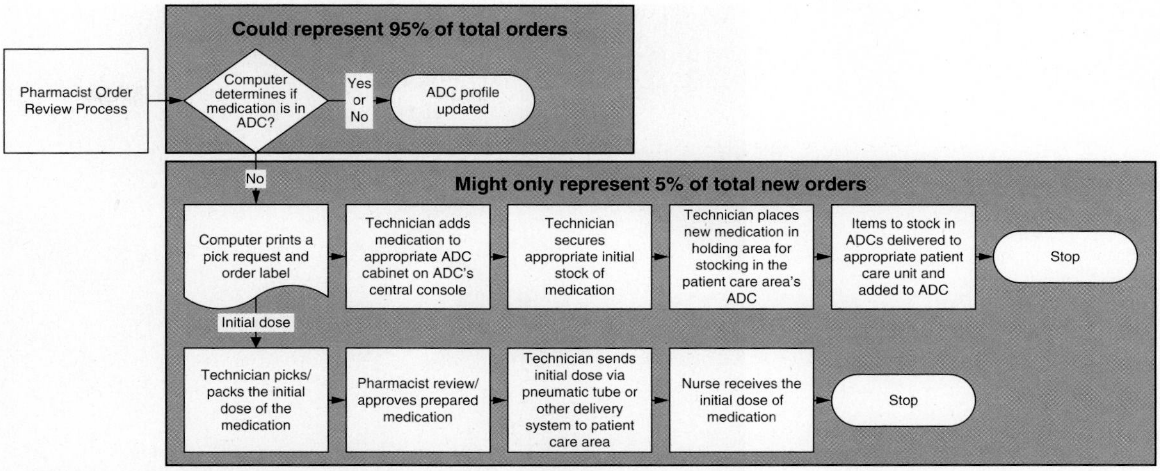

FIGURE 20-13 Flowchart of the basic activities that need to be accomplished to ensure the proper medications are available in the patient care area.

limited to only that small percentage of orders where the required medication is not in the appropriate ADC. Turnaround time is essentially limited to the length of time that it takes a pharmacist to review and clear a new medication order into production. **Figure 20-13** describes the basic activities that are required to ensure that ordered medications are available in patient care.

In this system, the drug distribution process is transformed into a materials management process that restocks a supply area rather than fills a patient-specific order for the majority of medication orders. The flowchart depicts the process used to supplement medications initially not available in the ADC, but ensures that the next time that same medication is needed, it will be readily available for the same patient or any other patient in that same patient care area. The profile-enabled ADC system provides a solution to the three largest challenges that have faced pharmacies using the unit-dose drug distribution system: (1) turnaround time for new medication orders, (2) missing doses, and (3) managing credits.

Patient medications that are not stocked in the ADC can be issued to a specific patient and still stored in the ADC for retrieval and documentation of usage. Some medications such as creams, ointments, lotions, and IV admixtures may be stocked in other locations. The medication profile on the ADC can direct the caregiver to those locations.

The pharmacy technician's role in interacting with an ADC approach to drug distribution may include the following tasks:

- Prepare the initial supplies for new medication orders for specific patients.
- Transport the initial supplies for new medication orders when released by the pharmacist.
- Modify the ADC stock to add new medications to appropriate locations.
- Ensure that the next replenishment cycle for the ADC incorporates the new medication.

Medication Labeling Considerations

Medications distributed through any of the drug distribution system models may be subject to either routine labeling or special labeling. The technician, in most cases, will be responsible for labeling medications. Labels may be computer generated,

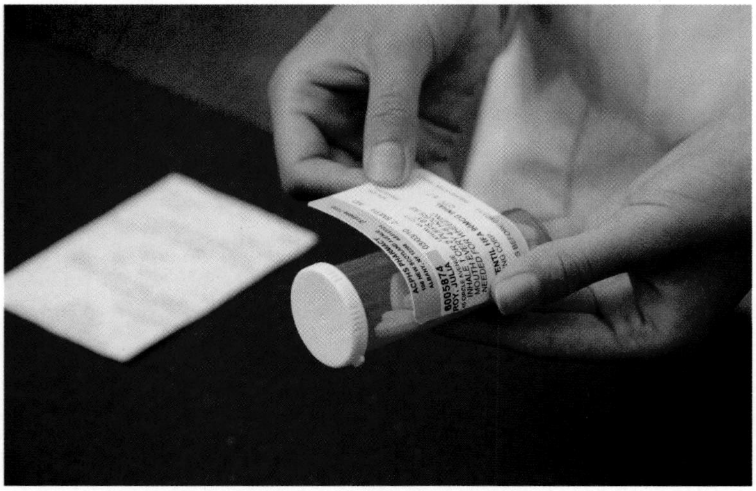

FIGURE 20-14 A primary responsibility of the pharmacy technician is to properly and neatly adhere the prescription label to the medication.

typed, or machine printed. Handwritten labels with pen, pencil, or marker are absolutely prohibited. One label should never be superimposed over a previous label. The label should be clear, legible, and free from erasures and strikeovers. It should be firmly affixed to the container (**Figure 20-14**). The pharmacist must always confirm the original prescriber's order with the drug and label prior to dispensing.

The appearance of the label may also affect how the patient views the hospital and the medication being used. A neat label demonstrates care in the handling of the medication. It may also signify to the patient that the drug is effective and will be beneficial. A sloppily printed label tends to reflect a lack of concern by the pharmacy and poor quality control. The patient, nurse, and prescriber could interpret this indifference as a lack of effectiveness of the drug or lack of concern for the patient's well-being.

With the exception of unit-dose or unit-of-use products, the label should bear the name, address, and the telephone number of the hospital or pharmacy. Medications should never be relabeled by nursing personnel or anyone other than personnel supervised by a pharmacist.

Changing the labeling on commercially packaged products must be accomplished with the same care that was used by the manufacturer. Appropriate records must be created for each product that undergoes relabeling for a specific patient. For more information on labeling, relabeling, or prepackaging, see Chapter 27 "Pharmaceutical Supply Chain."

Here are some important points to consider in labeling:

- The metric system, rather than the apothecary system, should be utilized (e.g., 65 milligrams rather than 1 grain).
- When dispensing medications, the technician should be aware of any needed auxiliary labels, which should be attached to the container. These may include, but are not limited to, the following:
  - "For the Eye"
  - "Keep in the Refrigerator"
  - "Shake Well Before Use"
  - "Swallow Whole: Do Not Crush, Break, or Chew"
  - "For the Ear"

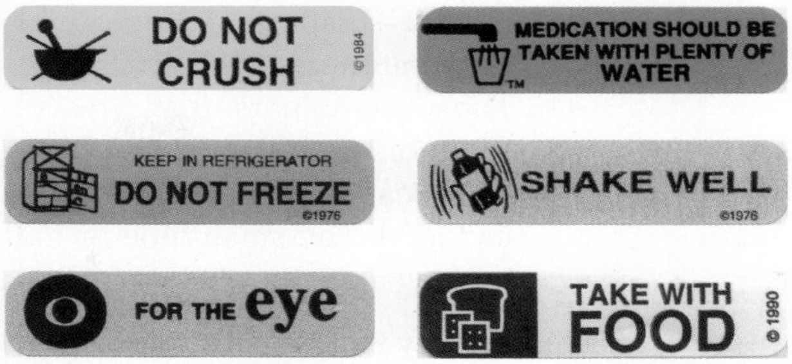

FIGURE 20-15 Examples of auxiliary labels.

  - "Poison: Not for Internal Use"
  - "Take with a Full Glass of Water"
- A multitude of auxiliary labels are available, and every pharmacy should have a representative supply on hand to assist patients or caregivers in understanding the appropriate use of the medication (**Figure 20-15**).
- When labeling a compounded prescription for inpatient use, the name and amount or percentage of each active ingredient should be indicated on the label. Prescriptions for outpatients should indicate the name of each therapeutically active ingredient.
- In the event the medication being labeled requires further dilution or reconstitution, the label should provide the appropriate directions. (*Note:* Effective unit-dose distribution systems should not require the nurse to conduct these operations; only in cases of extremely limited stability should this be allowed.)
- Expiration dates should always appear on both unit-dose and prescription labels. Little scientific information is available to assist the pharmacist in determining how long the effectiveness of a medication can be ensured once it is removed from the manufacturer's original container. Many hospitals will apply a 12-month expiration date, unless the manufacturer's date is shorter. In *no* case should the expiration date exceed that of the original container. Special circumstances will require that a specific expiration date be assigned. For example, many antibiotics for oral suspension when reconstituted are stable for no longer than 7 to 14 days. Packaging materials, storage conditions, light conditions, and other factors must be considered in assigning an appropriate expiration date. The primary or a secondary label should indicate the following: "Expiration Date: ________" or "Use Before ________."
- Parenteral medications may require special labeling in that the route of administration should be indicated (e.g., "For IM Use Only" or "Not for IV Use").
- Labels for large- and small-volume intravenous solutions should be placed on the container to allow visual inspection of the solution, and they should not cover the original solution (carrier) labeling. Remember to place the label so that it is readable in the hanging position of the container.
- If the medication is an oncology or chemotherapeutic medication, an auxiliary label must be attached indicating "Special Handling—Chemo

Hazard—Dispose of Properly." This label should be applied to all forms of chemotherapeutic drugs, whether they are oral, topical, or injectable.
- Those containers that present difficulty in labeling, such as small tubes or bottles, must be labeled with a minimum of the patient's name and location. If possible, the drug name and strength should also be included. The small tube or bottle can be placed in a larger container bearing another label with all of the pertinent information.

The pharmacy technician's role in labeling medication may include the following tasks:

- Identify medications to be labeled and what labeling is required.
- Generate labels and obtain product to be labeled.
- Complete appropriate information in the relabeling log.

Nonsterile Medication Compounding Considerations

Qualified pharmacy technicians may be allowed to conduct compounding and manufacturing under a pharmacist's direction and supervision. The term *compounding* is used if two or more drugs are mixed together. The term *manufacturing* is used if more than a single dose of a compounded product is prepared for future dispensing.

The first step of manufacturing is the recording of the process in the manufacturing log and obtaining a lot number for the product. A manufacturing worksheet is initiated and the lot number is recorded. All components are identified by name, manufacturer, lot number, and quantitative amounts on the manufacturing worksheet. Medications that are routinely manufactured generally have a formulation card similar to a recipe that describes how the product is made. Samples of labels and any required accessory labels are attached to the formulation card. A formulation card is created if one does not already exist. The formulation card should contain at least the lot number for the batch, the name of the finished product, the strength of the finished product if appropriate, the date of manufacture, the compounding directions, a complete listing of all ingredients with their quantity and a copy of the sample label and required accessory labels. A specific time, not to exceed 5 years, must be determined for when the product will expire and no longer be acceptable for use in patient care. This is usually determined by individual State Boards of Pharmacy.

The technician generally assembles all of the components to be used in the process. The technician records all of the appropriate information on the manufacturing sheet noting the amount that will be prepared and notifies the pharmacist. The pharmacist verifies the components, the quantity of each, and the information recorded on the formulation card for accuracy. The technician measures, weighs, and mixes the components according to the directions provided on the formulation card. The manufactured product is packaged in the appropriate containers and labeled. The finished product is inspected by the pharmacist.

Individual hospital's policies may differ some from the description above but probably will be similar.

The pharmacy technician's role in the nonsterile compounding may include the following tasks:

- Determine what needs to be manufactured.
- Obtain a lot number and formulation card for the product.
- Initiate the manufacturing sheet.

- Assemble the ingredients and measure out the appropriate amounts of each.
- Mix the ingredients in the appropriate sequence as described on the formulation card.
- Measure out the product into appropriate containers and note on the manufacturing sheet.
- Label all filled containers and add all appropriate accessory labels.

Use of Bar Codes

Bar code technology was first used in the general retail industry to assist in keeping up with inventory. Since it worked so well in inventory management, bar code technology was adopted as a method of ensuring that all retail items were sold for the right price. Early applications in health care were limited to charge recovery applications. Today, bar codes have become an essential component of many drug distribution systems. Reading small print in dim light and sometimes in bright light is problematic for the caregiver. Labeling space on many medications is very small and medication names are complicated. Bar codes help the caregiver ensure that they have the right medication when it comes time to administer that medication to a patient. Today's bar codes on pharmacy-dispensed products can tie the product to the patient through computer software programs to eliminate the majority of opportunity errors in the delivery of medications. Health care has embraced the use of bar codes. In many hospitals bar codes are used by a caregiver to validate that they have the right medication, in the right dose, for the right patient.

The volume of information contained in the bar code depends on the type of bar code that is used. Many different formats are currently in use. They range from being able to represent a single short reference number to pages of text. A Food and Drug Administration (FDA) rule change in 2003 required bar-coded labels on all manufactured human drugs and biologicals. As of 2011 many manufacturers have complied with this requirement on their unit-of-sale packages (i.e., packages of 100 unit-of-use packages). However, for a **bar code medication administration (BCMA)** program to work effectively, all medications delivered to the patient care area must have a bar code. The lack of bar codes on all commercial unit-of-use packaging creates a substantial challenge to pharmacy drug distribution systems. As discussed in Chapter 27 "Pharmaceutical Supply Chain," significant changes must occur in the receiving processes associated with pharmacy practice to effectively use bar codes in patient care.

bar code medication administration (BCMA) is a barcode system designed to prevent medication errors in healthcare settings and improve the quality and safety of medication administration. The overall goals of BCMA are to improve accuracy, prevent errors, and generate online records of medication administration.

When medications are not available from a manufacturer in an appropriate unit-of-use package, then the pharmacy must have a process in place for applying a suitable bar code to the product. The process generally uses unit-dosing packaging equipment (either manual or automated) that packages the product and adds a readable bar code to the label. The bar code must be compatible with existing systems already in use throughout the health care system, such as bar code scanners. Hospitals can overwrap products with a manual bar code, package products with bar codes, or outsource some medications to be bar coded by an external vendor. Bottom line, all products must have a readable bar code that is used to support patient care if the hospital has decided to implement BCMA.

There is no question that the use of bar codes can reduce the opportunity for errors and strengthen the overall drug distribution system. The challenge for

radio-frequency identification device (RFID) is the wireless noncontact use of radio-frequency electromagnetic fields to transfer data, for the purpose of automatically identifying and tracking tags attached to objects. The tags contain electronically stored information

pharmacy is the effective implementation of a BCMA program. **Radio-frequency identification devices (RFIDs)** are emerging as a possible substitute for the traditional bar code. Retail merchandising has already adopted this emerging technology to reduce its theft problems. These devices can be imbedded in a label eliminating the need for space on the printed label. These devices could support a passive form of documentation of who gave the med, what they gave, when they gave it, and who they gave it to. The elimination of a handheld scanner and the need for action should move this process to the next level of safety and accountability.

The pharmacy technician's role in using bar code technology may include the following tasks:

- Determine what products require relabeling with a bar code.
- Complete appropriate batch records for each group of products undergoing relabeling.

Collateral Areas of Responsibilities

The pharmacy technician is responsible for ensuring that all work areas are kept clean and orderly. Telephones act as the primary connection between patient care areas and the pharmacy. Courteously answering the telephone in a timely manner is another important function of the technician. Telephone courtesy can go a long way toward building better relationships with the members of other departments in a hospital. The interaction during a telephone call may be other staff members' only way to determine how focused pharmacy is on the quality of patient service. Thus it is important to always remain courteous and helpful during those conversations (**Figure 20-16**). The technician generally screens phone calls and refers callers to the appropriate individuals. All questions of a clinical or drug-action nature must be directed to the supervising pharmacist for his or her professional judgment.

The many areas that support the drug distribution system are discussed in other chapters.

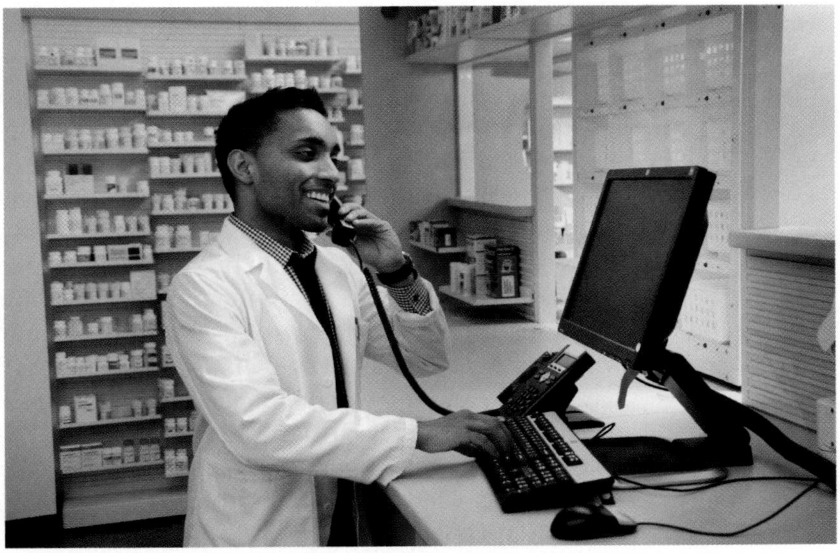

FIGURE 20-16 Exhibiting polite and courteous behavior during phone conversations is an important area where pharmacy technicians should try to excel.

The Future

The reduction of medication errors is an important goal in health care today. The proper use and implementation of automation will help the pharmacy team manage many of the redundant tasks associated with drug distribution that could otherwise generate errors. However, automation by itself without thoughtful implementation can lead to errors. The entire pharmacy team of pharmacists and technicians should be involved in the design of how automation is assembled in their hospitals to effectively remove the opportunities for errors. The use of CPOE will continue to expand and undergo refinements. Expert systems that aid the prescriber to generate more refined and appropriate medication orders will remove a lot of rework from future processes. As pharmacy fully implements the use of bar codes in their operations, the overall management of medications will become more precise and predictable. The future use of RFID technology to identify products will convert the manual process of scanning into the passive management of identification. The use of profile-enabled ADC systems will continue to expand and become more intelligent with the incorporation of RFID packaged medications. The goal of providing a safer environment for patients will continue to be the focus of health care systems because it is also the least expensive type of care.

The pharmacy profession will look to technicians to assume more of the distribution workload and responsibilities, thus freeing time for the pharmacist to be more involved in the clinical management of patients. The pharmacy technician may be called on to assist pharmacists as they assume their new clinical roles. For example, technicians could be trained to:

- Follow the pain management therapy of patients and provide information to the pharmacist to support their clinical role of medication management.
- Assist the pharmacist in spotting the potential diversion of controlled substances or other high-value medications.
- Identify patients on IV therapy who might be switched to an oral medication, resulting in both a less hazardous type of care and potential cost containment.
- Interview a patient at the time of his admission to document previous medical history. The resulting information could be used by the pharmacist to analyze what therapy might be appropriate during the patient's hospital stay.

As the procurement of medications becomes more challenging, the technician participating in the analysis of drug use and alternative therapies could assist the pharmacy's buyer in making purchasing decisions that could result in significant cost savings.

An underlying factor that can impede the growth of the pharmacy technician's capabilities and responsibilities is the current lack of standards for technician education and training. An important remedy to this challenge is the formation of a nationally recognized organization that sets the standards, supports continuing education, and provides for some level of certification of competency. An organization similar to the Accreditation Council for Pharmacy Education (ACPE), which performs similar functions for pharmacist education, could benefit the technician. Once pharmacy technician education has been standardized and meaningful testing of the required knowledge accomplished, then and only then will the role of the pharmacy technician be allowed to move forward. This will also increase the confidence and respect of pharmacists toward technicians and their profession.

Summary

In this chapter, the technician's role in drug distribution has been generally described. The functions depicted are broad in nature and not all inclusive. Only a small segment of the actual duties have been outlined. Each hospital pharmacy defines its operational requirements with the aid of the P&T Committee in policies and procedures. These policies and procedures should be covered in the initial orientation and training provided to new employees. The pharmacy should also have an ongoing continuing education program to ensure that all pharmacy technicians have access to the most current requirements at that hospital.

Because pharmacy is a dynamic profession, the roles of pharmacists and technicians are evolving from a product-oriented profession to a patient-oriented profession. The technician must be willing to continue the learning process, be open to innovative ideas, and be willing to assume newer responsibilities, which may be required as the profession of pharmacy advances.

TEST YOUR KNOWLEDGE

Multiple Choice

1. All of the following are acceptable ways to distribute medications to nursing stations *except*
   a. pharmacy courier.
   b. dumbwaiter.
   c. patients picking up their own medications.
   d. pneumatic tube system.

2. When using a pneumatic tube system, what precautions should first be considered?
   a. weight of item being sent
   b. possibility of breakage
   c. a and b
   d. none of the above

3. Telephone medication orders should be handled by
   a. the senior technician.
   b. a pharmacist.
   c. a and b.
   d. none of the above.

4. Identify the tool that allows the data from one computer system to be processed by a different computer system.
   a. modem
   b. mouse
   c. Internet connection
   d. interface

5. Which of the following is not a major vendor in pharmacy automation?
   a. Omnicell
   b. Pyxis
   c. Novation
   d. McKesson

6. The organization that sets practice standards and evaluates accreditation of health care facilities is the
   a. FDA.
   b. Joint Commission
   c. DEA.
   d. EPA.

7. Dumbwaiters are limited in their usefulness because of their
   a. horizontal movement only.
   b. vertical movement only.
   c. weight restrictions.
   d. noisiness during operation.

8. Compounding may only be performed by a
   a. registered pharmacist.
   b. a pharmacy technician under the supervision of a pharmacist.
   c. a and b.
   d. none of the above.

Matching

Match the terms with its definition:

1. ______ ASHP
2. ______ robotics
3. ______ MAR
4. ______ technician order entry
5. ______ pneumatic tube
6. ______ dumbwaiter
7. ______ NCR
8. ______ facsimile equipment

a. used by banks and hospitals for transportation
b. national organization for pharmacists and technicians
c. computerized robot for cassette filling
d. medication administration record
e. must be validated by a pharmacist
f. elevator for transporting medications or orders
g. fax
h. no carbon required

Fill in the Blank

1. The type of distribution system in which all medications are stocked on each nursing unit is called the ______________ system.
2. The elimination of errors resulting from illegible information, automatic dose calculation, and clinical decision-making support at the point of care are all benefits of ______________.
3. All information about a patient is maintained in the ______________.
4. “Shake Well Before Use,” “For the Eye,” and “Keep Refrigerated” are all examples of ______________.

Suggested Readings

Desselle, S. (2005). Certified pharmacy technician's views on their medication preparation errors and educational needs. *American Journal of Health-System Pharmacy, 62*, 1992–1997.

Keresztes, J. (2006). Role of pharmacy technicians in the development of clinical pharmacy. *Annals of Pharmacotherapy, 40*, 2015–2019.

Lefkowitz, S., Cheiken, H., & Barnhart, M. R. (1991). A trial of the use of bar code technology to restructure a drug distribution and administration system. *Hospital Pharmacist, 26*, 239–242.

Mansfield, B. (2007). The role of pharmacy technicians with reducing medication errors. *RXinnovate Healthcare Consulting*. Retrieved from http://www.continuingeducation.com

Paoletti, R., Suess, T., et al. (2007). Using bar-code technology and medication observation methodology for safer medication administration. *American Journal of Health-System Pharmacy, 64*, 536–543.

Poon, E., Cina, J., et al. (2006). Medication dispensing errors and potential adverse drug events before and after implementing bar code technology in the pharmacy. *American College of Physicians, 145*, 426–434.

Skibinski, K., White, B., et al. (2007). Effects of technological interventions on the safety of a medication-use system. *American Journal of Health-System Pharmacy, 64*, 90–96.

Weber, E., Hepfinger, C., & Koontz, R. (2005). Pharmacy technicians supporting clinical functions. *American Journal of Health-System Pharmacy, 62*, 2466–2472.

Manufacturers

Automed, 875 Woodlands Parkway, Vernon Hills, IL 60061. Phone: (888)537-3102; www.automedrx.com

McKesson Automation, 700 Waterfront Drive, Pittsburgh, PA 15222. Phone: (412)209-1400; www.mckesson.com

Omnicell, 1101 East Meadow Dr., Palo Alto, CA 94303. Phone: (800)850-6664; www.omnicell.com

Pyxis Corporation, 3750 Torrey View Ct., San Diego, CA 92130. Phone: (800)367-9947; www.pyxis.com

CHAPTER

21

Infection Control and Prevention in the Pharmacy

Competencies

Upon completion of this chapter, the reader should be able to:

1. List four general causes of contamination of pharmaceuticals and sterile pharmacy products.
2. Describe three principal goals for infection control and prevention programs.
3. List three basic principles of asepsis.
4. Name the precautions used by health care workers to protect themselves and others from exposure to bloodborne and other pathogens.
5. Cite three bloodborne pathogens of most concern to health care workers and for which OSHA exposure control plans are designed.
6. Recognize and describe the routes of transmission of microorganisms.
7. List components of the routine precautions used by health care workers to protect themselves and others from infections.
8. Explain what health care workers do when a possible occupational exposure to bloodborne pathogens occurs.

Key Terms

agent
airborne droplet nuclei
airborne transmission
asepsis
bacteria
bloodborne pathogen
chain of infection
cohorting
colonized
contact transmission
direct-contact transmission
droplet transmission
exposure control plan
fungi
indirect-contact transmission
infection
mode of transmission
multidrug-resistant organism (MDRO)
pathogen
personal protective equipment (PPE)
portal of entry
portal of exit
protozoa
reservoir
rickettsia
standard precautions
susceptible host
tuberculin skin test (TST)
vector-borne transmission
vehicle transmission
virus

Introduction

infection the state or condition in which the body (or part of it) is invaded by an agent that multiplies and produces an injurious effect

pathogen disease-causing organism

bacteria small, one-celled microorganisms that need a nourishing environment to survive

virus a submicroscopic agent of infectious disease that is capable of reproduction

fungi yeasts or molds that obtain food from living organisms

protozoa single-celled parasitic organisms with the ability to move

The infection control and prevention practices essential to ensure safe pharmaceuticals for patients are fundamentally rooted in good hygiene and sanitary practices. For example, hand hygiene is considered the single most important infection control measure practiced by health care workers. To prevent the spread of infection to themselves and to others, however, pharmacy workers need additional infection control education. Fortunately, the principles of infection control and prevention, once learned, are relevant to any health care setting. The information presented here is applicable to a freestanding pharmacy, acute care hospital, skilled nursing facility, home care program, or any other setting where pharmacy personnel work. Pharmacy personnel are responsible for ensuring that drugs and solutions are handled in a manner that prevents contamination and protects sterility when indicated. The pharmacy is responsible for the preparation and storage of most sterile medications and, in more and more instances, for managing intravenous therapy admixtures and enteral nutritional products. The pharmacist and pharmacy staff need knowledge of infection control and prevention first and foremost because patient morbidity (sickness) and mortality (death) can result from contaminated pharmaceuticals. Meticulous attention is needed to prevent the introduction and transmission of germs.

Infections

rickettsia intercellular parasites that need to be in living cells to reproduce

chain of infection the elements needed in order for an infection to occur

agent disease causing; may be biological, such as a bacteria or virus; chemical, such as medications or pesticides; or physical, such as radiation or heat

reservoir a place where a disease-causing agent can survive

portal of exit the route by which an agent moves from a reservoir to a susceptible host; may be through body secretions such as saliva, blood, and urine

mode of transmission the way in which the disease-causing agent is moved between the portal of exit and the portal of entry to a susceptible host

An **infection** is the damaging of body tissues or organs by the introduction of a **pathogen** (disease-causing organism). Five types of pathogenic organisms cause disease:

- **Bacteria:** small, one-celled microorganisms that need a nourishing environment to survive. Examples of diseases caused by bacteria are pneumonia and urinary tract infections.
- **Viruses:** organisms that can only live within another cell. Examples of viruses are the common cold, hepatitis, and genital herpes.
- **Fungi:** yeasts or molds that obtain food from living organisms. An example of a fungus is athlete's foot.
- **Protozoa:** single-celled parasitic organisms with the ability to move. An example of a protozoal infection is malaria.
- **Rickettsia:** intercellular parasites that need to be in living cells to reproduce. Lyme disease and Rocky Mountain spotted fever are caused by rickettsia.

Infection is an interactive process involving the agent, host, and environment. For an infection to occur, several essential elements need to take place; this process is often referred to as the **chain of infection** (**Figure 21-1**):

- A disease-causing agent must be present. An **agent** may be biological, such as a bacteria or virus; chemical, such as medications or pesticides; or physical, such as radiation or heat.
- A **reservoir** where the agent can survive must be present. This reservoir must contain the proper nutrients to keep the agent alive.
- A **portal of exit** from the reservoir to the susceptible host must be available. This can occur through body secretions such as saliva, blood, and urine.

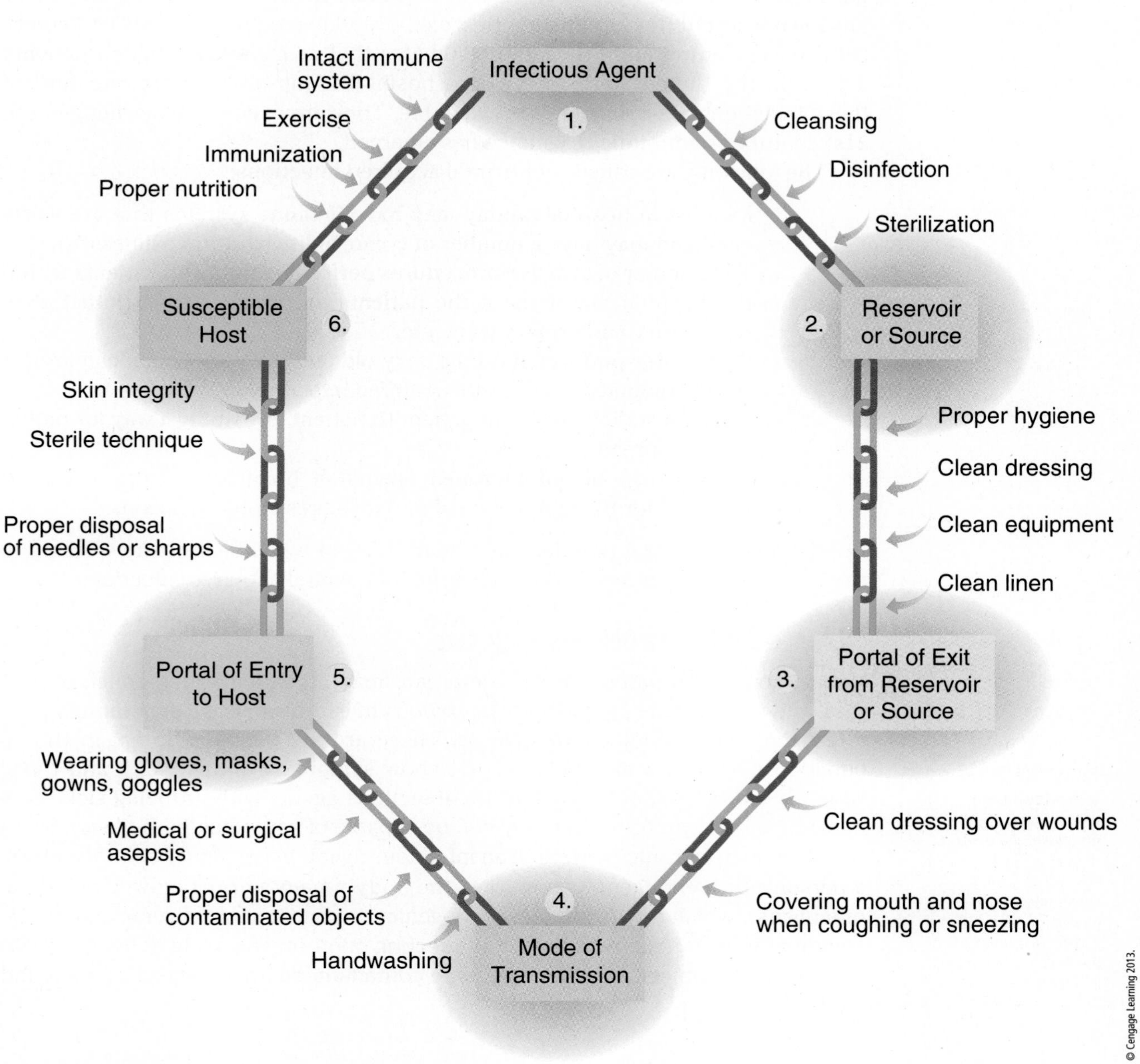

FIGURE 21-1 Chain of infection.

portal of entry
the route by which a disease-causing agent enters a host; may be through breaks in the skin, inhalation of contaminants, or insect bites

susceptible host
must be present for the agent to be transferred; the host is usually vulnerable to disease due to lack of resistance

- A **mode of transmission** between the portal of exit and the portal of entry to the susceptible host must exist.
- A **portal of entry**, the route by which the agent enters the host, must be available. This may be through breaks in the skin, inhalation of contaminants, and through insect bites.
- A **susceptible host** must be present for the agent to be transferred. The host is usually vulnerable to disease due to lack of resistance.

Hospital-acquired infections are infections that were not present at the time of hospital admission or part of the patient's original condition. They result from a procedure or form of treatment the patient received while in the hospital. Infections are considered hospital acquired if they first appear after 48 hours of the patient's hospital admission, within 30 days after a surgical procedure has been performed, or within 1 year of a surgical procedure in which an implantable device has been inserted (for select surgeries; e.g., a hip/knee replacement). The Centers for Disease Control and Prevention estimates that as many as 2 million patients a year, in the United States, develop a hospital-acquired infection; one-third of these infections are considered preventable. They are even more alarming in the 21st century as antibiotic resistance has emerged.

The following are causes of hospital-acquired infections:

- Patients in hospitals today may have immune systems that are weakened and may have a number of comorbidities (chronic illnesses).
- The number of invasive procedures performed today on patients within the hospital may bypass the patients' normal defenses (intact skin, respiratory and urinary tract, etc.).
- Procedures performed on the very old and the very young can impact the development of hospital-acquired infections.
- Hospital staff moves from patient to patient, providing a way for pathogens to spread.
- Routine use of antimicrobial agents in hospitals creates selection pressure for the emergence of multidrug-resistant organisms.

Good infection control practices and hand hygiene by all health care workers in the hospital setting is key to the prevention of hospital-acquired infections.

Sources of Infectious Agents

Human sources of pathogens in health care may be patients, personnel, or visitors, and may include people with an obvious infectious disease or, although rare, a less-than-obvious infectious disease. These are the people who are in the incubation period of a disease (may not show symptoms of infection); and those who are **colonized**, or living with the infectious agents without being sick (they may not show symptoms, but may still be capable of spreading pathogens). Some people may be chronic carriers of an infectious agent. In particular circumstances, a person's own endogenous flora (i.e., the body's many normal indwelling microorganisms), which are mostly nonpathogenic, can become pathogenic and be the source of infection. Other sources of infecting microorganisms may be inanimate environmental objects that have become contaminated, including equipment and medications.

colonized term used to describe the result when a group of microorganisms has grown from a single infectious microorganism within a particular part of the body, causing an infection

Susceptible Host

Resistance and susceptibility among people to pathogenic microorganisms vary greatly. Some people may be immune to an infection. Vaccines help the health care worker to be immune to some pathogens. For example, all hospital health care workers are offered the hepatitis B vaccine (unless they already have natural immunity from having had the disease hepatitis B).

Some people are naturally able to resist colonization by an infectious agent. Others exposed to the same organisms may establish a balanced relationship with the infecting microorganism and become asymptomatic carriers (i.e., pathogens adapt to grow on the skin and mucous surfaces of the host, forming part of the normal flora without making the person sick). Still others may develop a clinical disease.

Host factors may make people more at risk for infection. For example, an individual's age affects that person's ability to fight off infection. Children are known to be more susceptible, and babies born prematurely are especially vulnerable. The elderly are also less able to fight off infections. Other conditions that disrupt the body's ability to fight infection include underlying diseases like diabetes and cancer, and particular treatments including the use of antimicrobials, corticosteroid therapy, other immunosuppressive agents, and radiation therapy.

Procedures performed for diagnosis and treatment of disease often place the patient at higher risk and can contribute to infection. For instance, the patient is at risk for infection when there are breaks in the skin or other natural body defenses that occur during surgical operations, anesthesia, and when indwelling catheters are used.

Modes of Transmission

Microorganisms are spread via five ways, or routes, and the same microorganism may be transmitted in more than one way.

Contact Transmission

contact transmission a mode of transmission for microorganisms; divided into two subgroups: direct-contact transmission and indirect-contact transmission

direct-contact transmission infection through body surface–to–body surface contact with an infected person

indirect-contact transmission infection through contact with a contaminated object

Contact transmission, the most important and frequent mode of transmission of infections, is divided into two subgroups: direct-contact transmission and indirect-contact transmission. **Direct-contact transmission** involves direct body surface–to–body surface contact and physical transfer of microorganisms between a susceptible host and an infected or colonized person, such as occurs when nursing personnel bathe a patient or when physicians perform invasive procedures on patients who require direct personal contact. Direct-contact transmission can also occur between two patients, with one serving as the source of the infectious microorganisms and the other as a susceptible host.

Indirect-contact transmission involves contact of a susceptible host with a contaminated intermediate object, usually inanimate, such as contaminated instruments, needles, or dressings, or contaminated, improperly washed hands, and gloves that are not changed between patients. With the advent of multidrug-resistant organisms, many of which can live on patient care equipment for several days, environmental cleaning practices play an important role in the prevention of transmission of transmissible organisms through indirect contact.

Droplet Transmission

droplet transmission infection through contract with microscopic liquid particles coming from an infected person

Droplet transmission, theoretically, is a form of contact transmission. However, because the mechanism of transfer of the pathogen to the host is quite distinct from either direct- or indirect-contact transmission, the Centers for Disease Control and Prevention (CDC) considers droplet transmission a separate route of transmission. Droplets are generated from the source patient, primarily during coughing, sneezing, and certain procedures such as suctioning and bronchodilator treatments. Transmission occurs when droplets containing microorganisms generated from the infected person are propelled a short distance through the air and deposited on the host's conjunctivae (eye surface), nasal mucosa, or mouth. Because droplets do not remain suspended in the air, special air handling and ventilation are not required to prevent droplet transmission. Droplet transmission must not be confused with airborne transmission.

Airborne Transmission

airborne transmission infection by contact with airborne particles that contain infectious organisms

airborne droplet nuclei small-particle residue (5 microns or smaller in size) of evaporated droplets, containing microorganisms that remain suspended in the air for long periods of time

Airborne transmission occurs by dissemination of either **airborne droplet nuclei** (small-particle residue—5 microns or smaller in size—of evaporated droplets, containing microorganisms that remain suspended in the air for long periods of time) or dust particles containing the infectious agent. Microorganisms carried in this manner can be widely dispersed by air currents and may become inhaled by a susceptible host within the same room or over a longer distance from the source patient, depending on environmental factors. Therefore, special air handling and ventilation are required to prevent airborne transmission. Microorganisms transmitted by airborne transmission include *Mycobacterium tuberculosis*, varicella (chickenpox) virus, and zoonotic diseases (diseases transferred from animal to people) such as SARS (severe acute respiratory syndrome) and avian influenza (bird flu).

vehicle transmission infection through contact with contaminated food or water

vector-borne transmission infection through contact with infection-carrying insects or animals

Vehicle Transmission

Common **vehicle transmission** applies to contaminated items such as food (salmonellosis), water (cholera, *E. coli*), medications, devices, and equipment.

Vector-Borne Transmission

Vector-borne transmission occurs when vectors such as mosquitoes (malaria, West Nile encephalitis), flies, rats, ticks (Lyme disease), or other vermin transmit microorganisms. This route of transmission is less significant in hospitals in the United States than in other regions of the world, but it certainly does exist.

Control of Infections

Infection control and prevention programs have three principal goals:

1. Protect and provide a safe environment for the patient.
2. Protect the health care worker, visitors, and others in the health care environment from possible exposure to a communicable disease.
3. Accomplish the previous two goals in a cost-effective manner, whenever possible.

Because host and agent factors are difficult to control, interruption of the transfer of microorganisms in health care facilities is the primary goal of infection control and prevention programs. The greatest opportunity for health care workers to prevent infections comes from eliminating the transmission of pathogenic organisms.

The Principles of Aseptic Techniques

asepsis free from germs; sterile

To protect the patient and to prevent contamination, the basic principles of **asepsis** and the practices of aseptic techniques need to be understood and practiced:

- Microorganisms (germs) are capable of causing illness in humans.
- Microorganisms that are harmful to humans can be transmitted by direct or indirect contact.
- Interrupting the transmission of microorganisms from reservoirs (i.e., infected people, whether patients, other staff members, or visitors and the environment) to susceptible hosts (other patients, health care workers, visitors) can prevent illness.

Aseptic techniques (clean practices) are used to reduce the number of microorganisms or to eliminate their transmission from one person or environment to another. The practices of aseptic technique include hand hygiene to reduce the number of skin microorganisms, the use of barriers such as gloves and gowns to avoid skin and clothing contact with contaminated surfaces, and environmental controls, ranging from routine environmental cleaning and disinfection to the use of controlled airflow hoods.

Standard Precautions

standard precautions infection control safety measures developed by OSHA; designed to protect health care workers and patients from infections; also called *universal precautions*

For many years, universal precautions and procedures for universal precautions developed by the Occupational Safety and Health Administration (OSHA) referred to infection control safety measures designed to protect health care workers from infections. The CDC, which is responsible for both health care workers and patients, expanded universal precautions to protect both health care workers and patients and used the term **standard precautions**. Today, a facility may use either term or a combination of the two to name the infection control and prevention principle practices needed for all exposures to blood and body fluids and to equipment potentially contaminated by blood and body fluids. **Figure 21-2** lists the standard precautions for infection control.

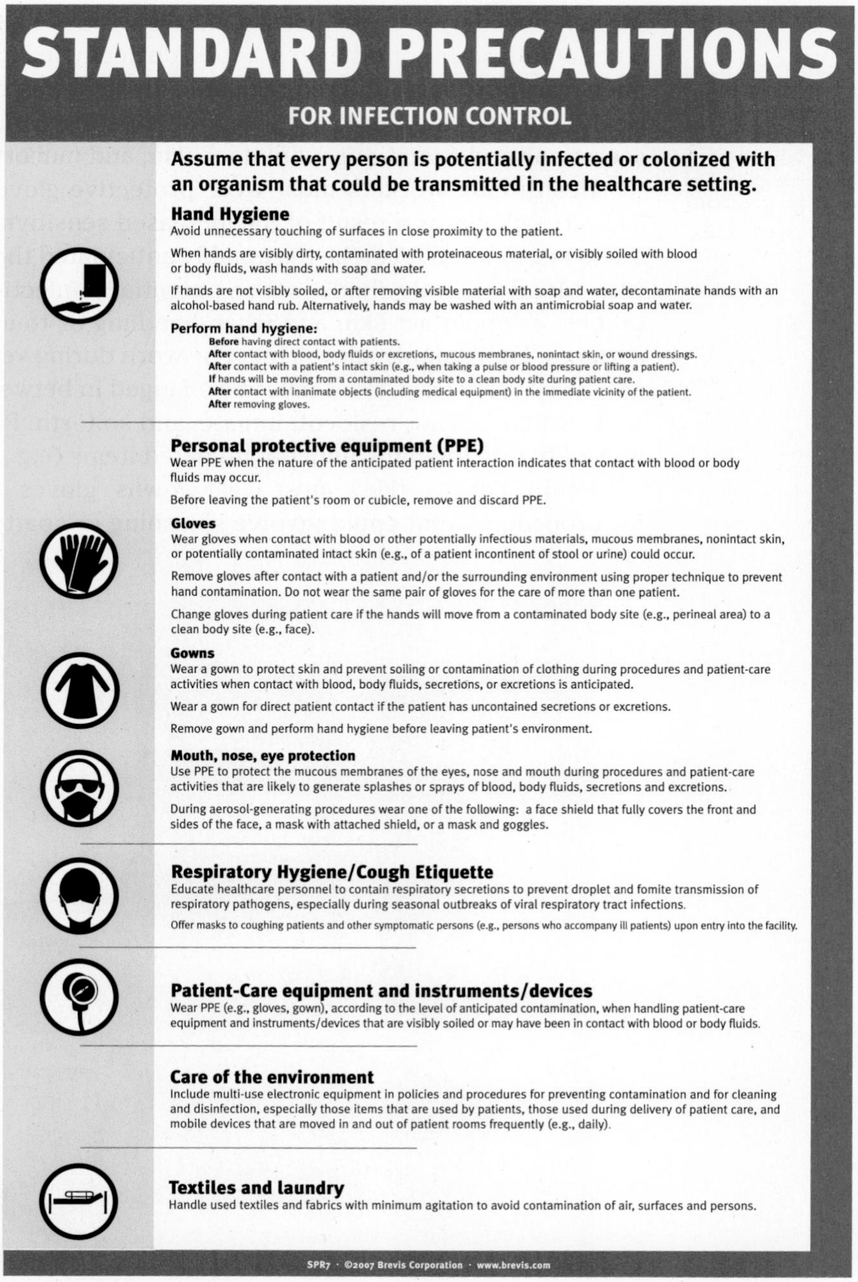
STANDARD PRECAUTIONS
FOR INFECTION CONTROL
Assume that every person is potentially infected or colonized with an organism that could be transmitted in the healthcare setting.
Hand Hygiene
Avoid unnecessary touching of surfaces in close proximity to the patient.
When hands are visibly dirty, contaminated with proteinaceous material, or visibly soiled with blood or body fluids, wash hands with soap and water.
If hands are not visibly soiled, or after removing visible material with soap and water, decontaminate hands with an alcohol-based hand rub. Alternatively, hands may be washed with an antimicrobial soap and water.
Perform hand hygiene:
Before having direct contact with patients.
After contact with blood, body fluids or excretions, mucous membranes, nonintact skin, or wound dressings.
After contact with a patient's intact skin (e.g., when taking a pulse or blood pressure or lifting a patient).
If hands will be moving from a contaminated body site to a clean body site during patient care.
After contact with inanimate objects (including medical equipment) in the immediate vicinity of the patient.
After removing gloves.
Personal protective equipment (PPE)
Wear PPE when the nature of the anticipated patient interaction indicates that contact with blood or body fluids may occur.
Before leaving the patient's room or cubicle, remove and discard PPE.
Gloves
Wear gloves when contact with blood or other potentially infectious materials, mucous membranes, nonintact skin, or potentially contaminated intact skin (e.g., of a patient incontinent of stool or urine) could occur.
Remove gloves after contact with a patient and/or the surrounding environment using proper technique to prevent hand contamination. Do not wear the same pair of gloves for the care of more than one patient.
Change gloves during patient care if the hands will move from a contaminated body site (e.g., perineal area) to a clean body site (e.g., face).
Gowns
Wear a gown to protect skin and prevent soiling or contamination of clothing during procedures and patient-care activities when contact with blood, body fluids, secretions, or excretions is anticipated.
Wear a gown for direct patient contact if the patient has uncontained secretions or excretions.
Remove gown and perform hand hygiene before leaving patient's environment.
Mouth, nose, eye protection
Use PPE to protect the mucous membranes of the eyes, nose and mouth during procedures and patient-care activities that are likely to generate splashes or sprays of blood, body fluids, secretions and excretions.
During aerosol-generating procedures wear one of the following: a face shield that fully covers the front and sides of the face, a mask with attached shield, or a mask and goggles.
Respiratory Hygiene/Cough Etiquette
Educate healthcare personnel to contain respiratory secretions to prevent droplet and fomite transmission of respiratory pathogens, especially during seasonal outbreaks of viral respiratory tract infections.
Offer masks to coughing patients and other symptomatic persons (e.g., persons who accompany ill patients) upon entry into the facility.
Patient-Care equipment and instruments/devices
Wear PPE (e.g., gloves, gown), according to the level of anticipated contamination, when handling patient-care equipment and instruments/devices that are visibly soiled or may have been in contact with blood or body fluids.
Care of the environment
Include multi-use electronic equipment in policies and procedures for preventing contamination and for cleaning and disinfection, especially those items that are used by patients, those used during delivery of patient care, and mobile devices that are moved in and out of patient rooms frequently (e.g., daily).
Textiles and laundry
Handle used textiles and fabrics with minimum agitation to avoid contamination of air, surfaces and persons.
SPR7 · ©2007 Brevis Corporation · www.brevis.com

FIGURE 21-2 Standard precautions for infection control.

Because people harboring infectious agents may not look sick, health care personnel must use precautions during the care of all patients, and for all contact with patients, clients, residents, and inmates, regardless of the diagnosis or presumed infection status. Standard precautions apply to any contact with blood, all body fluids, secretions and excretions except sweat (regardless of whether or not they contain visible blood), nonintact skin (e.g., open cuts, wounds, surgical sites), and mucous membranes (e.g., surface of the eye, inside of the nose and mouth).

Personal Protective Equipment

personal protective equipment (PPE) protective gear worn by health care workers, made up of barriers used to prevent skin and mucous membrane exposure when contact with blood or other potentially infectious materials is anticipated

Personal protective equipment (PPE) is made up of barriers used to prevent skin and mucous membrane exposure when contact with blood or other potentially infectious material is anticipated. PPE includes impermeable gowns or aprons, disposable nonsterile gloves, masks, masks with eye shields, goggles, resuscitation bags, mouthpieces or other ventilation devices used for patient resuscitation, specimen transport bags, and red regulated medical waste garbage bags (**Figure 21-3**). Health care workers use PPE when anticipating contact with blood, body fluids, secretions and excretions, nonintact skin, and mucous membranes.

Health care workers must wear protective gloves (most facilities today use latex-free gloves as a result of the increased sensitivity by many health care workers to latex) when it can be reasonably anticipated that there may be hand contact with blood or body fluids, other potentially infectious material, mucous membranes, or nonintact skin and when handling or touching contaminated items or surfaces. For example, gloves must be worn during venipuncture or other vascular access procedures. Gloves must be changed in between the care and contact with each patient, client, resident, inmate, and so forth. Protective gloves are to be removed before touching noncontaminated items (e.g., telephones, doorknobs).

Health care workers must wear gowns, gloves, and masks with eye shields for procedures that could involve splashing or spattering of blood or other body

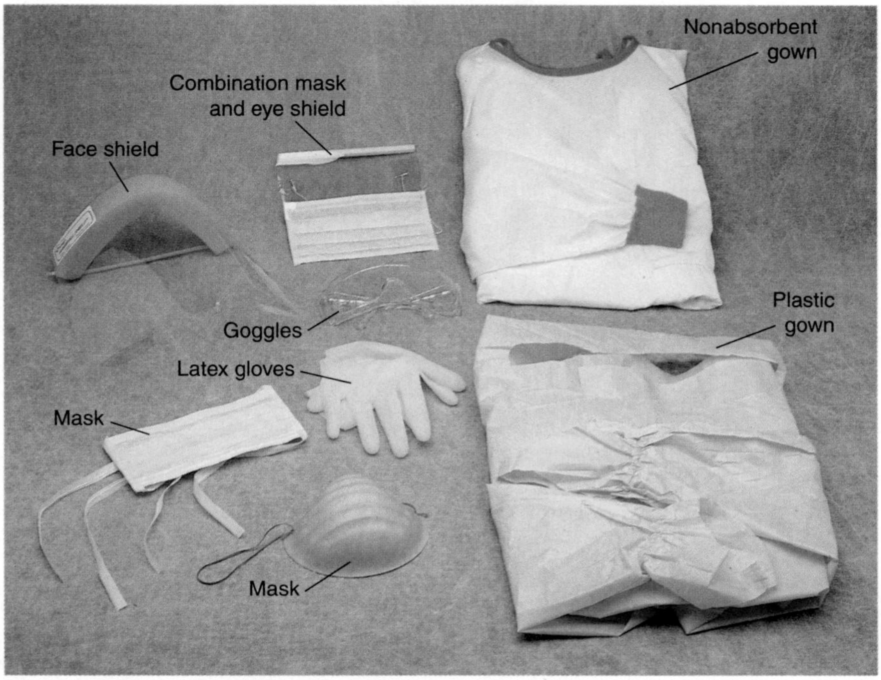

FIGURE 21-3 Personal protective equipment (PPE).

fluids or other potentially infective materials that may be transmitted to one's eyes, nose, or mouth.

The following procedures must be observed with PPE:

- Wash hands prior to application of PPE and immediately, or as soon as feasibly possible, after removal of gloves or other PPE.
- Remove PPE after it becomes contaminated and before leaving the work area.
- Remove PPE either before leaving a contaminated area (e.g., a lab) or right after leaving (e.g., a TB [*Mycobacterium tuberculosis*] airborne isolation room).
- Remove immediately, or as soon as feasible, any garment contaminated by blood or body fluids in such a way as to avoid contact with the outer surface.

Prevention of Needlestick and Other Sharps Injuries

Precautions must be taken to prevent injuries caused by needles, scalpels, and other sharp instruments or devices during and after use. To prevent needlestick injuries, needles should *not* be recapped, purposely bent or broken by hand, removed from disposable syringes, or otherwise manipulated by hand. In the event a needle must be recapped, a "one-hand scoop" method must be employed. After use, disposable syringes and needles and all other sharp items, both used and unused, should be discarded in appropriate puncture-proof sharps biohazard containers (**Figure 21-4**). In today's health care system, a number of safety devices are available for use with needles. For example, needles that retract into the syringe (or a sheath that will cover the needle) after the injection is given prevent the health care worker from being stuck.

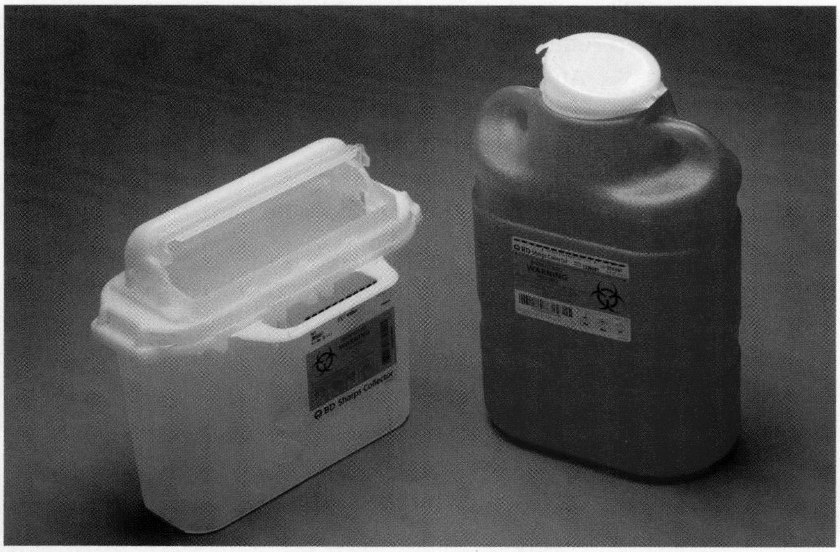

FIGURE 21-4 Sharps containers are used to dispose of needles or any other sharp objects that penetrate the skin.

Hand Hygiene

Hands and other skin surfaces must be washed immediately and thoroughly if contaminated with blood or other body fluids. Hand washing significantly reduces the transmission of pathogens in hospitals and is considered the most important infection control and prevention measure that the health care worker can perform. Health care workers must wash their hands frequently. Hands must be washed before putting on gloves and immediately after gloves are removed, before entering a patient's room, between patient contacts, and when otherwise indicated to avoid transfer of microorganisms to other patients or environments.

To properly wash hands, wet the hands with warm water and then add soap. Use friction to generate lather and wash hands (**Figure 21-5**). Use a vigorous 10- to 20-second rub to remove transient microorganisms (wash longer for more heavy contamination or after a possible exposure to **bloodborne pathogens** and other potentially infectious material). Follow with a thorough rinsing with warm water. In certain work areas a counted scrub is used for hand washing (e.g., operating room, neonatal intensive care). A counted scrub is a surgical scrub technique in which a counted brush stroke method is used for each finger, palm, back of the hand, or arm. Health care workers need to wash hands before beginning work, before and after giving treatments or handling used equipment, before eating, and before and after using the bathroom.

bloodborne pathogen a microorganism that is transmitted through exposure to contaminated blood products

Waterless alcohol-based hand hygiene products are now available in most health care facilities for hand washing procedures. Health care workers appreciate these products because they are easy to use and because they contain emollients, so they do not dry the skin. Especially important when sinks are not available, dispensers for waterless hand cleaners can be located anywhere hand hygiene might be needed. In some instances health care workers may carry the hand hygiene product with them to use as needed. Soap and water must still be used when the hands are visibly soiled, because alcohol will not disinfect the hands through the soil. Waterless products are used for routine hand hygiene procedures, but do not replace counted or timed scrubs. Waterless alcohol-based hand rubs are not to be used when caring for a patient with *Clostridium difficile* (a gram positive bacteria). The actual action of washing with an antimicrobial soap and warm water is needed to remove *C. difficile* from an individual's hands.

An important aspect of the CDC recommendations for good hand hygiene is the maintenance of clean, short fingernails, which are to be free of artificial extenders or nails. This includes fingernail wraps and all forms of acrylic nails. Fashionable fingers and health care may be a recipe for infected nails, and extensive scientific studies have revealed that nail beds harbor a high bacterial count.

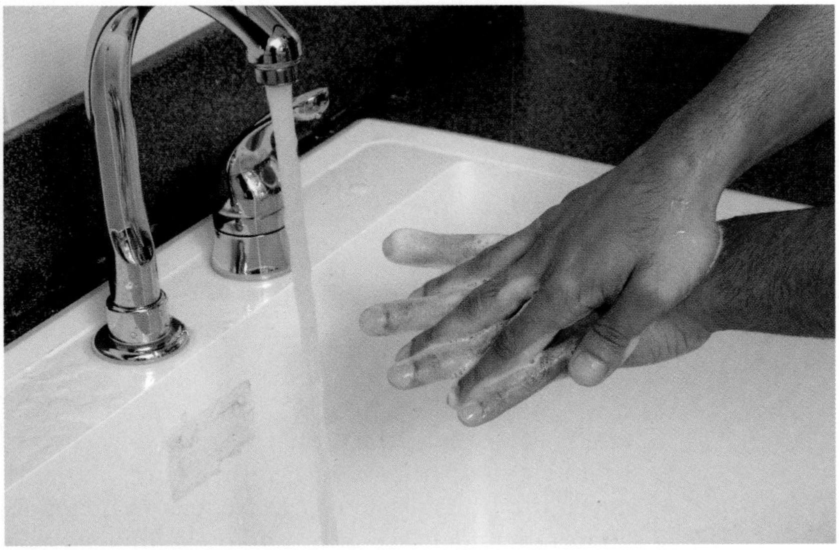

FIGURE 21-5 Hand hygiene is the single most important method of infection control.

Respiratory Hygiene/Cough Etiquette

The following measures to contain respiratory secretions are recommended for all individuals with signs and symptoms of a respiratory infection:

- Cover your mouth and nose with a tissue when coughing or sneezing.
- Use the nearest waste receptacle to dispose of the tissue after use.
- Perform hand hygiene (e.g., hand washing with nonantimicrobial soap and water, alcohol-based hand rub, or antiseptic handwash) after having contact with respiratory secretions and contaminated objects/materials.

Health care facilities should ensure the availability of materials for adhering to respiratory hygiene/cough etiquette in waiting areas for patients and visitors:

- Provide tissues and no-touch receptacles for used tissue disposal.
- Provide conveniently located dispensers of alcohol-based hand rub.
- Where sinks are available, ensure that supplies for hand washing (i.e., soap, disposable towels) are consistently available.

Cleaning and Decontamination of Surfaces and Spills

Environmental contamination is an effective method of disease transmission for microorganisms and particularly for the hepatitis B virus (HBV). The CDC states that HBV can survive for at least 1 week in dried blood on environmental surfaces. Cleaning of contaminated work surfaces after completion of procedures or after spills is required to ensure that employees are not inadvertently exposed to blood or other potentially infectious material remaining on a surface from previous procedures or from a spill. All cleaning should be done with institutionally approved disinfectants.

Specific procedures are used for spills of blood or other potentially infectious material. If the pharmacy technician encounters a spill, he or she should call for help from the professional staff. Biohazard symbols (**Figure 21-6**) or red bags are used to warn employees of the potential hazard posed by their contents.

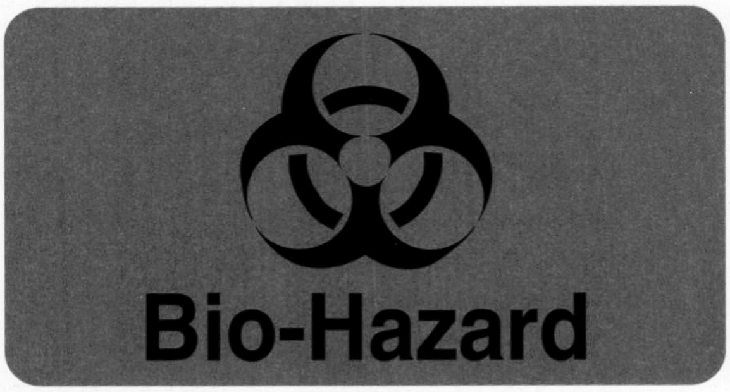

FIGURE 21-6 Biohazard symbol.

The storage of food, as well as eating, drinking, smoking, applying cosmetics or lip balm, and handling contact lenses, is prohibited in patient care areas and in other work areas where there is the likelihood of occupational exposure.

Blood and other potentially infectious materials must be handled carefully in order to minimize the potential for splashing and spraying.

Engineering and Workplace Controls

Engineering controls reduce the risk of employee exposures either by removing, eliminating, or isolating hazards.

Regulated Medical Waste Handling

Most hospital waste is not any more infective than residential waste. Consistent with most current state and local regulations, regulated medical waste (RMW) is defined as sharps, culture/stocks, human pathological waste, animal research waste, and human blood or blood products. State regulations for proper handling and disposal of these wastes may vary and need to be checked on a state-by-state basis.

Containers with free-flowing blood or blood products, or discarded material saturated or dripping with blood (e.g., dressings, blood transfusion bags, or tubings), should be considered RMW. Materials that produce free-flowing fluid when compressed or squeezed are considered RMW. All other hospital-related items are to be disposed of as regular waste. RMW is placed in closable containers constructed to hold all contents and prevent leakage. The containers are appropriately labeled as a biohazard or color coded, and closed prior to removal to prevent spillage or protrusion of contents during handling.

Because pharmaceuticals are considered chemicals, the Environmental Protection Agency (EPA), the American Hospital Association (AHA), and The Joint Commission (JC) have been working together to set guidelines for the disposal of certain hazardous pharmaceuticals that must be disposed of appropriately. This is a result of the Resource Conservation and Recovery Act (RCRA) enacted by Congress in 1976. This regulation is now being enforced, and health care facilities must incorporate a proper disposal program for these select pharmaceutical agents within their medical waste programs. Pharmaceutical hazardous waste has been divided into three categories by the RCRA: the P-List, the U-List, and the D-List.

P-List wastes are considered acutely hazardous and are the most dangerous chemicals for acute exposure if they present as the sole active ingredient of a product. Examples are arsenic and epinephrine. U-List wastes are considered toxic and involve the majority of chemotherapy agents. Items on the D-List are considered hazardous waste as a result of their ability to ignite and their toxicity, corrosiveness, and reactivity. All health professional organizations must identify, segregate, document, properly store, manifest, transport, and dispose of RCRA hazardous waste according to specific procedures. Each health care facility will have a very specific plan to address this issue.

Sharps Disposal Containers

Leakproof, puncture-resistant sharps disposal containers labeled with a biohazard label are located in all patient rooms, all patient care areas, and all other areas where contaminated sharps might be encountered. All sharps must be discarded into such containers as soon as possible.

Safety Devices and Proper Work Practices

Needlestick-prevention devices with engineered safety features are part of the comprehensive program to reduce the risk of bloodborne pathogen exposures. Safer medical devices used to prevent percutaneous injuries before, during, or after use, through safer design, are becoming increasingly available on the market and are being evaluated throughout the United States in response to a recent OSHA rule. Examples of safer devices include shielded-needle devices, blunt needles, needleless IV connectors, and IV access devices.

Proper work practices, such as reducing hand-to-hand instrument passing in the operating room and no-hands procedures in handling contaminated sharps (including broken glassware picked up using mechanical means, such as a brush and dustpan), reduce the risk of bloodborne pathogen exposure. Examples of engineered devices that are used as part of proper work practices include mechanical pipetting devices, centrifuge safety cups, splashguards, and biological safety cabinets.

Hospital Isolation Precautions

Isolation precautions are used in hospitals for patients known or suspected to be infected with highly transmissible microorganisms, for which additional precautions beyond universal/standard precautions are needed to interrupt the transmission of disease. The particular isolation precautions used are based on the way the infectious disease or microorganism is transmitted. These precautions might also be used in other parts of the health care system where the infectious disease is diagnosed prior to admission to the hospital.

Hospitals modify isolation systems to meet the needs of the patient population served and to meet federal, state, or local regulations. Each hospital isolation system, however, must preserve the principles of infection prevention and control and include precautions to interrupt the spread of infection by all routes (contact, airborne, droplet) likely to be encountered. Most hospitals use standard precautions (the use of good hand washing practices and the use of PPE when contamination is anticipated) and transmission-based precautions.

Communicable diseases and conditions require different types of transmission-based precautions (isolation). In most hospitals, a color-coded transmission-based precaution/isolation sign or card is placed outside of the patient's room to alert health care workers and visitors to the procedures required to prevent transmission of the disease or condition the patient is harboring. The isolation sign lists the requirements of the isolation (e.g., whether masks or gowns are required). Before entering any hospital room, be sure to check for these signs.

Pharmacy personnel, when in direct contact with patients, must be aware and trained in transmission-based isolation precautions. Those not trained in hospital isolation precautions are considered visitors and need to follow the instructions printed on the sign outside the patient's door: "Report to the Nurses' Station Before Entering the Room." The nurse will instruct visitors on what precautions are required to prevent transmission.

The three types of transmission-based precautions are airborne precautions, droplet precautions, and contact precautions. They may be combined for diseases that have multiple routes of transmission. When used either singly or in combination, they are to be used in addition to standard precautions (good hand washing and the use of PPE).

Standard precautions are designed to reduce the risk of transmission of microorganisms from both recognized and unrecognized sources of infection in hospitals. Since people harboring infectious agents may not look sick, health care personnel must use precautions during the care of all patients and for all contact with patients, clients, residents, and inmates, regardless of the diagnosis or presumed infection status.

Airborne Precautions

Airborne precautions require the use of a private room with a special air-handling system that creates negative air pressure (a technique that allows air to flow into the isolation room but not escape from the room) and discharges room air to the outdoors or out through a high-efficiency filter before the air is circulated to other areas in the hospital (**Figure 21-7**). Those entering the room are required to wear National Institute of Occupational Safety and Health (NIOSH)-approved respirators, unless they are immune to the disease. To safely use these respirators, annual fit testing must be performed by each employee, per OSHA recommendations.

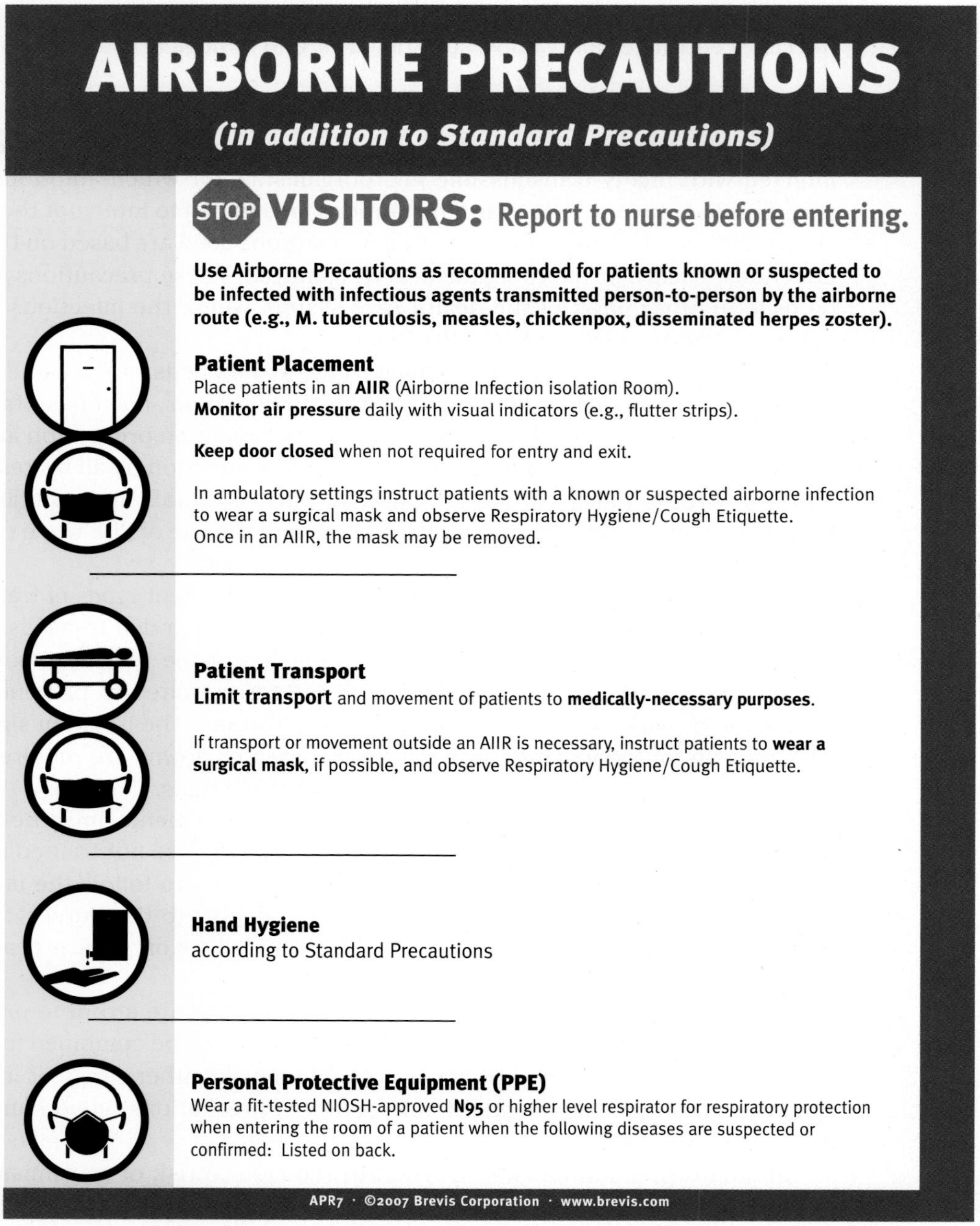
AIRBORNE PRECAUTIONS
(in addition to Standard Precautions)
STOP
VISITORS: Report to nurse before entering.
Use Airborne Precautions as recommended for patients known or suspected to be infected with infectious agents transmitted person-to-person by the airborne route (e.g., M. tuberculosis, measles, chickenpox, disseminated herpes zoster).
Patient Placement
Place patients in an AIIR (Airborne Infection isolation Room).
Monitor air pressure daily with visual indicators (e.g., flutter strips).
Keep door closed when not required for entry and exit.
In ambulatory settings instruct patients with a known or suspected airborne infection to wear a surgical mask and observe Respiratory Hygiene/Cough Etiquette.
Once in an AIIR, the mask may be removed.
Patient Transport
Limit transport and movement of patients to medically-necessary purposes.
If transport or movement outside an AIIR is necessary, instruct patients to wear a surgical mask, if possible, and observe Respiratory Hygiene/Cough Etiquette.
Hand Hygiene
according to Standard Precautions
Personal Protective Equipment (PPE)
Wear a fit-tested NIOSH-approved N95 or higher level respirator for respiratory protection when entering the room of a patient when the following diseases are suspected or confirmed: Listed on back.
APR7 · ©2007 Brevis Corporation · www.brevis.com

FIGURE 21-7 Airborne precautions.

Airborne precautions are used for patients diagnosed with or suspected of having measles, varicella (chickenpox), suspected or diagnosed pulmonary tuberculosis, and other possible airborne diseases. The door to the room used for airborne precautions must remain closed to maintain negative air pressure in the room in relation to surrounding areas and to contain microorganisms that remain suspended in the air for long periods of time to prevent them from being widely dispersed by air currents. The integrity of air handling for negative pressure must be evaluated daily to ensure protection.

Droplet Precautions

Droplet precautions require the use of a private room, or that the patient be placed in a room with a patient who has active infection or colonization with the same

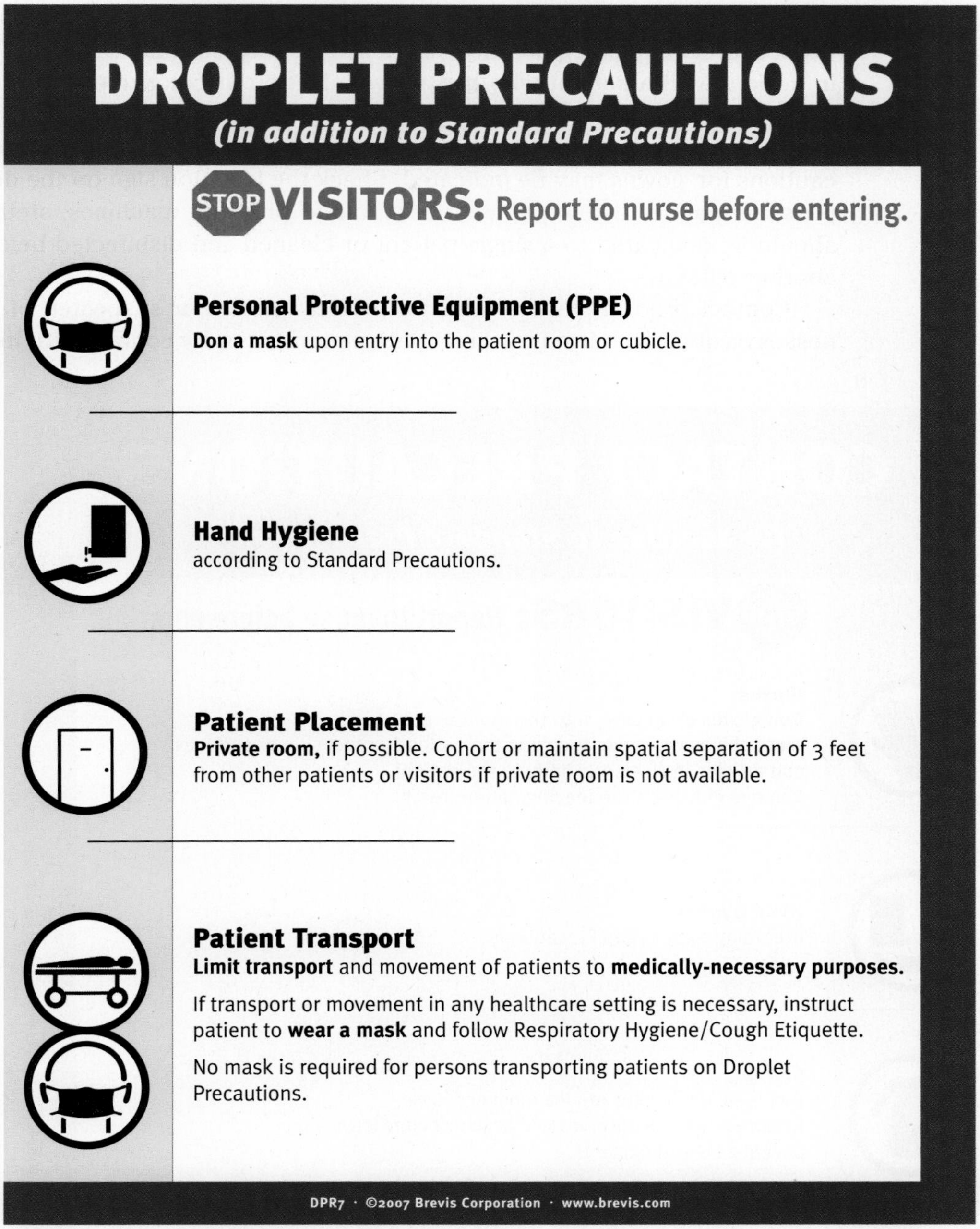

FIGURE 21-8 Droplet precautions.

> **cohorting** infection control process in which a patient is placed in a room with another patient who has an active infection or colonization with the same microorganism but with no other infection

microorganism but with no other infection (**Figure 21-8**). This is called **cohorting**. Surgical masks with or without eye protection are used when entering the room or when within a certain distance of the patient.

Droplet precautions are used for patients diagnosed with or suspected of having some types of meningitis, serious bacterial respiratory infections such as pertussis (whooping cough), influenza (flu), streptococcal pharyngitis, pneumonia or scarlet fever in infants and young children, and serious viral infections. Transmission occurs when droplets are propelled a short distance through the air, but because droplets do not remain suspended in the air, special air handling and ventilation are not required to prevent droplet transmission. Droplet transmission must not be confused with airborne transmission.

Contact Precautions

Contact precautions require the use of a private room, or that the patient be placed in a room with a patient who has active infection or colonization with the same microorganism, but with no other infection (cohorting) (**Figure 21-9**). Gloves are used when entering the room. Depending on what the patient is on contact precautions for, gowns may be indicated. Check the isolation sign on the door. When possible, patient care equipment (e.g., blood pressure machines, stethoscopes) should be dedicated to a single patient or cleaned and disinfected before use on another patient.

Contact precautions are used for patients known or suspected of having illnesses easily transmitted by direct patient contact or by contact with items in the

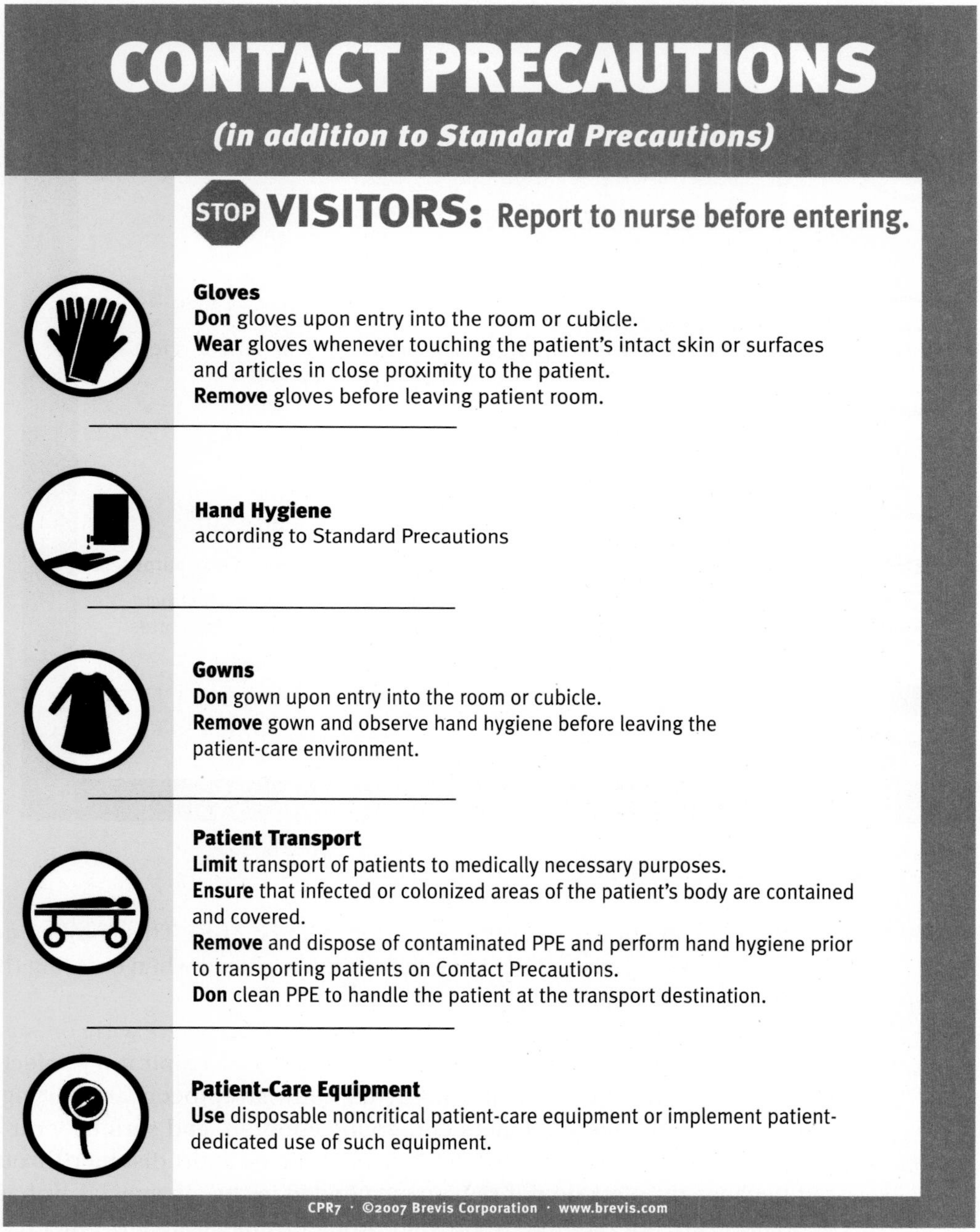
CONTACT PRECAUTIONS
(in addition to Standard Precautions)
STOP VISITORS: Report to nurse before entering.
Gloves
Don gloves upon entry into the room or cubicle.
Wear gloves whenever touching the patient's intact skin or surfaces and articles in close proximity to the patient.
Remove gloves before leaving patient room.
Hand Hygiene
according to Standard Precautions
Gowns
Don gown upon entry into the room or cubicle.
Remove gown and observe hand hygiene before leaving the patient-care environment.
Patient Transport
Limit transport of patients to medically necessary purposes.
Ensure that infected or colonized areas of the patient's body are contained and covered.
Remove and dispose of contaminated PPE and perform hand hygiene prior to transporting patients on Contact Precautions.
Don clean PPE to handle the patient at the transport destination.
Patient-Care Equipment
Use disposable noncritical patient-care equipment or implement patient-dedicated use of such equipment.
CPR7 · ©2007 Brevis Corporation · www.brevis.com

FIGURE 21-9 Contact precautions.

patient's environment, including gastrointestinal, respiratory, skin or wound infections, or colonization with multidrug-resistant bacteria judged by the institution to be significant.

Preventing Infections in Health Care Workers

Following the AIDS epidemic that began in the early 1980s, and in response to the threat of other serious on-the-job infections, federal and state legislatures have written into law the requirement for institutions to give all their health care workers infection control and prevention education. Such education should encompass safe infection control practices as well as preventive measures the health care worker is required to take within the institutional environment, and what to do if the health care worker has been exposed to a communicable disease. In the past number of years, the health care industry has been charged with the task of evaluating all occupational exposures and adopting safety practices and devices to prevent health care worker injuries and exposures to bloodborne pathogens and airborne infectious diseases. Some possible bloodborne infectious diseases are hepatitis B, hepatitis C, and HIV (human immunodeficiency virus), which causes AIDS. Some airborne infectious diseases are pulmonary TB and varicella (chickenpox).

Hepatitis B Vaccination

Employees found to be nonimmune to hepatitis B must be encouraged to receive the hepatitis B vaccination, which must be available at no charge to the employee. Nonimmune employees choosing to decline the hepatitis B vaccination must sign a declination form. The employee may rescind a declination at any time.

Infection Control Education

All health care facilities are required to have infection control programs that establish infection control and prevention standards of care. Hospital staffs are required to review these infection control policies and procedures, some of which are specific to a department (such as the pharmacy), and others that relate to all members of the health care team on a yearly basis.

Pharmacy personnel are not at high risk for occupational exposure to infectious diseases unless they are involved in direct patient care and have contact with body fluids or patients with an airborne communicable disease. In some situations, the pharmacist might assist the medical team (e.g., during cardiac arrest response) and could possibly have contact with body fluids or a patient with an airborne disease. Other situations with less potential for pharmacy staff occupational exposure might nonetheless be harmful if basic infection control principles are not followed. For instance, during the delivery and distribution of pharmaceuticals to patient care areas, there could be an unexpected encounter with patients, patient linens, or with soiled patient care equipment. Health care worker duties requiring contact with blood or body fluids, or with equipment that is contaminated with blood and other potentially infectious materials such as body fluids, create the most risk for exposure to serious infections.

To protect themselves and others from infection, all health care workers use universal/standard precautions whenever they are in a health care environment. The details of these precautions are mandated by OSHA and the Public Employee Safety and Health Administration (PESH) and are based on recommendations from the CDC.

exposure control plan guidelines to follow in the event of an exposure to an infectious disease; includes infection control training

Through the Bloodborne Pathogen Standard, a federal law, OSHA and PESH ordered that all health care facilities have in place **exposure control plans** to protect workers from exposure to infectious diseases. These plans must include infection control training for health care workers at risk for occupational exposure to blood and other potentially infectious material, because these may contain bloodborne pathogens, or to patients who are harboring an airborne pathogen. The tuberculosis control plan must be reviewed because some health care workers may be at risk for exposure to this disease.

The bloodborne pathogens of most concern in health care include but are not limited to the hepatitis B virus (HBV), which causes hepatitis B infection; the human immunodeficiency virus (HIV), which causes acquired immunodeficiency syndrome (AIDS); and the hepatitis C virus (HCV), which causes hepatitis C infection. Other bloodborne pathogens include microorganisms that are considered less of a risk to health care workers from exposures, but can potentially cause diseases like syphilis, malaria, and viral hemorrhagic fever.

Not all tasks within the health care setting carry the same chance of contact with blood, potentially infectious body fluids, or an airborne communicable disease. Tasks that carry a high risk of exposure require that the health care worker wear appropriate clothing (PPE), including cover gowns, gloves, masks, and protective eye wear. OSHA requires the health care facility to provide all protective equipment free of charge to their employees.

Pulmonary Tuberculosis Testing

tuberculin skin test (TST) a test performed to identify exposure to the tuberculosis bacillus

All new employees in hospitals and other health care facilities must have a baseline evaluation for evidence of tuberculosis infection, consisting of a two-stage **tuberculin skin test (TST)**, unless they have a history of positive TSTs. Health care workers with negative TSTs must be retested at periodic intervals—annually in most cases, but every 6 months or more frequently for employees in work areas that are at high risk for tuberculosis. Health care workers with positive TSTs are evaluated to rule out active disease and must receive counseling regarding current recommended treatments and the symptoms of tuberculosis disease (including coughs and fevers that last 2 weeks or longer, night sweats, weight loss, blood in sputum). People with positive TSTs but without active disease have TB infection and may require treatment.

TB infection is not the same as having pulmonary TB disease. Pulmonary TB infection is a condition in which living tuberculosis organisms are present in a person without causing continuing destruction of tissue. The healthy immune system usually keeps the infection in check, but prophylactic treatment with INH (isoniazid) is needed to kill the *Mycobacterium tuberculosis* organism. If not treated and the immune system fails, TB disease may develop. Pulmonary TB disease is a condition in which living tuberculosis organisms produce progressive destruction of tissue. Pulmonary TB disease is contagious. TB infection is not contagious.

Multidrug-Resistant TB

Some strains of TB have developed resistance to the drugs used to treat tuberculosis disease. The main reason that multidrug-resistant strains of TB have developed is that TB patients have not followed their prescribed drug treatment. The drugs used to treat TB usually alleviate the symptoms within 2 to 3 weeks; however, they do not eliminate the underlying infection unless they are taken for at least 6 months. When patients do not adhere to their prescribed drug regimen, the bacteria can become resistant to the drugs being used. Symptoms can return and the patient can transmit these resistant organisms to others, including health care workers. Employees exposed to pulmonary tuberculosis in the workplace are evaluated for evidence of infection by means of a postexposure evaluation.

Occupational Exposures

Infectious body substances that carry a risk for bloodborne pathogen transmission include blood, bloody fluid, semen, vaginal secretions, and synovial, pleural, peritoneal, pericardial, cerebrospinal, or amniotic fluid. Exposures that may place a health care worker at risk for bloodborne pathogen infections include a percutaneous injury (e.g., a needlestick or cut with a sharp object); contact with mucous membrane, conjunctivae, or nonintact skin (e.g., when the exposed skin is chapped, abraded, or afflicted with dermatitis) with blood, tissue, or other body fluids; and contact with intact skin when the duration of contact is prolonged (i.e., several minutes or more) or involves an extensive area with blood, tissue, or other body fluids.

What to Do If Exposed

Clean the affected area *immediately*. Wash with soap and water.

- For needlesticks, cuts, or skin contact, wash the area with soap and running water for several minutes. Do not vigorously disrupt the skin, and do not use bleach or other strong chemicals, since these can increase chances of infection through skin damage.
- For eye contact, flush the eyes with copious amounts of running water for several minutes.

Notify the area supervisor *immediately*. Complete an employee accident form. Report to the emergency department or to the employee health service as directed by the hospital *immediately*. Smaller hospitals and other institutions may make arrangements with area hospital emergency departments for their staff to be seen for occupational exposures.

Postexposure prophylaxis (PEP) is recommended for individuals exposed to potentially infectious body substances within 1 to 2 hours of a reported event, ideally within 1 hour. Health care workers must not delay seeking evaluation and treatment. (CDC-specific antiretroviral recommendations may vary from your state's department of health recommendations.)

The risk of HBV infection following a needlestick with infected blood appears to be approximately 6% to 30%. The risk of HCV infection following a needlestick with infected blood appears to be approximately 3%. The risk of HIV infection following a needlestick with infected blood appears to be 0.3% to 0.5%.

Postexposure services must be available 24 hours a day, every day, in a designated center to any employee who sustains an occupational exposure. All expenses for medical evaluations and procedures, vaccines, and PEP must be at no cost to the employee.

Bloodborne Pathogen Exposure Evaluation and Follow-Up

After possible exposure to a bloodborne pathogen, health care workers need to be tested for hepatitis B, hepatitis C, and HIV and referred for follow-up care. Laws may vary by state, but usually the health care worker will be asked to consent to HIV testing. If consent is given, the source individual's blood will be tested as soon as feasible, and after consent is obtained in accordance with state and local laws relating to this matter. If the health care worker has never been infected with hepatitis B or has not been vaccinated against hepatitis B, the vaccine will be offered along with hyperimmune gamma globulin (HBIG), if indicated.

The source patient will be requested to sign an informed consent authorizing disclosure of his or her HIV status information to the exposed worker or to undergo consented HIV testing with disclosure of the test results to the exposed worker. Follow-up care is offered to the health care worker or person exposed, either through the employee health services or by a physician.

Health Care Worker Work Restrictions

Health care workers with infections can infect patients and other health care workers. Personnel with open draining lesions such as abscesses or wounds must remain away from their jobs in the hospital and other health care settings and are to return only after cleared for work by the employee health service. Employees with herpetic lesions (herpes infections) should not care for patients in high-risk categories, including those in the nursery, oncology department, and ICU, until cleared by employee health clinic. Health care workers with rashes (especially if susceptible to varicella/chickenpox and after known exposure to chickenpox) or conjunctivitis should not work until they have seen or spoken with their physician or employee health clinic.

Contamination of Pharmaceuticals

Contamination of pharmaceutical preparations has led to epidemics. Pharmacy personnel are required to know how to prevent contamination in the first place and must be prepared to participate in curtailing disease when contamination does occur. For example, if the possibility of an incident has occurred, the pharmacy staff will be a key part of a multidisciplinary team that will perform a complete investigation. Other important members of the team will be the infection control professional, the director of medical services, the nursing services representative, and other team members who may glean insight into all the medications that are involved, whether the medications were intrinsically contaminated (i.e., occurred during the manufacturing process) or extrinsically contaminated (i.e., occurred subsequent to manufacturing, during the admixture process or while the infusate was in use), and to whom the contaminated medications were administered. The pharmacy technician will be involved in aiding in the coordination process for all recalls that occur in cases of manufacturer contamination.

Intravenous Products

Preparation of intravenous (IV) products in areas outside of the pharmacy (in areas not providing a Class 100 environment—for example, preparation of IVs outside a laminar airflow hood) may lead to contamination. IV solution contamination rarely occurs, but when it does, bloodstream infections can cause bacteremia or fungemia, resulting in patients becoming critically ill and possibly developing septic shock. Also, IV solution contamination has the potential to result in outbreaks and possibly an epidemic because of the likely wide distribution and use of the contaminated solutions.

Solutions intrinsically contaminated during production have caused widespread outbreaks of bloodstream infections in different facilities, extending at times to different states, which may escalate to epidemic proportions, increasing patient mortality and morbidity. Extrinsic contamination is a constant threat during the admixture process or while the infusate is in use. The threat of extrinsic contamination is always possible when aseptic technique is improperly used. Recommendations for the prevention of contamination of intravenous infusions include the following:

- Compound all admixtures in the pharmacy. The CDC and the Intravenous Nursing Society Standards of Practice both recommend that all parenteral fluids be prepared in the pharmacy using a laminar airflow hood.
- Prepare sterile products using facilities and equipment recommended by the American Society of Health-System Pharmacists (ASHP) and the standards implemented by U.S. Pharmacopeia Chapter <797>.
- The sterile product preparation area should have directly adjacent to it a hand washing facility with hot and cold running water and a facility-approved antimicrobial soap. The ASHP recommends that personnel preparing sterile products wear clothing covers or gowns that generate low numbers of particles, and masks and coverings for head and facial hair. All hair, whether on your head, face, or arms, holds particles that may contaminate the sterile product during preparation. It is important to ensure this safety practice is utilized at all times during the preparation process.
- All sterile products should be prepared in a Class 100 environment with the use of a vertical or horizontal laminar airflow hood. The area is to be separate from other areas, with limited personnel traffic. Particle-generating items such as cardboard boxes are not to be stored in the sterile preparation room. Opening cardboard boxes generates dissemination of possible contaminated particles into the air, which in turn can contaminate stored pharmaceutical products. Solutions and medications should be removed from the boxes prior to storage within the pharmacy area. Note that the pharmacy technician is typically the first person within the pharmacy to visualize IV solutions and medications that enter the pharmacy. This professional should carefully inspect solutions and medications for defects, expiration dates, and product integrity. For example, if the pharmacy technician notes that IV solutions appear cloudy or sees abnormal particles within the solution, the technician must remove the product and alert the pharmacist immediately.

Use the following aseptic techniques to prevent contamination of pharmaceuticals:

- Perform hand and forearm hygiene before preparing sterile products. Use an antimicrobial or detergent, facility-approved soap with warm running water, or use a waterless alcohol skin hygiene product if no organic matter is present on your hands or forearms, as directed by the latest CDC hand hygiene guidelines.
- Abstain from eating, drinking, and smoking in the preparation area.
- Wipe or spray the rubber stoppers of containers with a 70% alcohol preparation before accessing the container.
- Disinfect the entire surface of ampoules, vials, and container closures, including automated devices used for compounding sterile products, before placing them in the laminar airflow hood, as recommended by the ASHP.

- Avoid touching sterile supplies, which may result in contamination of the product.
- Contaminated multidose vials (MDVs) are excellent vehicles for the transmission of bacteria into the patient and the possible development of an infection. Although contamination of in-use vials is rare according to several well-controlled studies, epidemics have been traced to their use. In the past, most hospitals established policies to discard MDVs after a set period of time, usually 28 days, although some hospitals continue to use the manufacturer's expiration date on the vial.

Recommendations for the prevention of contamination of MDVs include the following:

- When MDVs are used, the vial is dated once opened, and CDC recommendations call for the refrigeration of the vial after opening *ONLY if recommended by the manufacturer.*
- Each time a vial is accessed, the rubber diaphragm of the vial must be cleaned carefully with an alcohol wipe, allowing the alcohol to dry (this is key to ensure the effectiveness of the antiseptic) before inserting a sterile needle into the vial. Avoid hand contamination of the device before penetrating the rubber diaphragm.
- Discard the MDV when empty, when suspected or visible contamination (e.g., cloudiness) is present, or when the manufacturer's stated expiration date has been reached.
- Inadequate quality control practices may lead to contamination of pharmaceuticals. The pharmacy is responsible for the storage of all pharmaceuticals, for monitoring for expiration dates (rotation of stock may be indicated for items that do not move quickly), and for monitoring the temperature of refrigerators and freezers used to store pharmaceuticals in all locations.

Recommendations for the prevention of contamination include the following:

- Sterile products should be examined for leaks and cracks and for turbidity or particulate matter that could indicate contamination. Keep in mind the growth of microorganisms, even in high numbers, may not be evident.
- Labeling all admixed parenterals according to ASHP recommendations provides for patient safety, and the use of control or lot numbers for batch-prepared items should assist with recalls, if needed.
- Admixed parenterals may be stored in the refrigerator for up to 1 week, providing that refrigeration begins immediately after preparation and is continuous, unless stability of ingredients dictates a shorter storage time. According to the ASHP, some admixed parenterals may be stored longer, depending on the sterile product preparation procedures used and the storage temperature.

Multidrug-Resistant Organisms

Microorganisms, predominantly bacteria, that are resistant to one or more classes of antimicrobial agents (antibiotics) are known as **multidrug-resistant organisms (MDROs)**. During the past 20 years, MDROs have steadily impacted the direct care of patients. In most instances, patients with MDROs have clinical symptoms

multidrug-resistant organisms (MDROs) microorganisms, predominantly bacteria, that are resistant to one or more classes of antimicrobial agents (antibiotics)

similar to infections caused by susceptible microorganisms; however, options for treating patients with infections caused by MDROs are often extremely limited. For example, at one point we had only one antibiotic that would treat methicillin-resistant *Staphylococcus aureus* (MRSA), which is an invasive skin bacterium that can cause a raging infection. Today, we have a number of MDROs within the health care system. Patients who are colonized with these organisms can transmit them to other patients and cause an infection to occur. Many of these organisms are transmitted from person to person and from inanimate object to person if cleaning practices are not adequate. Once again, good hand hygiene practices are the key to the prevention of transmission of these pathogenic organisms.

The role of the pharmacy in infection control and prevention extends beyond assuring the integrity of pharmaceuticals. The dramatic increase in the past several decades of the loss of activity of standard antibiotics to common bacteria has led to an incredible challenge. There is a demand for a pharmacy leadership role in the selection, use, and control of antibiotics as hospitals and other health care facilities deal with infections caused by bacteria that are resistant to multiple antibiotics. Working together with physicians, microbiologists, and infection control professionals, pharmacists participate in programs that limit unnecessary antibiotic use and seek to prevent the spread of MDROs. These programs attempt to influence practitioner antimicrobial prescribing practices and the antibiotic habits of the public.

Summary

The prevention and control of infection is a high priority in all health institutions. The pharmacy is an integral part of the health care system. The pharmacist and pharmacy technician are key players on the health care team. This chapter identifies areas of concern and methods to be employed to prevent and control the spread of infection in institutions where people with infections are routinely treated. Two areas of major concern that are addressed is preventing contamination of pharmaceuticals and ensuring the sterility of all injectable medications.

TEST YOUR KNOWLEDGE

Multiple Choice

1. Some of the general causes of contamination of IV fluids during preparation include
   a. not cleaning the rubber stopper of the medication vial with alcohol prior to entry with the needle.
   b. touching the sterile ports of IV fluids with sterile gloves.
   c. preparing parenteral nutrition solutions under the laminar airflow hood.
   d. examining fluids for turbidity.

2. Good hand washing practices are
   a. used by pharmacy personnel mainly while handling sterile medications and solutions.
   b. important in health care mostly when caring for patients in isolation rooms.
   c. used by medical personnel primarily to protect themselves from infections.
   d. considered the single most important infection control measure practiced by health care workers.

3. The principles of asepsis include the idea that
   a. microorganisms can be completely eliminated from humans.
   b. pathogens can be transmitted by direct or indirect contact.
   c. pathogens do not cause infection in health care workers.
   d. microorganisms cannot be spread in clean hospitals.

4. Aseptic techniques
   a. are used to reduce the transmission of germs.
   b. are not used routinely by pharmacy personnel.
   c. are needed only when working with items that are obviously soiled.
   d. decrease the number of bloodborne pathogens in blood and body fluids.

5. Pharmacy personnel
   a. are at great risk for infection at work.
   b. face no threat of infection on the job.
   c. are not included in infection control education programs because they do not have direct contact with patients.
   d. need to know how to protect themselves from contact with blood or body fluids, from airborne diseases, and from contaminated equipment.

6. For an infection to develop,
   a. organisms have to be transmitted from people who have obvious infections.
   b. microorganisms are transmitted from an infected or contaminated source to a susceptible host (person).
   c. health care workers have to be very young or very old.
   d. pathogens have to be contacted by hand.

7. In hospitals, microorganisms are most frequently spread
   a. by mosquitoes and flies.
   b. by contaminated food and water.
   c. by contact with contaminated people or objects.
   d. by droplets.

8. Standard precautions are used
   a. by physicians when shaking hands with patients and visitors.
   b. by some health care workers in the laboratory.
   c. by health care workers when they anticipate possible contamination with a patient's blood, body fluids, and/or wounds.
   d. by health care workers when they have contact with a patient who is sweating profusely.

9. Hospitalized patients are placed on isolation precautions
   a. to prevent the spread of microorganisms that are highly transmissible or resistant to multiple antibiotics.
   b. to alert hospital staff to the special precautions required to prevent infection from the disease or condition being isolated.
   c. to alert pharmacy personnel and other visitors that there is a need to check with the nursing staff for special instructions before entering the room.
   d. all of the above.

10. An occupational exposure that might place a pharmacy worker at risk for exposure to a bloodborne pathogen includes
   a. a needlestick from a needle that was used to inject medication into IV solution.
   b. a needlestick from a needle that was used to draw blood from a vein.
   c. a needlestick from an unused needle.
   d. a finger skin cut from paper in the pharmacy.

11. In the event of possible or actual exposure to a patient's blood or body fluids,
   a. wash the area with bleach and call for help.
   b. cover the area thoroughly with a dressing.
   c. wash skin area immediately with soap and water, or flush the eyes with copious amounts of running water for several minutes.
   d. report to your supervisor during your next scheduled evaluation session.

12. Pulmonary tuberculosis
   a. might be spread to or from a pharmacy worker; therefore, all pharmacy workers in hospitals must be screened.
   b. does not exist in pharmacy personnel; therefore, screening is not required.
   c. is spread by people with tuberculosis infection as evidenced only by a positive tuberculin skin test.
   d. is a disease of underdeveloped countries and not a problem in the United States.

13. Health care workers can infect others
   a. if they work while they have an open, draining wound or abscess.
   b. if they have never had chickenpox and come to work with a rash.
   c. if they have pinkeye or conjunctivitis.
   d. all of the above.

Matching

Match the disease with the type of pathogen causing that disease.

1. ______	athlete's foot	a. bacteria
2. ______	malaria	b. virus
3. ______	Lyme disease	c. fungi
4. ______	hepatitis	d. protozoa
5. ______	pneumonia	e. rickettsia

Fill in the Blanks

1. The single most important infection control measure practiced by health care workers is ______________.

2. The ______________ must contain the proper nutrients to keep the agent alive.

3. ______________ transmission occurs as a result of coughing and sneezing.

4. Gloves, gowns, and masks are all examples of ______________.

5. Placing patients with the same active infection in the same room for treatments is called ______________.

Suggested Readings

American Society of Health-System Pharmacists. (2000). *ASHP technical assistance bulletin on quality assurance for pharmacy-prepared sterile products* (Best Practices for Health System Pharmacy Positions and Guidance Documents). Bethesda, MD: Author.

Association for Professionals in Infection Control and Epidemiology. (2008). *Guide to the elimination of* Clostridium difficile *in healthcare settings.* Washington, DC: Author.

Boyce, J. M., & Pittet, D. (2002). Guideline for hand hygiene in health-care settings: Recommendations of the Hospital Infection Control Practices Advisory Committee and the HICPAC/SHEA/APIC/IDSA Hand Hygiene Taskforce. *Morbidity and Mortality Weekly, 51*(RR16), 1–44.

DeCastro, M. A. (2000). Aseptic technique. In *APIC text of infection control and epidemiology* (p. 27). Washington, DC: Association for Professionals in Infection Control and Epidemiology.

Hospital Infection Control Practices Advisory Committee. (1996). Recommendations for isolation precautions in hospitals. *American Journal of Infection Control, 24*, 24–52.

Hospital Infection Control Practices Advisory Committee. (1996). Recommendations for the prevention of nosocomial intravascular device related infections. *American Journal of Infection Control, 24*, 262–293.

Hospital Infection Control Practices Advisory Committee. (1998). Guidelines for infection control in health care personnel. *American Journal of Infection Control, 26*, 289–454.

Hospital Infection Control Practices Advisory Committee. (2007). *Guidelines for isolation precautions: Preventing transmission of infectious agents in health care settings.* Atlanta, GA: Centers for Disease Control and Prevention.

Hospital Infection Control Practices Advisory Committee. (2011). *Guidelines for the prevention of intravascular catheter-related infections.* Atlanta, GA: Centers for Disease Control and Prevention.

Intravenous Nurses Society. (1998). Intravenous nursing standards of practice. *Journal of Intravenous Nursing, 21*, S1–S95.

Montgomery, P. A., & Cornish, L. A. (2000). Pharmacy. In *APIC text of infection control and epidemiology* (p. 68). Washington, DC: Association for Professionals in Infection Control and Epidemiology: A Consensus Panel Report. *Infection Control and Epidemiology*, 19, 114–124.

Montgomery, P. A., & Cornish, L. A. (2004). Pharmacy: Diagnostic and therapeutic services. In *APIC text of infection control and epidemiology, 68*, 1–8. Washington, DC: Association for Professionals in Infection Control and Epidemiology.

Occupational Safety and Health Administration. (2001). Occupational exposure to bloodborne pathogens: Needlesticks and other sharps injuries. *Final Rule*, 29 C.F.R. § 1910. 1030(b).

Saljoughian, M. (2004). Disposal of hazardous pharmaceutical waste. *U.S. Pharmacist*. HS-22-HS-24.

Siegel, J. D., Rhinehart, E., Jackson, M., Chiarello, L., & Healthcare Infection Control Practices Advisory Committee. (2006). *Management of multidrug-resistant organisms in the healthcare setting*. Atlanta, GA: Centers for Disease Control and Prevention.

Siegel, J. D., Rhinehart, E., Jackson, M., Chiarello, L., & Healthcare Infection Control Practices Advisory Committee. (2007, June). *CDC guideline for isolation precautions: Preventing transmission of infectious agents in healthcare settings*. Retrieved from http://www.cdc.gov/ncidod/dhqp/pdf/isolation2007.pdf

U.S. Pharmacopeial Convention. (2013). Chapter 797: *Pharmaceutical compounding—Sterile preparations*. In *U.S. pharmacopeia, 36th ed./National formulary, 31st rev., second supplement*. Rockville, MD: Author.

PART

IV

Clinical Aspects of Pharmacy Technology

CHAPTER

22

Introduction to Biopharmaceutics

Competencies

Upon completion of this chapter, the reader should be able to:

1. Describe key factors that can affect the absorption of a drug.
2. Define bioavailability, and calculate it given the appropriate information.
3. Describe the processes of drug distribution, metabolism, and elimination.
4. List factors that could decrease the bioavailability of a drug administered orally.
5. Explain the three parameters obtained from drug plasma concentration time data to assess bioequivalence.
6. Identify a current reference for obtaining information on bioequivalence of drug products, and use this reference to determine whether two products may be legally substituted.

Key Terms

absorption
area under the plasma concentration–time curve (AUC)
bioavailability
bioequivalence
C_{max}
distribution
elimination
elimination half-life
first-pass metabolism
metabolism
T_{max}

Introduction

absorption a process by which drugs move from the site of administration into the body's systemic circulation

bioavailability the fraction of an administered dose that ultimately reaches the systemic circulation

Biopharmaceutics focuses on the interrelationship between the rate and extent of systemic drug **absorption** (method for drugs to enter the body's circulation) and the physiochemical properties of the drug molecule, the drug dosage form, and the route of administration of the dosage form. **Bioavailability** is the extent of drug absorption, and it is defined as the fraction of an administered dose that ultimately reaches the systemic or whole body blood circulation. The rate of drug absorption is evaluated by the magnitude of the maximum drug concentration (C_{max}) and by how long it takes to reach that maximum concentration (T_{max}). Many factors can affect the rate and extent of drug absorption from a particular dosage form and, consequently, the therapeutic effect of the drug. These factors include the route of administration and various anatomical and physiological factors.

Routes of Administration

C_{max} the maximum plasma concentration of a drug

T_{max} time required to reach maximum plasma drug concentration

Drugs are given by many different routes of administration. These routes can be divided into two categories: intravascular and extravascular administration. *Intravascular administration* refers to the direct administration into the vasculature or bloodstream by an intravenous or intra-arterial route. *Extravascular administration* includes all routes of administration in which the drug is not delivered directly to the bloodstream. These routes include oral, sublingual, buccal, intramuscular, subcutaneous, transdermal or percutaneous, pulmonary or inhalation, rectal, and intranasal. Any drug administered extravascularly must first be absorbed from its site of administration to subsequently enter the bloodstream.

Many factors must be considered when determining the best route of administration for a particular drug in an individual patient. These factors range from the physiochemical properties of the drug, severity of the disease state, and concurrent disease states to anticipated patient adherence and cost. There are numerous benefits of oral administration, including ease of administration, patient acceptance, cost, and the ability to formulate sustained-release dosage forms. Therefore, the most common route of administration is oral and, consequently, a complete understanding of factors affecting absorption from oral dosage forms is very important.

Factors Affecting Drug Absorption from an Extravascular Route

A drug administered by an extravascular route must overcome a number of barriers before it can reach the bloodstream. These barriers can affect both the amount of drug reaching the bloodstream and the rate at which the drug reaches the bloodstream. These barriers include drug release from the dosage form, dissolution of the drug in the surrounding fluid, and diffusion of the drug into the bloodstream. A simple diagram of this process for an oral tablet is presented in **Figure 22-1**.

Drug Release from the Dosage Form

A solid drug product, such as a tablet, normally must disintegrate into smaller particles so the drug can be released from the formulation. Other dosage forms can release the drug without disintegrating. These include depot injections, implants, patches, creams, and ointments. The rate and extent to which the drug is released

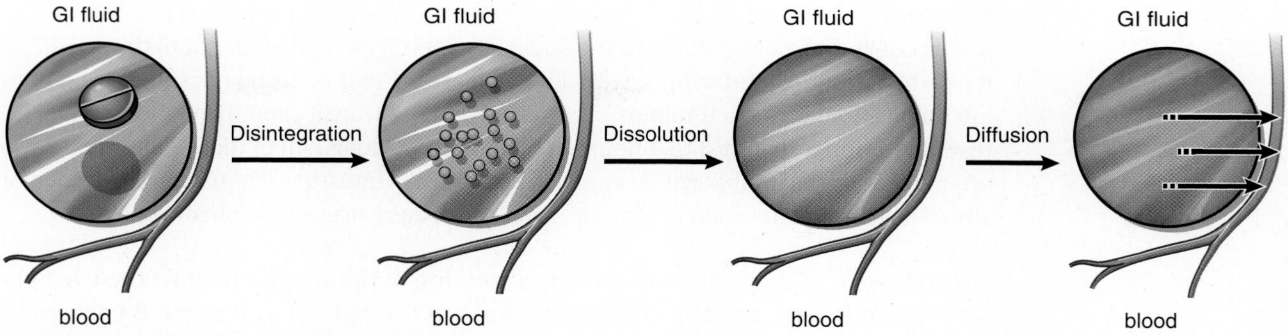

FIGURE 22-1 Extravascular drug absorption.

from the dosage form directly influences the rate and extent of drug absorption into the bloodstream.

Dissolution

Unless the drug is already in solution when it is released from the dosage form, it must dissolve in the aqueous fluid surrounding it before diffusion can occur. In general, compared to drugs with good solubility in the surrounding biological fluid, a drug with poor solubility will be absorbed more slowly or incompletely.

Diffusion

Once the drug is in solution, it is able to diffuse across biological membranes. However, particular substances in gastrointestinal fluid, including some drugs, may then bind or adsorb the drug and prevent its diffusion. To avoid this type of interaction, the administration of certain combinations of drugs must be separated by several hours (e.g., levothyroxine and cholestyramine). For an oral dosage form, the drug must diffuse across the gastrointestinal epithelium. The lipid nature of biological membranes, including the gastrointestinal epithelium, results in their being more permeable to lipid-soluble substances.

Anatomical and Physiological Considerations

Because orally administered drugs must diffuse across the epithelium of the gastrointestinal tract, the anatomical and physiological features of the gastrointestinal tract are very important in determining how much of a drug diffuses. The amount of drug that will diffuse across the epithelium of the gastrointestinal tract is dependent on various factors including the permeability of the epithelium, the surface area, the amount of time the drug is in the area of the epithelium, the blood supply, and the pH and nature of the gastrointestinal contents.

Stomach

The stomach has a relatively small surface area, so diffusion is usually limited in the stomach. Parietal cells in the stomach secrete hydrochloric acid that yields a very acidic environment with a fasting pH of 2 to 6 and decreasing to a pH of 1 to 2 in the presence of food. Food, especially fatty food, inhibits the emptying of gastric contents into the small intestine. Therefore, if a rapid onset of action is desired, the drug should be taken on an empty stomach so it will reach the small intestine more quickly.

Small Intestine

The small intestine consists of the duodenum, jejunum, and ileum. The average total length of the small intestine is approximately 3 meters. The total surface area of the small intestine has been estimated to be about 200 m^2, or approximately the area of a singles tennis court. The permeability of the small intestine is greater than that of the stomach. It also has a large blood supply, with approximately 1 liter of blood passing through the intestinal capillaries each minute. The total travel or transit time through the small intestine is approximately 3 to 4 hours in healthy individuals. All of these factors contribute to the enormous absorptive capacity of the small intestine. Therefore, the principal site of absorption for most orally administered drugs is the small intestine.

Duodenum. The duodenum is the first section of the small intestine. Gastric contents are released into the duodenum through the pyloric sphincter. Bicarbonate from the pancreas buffers the contents coming from the stomach to a pH of 4 to 6. The anatomical structure of the duodenum includes villi and microvilli. These are small finger-like processes that project from the surface of the epithelium, yielding a very large surface area. Due in part to this large surface area, the duodenum is the primary site of diffusion for many drugs into the bloodstream.

Jejunum. The jejunum is the center section of the small intestine. Although there is a gradual decrease in the diameter of the small intestine and the number of villi and microvilli along its length, the jejunum still has a large surface area. The normal pH of the jejunum is in the range of 5 to 7. Due to these continuing favorable conditions, a significant amount of drug diffusion still occurs in the jejunum.

Ileum. The ileum is the terminal section of the small intestine. The diameter and number of villi and microvilli continue to decrease. However, the ileum still has a relatively large surface area. The normal pH of ileum is in the range of 7 to 8. The blood supply to the ileum is much less than the blood supply to the duodenum and jejunum. Drug absorption continues to occur in the ileum, but not the extent that occurs in the duodenum and jejunum.

Large Intestine

The large intestine is, on average, slightly more than 1 meter in length and consists of the cecum, colon, and rectum. The contents of the small intestine are released into the cecum through the ileocecal valve. Due to a lack of villi and microvilli, the large intestine has a much smaller surface area than the small intestine. The contents of the large intestine are also more viscous and begin to take on a semisolid to solid form. These factors limit the capacity for the diffusion of drugs in the large intestine. The pH of the large intestine can vary widely from 4 to 8. The rectum and anal canal consist of a straight, muscular tube that begins at the terminal colon and extends to the anus. Drug absorption by rectal administration can occur in the rectum via the hemorrhoidal veins.

First-Pass Metabolism in the Liver

Once an orally administered drug diffuses across the gastrointestinal epithelium into the blood of the hepatic portal vein, the drug is delivered directly to the liver before it can pass into the rest of the body (**Figure 22-2**). The liver then has the opportunity to metabolize the drug before it reaches the systemic or whole body circulation. This initial **metabolism** is known as **first-pass metabolism** because it occurs during the first pass of the drug through the liver. First-pass metabolism can significantly reduce the total amount of an orally administered drug reaching the systemic circulation, even if the drug diffuses completely from the gastrointestinal tract into the blood. A drug with a very large first-pass effect cannot be administered orally because not enough of the drug will make it into the systemic

metabolism the process by which an organism converts food to energy needed for anabolism

first-pass metabolism occurs when a drug is rapidly metabolized in the liver after oral administration with minimum bioavailability

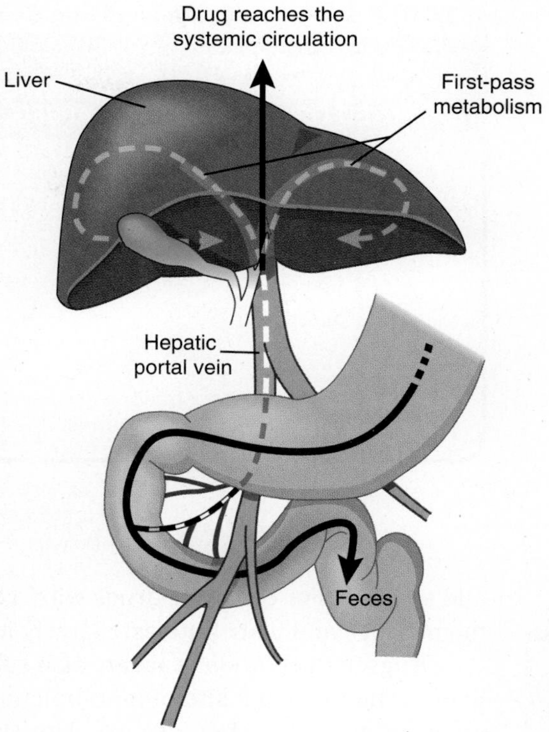

FIGURE 22-2 First-pass metabolism.

circulation to achieve its desired therapeutic effect (e.g., nitroglycerin). The drug would have to be administered by routes not subject to first-pass metabolism (e.g., sublingually, transdermally, intravenously).

Bioavailability

The amount of drug in the dosage form that ultimately clears all of the body's anatomical and physiological barriers and reaches the systemic circulation unchanged is considered to be bioavailable. The bioavailability (*F*) of a dosage form can be defined by the following equation:

$$F = \frac{\text{amount of drug reaching the systemic circulation unchanged}}{\text{amount of drug in the administered dosage form}}$$

Because intravenous doses are administered directly into systemic circulation, the bioavailability of an intravenous dose is always one, or 100%. However, the bioavailability of any drug given by an extravascular route can range from zero to one, or 0% to 100 %, depending on the amount of the dose that reaches the systemic circulation unchanged.

Drug Distribution, Metabolism, and Elimination

distribution the movement of a drug from the bloodstream to other body tissues

Once a drug reaches the bloodstream, it must then move to the site(s) where it exerts its pharmacological action(s). This movement of drug from the bloodstream to other body tissues is called **distribution**. Several characteristics of the tissue affect the distribution of a drug in and out of the tissue: regional pH, tissue composition and blood flow, lipid solubility of the drug, extent of drug bound to protein,

TABLE 22-1 Half-Life and Drug Concentration

TOTAL TIME NUMBER OF HALF-LIVES EXPECTED DRUG	AFTER MEASURED ELAPSED	AFTER CONCENTRATION MEASURED (mg/L)
0	0	10.0
6	1	5.0
12	2	2.5
18	3	1.2
24	4	0.6
30	5	0.3

The expected drug concentrations from a single dose of a drug with a half-life of 6 hours and a measured drug concentration of 10 mg/L.

elimination the removal of waste material from the body

elimination half-life the amount of time it takes to eliminate one-half of the total amount of a drug in the blood

and so forth. For example, drugs with a high lipid solubility easily cross biological membranes and distribute extensively into adipose or fat tissue.

Drugs in the bloodstream are also subject to metabolism and **elimination**. The liver is the principal site of metabolism in the body, although drug-metabolizing enzymes exist in other tissues. The typical purpose of drug metabolism is to convert the drug molecule to more water-soluble and inactive metabolites. However, metabolism can also convert drugs to active (e.g., codeine to morphine) or toxic metabolites (e.g., meperidine to normeperidine). Finally, the drug or metabolites can be excreted by the kidneys into the urine and eliminated from the body.

The amount of time it takes to eliminate one-half of the total amount of drug in the blood is the **elimination half-life**. For example, if the concentration in the blood is 10 mg/L and the half-life is 6 hours, then the concentrations presented in **Table 22-1** would result if no additional doses were administered. After five half-lives, the drug is clinically considered to be completely eliminated from the body, although a small residual amount would remain.

The half-life of a drug is also normally related to its duration of activity and therefore the allowable length of time between doses. Drugs with short elimination half-lives must be dosed more frequently to maintain an adequate amount of drug in the body to achieve the desired therapeutic effect. Alternatively, a sustained-release formulation, designed to slowly release the drug from the dosage form, can be developed for drugs with short half-lives. The drug can then be given less frequently, which should increase the consistency and accuracy with which a patient follows the directions for taking the medication. Patient adherence with four-times-a-day regimens has been shown to average about 40%, whereas patients receiving once-daily and twice-daily regimens have average adherence rates of approximately 70%.

Bioavailability Studies

Bioavailability studies are generally conducted to determine both the rate and the extent (i.e., absolute bioavailability) to which a drug is absorbed from the dosage form into the systemic circulation. The three measures of the rate and

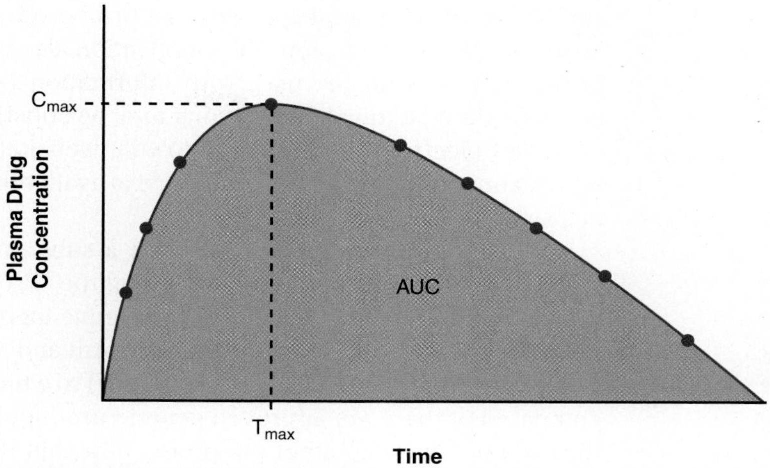

FIGURE 22-3 AUC (area under the plasma concentration–time curve).

area under the plasma concentration–time curve (AUC) the plasma drug concentration can be determined by calculating the rate and extent of systemic absorption, as visualized by the plasma concentration–time curve

extent of drug absorption are C_{max} (maximum plasma concentration achieved), T_{max} (time of the maximum plasma concentration), and **area under the plasma concentration–time curve (AUC)**. The rate and extent of systemic absorption from a dosage form can be visualized graphically by the plasma concentration–time profile (**Figure 22-3**).

During drug product development, bioavailability studies are routinely employed to compare different formulations of the same drug product. The formulation with the most desirable rate and extent of absorption can then be pursued. The desired rate and extent of absorption will depend on the therapeutic application of the drug in the dosage form. For example, it would be desirable for a dosage form of a drug used to treat acute pain to provide a fast rate of release and absorption of the drug to quickly relieve the pain. In contrast, a drug needed to control a patient's blood pressure around the clock would be appropriate for manufacture as a modified or slow-release product.

bioequivalence the comparison of the bioavailability of different drug products with the same active ingredient

Bioequivalence studies are bioavailability studies specifically comparing two or more formulations of the same dose of the same drug in the same dosage form. The purpose of bioequivalence studies is to determine if the concentration–time profiles produced by test, or generic, formulations are similar to an innovator's product that is or soon will be off-patent. If a test formulation is found to be statistically bioequivalent in terms of C_{max}, T_{max}, and AUC to the innovator's or a reference formulation, then it is considered to be bioequivalent. Since the innovator's product has already undergone extensive safety and efficacy testing to be approved by the Food and Drug Administration (FDA), it is assumed that the bioequivalent formulation will be unlikely to result in any clinically significant differences in therapeutic responses or adverse events. Bioequivalence studies are one of the requirements for pharmaceutical companies trying to gain FDA-approved generic status for their formulation of off-patent products.

Generic Substitution

To reduce drug costs, most private and public third-party formularies require the substitution of a trade name product with an appropriate generic product, when available. It is important for pharmacists and pharmacy technicians to know where to obtain accurate and current information on the therapeutic equivalence of drug products so that they may choose an appropriate generic product. The publication *Approved Drug Products with Therapeutic Equivalence Evaluations*, also known as the *Orange Book*, contains a list of all drug products approved by the FDA on the basis of safety and efficacy. This publication also contains therapeutic equivalence codes that provide the user with information regarding whether two products are considered equivalent and thus may be substituted. The *Orange Book* may be accessed electronically at the following website: www.fda.gov/cder/ob. Detailed information about using this reference is available at the same website in the preface section.

To use the *Orange Book* to identify a substitutable generic product, you may search the Electronic Orange Book using the "Proprietary Name" search to determine the ingredient(s). Then use the "Active Ingredient" Search to obtain a list of approved products grouped by dosage form and route of administration. For each group there is a reference listed drug (RLD) to which potential generic products are compared. If there are approved generic products from another manufacturer, the RLD will be "No" and all of the products within the group will have a therapeutic equivalence code (TE code). These TE codes are two-letter designations and can be divided into two general groups. Those that the FDA considers therapeutically equivalent, and that may be substituted, have a TE code that begins with the letter *A* (e.g., AB), and those that are not considered equivalent have a *B* as the first letter.

Summary

The therapeutic effect of a drug depends on many factors, including the rate and extent of drug absorption from a particular dosage form, the distribution of the drug into body tissues, the metabolism of the drug, and the rate of drug elimination. Drug absorption depends on the route of administration, the formulation of the dosage form, the physiochemical properties of the drug, and various anatomical and physiological factors. Bioavailability studies are commonly employed to assess the rate and extent of drug absorption from different dosage forms. Bioequivalence studies specifically examine the C_{max}, T_{max}, and AUCs of different formulations of the same drug in the same dosage form to determine if the two formulations are similar in their release of the drug from the dosage form. If they are not found to be significantly different, then no differences in clinical outcome from their substitution would be expected. The publication *Approved Drug Products with Therapeutic Equivalence Evaluations*, also known as the *Orange Book*, contains information regarding whether two products are considered equivalent by the FDA and thus may be substituted.

TEST YOUR KNOWLEDGE

Multiple Choice

1. Bioequivalence studies assess the similarity of plasma concentration–time profiles by comparing
   I. AUC.
   II. C_{max}.
   III. T_{max}.
   a. I only
   b. I and II only
   c. II and III only
   d. I, II, and III

2. Which of the following therapeutic equivalence (TE) codes indicate(s) a product appropriate for generic substitution?

I. AB
II. AT
III. BC

a. I only
b. III only
c. I and II only
d. I, II, and III

3. The bioavailability of a drug administered intravenously is

a. 0%.
b. 25%.
c. 50%.
d. 100%.

4. The elimination half-life of a drug is

a. the time required to completely eliminate the drug from the body.
b. the time required to eliminate one-half of the drug from the body.
c. the time required to absorb one-half of the drug from the dosage form.
d. the time required to completely absorb the drug from the dosage form.

5. If 1,000 mg of a drug is administered in an oral tablet and 400 mg of the drug is absorbed into the systemic circulation, then the absolute bioavailability (*F*) is

a. 20%.
b. 40%.
c. 60%.
d. 80%.

6. The bioavailability of an oral tablet could be decreased due to

I. incomplete dissolution.
II. incomplete diffusion.
III. first-pass metabolism.

a. I only
b. I and II only
c. II and III only
d. I, II, and III

7. Bioavailability is defined as

a. the amount of an administered dose that reaches the systemic circulation.
b. the fraction of an administered dose that fails to reach the systemic circulation.
c. the amount of an administered dose that fails to reach the systemic circulation.
d. the fraction of an administered dose that reaches the systemic circulation.

8. Which of the following is/are extravascular route(s) of administration?

I. oral
II. subcutaneous
III. intravenous

a. I only
b. III only
c. I and II only
d. I, II, and III

9. Which one of the following represents the correct order of events an oral dosage form must go through for the drug to reach the bloodstream?
   a. disintegration, dissolution, diffusion
   b. dissolution, disintegration, diffusion
   c. disintegration, diffusion, dissolution
   d. diffusion, dissolution, disintegration

10. The principal site of absorption for most orally administered drugs is the
   a. liver.
   b. stomach.
   c. small intestine.
   d. large intestine.

Matching

Match the appropriate term to the correct description.

1. ______ movement of a drug from the blood to other body tissues

2. ______ process that converts a drug molecule to more water-soluble and inactive metabolites

3. ______ method for drugs to enter the body's circulation

4. ______ term for two drugs that have comparable concentration–time profiles when administered by the same route

5. ______ one of the three measures of the rate and extent of drug absorption along with C_{max} (maximum plasma concentration achieved) and T_{max} (time of the maximum plasma concentration)

a. absorption
b. area under the plasma concentration–time curve (AUC)
c. bioavailability
d. bioequivalence
e. distribution
f. elimination
g. half-life
h. metabolism

Fill in the Blank

1. ______________ is the fraction of an administered dose that ultimately reaches the systemic or whole body circulation.

2. A ______________ drug product must disintegrate into smaller particles so the drug can be released from the formulation.

3. The liver has the opportunity to metabolize a drug before it reaches the systemic or whole body circulation; this is called ______________.

4. This movement of a drug from the bloodstream to other body tissues is called ______________.

5. ______________ studies are bioavailability studies specifically comparing two or more formulations of the same dose of the same drug in the same dosage form.

References

Allen, L., Popovich, N., & Ansel, H. (2011). *Pharmaceutical dosage forms and drug delivery systems* (9th ed.). Baltimore, MD: Lippincott Williams & Wilkins.

Burton, M., Shaw, L., Schentag, J., & Evans, W. (2006). *Applied pharmacokinetics & pharmacodynamics: Principles of therapeutic drug monitoring* (4th ed.). Baltimore, MD: Lippincott Williams & Wilkins.

Dipiro, J., Spruill, W., Wade, W., Blouin, R., & Pruemer, J. (2010). *Concepts in clinical pharmacokinetics* (5th ed.). Bethesda, MD: American Society of Health-System Pharmacists.

Seeley, R., Stephens, T., & Tate P. (2007). *Anatomy and physiology* (8th ed.). New York, NY: McGraw-Hill.

Shargel, L., Wu-Pong, S., & Yu, A. (2012). *Applied biopharmaceutics and pharmacokinetics* (6th ed.). New York, NY: McGraw-Hill.

CHAPTER

23

The Actions and Uses of Drugs

Competencies

Upon completion of this chapter, the reader should be able to:

1. Compare the advantages and disadvantages of the various routes of drug administration.
2. Recognize the standard abbreviations for the various routes of administration.
3. Describe the major factors that affect variability in drug response.
4. Explain the role of drug therapy in some common disease states.
5. Identify the therapeutic category for commonly prescribed drugs.
6. Match the generic and brand names of commonly prescribed medications.

Key Terms

adherence
extravascular
intravascular
pharmacogenetic polymorphism
prodrug

Introduction

Drugs are prescribed to treat a wide variety of medical conditions. Therefore, the knowledge of the action and use of individual drugs is critical because individual patient response to the actions of drugs can be highly varied. Many of the factors contributing to a drug's actions are addressed here. This chapter also describes the use of drugs by categorizing them by the major therapeutic classes and by both their trade and generic names.

Factors Affecting Drug Response

Once drug therapy is initiated in a patient, many factors affect the outcome of the drug therapy. All of these factors combined can result in large interpatient variability, which is the difference in drug response from patient to patient. The route of administration is one factor that can significantly affect drug response. Each route offers advantages and disadvantages that must be taken into consideration. Many patient-specific factors also affect drug response, including patient adherence with administration directions, drug-food interactions, drug-drug interactions, drug-disease interactions, and the age, weight, and genetics of patients.

Route of Administration

Drug dosage forms are given by various routes of administration. Although the pharmacological effect of the same drug administered by different routes should be similar, the route can affect both the speed at which the desired effect is attained and the intensity of the effect. These differences between the various routes of administration are covered in detail in Chapter 18.

Intravenous

intravascular injection into a blood vessel

extravascular outside of the blood vessels or lymphatic vascular channel

Directly injecting a sterile drug into a vein is known as the *intravenous* (or **intravascular**) *route* of administration, which is abbreviated as "IV" on a prescription. Advantages to intravenous administration of drugs include a more rapid onset of drug action—which can be extremely valuable in emergency situations—and allowing the use of drugs that might not be suitable for **extravascular** (outside the body vessels) administration due to poor absorption into the bloodstream or significant first-pass metabolism. Several disadvantages to intravenous administration include possible pain, irritation, and increased risk of infection at the injection site and in the bloodstream. Pantoprazole is an example of a drug that can be administered via the intravenous route as a treatment for increased stomach acid production.

Intra-Arterial

Drugs are occasionally injected into the arterial side of the bloodstream. This *intra-arterial route* is usually reserved for delivery of some anticancer drugs and diagnostic agents to a particular tissue or organ for localized effects. Otherwise, it offers the advantages and disadvantages of intravenous administration. Cisplatin is an example of a drug that can be administered via the intra-arterial route to treat various types of cancer.

Oral

For *oral administration*, the drug dosage form is placed into the mouth and swallowed, and it is abbreviated as "PO" or "po" on a prescription. This route is the most common, convenient, and economical route for delivery of many drugs. In addition, dosage forms can be designed to offer sustained or prolonged action of the drug, which decreases the frequency with which the drug must be taken. Disadvantages include limited absorption of some drugs, destruction of some drugs by digestive enzymes or the acidic pH of the stomach, and significant metabolism of some drugs during first-pass metabolism. When a drug is taken orally, it must pass through the liver before it can reach the systemic bloodstream. Therefore, the liver has the first chance to metabolize the drug before it reaches the rest of the body. Ibuprofen is an example of a drug that is often taken orally for pain relief and fever reduction.

Buccal, Sublingual, and Translingual

The *buccal*, *sublingual*, and *translingual routes* are types of drug dosage forms that are placed into the mouth without being swallowed. For buccal administration, the dosage form is placed between the cheek and gum. For sublingual administration, the dosage form is placed under the tongue to dissolve and is abbreviated as "SL" on a prescription. For translingual administration, the drug is sprayed directly onto the tongue or mouth tissue. These routes of administration offer several advantages, including rapid absorption and rapid onset of drug action.

Direct absorption into the bloodstream prevents the drug from encountering the acidic environment of the stomach and first-pass metabolism. One disadvantage is that unless properly instructed, patients may swallow the medication before it is completely absorbed. Nicotine gum is used for quick absorption through the cheek into the bloodstream. Nitroglycerin preparations are often administered sublingually and translingually for rapid relief of anginal chest pain, but if the dosage form is swallowed, nitroglycerin will undergo a very large first-pass metabolism and be ineffective.

Intramuscular

Intramuscular administration is the term used when a sterile drug is directly injected into a skeletal muscle, and it is abbreviated as "IM" on a prescription. Common sites include the deltoid (shoulder) and gluteus maximus (buttocks). Absorption of the drug occurs as the drug diffuses from the site of injection into surrounding muscle fibers and into the blood vessels in those fibers. The rate of absorption into the bloodstream depends on the blood flow to the muscle. For example, the deltoid has a higher blood flow than the gluteus maximus. Therefore, absorption is normally quicker from the deltoid muscle compared to the gluteus maximus. The rate of absorption is also dependent on the formulation of the injection. For example, aqueous or water-based injections are generally more rapidly absorbed than oil-based ones. Advantages include the potential for a sustained release while bypassing gastrointestinal absorption problems and first-pass metabolism. As with intravenous administration, disadvantages include pain, irritation, and risk of infection at the injection site. Tetanus vaccinations are administered as intramuscular injections.

Subcutaneous

Subcutaneous administration means the injection of a sterile drug just beneath the surface of the skin and should not be abbreviated, but "subc," "subq," "SC," or "SQ" may be seen on a prescription as an abbreviation for subcutaneous. This route can only be used for drugs that are not irritating to the tissue and can be given in a small volume. The rate of absorption varies with blood flow to the area of the injection and formulation of the product. Advantages include the potential for a sustained release while bypassing gastrointestinal absorption problems and first-pass metabolism. Disadvantages may include pain and irritation at the injection site. Insulin is injected under the skin, or subcutaneously.

Topical and Transdermal

Topical or *transdermal administration* involves applying a drug directly on the surface of the skin. Topical administration is abbreviated as "top." on a prescription and is used for local drug effects in the skin and is most commonly administered as a lotion, cream, or ointment. Triamcinolone cream is commonly used as a topical steroid cream. Transdermal administration is mainly used to deliver a drug into the bloodstream for systemic effects. However, transdermal patches can also be used for local action. A transdermal patch is designed to control the release of drug and provide a sustained absorption of the drug into the bloodstream. In addition to the potential for sustained effects, transdermal products bypass any problems with gastrointestinal absorption and first-pass metabolism. As an example, a selegiline patch can be used as an adjunct in the treatment of Parkinson's patients.

Inhalation

Inhalation administration delivers a sterile drug directly into the lungs. This route is mostly used for local effects in the lungs, but it is sometimes used for absorption of a drug into the bloodstream for systemic effects. The advantages of this route include a rapid onset of activity and avoidance of gastrointestinal absorption problems and first-pass metabolism. In addition, systemic side effects are uncommon when this route is used for local effects. Albuterol is often used via inhalation for the treatment of asthma and chronic obstructive pulmonary disease (COPD). There could be a slight increase in heart rate (systemic), but the key local effect is the bronchodilation.

Rectal

Rectal administration refers to insertion of a drug suppository directly into the rectum and is abbreviated as "rect." or "PR" on a prescription. This route is used for either local effects in the rectum or for absorption of drug into the bloodstream for systemic effects. This route is an inexpensive alternative to the oral route for unconscious or vomiting patients when a systemic effect is desired. Advantages include a relatively low cost while bypassing first-pass metabolism. The disadvantages of this route can include variable absorption and patients' dislike of inserting dosage forms into the rectum. The administration of prochlorperazine suppositories for the management of nausea and vomiting is a good example of the effective use of the rectal route of administration.

Vaginal

Vaginal administration involves the insertion of a drug directly into the vagina. This route is primarily used for local vaginal disorders, but some drugs administered vaginally can be absorbed into the bloodstream. Many vaginal preparations are antifungal agents in the form of creams, gels, ointments, and suppositories. Metronidazole is used as a vaginal cream and gel to treat vaginal bacterial infections.

Intranasal

Intranasal administration refers to administration of a drug directly into the nasal cavity. This route is used for either local effects in the nasal passages or for absorption of drugs into the bloodstream for systemic effects. The advantage of this route for systemic effects is the avoidance of gastrointestinal absorption problems and first-pass metabolism. When used for local effects, such as decongestant sprays, the systemic side effects are minimal. Phenylephrine is used as a nasal decongestant and causes constriction of the nasal blood vessels, decreasing congestion while only minimally causing an increase in heart rate.

Ophthalmic and Otic

Ophthalmic or *otic administration* refers to giving a sterile drug directly into the eye or ear, respectively. Both of these routes are used for local drug effects that minimize or eliminate any systemic side effects. Ciprofloxacin preparations to treat bacterial infections are available for the ears and eyes.

Patient Variability

In addition to variability in drug response due to the route of administration, many patient-specific factors can affect an individual's response to drug therapy. Patient-specific factors include adherence, drug-food interactions, drug-drug interactions, drug-disease interactions, age, weight, or genetics.

Adherence

adherence the act of complying with prescribed directions

Adherence is the consistency or accuracy with which patients follow the prescribed directions for taking their medication. A general lack of adherence is a serious public health problem with major health and economic implications. Studies report adherence rates in adults range from about 8% to 93%, depending on the medication and the frequency with which the medication should be taken. If not taken properly, the best possible therapeutic effect of the drug will not be achieved.

Drug-Food Interactions

Drug-food interactions occur when the presence of food results in altered absorption of orally administered drugs. Drug-food interactions can be a significant source of patient variability for certain drugs and can occur by several mechanisms. Some foods, particularly those high in fat, can significantly slow the rate of stomach emptying into the small intestine, thereby extending the drug's presence in the acidic pH of the stomach. The presence of food also influences the pH of the stomach. For these reasons, certain medications must be taken either with or without food, according to the instructions of the manufacturer. One example of a drug-food interaction is the intake of foods rich in vitamin K (e.g., spinach), which can counteract the blood-thinning effects of warfarin.

Drug-Drug Interactions

Drug-drug interactions occur when a patient taking two or more drugs concurrently has an altered response to one or more of these drugs caused by the other drug(s). The effect of drug-drug interactions can be insignificant, or it can decrease the therapeutic effect or increase the incidence and severity of side effects for one or more of the drugs the patient is taking. The interactions can be due to alterations in the absorption, distribution, metabolism, and elimination of one or more of the interacting drugs or a pharmacological interaction (i.e., additive, synergistic, or antagonistic effects).

Absorption. Altered drug absorption due to the interaction of two or more drugs can occur by several mechanisms. The rate and extent of absorption of drugs depend on many factors that can be altered by the presence of other drugs. Drugs administered to elevate the pH in the stomach can affect the absorption of certain drugs. Absorption can also be altered by the binding of two or more drugs in the gastrointestinal tract, thereby preventing the drug's absorption. Finally, drugs that alter stomach emptying rate or gastrointestinal motility can affect the absorption of certain drugs by affecting the amount of time the drug takes to be absorbed. For example, there can be a delay in onset of the analgesic effect of acetaminophen or aspirin when taken with a meal due to a delay in gastric emptying.

Distribution. Altered drug distribution due to the interaction of two or more drugs normally occurs due to changes in plasma protein binding of drugs. Some drugs are highly bound to proteins in the blood. Interacting drugs that are also highly bound to these same proteins can competitively displace the other drug from its protein binding sites. This displacement leads to more unbound drug in the bloodstream, which is free to diffuse out of the bloodstream into other tissue, which is the process of distribution. The net effect of this interaction is an increase in the distribution of the drug into tissues outside of the bloodstream. In addition, more unbound drug translates to more pharmacological activity, which can lead to increased side effects. Quinidine alters the distribution of digoxin, so more digoxin distributes into the bloodstream and can result in higher than normal digoxin concentrations.

Metabolism. Altered drug metabolism due to the interaction of two or more drugs can occur by two primary mechanisms: enzyme induction and inhibition. Most drugs are metabolized to some extent by various enzymes, including the cytochrome P450 system (abbreviated CYPs, are the major enzymes involved in drug metabolism accounting for about 75% of the total number of different metabolic reactions) in the liver and other parts of the body. These enzymes can have increased or decreased activity due to the presence of one or more drugs, as well as nondrug substances. These increases and decreases in metabolism due to other drugs are known as *enzyme induction* and *enzyme inhibition*, respectively. The drugs causing these changes in activity are generally known as *inducers* and *inhibitors*. Enzyme induction can lead to lower blood concentrations of drugs metabolized by that enzyme, which can result in a decreased or lack of therapeutic effect. Enzyme inhibition can lead to higher blood concentrations of drugs metabolized by that enzyme, which can result in an increased incidence of side effects. For example, fluconazole (Diflucan) inhibits the metabolism of phenytoin, which can lead to higher than normal concentrations of phenytoin.

Elimination. Altered drug elimination due to the interaction of two or more drugs can occur by several mechanisms. The kidney is the primary organ for drug elimination, and it is involved in both the elimination of the administered drug (i.e., parent drug) and its metabolites. Interacting drugs may increase or decrease the elimination of certain drugs by the kidneys. As with altered metabolism, these changes in elimination can lead to decreased drug concentrations in the blood and a corresponding decrease or lack of therapeutic effect, or increased drug concentrations and a corresponding increased incidence of side effects.

Additive, Synergistic, and Antagonistic Pharmacological Interactions. Two or more drugs can combine to exert their individual pharmacological effects in an additive manner. Two or more drugs can also combine to exert their pharmacological effects in a manner resulting in an overall effect that is more than what would result from a simple additive effect, analogous to "one plus one equals three." This type of interaction is known as a *synergistic interaction*.

An *antagonist interaction* results when one or more drugs inhibit the pharmacological effect of another drug. These interactions can be beneficial and used in the treatment of a patient's medical condition. For example the drug Methotrexate, a drug used in the treatment of cancer, whose adverse effects can be reversed by folinic acid (leukovorin) in a process known as "leukovorin rescue." But these interactions can also decrease the effectiveness of the patient's drug therapy if they are not recognized. All drug interactions should be carefully considered since the result can be dangerous. For example, the combination of sildenafil (Viagra) and nitrates (e.g., isosorbide dinitrate, isosorbide mononitrate, and nitroglycerin) can cause a severe and potentially deadly drop in blood pressure.

Drug-Disease Interactions

Drug-disease interactions occur when a patient's disease state results in altered drug response. Therefore, the overall health of the patient can significantly affect the response to drug therapy. The liver is the primary location for drug metabolism, so diseases such as hepatitis and alcoholic liver disease can result in decreased drug metabolism (e.g., procainamide). The kidney is the primary organ of drug elimination, so diseases such as acute and chronic renal failure can result in decreased drug elimination (e.g., gentamicin). Both of these examples would lead to higher concentrations of drugs in the blood, which can increase side effects and the drug's effectiveness.

Age and Weight

Weight progressively increases from birth through adolescence, increases more slowly through adulthood, and then gradually declines in the elderly. Body water, muscle mass, and organ mass are all related to body weight. In addition, many bodily functions, including organ blood flow and organ function, are related to body weight. Some individuals may be considerably underweight or overweight compared to normal individuals. All these factors can lead to the requirement of greatly different doses to achieve the desired therapeutic response, depending on an individual patient's age and weight. For example, elderly patients are normally started on lower than normal doses of many medications.

Genetics

Genetic variation can account for large variability in drug response. Genetic variation in drug-metabolizing enzymes usually results in severely decreased drug metabolism. These genetic variations are known as **pharmacogenetic polymorphisms**, and they have been identified in the cytochrome P450 system and other drug-metabolizing enzymes. The changes in drug metabolism due to pharmacogenetic polymorphisms can be very dramatic and can result in toxic concentrations of drugs when normal doses of the medications are taken.

Pharmacogenetic polymorphisms can also result in a lack of therapeutic effect if the administered drug is a **prodrug**, meaning it requires metabolic conversion in the body to an active compound. Codeine is a good example of a prodrug that requires conversion to morphine by cytochrome P450 2D6 to exert its analgesic activity. However, 8% to 14% of Caucasians have pharmacogenetic polymorphisms of this particular enzyme and, therefore, cannot convert codeine to the active analgesic, morphine. Unmetabolized codeine results in a lack of pain relief and may cause nausea and vomiting.

pharmacogenetic polymorphism a genetic variation accounting for changes in severely decreased drug metabolism, or when a normal dose is given, toxic concentrations can result

prodrug a class of drugs, the pharmacological action of which results from a chemical modification (or modifications) made by an organism on a chemical compound

Common Disorders and Associated Drug Therapies

This section provides information on drugs and their therapeutic category. It is divided into bone and joint disorders, cardiovascular disorders, endocrine disorders, gastrointestinal disorders, gynecological and obstetrical disorders, infectious diseases, neurological disorders, psychiatric disorders, and respiratory disorders. The list of medications is not all inclusive, but attention has been placed on the most prescribed drugs in each category. Some prescription drugs are available without a prescription, but are usually lower in strength compared to their prescription counterparts. These over-the-counter (OTC) products are marked with an asterisk (*) in the following sections.

Bone and Joint Disorders

Bone and joint disorders including osteoporosis, osteoarthritis, and pain can often be effectively treated with medication. What once was assumed to be simply associated with getting older can now be treated and increase patients' quality of life.

Osteoporosis

Osteoporosis is a condition of diminished bone density. Many factors can contribute to osteoporosis, but the result is bone mass being lost faster than it is being formed. This decrease in bone density leads to an increased risk of fractures. Osteoporosis is most common in elderly women, but also occurs in men. Treatment and prevention of osteoporosis includes bisphosphonates, calcium supplements, estrogens, and vitamin D therapy. A list of drugs used to treat osteoporosis can be found in **Table 23-1**.

Osteoarthritis and Pain

Almost 50 percent of individuals over age 65 are afflicted with osteoarthritis. Osteoarthritis is marked by a degeneration of cartilage, primarily in weight-bearing joints. The lack of cushioning between articulating bones results in inflammation, mild to moderate pain, and limited range of motion. Appropriate pain management is vital when treating osteoarthritis. It is best to begin therapy with an agent that will have the fewest side effects. These usually include aspirin, acetaminophen, and nonsteroidal anti-inflammatory drugs. Narcotic analgesics are rarely used in osteoarthritis, but are usually reserved for moderate to severe pain from other causes. Analgesics are often taken orally, although some are available as transdermal and injectable products. Anesthetics can also be used for acute and chronic pain. These agents can be injected or applied topically and work by blocking painful nerve impulses. Pain medications used in the treatment of osteoarthritis are found in **Table 23-2**

TABLE 23-1 Drugs Used to Treat Osteoporosis

GENERIC NAME	COMMON BRAND NAME(S)
Bisphosphonates	
alendronate and combinations	Fosamax, Fosamax Plus D
ibandronate	Boniva
risedronate and combinations	Actonel, Actonel with Calcium
Estrogens	
conjugated estrogens	Premarin, Enjuvia, Cenestin
esterified estrogens	Menest
esterified estrogens and methyl	Estratest, Estratest H.S.
micronized estradiol	Estrace
transdermal estrogen	Climara, Alora, Vivelle-Dot
Miscellaneous agents	
calcitonin	Miacalcin
calcium*	Tums, Viactiv, Os-Cal, Citracal
raloxifene	Evista
vitamin D*	Various

*Over-the-counter product.

TABLE 23-2 Pain Medication

GENERIC NAME	COMMON BRAND NAME(S)
Analgesics (non-narcotic)	
acetaminophen*	Tylenol
acetylsalicylic acid*	Aspirin
celecoxib	Celebrex
diclofenac	Voltaren, Voltaren Gel
ibuprofen*	Advil, Motrin
indomethacin	Indocin
meloxicam	Mobic
nabumetone	Relafen
naproxen sodium*	Aleve, Anaprox, Naproxen
Analgesics (narcotic)	
codeine (and combinations)	Tylenol with Codeine #3
fentanyl	Duragesic, Actiq
hydrocodone combinations	Lorcet, Lortab, Vicodin
hydromorphone	Dilaudid
meperidine	Demerol
methadone	Dolophine
morphine	MS Contin, MS IR
oxycodone (and combinations)	OxyIR, Percocet, Tylox, Endocet
oxycodone (extended release)	OxyContin
oxymorphone	Opana
pentazocine	Talwin, Talwin NX
pregabalin	Lyrica
tramadol (and combination with acetaminophen)	Ultram, Ultracet
Anesthetics	
bupivacaine	Marcaine
dibucaine	Nupercainal
halothane	Fluothane
lidocaine	Xylocaine
procaine	Novocain
propofol	Diprivan
tetracaine	Pontocaine
thiopental	Pentothal

*Over-the-counter product.

Cardiovascular Disorders

Cardiovascular disorders are the number one cause of death in the United States, according to the National Vital Statistics Report published by the Centers for Disease Control and Prevention. These disorders include arrhythmias, coronary artery disease, hyperlipidemia, and hypertension.

TABLE 23-3 Classifications of Antiarrhythmic Drugs

GENERIC NAME	COMMON BRAND NAME(S)
Type 1A	
disopyramide	Norpace
procainamide	Procanbid, Pronestyl
quinidine	Quinaglute, Quinidex
Type 1B	
lidocaine	Xylocaine
mexiletine	Mexitil
Type 1C	
flecainide	Tambocor
propafenone	Rythmol, Rythmol SR
Type 2	
beta-adrenergic blockers	(see table 23-6)
Type 3	
amiodarone	Cordarone, Pacerone
bretylium	Bretylium
dofetilide	Tikosyn
sotalol	Betapace, Betapace AF
Type 4	
diltiazem	Cardizem, Dilacor XR, Tiazac
verapamil	Calan, Covera, Isoptin, Verelan
Miscellaneous agents	
adenosine	Adenocard
digoxin	Lanoxin

Arrhythmias

An arrhythmia is a disruption in the heart's normal beating or rhythmic pattern. This abnormal electrical conduction can occur in different areas of the heart. Some common examples of arrhythmias are sinus bradycardia, sinus or ventricular tachycardia, atrial fibrillation, and ventricular fibrillation. Antiarrhythmic drugs are used to treat these arrhythmias (**Table 23-3**) and are classified into four types based on their electrophysiological properties.

Coronary Artery Disease

Coronary artery disease (CAD) develops as atherosclerotic plaques form on the inner walls of cardiac vessels. There are modifiable and nonmodifiable risk factors involved in the development of CAD. Angina pectoris is a common condition that is associated with coronary artery disease. When the vessels of the heart become blocked with plaque or fatty material, the oxygen demands of the body may not be met. Vasodilators, calcium channel blockers, and beta-adrenergic blockers are often used in the treatment of angina pectoris. A thrombus, or clot, can also form in vessels and block blood flow through those vessels. Antithrombotic agents can prevent platelet aggregation and reduce the likelihood of clot formation. Thrombolytic agents are used to dissolve previously formed clots. A list of agents used in the treatment of coronary artery disease can be found in **Table 23-4**.

TABLE 23-4 Agents Used in Coronary Artery Disease

GENERIC NAME	COMMON BRAND NAME(S)
Antithrombotic agents	
argatroban	Argatroban
dalteparin	Fragmin
enoxaparin	Lovenox
fondaparinux	Arixtra
heparin	Hep-Lock
Calcium channel blockers	
amlodipine	Norvasc
diltiazem	Cardizem, Dilacor, Tiazac
felodipine	Plendil
nifedipine	Adalat CC, Procardia XL
verapamil	Calan, Covera HS, Isoptin SR, Verelan
Coumadin thrombolytic agents	
alteplase	Activase
streptokinase	Streptokinase
urokinase	Abbokinase
Nitrates	
isosorbide dinitrate	Isordil
isosorbide mononitrate	Imdur
nitroglycerin	Nitrostat, Nitro-Bid

Hyperlipidemia

Hyperlipidemia is an abnormally high concentration of lipids, or cholesterol, in the blood. Cholesterol is synthesized in the liver and is contained in many foods. The human body can use cholesterol as an energy source or store it. Cholesterol and triglycerides are two major lipids found in the body. A total cholesterol level of less than 200 mg/dL is desirable. Hyperlipidemia increases patients' chances of developing coronary artery disease (CAD) and peripheral vascular disease (PVD).

Several classes of drugs with different mechanisms of action are used to treat hyperlipidemia. Bile acid resins bind with bile acid to inhibit cholesterol absorption and storage. Fibrates cause an increase in enzymes, which results in an increase in cholesterol metabolism. HMG-CoA reductase is an important enzyme that catalyzes in vivo cholesterol synthesis. HMG-CoA reductase inhibitors target this enzyme and inhibit its activity. Drugs used to lower cholesterol are listed in **Table 23-5.**

Hypertension

Hypertension, or high blood pressure, is a constant elevation in the systolic or diastolic blood pressure. Blood pressure is considered to be high when the systolic pressure is greater than 140 mmHg and the diastolic pressure is greater than 90 mmHg. Numerous mechanisms cause elevations in blood pressure. Drugs with different mechanisms of action can be utilized to reduce blood pressure effectively in individual patients. Alpha-adrenergic blockers hinder the nerve conduction to the heart and block nerve impulses that would make the heart beat faster. Angiotensin-converting enzyme inhibitors (ACE inhibitors) and angiotensin II receptor blockers (ARBs) work against the body's own mechanisms for raising

TABLE 23-5 Drugs Used to Treat Hyperlipidemia

GENERIC NAME	COMMON BRAND NAME(S)
Bile acid resins	
cholestyramine	Questran, Questran Light
colesevelam	Welchol
colestipol	Colestid
Fibrates	
fenofibrate	Tricor
gemfibrozil	Lopid
HMG-CoA reductase inhibitors	
atorvastatin	Lipitor
lovastatin	Mevacor
pravastatin	Pravachol
rosuvastatin	Crestor
simvastatin	Zocor
Miscellaneous agents	
amlodipine and atorvastatin	Caduet
ezetimibe	Zetia
ezetimibe and simvastatin	Vytorin
niacin*	Niaspan

*Over-the-counter product.

blood pressure. Beta-adrenergic blockers regulate the heart rate. Calcium channel blockers weaken muscle contractions and decrease the workload placed on the heart. Diuretics lower blood pressure by lowering the volume of the vasculature, and vasodilators relax the walls of blood vessels. All of these agents are commonly used in treating hypertension (**Table 23-6**).

TABLE 23-6 Drugs Used to Treat Hypertension

GENERIC NAME	COMMON BRAND NAME(S)
Alpha-adrenergic blockers	
doxazosin	Cardura
prazosin	Minipress
terazosin	Hytrin
Angiotensin-converting enzyme inhibitors	
benazepril	Lotensin
captopril	Capoten
enalapril	Vasotec
fosinopril	Monopril
lisinopril	Prinivil, Zestril
quinapril	Accupril
ramipril	Altace

TABLE 23-6 (Continued)

GENERIC NAME	COMMON BRAND NAME(S)
Angiotensin II receptor blockers	
candesartan	Atacand
irbesartan	Avapro
losartan	Cozaar
telmisartan	Micardis
valsartan	Diovan
Beta-adrenergic blockers	
atenolol	Tenormin
bisoprolol + hydrochlorothiazide	Ziac
carvedilol	Coreg, Coreg CR
labetalol	Trandate
metoprolol	Lopressor, Toprol XL
nadolol	Corgard
propranolol	Inderal, Inderal LA
Calcium channel blockers	
amlodipine	Norvasc
diltiazem	Cardizem, Dilacor, Tiazac
felodipine	Plendil
nifedipine	Adalat CC, Procardia XL
verapamil	Calan, Covera HS, Isoptin, Verelan
Diuretics	
bumetanide	Bumex
furosemide	Lasix
hydrochlorothiazide	Esidrix, HydroDIURIL, Oretic
spironolactone	Aldactone
triamterene and hydrochlorothiazide	Dyazide, Maxzide
Renin inhibitor	
aliskiren	Tekturna
Vasodilators	
hydralazine	Apresoline
sodium nitroprusside	Nitropress
Miscellaneous agents	
clonidine	Catapres, Catapres-TTS
methyldopa	Aldomet
potassium chloride	K-Dur, Klor-Con, Micro-K, Slow-K

Endocrine Disorders

Common endocrine disorders include diabetes and thyroid disorders. These disorders are the result of inappropriate hormone release. Drug therapy can help control these disorders and improve the patients' quality of life.

Diabetes Mellitus

Diabetes mellitus is the body's inability to either produce or efficiently use insulin, resulting in high blood sugar, or hyperglycemia. Type 1 diabetes is characterized by the inability to produce insulin. Type 2 diabetes differs in that the body cannot efficiently utilize the insulin that it makes. People with type 1 diabetes are usually diagnosed during adolescence, whereas type 2 diabetes usually manifests later in adulthood. The goal of therapy in diabetes mellitus is to maintain blood sugar levels within 80 to 120 mg/dL. Insulin is used more often by people with type 1 diabetes as compared to those with type 2 diabetes. However, both populations can utilize oral hypoglycemic agents to control blood glucose concentrations. Drugs used to treat diabetes are listed in **Table 23-7**.

TABLE 23-7 Drugs Used to Treat Diabetes Mellitus

GENERIC NAME	COMMON BRAND NAME(S)
Insulin preparations	
intermediate-acting insulin	Humulin N, Novolin N
long-acting insulin	Lantus, Levemir
NPH-regular combinations	Humulin 70/30, Novolin 70/30
rapid-acting insulin	Humalog, NovoLog, Apidra
short-acting insulin	Humulin R, Novolin R
Noninsulin Injectable Preparations	
exenatide	Byetta
liraglutide	Victoza
pramlintide	Symlin
Oral hypoglycemic agents	
acarbose	Precose
chlorpropamide	Diabinese
glimepiride	Amaryl
glipizide	Glucotrol, Glucotrol XL
glyburide	DiaBeta, Glynase PresTab, Micronase
metformin	Glucophage, Glucophage XR
nateglinide	Starlix
pioglitazone	Actos
repaglinide	Prandin
rosiglitazone	Avandia
saxagliptin	Onglyza
sitagliptin	Januvia
Combination oral agents	
glipizide and metformin	Metaglip
glyburide and metformin	Glucovance
pioglitazone and metformin	Actoplus Met
rosiglitazone and glimepiride	Avandaryl
rosiglitazone and metformin	Avandamet
sitagliptin and metformin	Janumet

TABLE 23-8 Drugs Used to Treat Thyroid Disorders

GENERIC NAME	COMMON BRAND NAME(S)
Hyperthyroidism agents	
methimazole	Tapazole
propylthiouracil	Propylthiouracil
Hypothyroidism agents	
levothyroxine	Levothroid, Levoxyl, Synthroid
liothyronine	Cytomel
liotrix	Thyrolar
thyroid USP	Armour Thyroid

Thyroid Disorders

The thyroid gland plays a crucial role in growth, body development, and metabolism. Thyroid disorders involve either producing excess thyroid hormone or failing to produce an adequate amount.

Hyperthyroidism is an increase in production of thyroid hormone. *Hypothyroidism* is a decrease in thyroid hormone production. Treatment consists of suppressing thyroid hormone production in hyperthyroidism, or supplying an exogenous source of thyroid hormone for hypothyroidism. Drugs used for this purpose are listed in **Table 23-8**.

Gastrointestinal Disorders

Common gastrointestinal disorders include diarrhea, constipation, and gastroesophageal reflux disease.

Diarrhea and Constipation

Diarrhea is an abnormally frequent occurrence of watery or semisolid stools. Diarrhea can be caused by disease, drugs, infection, and toxins. This increased frequency of watery defecation can lead to dehydration. Treatment consists of agents that can absorb the excess water or slow down the intestinal motility. Constipation is a decrease in stool frequency. This decreased frequency could be caused by certain medications. It is also often directly related to dietary fiber consumption. Common treatments of constipation are aimed at softening stools, increasing motility, and increasing bulk or volume of feces. Medications used to treat diarrhea and constipation are listed in **Table 23-9**.

Gastroesophageal Reflux Disease

Gastroesophageal reflux disease (GERD) is a condition in which gastric acid and other stomach contents come back up into the esophagus, causing pain and irritation. Common foods such as chocolate, coffee, and carbonated beverages can worsen GERD. Certain medications (such as prednisolone) can also worsen GERD. Treatment usually consists of over-the-counter antacids and histamine receptor (H_2) blockers, or prescription proton pump inhibitors (**Table 23-10**).

Gynecological and Obstetrical Disorders

Contraception and hormone replacement therapy are common treatments for gynecological patients. Contraception is simply the prevention of pregnancy or conception. There are various methods of contraception, but this section focuses on

TABLE 23-9 Drugs Used to Treat Diarrhea and Constipation

GENERIC NAME	COMMON BRAND NAME(S)
Absorbing agent for diarrhea	
polycarbophil*	Fiberall, Fibercon
Antimotility agents	
diphenoxylate	Lomotil
loperamide*	Imodium
Laxative and cathartic agents for constipation	
bisacodyl*	Dulcolax
docusate*	Colace
glycerin*	various
lactulose	Chronulac
mineral oil*	various
polyethylene glycol	GoLytely, MiraLAX*, HalfLytely, MoviPrep
psyllium*	Metamucil
saline*	various
senna and combinations*	Senokot, Senokot S

*Over-the-counter product.

TABLE 23-10 Drugs Used to Treat GERD

GENERIC NAME	COMMON BRAND NAME(S)
Antacids	
aluminum-containing*	Alterna-GEL
calcium-containing*	Rolaids, Tums
magnesium/aluminum combinations*	Gaviscon, Maalox, Mylanta
sodium bicarbonate*	various
Histamine receptor (H_2) blockers	
cimetidine*	Tagamet
famotidine*	Pepcid
nizatidine*	Axid
ranitidine*	Zantac
Proton pump inhibitors	
dexlansoprazole	Dexilant
esomeprazole	Nexium
lansoprazole*	Prevacid, Prevacid SoluTab
omeprazole*	Prilosec, Prilosec OTC
pantoprazole	Protonix
rabeprazole	AcipHex
Miscellaneous agents	
metoclopramide	Reglan
misoprostol	Cytotec
sucralfate	Carafate

*Over-the-counter product.

TABLE 23-11 Drugs Used for Contraception and Hormone Replacement

GENERIC NAME	COMMON BRAND NAME(S)
Estrogens	
conjugated estrogens	Premarin, Cenestin, Enjuvia
conjugated estrogens with medroxyprogesterone	Premphase, Prempro
esterified estrogens	Menest
micronized estradiol	Estrace
transdermal estrogen	Climara, Estraderm, Vivelle-Dot
Progestins	
medroxyprogesterone	Provera
norethindrone	Aygestin, Micronor, Nor-QD
norgestrel	Ovrette
progesterone	Prometrium
Combined oral contraceptives	
ethinyl estradiol and desogestrel	Desogen, Mircette
ethinyl estradiol and drospirenone	Yaz, Yasmin, Ocella
ethinyl estradiol and etonogestrel vaginal	NuvaRing
ethinyl estradiol and levonorgestrel	Lybrel, Quasense, Seasonale, Seasonique
ethinyl estradiol and norelgestromin transdermal	Ortho Evra
ethinyl estradiol and norethindrone	Estrostep FE, Ortho-Novum, Ovcon, Femhrt
ethinyl estradiol and norgestimate	Ortho-Cyclen, Ortho Tri-Cyclen, Ortho Tri-Cyclen
ethinyl estradiol and norgestrel	Ovral, Lo/Ovral, Low-Ogestrel-28

oral contraception. Oral contraception involves the manipulation of estrogen and its role in normal physiology. Most oral contraceptives contain a form of estrogen and a progestin component. Hormone replacement therapy usually begins during menopause to decrease associated symptoms. Drugs used as contraceptives and for hormone replacement are listed in **Table 23-11**.

Infectious Diseases

Infectious diseases can be bacterial, fungal, or viral. Antibiotics used to treat bacterial infections are classified as either bacteriostatic or bacteriocidal. Bacteriostatic drugs inhibit the growth of an infecting organism, and bacteriocidal drugs kill the infecting organism. Antibiotics also work by various mechanisms of action. Penicillins and cephalosporins disrupt the cell wall of the organism. Aminoglycosides, fluoroquinolones, macrolides, and tetracyclines move into the cell to inhibit RNA and protein synthesis. Antifungal agents are used to treat both topical and systemic fungal infections. Antiviral agents are reserved for the treatment of viral infections. Drugs used to treat infections are found in **Table 23-12**.

Neurological Disorders

Neurological disorders are disorders that affect the nervous system. Common neurological disorders that are often treated with prescription medications are epilepsy and numerous psychiatric disorders.

TABLE 23-12 Drugs Used to Treat Infections

GENERIC NAME	COMMON BRAND NAME(S)
Aminoglycosides	
amikacin	Amikin
gentamicin	Garamycin
neomycin	Mycifradin
streptomycin	various
tobramycin	Nebcin
Antifungal agents	
amphotericin B	Abelcet, Fungizone
clotrimazole*	Mycelex, Lotrimin
fluconazole	Diflucan
itraconazole	Sporanox
ketoconazole*	Nizoral
miconazole*	Monistat
nystatin	Mycostatin
voriconazole	Vfend
Antiviral agents	
acyclovir	Zovirax
amantadine	Symmetrel
didanosine	Videx
famciclovir	Famvir
ribavirin	Virazole
rimantadine	Flumadine
stavudine	Zerit
valacyclovir	Valtrex
zidovudine	Retrovir
Cephalosporins	
cefaclor	Ceclor
cefadroxil	Duricef
cefdinir	Omnicef
cefpodoxime	Vantin
cefprozil	Cefzil
ceftazidime	Fortaz
ceftriaxone	Rocephin
cefuroxime	Ceftin
cephalexin	Keflex
Fluoroquinolones	
ciprofloxacin	Cipro, Cipro XR
moxifloxacin	Avelox
levofloxacin	Levaquin

TABLE 23-12 (Continued)

GENERIC NAME	COMMON BRAND NAME(S)
Macrolides	
azithromycin	Zithromax, Z-Pack
clarithromycin	Biaxin, Biaxin XL
erythromycin	E.E.S., Ery-Tab
Penicillins	
amoxicillin	Amoxil, Trimox
amoxicillin/clavulanate	Augmentin, Augmentin XR
ampicillin	Principen
ampicillin/sulbactam	Unasyn
penicillin G	various
piperacillin	Pipracil
piperacillin/tazobactam	Zosyn
ticarcillin/clavulanate	Ticar
Penicillin-related agents	
aztreonam	Azactam
imipenem/cilastin	Primaxin
meropenem	Merrem
Tetracyclines	
doxycycline	Vibramycin
minocycline	Minocin
tetracycline	Sumycin
Miscellaneous anti-infectives	
isoniazid	INH
metronidazole	Flagyl, Flagyl ER
nitrofurantoin	Macrobid, Macrodantin
rifampin	Rifadin
sulfamethoxazole/trimethoprim	Bactrim, Bactrim DS, Septra, Septra DS

Epilepsy

Epilepsy is a term that encompasses various symptoms that can range from some alteration in consciousness to uncontrollable convulsions or seizures that result from altered brain function. Decreasing the frequency of these attacks or seizures greatly increases the quality of life of people with epilepsy. Drugs used to treat epilepsy are found in **Table 23-13**.

Psychiatric Disorders

Psychiatric disorders range from depression, anxiety, and sleep disorders to more severe illnesses. Depression is an overwhelming feeling of sadness or guilt. Numerous options are available for treating depression. Serotonin reuptake inhibitors are often used to treat depression. Anxiety disorders are characterized by abnormal restlessness and worry. Anxiety is commonly treated with benzodiazepines. With disruptions in mood, a lack of restful sleep often follows. Hypnotics are used to induce sleep in patients. Drugs used to treat psychiatric disorders can be found in **Table 23-14**.

TABLE 23-13 Drugs Used to Treat Epilepsy

GENERIC NAME	COMMON BRAND NAME(S)
Anticonvulsant agents	
carbamazepine	Tegretol
clonazepam	Klonopin
fosphenytoin	Cerebyx
gabapentin	Neurontin
lacosamide	Vimpat
lamotrigine	Lamictal
levetiracetam	Keppra, Keppra XR
phenobarbital	Luminal
phenytoin	Dilantin
topiramate	Topamax
valproic acid	Depakote
zonisamide	Zonegran

TABLE 23-14 Drugs Used to Treat Psychiatric Disorders

GENERIC NAME	COMMON BRAND NAME(S)
Antianxiety agents	
alprazolam	Xanax
buspirone	BuSpar
clonazepam	Klonopin
diazepam	Valium
hydroxyzine	Atarax, Vistaril
imipramine	Tofranil
lorazepam	Ativan
oxazepam	Serax
venlafaxine	Effexor, Effexor XR
Antidepressants	
amitriptyline	Elavil
bupropion	Wellbutrin SR, Wellbutrin XL
citalopram	Celexa
duloxetine	Cymbalta
escitalopram	Lexapro
fluoxetine	Prozac
mirtazapine	Remeron
nortriptyline	Pamelor
paroxetine	Paxil, Paxil CR
sertraline	Zoloft
trazodone	
venlafaxine	Effexor, Effexor XR
Hypnotic agents	
flurazepam	Dalmane
midazolam	Versed

TABLE 23-14 (Continued)

GENERIC NAME	COMMON BRAND NAME(S)
ramelteon*	Rozerem
temazepam	Restoril
triazolam	Halcion
zaleplon	Sonata
zolpidem	Ambien
Miscellaneous	
aripiprazole	Abilify
olanzapine	Zyprexa
quetiapine	Seroquel

*Only agent in class that is not a controlled substance.

Respiratory Disorders

Asthma and chronic obstructive pulmonary disease are two common respiratory disorders. Asthma is a condition that is characterized by inflammation of the airways. Wheezing, chest tightness, and coughing occur frequently with asthma. Environmental factors, exercise, and certain drugs can all be triggers of asthmatic episodes. Chronic obstructive pulmonary disease (COPD) has two main causes: chronic bronchitis and emphysema. COPD has an inflammatory component along with airway obstruction. Treatments of asthma and COPD are similar. Bronchodilators are used to relax the bronchial smooth muscle and assist in breathing. Mast cell stabilizers and steroids are used to treat the inflammatory components of asthma and COPD. Drugs used to treat asthma and COPD are listed in **Table 23-15**.

TABLE 23-15 Drugs Used to Treat Asthma and COPD

GENERIC NAME	COMMON BRAND NAME(S)
Anticholinergic agents	
ipratropium	Atrovent HFA
tiotropium	Spiriva Handihaler
Beta-2 adrenergic agonists	
albuterol	Proventil HFA, Ventolin HFA, ProAir HFA
ephedrine/guaifenesin	Primatene
levalbuterol	Xopenex, Xopenex HFA
metaproterenol	Alupent
pirbuterol	Maxair
salmeterol	Serevent
terbutaline	Brethine
Combination inhalation products	
fluticasone and salmeterol	Advair
ipratropium and albuterol	DuoNeb, Combivent
Leukotriene antagonists	
montelukast	Singulair
zafirlukast	Accolate

(Continued)

TABLE 23-15 (Continued)

GENERIC NAME	COMMON BRAND NAME(S)
Mast cell stabilizing agents	
cromolyn*	Intal, NasalCrom*
Steroids	
budesonide	Pulmicort
flunisolide	AeroBid
fluticasone	Flovent, Flonase
prednisone	Deltasone
triamcinolone	Azmacort

*Over-the-counter product.

Colds, Inflammation, and Allergic Reactions

Antihistamines block the activity of histamine that is released during colds, inflammation, and allergic reactions. Histamine receptors are found throughout the body, but this section focuses primarily on the H_1 receptor. Antihistamines block this receptor, which helps prevent the watering, redness, and swelling that is characteristic of a histamine reaction. Decongestants are often added to cold preparations to help alleviate a stuffy nose. Decongestants cause a constriction of blood vessels and allow for better breathing

TABLE 23-16 Antihistamines and Decongestants

GENERIC NAME	COMMON BRAND NAME(S)
Antihistamines	
brompheniramine combinations*	Dimetapp
cetirizine	Zyrtec*
chlorpheniramine*	Chlor-Trimeton
desloratadine	Clarinex
diphenhydramine*	Benadryl
fexofenadine*	Allegra
levocetirizine	Xyzal
loratadine*	Alavert, Claritin
meclizine*	Antivert, Bonine
promethazine	Phenergan
Decongestants	
ephedrine*	
phenylephrine*	Neo-Synephrine, Sudafed PE
pseudoephedrine*	Sudafed
Steroids	
budesonide	Entocort, Rhinocort Aqua
fluticasone	Flonase, Veramyst
mometasone	Nasonex
triamcinolone	Nasacort AQ

*Over-the-counter product.

through the nose. It is important to note that individuals who have high blood pressure should contact their pharmacist or physician before using any products containing decongestants. Drugs used as antihistamines and decongestants are listed in **Table 23-16**.

Summary

This chapter discussed the advantages and disadvantages of the various extravascular and intravascular modes of drug administration. Drug action is also affected by patient characteristics, such as adherence to directions for taking the drug, interactions of drugs with food and other drugs, and patient pathology, as well as age, weight, and genetic predispositions. The second major part of the chapter dealt with common disorders and the major therapeutic classes of drugs in use today to treat those disorders. The generic and trade names of the drugs in each category have been included. Both the actions and the uses of drugs have been described and noted to provide the pharmacy technician with a sound basis for understanding the basics of drug therapy.

TEST YOUR KNOWLEDGE

Multiple Choice

1. Which of the following route(s) of administration avoid first-pass metabolism?
I. oral
II. sublingual
III. intravenous
a. I only
b. III only
c. I and II only
d. II and III only

2. Which one of the following routes of administration is best when a rapid onset of systemic drug action is required in an emergency situation?
a. transdermal
b. rectal
c. intravenous
d. oral

3. Induction of drug-metabolizing enzymes is mostly likely to cause
a. increased drug concentrations and increased side effects.
b. increased drug concentrations and decreased therapeutic effects.
c. decreased drug concentrations and increased side effects.
d. decreased drug concentrations and decreased therapeutic effects.

4. Which of the following drugs is a beta-adrenergic blocker?
a. albuterol
b. captopril
c. metoprolol
d. fluconazole

5. Which of the following drugs is used to treat pain?
a. diltiazem
b. hydrocodone
c. minoxidil
d. atorvastatin

6. Albuterol, Spiriva, and Flovent are common treatments for
   a. coronary artery disease.
   b. respiratory disorders.
   c. hypertension.
   d. bacterial infections.

Matching

Match the abbreviation with its meaning.

1. ______	IM	a. intramuscular
2. ______	PO	b. sublingual
3. ______	PR	c. rectal
4. ______	SL	d. oral

Match the generic name with the brand name.

1. ______	digoxin	a. Lasix
2. ______	acetaminophen	b. Zoloft
3. ______	warfarin	c. Norvasc
4. ______	sertraline	d. Coumadin
5. ______	furosemide	e. Ambien
6. ______	amlodipine	f. Lanoxin
7. ______	zolpidem	g. Tylenol

Fill in the Blank

1. __________ administration means a sterile drug is directly injected into a skeletal muscle.
2. Two or more drugs can combine to exert their individual pharmacological effects in a/an __________ manner.
3. __________ is the consistency or accuracy with which patients follow the prescribed directions for taking their medication.
4. __________ is an abnormally high concentration of lipids, or cholesterol, in the blood.
5. A/An __________ is a disruption in the heart's normal beating or rhythmic pattern.

References

Brunton, L., Chabner, B., & Knollman, B. (Eds.). (2011). *Goodman & Gilman's the pharmacological basis of therapeutics* (12th ed.) New York, NY: McGraw-Hill.

DiPiro, J., Spruill, W., Wade, W., Blouin, R., & Pruemer, J. (2010). *Concepts in clinical pharmacokinetics* (5th ed.). Bethesda, MD: American Society of Health-System Pharmacists.

DiPiro, J., Talbert, R., Yee, G., & Matke, G. (Eds.). (2011). *Pharmacotherapy: A pathophysiologic approach* (8th ed.). New York, NY: McGraw-Hill.

Shargel, L., Wu-Pong, S., & Yu, A. (2004). *Applied biopharmaceutics and pharmacokinetics* (5th ed.). New York, NY: McGraw-Hill.

CHAPTER

24

Nonprescription Medications

Competencies

Upon completion of this chapter, the reader should be able to:

1. Define the term over-the-counter medication, and provide other common terms used to identify these agents.
2. Describe the various dosage formulations available as over-the-counter medications.
3. List the various therapeutic categories most commonly used for the purpose of self-care by patients.
4. Identify a specific nonprescription medication and recognize which therapeutic category it belongs to.
5. Explain common indications, adverse effects, and drug-disease interactions of select nonprescription medications.

Key Terms

allergies
analgesic
antacids
antihistamines
antitussives
cold
constipation
diarrhea
expectorant
gastroesophageal reflux disease (GERD)
nonprescription medications
over-the-counter medications (OTCs)
peptic ulcer disease (PUD)

Introduction

nonprescription medications drugs available to patients who have conditions that are considered self-treatable; also known as over-the-counter medications (OTCs)

over-the-counter medications (OTCs) drugs that can be sold without a prescription

Those practicing in a pharmacy environment must be familiar with the drugs that may be purchased by the consumer without a prescription from their health care provider. These **nonprescription medications**, also known as **over-the-counter medications (OTCs)**, are available for patients suffering from conditions that are considered self-treatable. Patients commonly come into the pharmacy seeking these medications to provide relief from various symptoms. Not only are they seeking relief, but often they have been exposed to direct-to-consumer advertising, which may result in their asking the pharmacy personnel for a specific brand name drug. The drug they come in asking for may not necessarily be the best drug for their condition. The pharmacist has the responsibility to offer consultation on the best drug option, depending on the patient's symptoms, other disease states, and medications.

An advantage of nonprescription medications is that they do not require patients to see their physician in order to gain access to them. This alleviates a substantial burden on the health care community, and because the pharmacy is so accessible, it allows opportunities for the pharmacist to provide direct patient care. It also allows individuals more control over their own personal health needs.

The disadvantage to nonprescription medications is that without their physician's guidance, patients may misdiagnose their condition, and a more serious condition may remain unrecognized. This can lead to inadequate treatment. For this reason, one of the roles of the pharmacist is to appropriately triage patients, either recommending self-treatment with nonprescription medications as appropriate or directing the patient to see a physician if the pharmacist thinks a more serious condition may be present.

In addition, OTCs have pharmacological activity. Thus, they have the potential to cause significant side effects and interact adversely with other medications a patient may be taking. Certain nonprescription medications may not be safe for those patients with specific disease states; therefore, it is important for the pharmacist and pharmacy technician to be aware of the OTCs a patient is taking to allow the pharmacist to effectively counsel a patient. For the reasons just stated, nonprescription medications are not benign, and all considerations used by the pharmacist when evaluating prescription medications should be applied when a patient purchases an OTC medication.

A technician can be of great assistance to the pharmacist in identifying patients who may require additional counseling by the pharmacist. When patients come into the pharmacy to purchase a nonprescription medication or to fill a prescription, the pharmacy technician may ask the patient about his or her nonprescription medication use so that it can be placed in the patient's profile. Information that a pharmacy technician obtains during a casual conversation with the patient should be communicated to the pharmacist and will aid in identifying potential problems that may have otherwise gone unrecognized. To be able to do this effectively, a technician should be familiar with the numerous available OTC products. It is important to note, though, that a technician should not offer the patient a diagnosis, counsel a patient, or make recommendations. This is beyond the scope of the technician's role. This chapter highlights the most common therapeutic agents that patients may purchase without a prescription.

Dosage Forms

OTCs are available in many different formulations, similar to prescription drugs. The most widely used agents are available as oral dosage forms and include capsules, chewable tablets, disintegrating tablets, compressed tablets, effervescent tablets, suspensions, and solutions. It is important for patients to shake a suspension well; solutions do not require this step. Effervescent tablets, such as Alka-Seltzer, need to be dissolved in water or another compatible liquid prior to ingesting. These agents also tend to have an increased amount of sodium, which becomes important in those patients who are on salt-restricted diets for disease states such as hypertension or heart failure. If an alternative dosage form is available, the pharmacist should make a recommendation that the patient take that rather than the effervescent tablet. Sugar-free and alcohol-free formulations are also more appropriate for certain patients, such as the children and people with diabetes.

Topical agents include creams, gels, ointments, and lotions. Other dosage forms include eardrops, eyedrops, suppositories, enemas, and shampoos. These dosage forms should never be taken by mouth since they are intended for external use only.

Nonprescription medications may contain multiple active ingredients. This is often the case with cough, cold, flu, and allergy products. The patient may end up taking a drug for which there is no indication, increasing the risk of side effects. When the patient's symptoms are known by the pharmacist, this scenario may be avoided. An additional important point to note about nonprescription product formulations is that the active ingredients in a brand may change. Sometimes this is done while keeping the same brand name, so it is always important to look at the active ingredients specified on the product label.

Pain

analgesic an agent that relieves pain without causing loss of consciousness (e.g., codeine)

Agents used to treat a patient's pain are known as **analgesics**. A patient may have pain for various reasons, and it may manifest as headaches, muscle pain, or bone or joint pain. Pain is often categorized as either *acute* or *chronic*. Acute pain is due to a recent, sudden occurrence such as an injury, medical procedure, or accident, while chronic pain is usually the result of an underlying disease state such as cancer, rheumatoid arthritis, or multiple sclerosis.

In general, nonprescription analgesics are most appropriately utilized in patients experiencing acute pain or as adjunctive agents in those with chronic pain. They are effective for mild to moderate pain. The pharmacist should direct the patient to see his or her physician for a complete evaluation if the pain has not resolved within 10 days of taking an OTC analgesic. Some analgesics are also commonly used as antipyretics to decrease a patient's fever. The pharmacist should direct the patient to see his or her physician for a complete fever workup if the fever has not subsided within 3 days of taking an OTC antipyretic.

Internal analgesics are those that can be taken by mouth (PO) and include salicylates (e.g., aspirin), acetaminophen, and nonsteroidal anti-inflammatory drugs (NSAIDs). See **Table 24-1** for examples of agents that are available without a prescription. OTC NSAIDs include ibuprofen, ketoprofen, and naproxen. The doses of OTC NSAIDs are considerably less than their prescription counterparts.

TABLE 24-1 Nonprescription Analgesic Agents

THERAPEUTIC CATEGORY	GENERIC NAME	BRAND NAME	FORMULATION
Salicylates	aspirin	Anacin, Ascriptin, Aspercin, Bayer, Bufferin, Ecotrin, St. Joseph Aspirin	Tablets, caplets, chewtabs
	magnesium salicylate	Doan's Extra Strength, Momentum	Tablets, caplets
	choline salicylate	Arthropan	Liquid
Nonsteroidal anti-inflammatory drugs	ibuprofen	Advil, Motrin, Nuprin	Tablets, chewtabs, caplets, capsules, geltabs, drops, suspension, liquid
	naproxen sodium	Aleve	Caplets, tablets
Other	acetaminophen	Acephen, Tylenol	Disintegrating tablets, effervescent tablets, tablets, chewtabs, caplets, capsules, geltabs, drops, elixir, suspension, liquid, suppositories
Counterirritants	menthol	Absorbine Jr., Bengay, Flexall, Icy Hot, Therapeutic Mineral Ice	Topical liquid, gel, cream
	capsaicin	Capzasin, Zostrix	Topical lotion, gel, cream

Common side effects of salicylates include bleeding and gastrointestinal irritation. These drugs should be avoided in pregnant patients. Children and adolescents are at increased risk of developing Reye syndrome, a fatal illness, especially if they have the flu or chickenpox. Therefore, salicylates are generally avoided in this population. An important drug interaction to consider with the salicylates is that they may cause increased risk of bleeding in those patients also taking warfarin. This interaction is also seen in patients taking NSAIDs and, to a lesser degree, acetaminophen.

Like salicylates, NSAIDs also cause significant stomach upset, dyspepsia, and heartburn. To help prevent stomach upset, the pharmacist should instruct patients to take these agents with food, milk, or antacids. The NSAIDs should be avoided in those patients who are allergic to aspirin or have asthma, ulcers, renal impairment, or heart failure.

Acetaminophen is also widely used for pain and is well tolerated, but may be damaging to the liver in higher doses, especially in those who are malnourished or drink heavily. Acetaminophen is available in several different dosage formulations and strengths for both the adult and pediatric populations. These include drops, syrups, suspensions, suppositories, chewable tablets, caplets, tablets, and gelcaps.

Combination products are available for the consumer to purchase as well. The most common combination products include caffeine, which may increase the analgesic activity of the primary ingredient. They may be found as part of combination products for cough, cold, flu, and allergy.

Topical OTCs are available and are applied externally to the affected area of pain. External analgesics, including topical NSAIDs, are of questionable efficacy. They may decrease pain, itching, and burning. Counterirritants produce mild pain and inflammation at a site close to the affected area and decrease the severity of the patient's pain. This masks the patient's pain to make it more tolerable. Camphor, menthol, capsaicin, and trolamine salicylate are the most commonly used counterirritants. See Table 24-1 for available formulations. The pharmacist should warn users not to apply counterirritants to wounded skin or in the eyes. Bandages should not be placed over these products. Patients should be made aware that these agents might cause a burning sensation when applied and are never to be ingested.

Cold and Allergy

cold a self-limiting viral infection of the respiratory tract

antitussive a drug used for relief of a cough

antihistamine a drug used to reduce runny nose and sneezing

allergy a disorder in which the body becomes hypersensitive to a particular antigen (called an *allergen*).

A **cold** is a self-limiting viral infection of the upper respiratory tract. The main goal in patients suffering from a cold is to alleviate their symptoms, because a cold cannot be cured by the administration of antibiotics. Decongestants are used for patients' nasal stuffiness, analgesics are used for fever and pain, and **antitussives** are used for coughs. **Antihistamines** can also be utilized to help control a runny nose and sneezing. Many combination products are available, because many patients experience one or more cold symptoms. Multiple medications used separately can be quite confusing and cumbersome for the patient, and the likelihood of mistakes is much higher.

Allergies are characterized by sneezing, itchy and watery eyes, and an itchy, runny nose. The person with allergies may also experience increased fatigue, irritability, and worsening moods. These symptoms are triggered by an allergen, such as mold, pollen, cigarette smoke, dust, or pet dander. The symptoms of allergies are treated with antihistamines, intranasal cromolyn, and topical decongestants.

OTC decongestants are available as eyedrops, nasal sprays/drops/inhalers, and various oral formulations. Eyedrops contain naphazoline, oxymetazoline, phenylephrine, and tetrahydrozoline, and are utilized most often in patients with allergies. Intranasal formulations contain naphazoline, oxymetazoline, phenylephrine, propylhexedrine, and xylometazoline. The oral decongestants, including pseudoephedrine and phenylephrine, are absorbed into the bloodstream and can result in cardiovascular and central nervous system stimulation. This results in increased blood pressure, palpitations, high heart rate, restlessness, tremors, anxiety, insomnia, and fear. The oral decongestants may worsen hypertension, hyperthyroidism, diabetes, coronary heart disease, ischemic heart disease, and benign prostatic hypertrophy. In general, patients with these conditions should avoid the oral decongestant agents.

As of September 2006, federal regulations mandated that pseudoephedrine be stored behind the pharmacy counter or in locked cabinets because of its abuse potential. It has been used to synthesize methamphetamine; therefore, its distribution needs to be limited. Purchasers must provide photo identification and sign a log for each purchase of pseudoephedrine. The pharmacy must keep records of the name, address, signature, product purchased, quantity purchased, and the date and time of the purchase. These records must be retained for 2 years and do not apply to the purchase of single-dose packages that contain less than 60 milligrams. A single individual cannot purchase more than 3.6 grams per day or 9 grams per month. Pharmacies must also submit a statement notifying the attorney general that all pharmacy staff members have been trained on these regulations.

As a result of this mandate, many manufacturers have reformulated their pseudoephedrine products to contain phenylephrine instead, which can remain OTC and cannot be used to synthesize methamphetamine. Some still make their pseudoephedrine products in addition to the reformulated products.

Antitussives are those agents that are approved to suppress a patient's cold-related cough. The generic names of the nonprescription antitussives are codeine and dextromethorphan. Some states sell OTC codeine with certain restrictions, while others do not allow the sale of codeine as a nonprescription medication. Common side effects of codeine include nausea, vomiting, sedation, dizziness, and constipation. Codeine should not be used in those who have respiratory problems or a history of addiction.

TABLE 24-2 Nonprescription Agents for Cold and Allergy

THERAPEUTIC CATEGORY	GENERIC NAME	BRAND NAME	FORMULATION
Topical nasal decongestants	naphazoline	Privine	Nasal spray
	oxymetazoline	Afrin, Anefrin, Dristan 12-Hour, Mucinex, Neo-Synephrine 12-Hour, Vicks Sinex 12-Hour	Nasal spray, pump, drops
	phenylephrine	Dristan Cold, Little Noses, Neo-Synephrine, Rhinall, Vicks Sinex	Nasal spray, drops
Oral decongestants	phenylephrine	Contac, Dimetapp, Sudafed PE, SudoGest PE	Tablets, caplets, liquid
	pseudoephedrine*	Sudafed	Tablets, capsules, liquid
Antitussives	dextromethorphan	Benylin, Creomulsion, Delsym, Robitussin, Sucrets, Vicks	Capsules, liquid, lozenges, strips
Antihistamines	diphenhydramine	Banophen, Benadryl, Compoz, Diphenhist	Caplets, capsules, chewtabs, tablets, liquid, strips
	chlorpheniramine	Aller-Chlor, Chlor-Trimeton	Tablets, syrup
	cetirizine	All Day Allergy, Zyrtec	Chewtabs, disintegrating tablets, tablets, solution, syrup
	fexofenadine	Allegra	Disintegrating tablets, tablets, suspension
	loratadine	Alavert, Claritin	Capsules, disintegrating tablets, tablets, solution, syrup
Expectorants	guaifenesin	Allfen, Altarussin, Guiatuss, Mucinex	Tablet, liquid, solution, syrup

expectorant a substance that promotes the ejection of mucus or an exudate from the lungs, bronchi, and trachea

Dextromethorphan is well tolerated and does not cause sedation or respiratory depression, or have addictive properties. Guaifenesin is an **expectorant** that loosens thick secretions to make a cough more productive and, therefore, should only be used in those patients suffering from a nonproductive cough. There is a popular nonprescription combination product that contains both guaifenesin and dextromethorphan. This product is irrational because it contains an agent that suppresses the cough and one that causes the cough to be more productive.

Antihistamines are also used to control symptoms of the common cold and allergies. Some OTC antihistamines can cause sedation, but some cause it to a greater degree than others. The first-generation antihistamines are sedating antihistamines and include chlorpheniramine, clemastine, diphenhydramine, and doxylamine. Of these, chlorpheniramine is the least sedating. First-generation antihistamines can cause dry mouth, blurred vision, decreased urination, constipation, and an increased heart rate. They may also impair a patient's ability to perform tasks, such as those required for driving or working. The pharmacist should instruct patients with glaucoma or benign prostatic hypertrophy to avoid these antihistamines. Nonsedating or second-generation antihistamines were traditionally only available by prescription; however, because of their favorable safety profile, cetirizine, fexofenadine, and loratadine were made available OTC. These agents need to be used with caution in patients with liver or kidney disease and should be used at recommended doses, because going above the recommended dose makes the drug more likely to be sedating.

Cromolyn is used to treat the symptoms of allergies and is available as an intranasal spray. The pharmacist should inform the patient that it may take 3 to 7 days to begin to take effect and up to a month for maximum benefit. The most common side effects include sneezing and nasal burning and stinging, primarily due to its administration. See **Table 24-2** for a list of commonly used nonprescription cold and allergy products.

Constipation

constipation difficult, incomplete, or infrequent bowel evacuation

A decrease in the frequency of stool to below that of the patient's normal frequency is known as **constipation**. Constipated patients may experience abdominal discomfort, lower back pain, difficult passage of stool, bloating, and flatulence. Constipation is usually the result of inadequate exercise and the inadequate intake of water or fiber. It can also be drug induced in patients who are taking opioids for chronic pain relief. This can be prevented by giving the patient a proper regimen containing a stool softener and stimulant laxative. Nonprescription treatment options that facilitate the elimination of stool include bulk laxatives, hyperosmotic laxatives, lubricants, saline laxatives, and stool softeners.

Bulk-forming laxatives are used for fiber replacement therapy and are usually mixed with a liquid and taken by mouth. These include methylcellulose, polycarbophil, psyllium, and malt soup extract and are the safest of the laxatives. Bulk laxatives can be utilized for both prevention and treatment of constipation. These agents take as long as 3 days to work; therefore, patients who take these should not expect a bowel movement until then. The pharmacist must also instruct the patient to drink sufficient water with these agents to avoid blockage. They should also take the medications 2 hours prior to or 2 hours after taking other medications by mouth, because they can bind/interact with medications such as digoxin, warfarin, and salicylates.

Saline laxatives may be used to treat more severe constipation and should be used with caution in those who are dehydrated because these agents pull a significant amount of water into the intestine to soften the stool. Magnesium- and sodium-containing saline laxatives are available. The sodium-containing laxatives should be avoided in those patients on a low-salt diet, such as patients with hypertension or heart failure. Sodium-containing laxatives are most commonly used as enemas. Also, many sodium-containing laxatives contain phosphate; therefore, they should not be used in patients with kidney impairment. Patients with kidney impairment must also avoid magnesium-containing laxatives. The oral saline laxative will take effect in 30 minutes to 3 hours, whereas the enemas will take 2 to 5 minutes to work.

Hyperosmotic laxatives include glycerin and sorbitol. They can be given rectally in the form of suppositories and enemas, which may cause mild discomfort for the patient. The laxative effects usually occur within 15 to 60 minutes.

Stool softeners allow for easier and less painful passage of the stool by softening it. Docusate is the only available OTC softener. It is available as sodium or calcium salt and takes 12 to 72 hours to take effect. Docusate is well tolerated and has minimal side effects.

Mineral oil is the only available lubricant laxative and is available as an enema or an oil that is taken by mouth. Mineral oil takes about 6 to 8 hours to work. It should not be used as a first-line laxative because of its many adverse

TABLE 24-3 Nonprescription Agents for Constipation

THERAPEUTIC CATEGORY	GENERIC NAME	BRAND NAME	FORMULATION
Bulk-forming laxatives	polycarbophil	Equalactin, FiberCon, FiberGen, Fiber-Lax, Konsyl Fiber	Chewtabs, tablets
	methylcellulose	Citrucel	Powder
	psyllium	Genfiber, Geri Mucil, Konsyl, Metamucil	Capsules, granules, powder, wafers
	malt soup extract	Maltsupex	Powder
Saline laxatives	magnesium citrate	Citroma	Solution
	sodium phosphate	Fleet Saline Enema and Fleet Enema Extract	Enema
	magnesium hydroxide	Milk of Magnesia, Pedia-Lax	Chewtabs, suspension
Hyperosmotic laxatives	glycerin	Fleet Babylax, Fleet suppository, Pedia-Lax, Sani-Supp	Suppositories
Stool softeners	docusate sodium	Colace, Correctol, Diocto, Doc-Q-Lace, Silace	Liquid, capsules, tablets, syrup
Lubricant laxative	mineral oil	Fleet Mineral Oil Enema, Kondremul	Oil, enema
Stimulant laxatives	bisacodyl	Alophen, Correctol, Dulcolax, Fleet Stimulant Laxative	Chewtabs, tablets, caplets, suppositories
	sennosides	Evac-U-Gen, Ex-Lax, Medi-Lax, Senokot	Chewtabs, tablets, syrup
	castor oil		Oil

effects and interactions. Patients may aspirate the mineral oil; therefore, the pharmacist should warn the patient to remain upright when taking it and to take it at least 30 minutes prior to going to bed. Because mineral oil prevents the absorption of the fat-soluble vitamins, it should be taken 2 hours prior to or 2 hours after a meal.

Stimulant laxatives are available as liquids, tablets, granules, or suppositories. These laxatives force the bowel to expel its contents within 6 to 12 hours. Taking stimulants for an extended period of time may result in damage to the intestines. Senna, cascara, and casanthranol are known as the *anthraquinones*. These agents turn urine a pink to red or brown to black color. It is important to warn the patient about this effect. Diphenylmethanes include bisacodyl, which is the only bowel stimulant available as a suppository as well as a tablet. Castor oil is also a stimulant laxative. In most cases the stimulant laxative should be combined with a stool softener, such as docusate. The stimulant alone may not soften the stool adequately, leading to pain and discomfort when the stool is passed. See **Table 24-3** for a list of commonly used nonprescription products for constipation.

Diarrhea

diarrhea increased frequency of stool that is loose and watery

An increased frequency of stools with loose and watery consistency is known as **diarrhea**, which can be the result of diet, infection, or medications. A pharmacist should always instruct parents or guardians of pediatric patients who have had persistent diarrhea or have a fever associated with their diarrhea to consult with a physician. Children under 3 years old are more prone to the effects of fluid losses, and their parents should consult with a pediatrician. Dehydration and electrolyte abnormalities can manifest from just 2 days of diarrhea depending on the severity; therefore, these patients should see a physician. They may require the administration of intravenous fluids to correct the abnormalities. Patients with a fever may have an infectious cause of diarrhea and should be put on appropriate therapy, such as antibiotics, rather than OTC products. Patients with infectious diarrhea should generally avoid OTC antidiarrheal agents because they inhibit the removal of the pathogen by slowing the gastrointestinal transit time, which could result in longer duration or increased severity of diarrhea. The nonprescription agents used to treat diarrhea include polycarbophil, attapulgite, bismuth subsalicylate, kaolin, loperamide, lactobacillus, and oral rehydration solutions.

Calcium polycarbophil is a bulk laxative that was discussed earlier in the constipation section. It can be utilized for both constipation and diarrhea. It absorbs up to 60 times its weight in water to help "bulk up" the consistency of the stool. The pharmacist must inform patients that they should maintain adequate fluid intake and to chew the tablets before swallowing them. Patients who are on tetracycline should stagger their dose to minimize the effect of calcium binding to the tetracycline. Adsorbents include attapulgite, kaolin, pectin, and bismuth subsalicylate. These agents work by binding to toxins, bacteria, and noxious materials that can cause diarrhea. Because these agents work by binding to substances, which can result in decreased amount of drug available for activity, they should generally be given at least 2 hours prior to or 2 hours after other medications. Kaolin alone may be effective, but has not been proven to be effective when given with pectin and was therefore removed from older products containing the combination. Older kaolin-pectin combination products

TABLE 24-4 Nonprescription Agents for Diarrhea

THERAPEUTIC CATEGORY	GENERIC NAME	BRAND NAME	FORMULATION
Bulk laxative	calcium polycarbophil		
Adsorbents	attapulgite	Diarrest, Kao-tin	Tablets, liquid
	bismuth subsalicylate	Bismatrol, Diotame, Pepto-Bismol, Kaopectate	Chewtabs, tablets, suspension
Motility agent	loperamide	Diamode, Imodium AD	Capsules, chewtabs, liquid, tablet

were reformulated to contain attapulgite, which is effective in treating diarrhea. Some attapulgite products, like Kaopectate, were later reformulated to contain bismuth subsalicylate. Bismuth subsalicylate is available as a suspension and contains salicylate. For this reason, caution should be used in the pediatric population, those who are allergic to aspirin, and in those who are taking other salicylates or anticoagulants such as warfarin. Bismuth subsalicylate may darken the tongue and stool.

Loperamide helps with the symptoms of diarrhea by slowing gastrointestinal motility and is available as caplets or a solution. Adverse effects are rare and include drowsiness, dizziness, and constipation.

Lactobacillus has not been proven effective, but may promote regrowth of normal flora in the bowel. This agent must be refrigerated and may cause flatulence. Activated charcoal is not proven to be effective and is not recommended for the treatment of diarrhea. Oral rehydration solutions may be helpful while a patient is waiting to see a physician.

See **Table 24-4** for a list of select antidiarrheal agents and their brand names.

Acid/Peptic Disorders

gastroesophageal reflux disease (GERD) disease in which excess stomach acid causes a burning sensation in the esophagus due to eructation of small amounts of acid into the esophagus

peptic ulcer disease (PUD) ulceration of the stomach or duodenal lining

This section emphasizes the common gastrointestinal disorders that can be controlled with OTC medications. These include **gastroesophageal reflux disease (GERD)** and **peptic ulcer disease (PUD)**. PUD is ulceration of the stomach or duodenal lining. Patients must be seen by a physician and diagnosed with PUD before the pharmacist can aid in the selection of a nonprescription medication. Nonprescription medications used for patients with PUD are used as adjunctive agents in addition to prescription medications. Antacids can be used for pain relief, and bismuth subsalicylate can be used as part of a regimen including prescription medications to treat *H. pylori*, an infectious cause of PUD.

GERD, also called heartburn, causes a burning sensation in the chest area. This burning is the result of reflux of the acidic contents of the stomach up into the esophagus. The reflux causes irritation to the lining of the esophagus that can lead to discomfort and ulceration. Dietary and lifestyle modifications are key to the management of a patient suffering from heartburn. These measures include elevating the head of the bed, eating smaller meals, eating meals at least 3 hours before bedtime, and avoiding trigger foods such as mints, chocolates, citrus juices, spicy foods, foods with tomatoes, and coffee. It may also be helpful to lose weight, quit smoking, and avoid alcoholic beverages. Agents for heartburn that are available without a prescription include alginic acid, antacids, histamine$_2$ receptor antagonists (H_2RAs), and, most recently, proton pump inhibitors (PPIs). If patients have symptoms of gastric distress for longer than a 2-week period the pharmacist should advise the patient to see their physician.

antacid an agent that neutralizes gastric acid

Antacids neutralize the acid in the stomach to produce minimal irritation to the lining of the gastrointestinal tract. Calcium carbonate, sodium bicarbonate, aluminum hydroxide, aluminum phosphate, magnesium hydroxide, and magnesium chloride are OTC antacids. Suspensions allow for quicker dissolution than tablet formulations; therefore, suspensions usually have a quicker onset of action. Calcium carbonate and aluminum hydroxide dissolve more slowly than sodium bicarbonate and magnesium hydroxide and take about 10 to 30 minutes to produce an effect. Magnesium-containing antacids can cause diarrhea, while aluminum-containing antacids may cause constipation. For this reason, combination products are available to negate the effects of either agent. Magnesium can accumulate to cause central nervous system depression in patients with renal failure; therefore, the pharmacist should recommend an alternative antacid for these patients. Aluminum and sodium bicarbonate antacids should also be avoided in patients with renal impairments due to accumulation. Alginic acid has been combined with sodium bicarbonate. This combination forms a viscous solution that floats on the acidic contents of the stomach, and instead of acid refluxing into the esophagus, the viscous solution is refluxed, which decreases irritation and symptoms. Antacids interact with many medications, and the pharmacist should be aware of these in order to counsel the patient.

Histamine$_2$ receptor antagonists are available in prescription and nonprescription strength. The nonprescription strength is available in a lower dosage form. The H_2RAs that are available over the counter are cimetidine, famotidine, nizatidine, and ranitidine. These agents decrease gastric acid secretion, which decreases damage done to the gastrointestinal mucosa. The nonprescription strength of these agents is not adequate to heal gastrointestinal ulcers due to GERD and PUD. The patient should be notified that these agents may not result in relief of symptoms for 1 to 2 hours; therefore, they should be taken 1 hour before a meal rather than at the time of symptoms. Common side effects from nonprescription doses of H_2RAs include headache, dizziness, constipation, nausea, and vomiting. Significant drug-drug interactions may occur with the H_2RAs. Of the drugs in this category, cimetidine is associated with the most drug interactions.

Proton pump inhibitors prevent acid production and are also available with or without a prescription. Currently, lansoprazole and omeprazole are the only PPIs available without a prescription. The patient should be notified that PPIs do not provide immediate relief and that relief of symptoms may not occur for 1 to 4 days. Significant drug-drug interactions may occur with lansoprazole and omeprazole, and patients taking certain medications should consult their physician prior to taking omeprazole. Patients should not take this drug for more than a 14-day course or more than one course every 4 months, unless directed by their physician. **Table 24-5** lists common agents for use in acid/peptic disorders.

TABLE 24-5 Nonprescription Agents for Acid/Peptic Disorders

THERAPEUTIC CATEGORY	GENERIC NAME	BRAND NAME	FORMULATION
Antacids	magnesium hydroxide		
	aluminum hydroxide	Alternagel	Suspension
	aluminum/magnesium hydroxide	Mag-Al, Alamag	Chewtabs, liquid, suspension
	calcium carbonate	Alka-Mints, Calci-Chew, Tums	Chewtabs, liquid
	calcium carbonate/ magnesium hydroxide	Rolaids, Mylanta	Chewtabs, gelcaps, liquid
	aluminum hydroxide/ magnesium trisilicate	Gaviscon	Chewtabs
H_2 receptor antagonists	cimetidine	Acid Reducer, Tagamet HB	Tablets
	famotidine	Acid Controller, Heartburn Relief, Pepcid AC	Chewtabs, tablets
	nizatidine	Axid	Tablets
	ranitidine	Acid Reducer, Zantac	Tablets
Proton pump inhibitors	lansoprazole	Prevacid 24HR	Capsules
	omeprazole	Prilosec OTC	Capsules, tablets

Summary

Pharmacy technicians working in a pharmacy environment must be familiar with over-the-counter agents sold to patients. These products have significant interactions and adverse effects and should be treated much like prescription medications. The technician can aid the pharmacist in identifying those patients who may require further pharmacist counseling on nonprescription products. Knowledge of over-the-counter agents can help the technician do this effectively and with greater confidence. This chapter covers some of the most common problems that are self-treated with over-the-counter drugs.

TEST YOUR KNOWLEDGE

Multiple Choice

1. All of the following are true statements regarding nonprescription medications *except*
   a. OTCs are available for conditions that are considered to be self-treatable.
   b. OTCs allow the patient more control over health care needs.
   c. OTCs have pharmacological activity.
   d. OTCs do not have the potential to cause adverse reactions.

2. Which of the following products is an option for the patient with hypertension?
   a. Alka-Seltzer
   b. Fibercon
   c. Sudafed
   d. Fleet's Enema

3. All of the following are examples of NSAIDs *except*
   a. naproxen.
   b. ketoprofen.
   c. acetaminophen.
   d. ibuprofen.

4. Which of the following should be shaken well prior to administration?
   a. solution
   b. suspension
   c. elixir
   d. lotion

5. All of the following are topical dosage forms *except*
   a. Doan's.
   b. Capzasin.
   c. Mineral Ice.
   d. Icy Hot.

6. Dextromethorphan belongs to which of the following therapeutic categories?
   a. decongestant
   b. antitussive
   c. antihistamine
   d. expectorant

7. Which of the following antihistamines is *not* available OTC?
   a. diphenhydramine
   b. chlorpheniramine
   c. fexofenadine
   d. desloratadine

8. In most cases, senna should be given with which of the following nonprescription agents to decrease the pain and discomfort of constipation?
   a. Citroma
   b. Colace
   c. Maltsupex
   d. Milk of Magnesia

9. Which of the following can be used for the treatment of both constipation and diarrhea?
   a. polycarbophil
   b. docusate
   c. loperamide
   d. senna

10. Which of the following agents can be safely used in a patient with renal impairment?
   a. Alu-Tab
   b. Tums
   c. Milk of Magnesia
   d. Amphojel

Matching

Match the drug category with what it is used to treat.

1. ______ analgesic		a. cough
2. ______ antacid		b. excess stomach acid
3. ______ antitussive		c. pain
4. ______ antihistamine		d. runny nose and sneezing
5. ______ laxative		e. constipation

Fill in the Blank

1. Tablets, suspensions, and solutions are examples of ____________ dosage forms.

2. ____________ agents include creams, ointments, and lotions.

3. A ____________ is a self-limiting viral infection of the respiratory tract.

4. ____________ are characterized by sneezing, itchy, and watery eyes, and an itchy, runny nose.

5. ____________ is defined as a decrease in the frequency of stool to below that of the patient's normal frequency.

Suggested Readings

AHFS drug information. Bethesda, MD: American Society of Health-System Pharmacists.

Krinsky, D. L., Berardi, R. R., Ferreri, S. P., et al. (Eds.) (2010). *Handbook of nonprescription drugs* (17th ed.). Washington, DC: American Pharmacists Association.

Pray, W. S. (2006). *Nonprescription product therapeutics* (2nd ed.). Philadelphia, PA: Lippincott Williams & Wilkins.

CHAPTER 25

Natural Products

Competencies

Upon completion of this chapter, the reader should be able to:

1. Describe what makes a product an herbal (or botanical) versus a drug.
2. Describe how herbals are regulated by the U.S. Food and Drug Administration.
3. Explain the preparation and administration routes of most herbals.
4. Explain the potential for possibly dangerous interactions between herbals and standard drug therapy.
5. Be able to find reliable sources of current information on herbal safety and effectiveness.
6. List some common traditional uses of the major herbals.

Key Terms

dietary supplement
GRAS list
Herb Contraindications and Drug Interactions
herbal
hypersensitivity reaction
metabolite
secondary plant metabolite

Introduction

During the past two decades, the use of herbal natural products and dietary supplements in the United States has grown dramatically. The annual sales for the dietary supplement market in the United States for 2010 was estimated to be over $28 billion (Nutrition Business Journal, 2011). This is a significant increase from the year 2001, when the dietary supplement market was estimated to be about $18 billion (Nutrition Business Journal, 2002). Exactly how many of these sales are due to natural products is difficult to determine because of the overlap between the different categories of dietary supplements (such as herbal medicines and functional healthy foods). However, a number of clinical surveys during the past few years have demonstrated that upwards of 30% of all patients taking prescription drugs are also taking a dietary supplement or herbal. Therefore, it is important for the pharmacy technician to be familiar with benefits and potential hazards of herbal natural products. First, some terms must be defined.

By definition, a *drug* is "any substance or mixture of substances intended for the cure, mitigation, diagnosis, or prevention of disease." This definition comes, in large part, from the Pure Food Act of 1906 which formed the basis of what is now the U.S. Food and Drug Administration (FDA). Regulation of drugs in the United States is discussed elsewhere in this textbook and summarized in a subsequent section in this chapter.

herbal a plant with therapeutic properties that can be used for nutritional or medicinal purposes

dietary supplement any product containing a vitamin, mineral, amino acid, or herb that is intended to supplement the diet by increasing overall intake of a particular substance

When most people talk about "natural products" for medicinal use, they are referring to herbal preparations. An **herbal** substance is defined in the 1994 Dietary Supplement Health and Education Act (DSHEA) as a **dietary supplement**, not a drug. The DSHEA definition of a *dietary supplement* is any "product that contains a vitamin; mineral; amino acid; an herb or other botanical; a dietary substance for use by man to supplement the diet by increasing total daily intake; or a concentrate metabolite constituent, extract, or combinations of these ingredients."

Because they are not drugs, herbals and other dietary supplements cannot claim to cure, prevent, treat, or diagnose disease. They can claim to have a health action such as promoting healthy digestion. However, it is important to recognize that as a dietary supplement, herbal products are not evaluated by the FDA for either safety or effectiveness in the same manner that prescription drugs are evaluated. The reasons for this situation are discussed in the next section. In addition, the regulatory oversight that we have come to expect from the FDA with regard to drug manufacture has not necessarily been followed for the production of herbal products. In June 25, 2007, the FDA released revised regulations that set forth Good Manufacturing Practice (GMP) guidelines for dietary supplements. These guidelines came into force in June 2008 for large manufacturers (500 or more employees) and began to be phased in for small companies in 2010. They are now mandatory for all businesses that manufacture, label, or package dietary supplements for sale in the United States, including foreign businesses who ship into the United States (21 CFR Part 111).

Although these regulatory changes are helpful, there continues to be a lack of enforcement and assurance as to the safety, quality, and effectiveness of herbal preparations. In turn, this often places the pharmacy in a difficult position when asked for recommendations about herbal products. One of the goals of this chapter is to provide some guidelines for the review of herbal preparations and sources of reliable safety information.

History of Herbal Preparations

The use of natural products, especially plant products (herbals), for medicinal purposes predates recorded human history. Early humanoids would have used any materials available to try to treat illness, often mimicking nature in their attempts. When they achieved any success, it was likely they that they passed on the knowledge gained via oral tradition. The healing arts were likely an important tradition carefully guarded and maintained within various human groups. Learning these traditions probably took a great deal of time and commitment on the part of both the master and the apprentice. It is also likely the knowledge of which plants in a region produced beneficial effects was often lost with the death of one of these early herbalists if that person had not passed on his or her knowledge to an apprentice.

The invention of writing helped correct the loss of empirical herbal knowledge because now a more permanent record of observations could be made. As soon as written records appear in a culture, texts devoted to the recognition and preparation of medicines (*materia medica*) begin to appear. Indeed, it appears that one important reason for developing a system of writing was to record a *materia medica*, a set of recipes for preparing medicines.

In Europe, the invention of the movable type printing press in the mid-fifteenth century expedited the process and numerous herbal texts and *materia medica* were published from 1500 through the 1800s. Although these texts made the basic knowledge of natural products more available to the public, their use still required skillful interpretation and application. These skills were usually the purview of the apothecary or early pharmacist.

One of the primary roles of the apothecary or pharmacist was the compounding or mixing of medicines. However, pharmacists were not alone in this function. Several competing groups were seeking the revenue that came from the preparation of medicinal products. These groups included not only physicians and members of other medical professions, but also the grocers. Actually in England, the apothecaries originated as part of the Guild of Grocers in the late 1300s. In 1617, King James chartered a separate Apothecaries Guild separate from the Guild of Grocers. This separation of functions (and revenue) did not please the Grocers Guild. While the recognition of the specialized skills needed for correct medicine preparation did much to establish the professional identity of pharmacy, the battle for the monies generated continued well into the twentieth century. In the early twentieth century, numerous physicians not only diagnosed but also compounded and dispensed medicines. Also unlike today, patients did not have to go to a physician to get a prescription to buy medicines. Indeed, as late as the 1920s, less than 25% of all medicines and drugs purchased in drugstores were bought using prescriptions.

Most of the early medicines compounded were based on plant materials. One important example of such a medicine is digitalis, which was used to treat congestive heart failure. The active ingredients were usually harvested from the purple foxglove (*Digitalis purpurea*) or from the white foxglove (*Digitalis lanata*). In fact, the medicine derived its name from the genus name of the plants from which it was harvested. This medication was popularized by William Withering, a British physician, who published a monograph in 1785 on the use of extract of foxglove and the beneficial effects of digitalis on dropsy (the old name for congestive heart failure). Withering's treatise was one of the first published scientific studies of an herbal compound. Although crude digitalis extract is no longer used in the United States, digoxin and digitoxin (members of the cardiac glycoside drug class), which are the main components of the extract, are currently available.

To aid pharmacists in preparing compounds in a more a consistent manner, several national publications arose. The U.S. Pharmacopeia (USP) started in 1820 and the National Formulary (NF) started in 1888 by the American Pharmaceutical Association are two publications that have taken on the status of being official compendiums that set national standards. The USP describes standards for drug identity, strength, quality, purity, packaging, and labeling. The NF sets standards for excipients, botanicals, and other similar products. The NF was purchased by the USP in 1975, combining the two publications under one cover entitled the USP-NF.

Early on, these publications had numerous monographs on the preparation of botanical products. At its peak, the USP published over 600 monographs on botanicals. By 1900, that number had decreased to 169 monographs. Between 1900 and 1990, the increasing use of synthetic organic drugs resulted in a further reduction in attention to plant-derived medicines. Thus, in the latter quarter of the twentieth century, the USP-NF had few monographs on botanicals. Fortunately, that situation is changing and the USP-NF has reenergized its efforts to review botanicals and herbal products and publish appropriate monographs.

Thus, the use of natural products has been intimately connected to the profession of pharmacy since its inception. In the early twentieth century, the pharmacist was usually the individual collecting and preparing the natural product for use by the patient. The growth of large corporate pharmaceutical companies profoundly changed this process. Drugs prepared by the large pharmaceutical companies to relatively exacting standards came to be thought of as more uniform and therefore safer than the older, individually compounded preparations. Thus, by the late twentieth century, pharmacists were often viewed as having only a dispensing role providing prepackaged drugs for patient treatment.

Historical Review of Drug Regulations

At this point, a brief history of drug regulation in the United States is useful. Prior to the early 1900s, the United States had few enforceable laws pertaining to medicines or what we would now call drugs. In 1906, the Pure Food Act was passed by Congress and signed into law. The legislation was enacted largely due to public concern over adulteration of foods as described by authors such as Upton Sinclair. Sinclair's book *The Jungle* described horrific practices at some meat packing plants and sparked public outrage demanding regulatory oversight over the production of food and medicines.

Although the title of the 1906 Pure Food Act suggests that it was about purity and food safety, in reality the law focused on making sure only that foods and drugs were truthfully and accurately labeled. The 1906 law had several important impacts on pharmacy. The law defined what constituted a drug and prohibited adulterated or misbranded drugs. However, it did not require that a drug be proven safe or effective. The 1906 law also converted the USP and NF from private publications into the official standards for the manufacture and compounding of drugs. And finally, the law essentially triggered creation of what has become the Food and Drug Administration.

To enforce the provisions of the 1906 legislation, the Department of Agriculture's Division of Chemistry headed by Harvey W. Wiley was enlarged and renamed the Bureau of Chemistry. The Bureau of Chemistry was charged with assaying and checking the accuracy of content labels. By 1927, the regulatory aspects of the

Bureau of Chemistry had become so large that they were moved to a new agency named the Food, Drug, and Insecticide Administration. In 1931, the name was shorted to the Food and Drug Administration (FDA).

As described earlier, the 1906 act was primarily concerned with truth in labeling. The Bureau of Chemistry could only act if a drug was misbranded or adulterated. There were no requirements that a drug be proven effective or even safe before being sold to the public. Then in 1937, the "elixir of sulfanilamide" tragedy occurred. A pharmaceutical company mixed sulfanilamide with diethylene glycol because it dissolved well and had a reasonable taste. Unfortunately, diethylene glycol, like ethylene glycol (the main component in automobile antifreeze), is poisonous to humans, causing potentially fatal central nervous system and kidney (renal) damage. More than 100 of the patients who ingested the mixture died due to renal failure. Because there was no requirement that drugs be proven safe prior to sale, the FDA could only charge the pharmaceutical company with misbranding because it had used the term *elixir* in the drug's name. Elixir is used to indicate an alcohol solution and there was no alcohol in the mixture. A fine of slightly more than $26,000 was levied on the company, but no other action could be taken.

Once again, public outrage led to enactment of new legislation. In 1938, the Federal Food, Drug, and Cosmetic Act was signed into law. This legislation focused on demonstration of drug safety. The law spelled out procedures for how applications for new drug approval had to occur. For the first time medical devices were included in FDA regulations. Perhaps most importantly, the regulations gave special treatment to prescriptions written by physicians, veterinarians, and dentists. They distinguished between prescription and over-the-counter (OTC) drugs, which led to the prescription-only method of drug acquisition that is common today. The 1938 Federal Food, Drug, and Cosmetic Act is the foundation of drug regulation as it exists in the United States.

However, the 1938 legislation still did not require a drug to be effective. This was corrected by the Drug Amendments of 1962 (often called the Kefauver-Harris Amendments), which required that all drugs marketed after 1962 in the United States be proven both safe and effective. Although already in committee in the Congress, enactment of this legislation was spurred by the thalidomide tragedy. Although never approved for sale in the United States, use of thalidomide in pregnant women often led to phocomelia, a birth defect in which the child is born missing one or more limbs. Although nothing in the 1962 Drug Amendments would have specifically prevented clinical testing of thalidomide in the United States, it did encourage the mentality that the FDA should decide what drugs would be allowed on the market and then tightly regulate how they should be used.

To determine which drugs were effective, the FDA worked with the National Academy of Sciences' National Research Council to organize a drug efficacy study. This study examined the effectiveness of some 4,000 drugs that contained about 300 different chemicals. A final report was made in 1969. This report established much of how we think about prescription drugs in pharmacy today.

The drugs that could be purchased without a physician's prescription, the OTC drugs, were not examined (to any great extent) in the drug efficacy study. To deal with this oversight, the FDA set up 17 panels in 1972 to evaluate the effectiveness of the active ingredients of OTC drugs. However, lack of sufficient data and resources to evaluate many of the OTCs led to a less than satisfactory result. The panels only examined ingredients if they were asked to do so and then only evaluated evidence presented to them. In 1990, when the final OTC study was released to the public, the safety and efficacy of many herbals was still in question.

A few botanicals, such as senna leaves (which act as a laxative), were found to be safe and effective and classed as Category I (safe and effective). Almost 150 herbals were classed as Category II (unsafe or ineffective). However, over 100 herbals were classed as Category III (insufficient evidence to evaluate). Note that a Category III designation does not mean that an herbal was not safe or effective; it merely means that no decision was made because of lack of supporting evidence. For those looking for more direction on the use of herbals in medical practice, this was a disappointing outcome. This classification system certainly did not provide pharmacy with much guidance in dealing with herbals.

Regulation of Herbals in the United States

GRAS list a list of food additives generally recognized as safe by the Food and Drug Administration

One approach to address the concerns over herbals was to use the GRAS list. A number of herbals are on a 1958 list of Generally Recognized As Safe food additives, known as the **GRAS list**. However, as the name indicates, this list is directed primarily at food and flavoring agents and not at therapeutic actions. Thus, little reliable information was available to pharmacies for evaluating the safety and effectiveness of herbals as compared to prescription drugs.

Finally, in 1994 the Dietary Supplement Health and Education Act (DSHEA) was signed into law. This law treats herbals as dietary supplements, not drugs, and allows them to make claims with regard to general health promotion but not treatment of disease claims (like drugs). Much like the 1906 Pure Food Act, DSHEA focuses on the labeling of herbals (as well as other dietary supplements), spelling out what constitutes a misbranded or adulterated botanical (herbal).

According to DSHEA, an herbal must (1) be labeled as a dietary supplement, (2) identify all ingredients by name, (3) list the quantity of each ingredient, (4) identify the plant and the plant part from which the ingredient is derived, (5) comply with any standards set by an official compendium (such as the USP and the NF), and (6) meet the quality, purity, and compositional specifications as established by validated assays. Failure to comply with these regulations means that an herbal is misbranded. The DSHEA also sets guidelines to prevent adulteration of dietary supplements. The DSHEA even states that a botanical or herbal must be "prepared, packed or held" under Good Manufacturing Practices (GMP) protocols. Mandating GMP is meant to ensure quality at the manufacturing (or preparation) stage of herbal production. As noted earlier, although mandated in 1994, the final guidelines for GMP standards were not published until June 25, 2007 (FDA 21 CFR Part 111). The regulations were to be phased into practice between June 2008 (for manufacturers with 500 or more employees) and June 2010 (for small companies). The expectation was that these GMP guidelines would result in enhanced quality assurance and safer herbal products. A summary review of FDA's final GMP guidelines for dietary supplements was published in the journal of the American Botanical Council (Cavaliere & Blumenthal, 2007).

However, to follow GMP during manufacture or preparation requires absolute standards that do not currently exist for many herbals. The new GMP guidelines require only that the methods be "scientifically valid" while allowing the manufacturers to establish their own specifications for identity, purity, potency and relative composition. Furthermore, the DSHEA regulations say that the FDA may not "impose standards for which there is no currently and generally available analytical methodology."

For example, in the preparation of St. John's wort (an herbal often used for depression), which of the many components of the plant should be used by a manufacturer to standardize its manufacturing process? Two major components in St. John's wort are hypericin and hyperforin. Currently, many companies use hypericin levels as their assay standard for preparation of St. John's wort extract. However, there is no direct evidence that hypericin is the active ingredient in St. John's wort. Indeed, recent evidence suggests that if St. John's wort is effective in depression that the active ingredient may be hyperforin, not hypericin. Until the exact efficacious ingredients have been determined for a particular herbal, exact potency (and therefore dosage) will be problematic.

In summary, as this brief history of the regulation of herbals indicates, herbals have a unique status in the United States. Manufacturers can only market them with health claims and may not make any claims as to their use in treating disease (i.e., disease claims). However, millions of consumers (and patients) are purchasing these preparations to treat disease. While health care professionals at many levels are concerned about the safety and effectiveness of these preparations, current limitations on the FDA make it unlikely that this agency will be able to readily address these concerns in the near future. This leaves pharmacies in the difficult position of trying to counsel the consumer (patient) without adequate information. Certainly, the easiest, most conservative advice would be to not purchase or use herbals unless advised to do so by a physician. However, without specific warnings (e.g., "Use of this preparation has caused liver failure in patients with your condition!"), the "do not use" advice is likely to be ignored. Annual sales of dietary supplements are estimated to be more than $28 billion. More and more people are turning to herbals as part of their health care. Thus, the rest of this chapter is directed toward helping pharmacy technicians understand and obtain up-to-date, useful information on herbals.

Chemical Structure: Most Herbals Are Secondary Plant Metabolites

secondary plant metabolite derived from primary plant metabolites

metabolite a chemical synthesized within cells as part of a metabolic pathway

Although the term *herbal* has been applied to any plant substance used for health purposes, most herbals are **secondary plant metabolites**. The term **metabolite** refers to a chemical synthesized within cells as part of a metabolic pathway. Primary plant metabolites are compounds that are essential for basic plant cell function and life. Primary metabolites fall into five general classes: proteins, nucleic acids, carbohydrates (sugars), simple organic acids, and lipids (fats). Secondary metabolites are derived from the primary metabolites, but have their own specialized pathways of synthesis. Secondary metabolites may be important for the success and health of the plant, but they are not as essential to basic plant cell survival as primary metabolites.

The functions of secondary metabolites in plants are quite varied. It is important to recognize that plants face many of the same environmental challenges that humans do, except they cannot change their location in response to these challenges. Thus some secondary metabolites evolved to help conserve moisture for the plant (e.g., the suberins and waxes), some evolved to help ward off herbaceous animals (predators) as a form of chemical self-defense (e.g., various plant toxins such as nicotine), and some evolved to fight fungal, bacterial, and viral infections in plants. It is this last group of substances that is of particular interest to modern medicine and pharmacy because some of these compounds can also be used to fight infections in humans.

For simplicity, secondary plant metabolites can be divided into three major groups or classes of compounds: (1) the terpenoids, (2) the alkaloids, and (3) the phenylpropanoids (including the flavonoids) and allied phenolics. Of these, the terpenoids are by far the most numerous in occurrence with more than 25,000 identified chemically. By comparison, about 12,000 alkaloids have been identified and approximately 8,000 plant phenolics characterized. The chemical characteristics of secondary plant metabolites have been reviewed and summarized in numerous texts such as those of Bowsher et al. (*Plant Biochemistry*), Dewick (*Medicinal Natural Products*), Gleason and Chollet (*Plant Biochemistry*), and Buchanan et al. (*Biochemistry & Molecular Biology of Plants*). Although these secondary metabolites have been extensively characterized chemically, only a fraction of them have been tested for possible medicinal benefit.

Preparation and Routes of Administration of Herbals

Up until the mid-twentieth century, much of the work in the pharmacy was focused on preparation and compounding of plant material into herbal medicines. Today, however, most herbal preparations will enter the pharmacy already packaged. One reason for this is because few pharmacists are currently trained in pharmacognosy. *Pharmacognosy* is the science of selecting and preparing plant materials for medical use (see Robbers et al. entry in the Suggested Readings section at the end of this chapter). Note that the selection and harvesting of plant material for herbal preparation should only be performed by trained and experienced professionals. There is significant risk of plant misidentification and subsequent toxicologic misadventure. Use of published identification standards is recommended (e.g., see Applequist entry in the Suggested Readings section).

A second reason is economic; that is, it is cheaper to purchase the material ready to sell rather than to have to prepare and package it. This is certainly the case with many OTC preparations. However, compounding of an herbal product may be the only way to get it into a form usable to a patient. Even with prepackaged materials, there is still the matter of product safety, which is more complicated for herbals than for drugs (see later discussion).

Many retail herbal preparations are supplied as tablets, capsules, lozenges, liquids, or tinctures to be taken orally (PO). Some herbals are supplied in a dry form to be taken PO as a powder or made into a tea or similar drink. A number of herbals are for external skin or topical use only and are supplied as a gel, cream, or ointment. It is difficult to obtain herbal products that meet the microbiological and particulate safety standards needed for injection of a product in the human body. Thus, *for safety reasons, herbal products should not be given by injection*, that is, by intravenous (IV), intramuscular (IM), or intra-arterial routes.

The Safety of Herbals

Advocates for herbals often state that they are safer than modern drugs because they have been used by humans for a long time. In some instances, herbals have been used as a food or dietary supplement for generations. In general, most herbals are safe at low to moderate dosages. However, a number of issues remain that must be considered by the pharmacy. The most important of these issues are (1) the potential of a hypersensitivity (i.e., allergic) response to an herbal, (2) that the product actually contains the herbal claimed, (3) the potential contamination or adulteration of the herbal product with toxic material, and (4) the potential for an herbal-drug interaction.

Hypersensitivity (Allergic) Reactions

hypersensitivity reaction a reaction that occurs after a person is exposed to a compound and has generated antibodies against the compound

Just as with any newly administered drug or food, attention must be paid to the possibility of a hypersensitivity reaction to a component of the herbal product by the patient. A **hypersensitivity reaction** occurs when a patient has been exposed to a compound previously and has made antibodies against the compound. When the patient takes the compound again, a "hyper" or larger than normal immune response occurs and the patient's own antibodies or immune cells begin to cause problems. Examples of hypersensitivity reactions are a pollen allergy or a food allergy such as to peanuts. Hypersensitivity reactions can range in intensity from an immediate allergic reaction such as anaphylactic shock that can lead to death to the skin rashes common in delayed hypersensitivity. Unfortunately, there is no easy way to predict which patients will have a hypersensitivity response to a particular food, compound, or drug. With herbal products, the concern about potential allergic responses is heightened because of the complex chemical natural of herbals. An herbal product may contain dozens to hundreds of compounds that might react with the immune system. On the other hand, immune tolerance can be induced by a number of food components and certain herbals may be better tolerated because of a cross-tolerance effect.

In summary, given the potential severity and unpredictability of hypersensitivity reactions, the patient should be counseled to be on the lookout for the signs and symptoms of hypersensitivity not just the first time they take an herbal but also with each subsequent use. The pharmacy personnel should also be on the lookout for such reactions. *If there is an indication that a patient is having an allergic response to an herbal product, the person should immediately discontinue use of the product and seek appropriate medical treatment at once.*

Content and Concentration of the Herbal Product

The concern that the product may not contain the herbal listed on the label or may have varying concentrations of the herbal is still a significant problem. Several analytical testing laboratories have examined herbal products from a number of manufacturers or producers and found a wide disparity in the contents of the product. Indeed, different batches of a product from the same manufacturer may vary significantly in content and concentrations. An important next step in the herbal industry will have to be the standardization of various products. According to the new GMP guidelines, starting in 2008 manufacturers were required to establish and maintain records of identity, purity, strength, and relative composition of components in their product. There is no requirement that an expiration date be placed on an herbal product. However, if a date is provided, the manufacturer must maintain records that support the choice of date (i.e., shelf life of the product). Quality assurance for the new GMP regulations requires that each manufacturer test subsets of each batch of finished herbal product in a manner that is consistent with currently accepted statistical sampling methods. The resultant data must be maintained for at least 1 year after the product's expiration date (if one is used) or for 2 years beyond the date of distribution of the last batch of an herbal product. The new regulations and the increased involvement of the FDA should clarify some of the issues about quality and content in herbals.

However, as pointed out earlier, nationally recognized absolute standards for many herbals do not exist at this time. In many cases, no single active ingredient has been identified. This leaves the question of content of an herbal open ended. In the end, a pharmacy (or parent organization such as a retail chain or hospital) must investigate to determine how well an herbal manufacturer is meeting the required GMP standards. In addition to the FDA's involvement, several other organizations are offering verification programs to assist the pharmacy in this regard (see later discussion).

Potential Contamination or Adulteration of an Herbal Product

In addition to the question of how much of a desired herbal may be in a finished product, there is also concern that undesired plant materials or heavy metals or other toxic contaminants may be present in the product. In particular, if an herb is harvested from a wild or uncultivated field, the possibility of undesired plant contamination is significant.

This issue has taken on a heightened concern with the reported incidents of toxic contamination on the increase. In one case in Europe, an herbal product for weight reduction was found to be adulterated with the plant contaminant aristolochic acid. This compound has been reported to be nephrotoxic in laboratory animals. In an investigation reported in 2000, this compound was also associated with the development of urothelial carcinoma in a number of Belgian consumers of the weight-reduction herbal. These observations have been confirmed and expanded. In 2008, the International Agency for Cancer Research concluded that aristolochic acids are carcinogenic in humans (Grosse et al., 2009). Concern about aristolochic acid contamination in herbals is significant enough that they are now listed in the annual *Report on Carcinogens* published by the U.S. Department of Health and Human Services (U.S. National Toxicology Program, 2011).

In another case, an herbal product was found to be contaminated with *Digitalis lanata* (white foxglove). The contamination was discovered when a consumer of the herbal was admitted to hospital with what was found to have been digitalis poisoning. After an investigation by the FDA, the manufacturer voluntarily removed the product from the market. Although the manufacturer responded appropriately to protect the public safety, note that this contamination was only discovered after consumers had been exposed to the risk. Similar incidents have been reported with regard to heavy metal contamination (e.g., lead, mercury, and cadmium) of glucosamine products derived from mollusks. The only solution to such situations is extensive screening and testing for toxic contaminants by the manufacturer or producer of an herbal. Unfortunately, many small manufacturers do not currently have the expertise or equipment for such screening. This issue has been a major problem in determining the safe use of herbals.

The new GMP regulations require manufacturers to determine if there are any contaminants in their finished herbal products and to determine the identity of any such contaminants. However, the FDA regulations do not specify upper limits for any contaminants. This suggests that there may be a range of responses to this particular section of the guidelines. Therefore, it will probably take some time before the FDA clarifies this aspect of the regulations to the satisfaction of health care providers.

Meanwhile, several third-party organizations can assay and report on potential contaminants in herbal products. Some of these are trade-associated organizations or for-profit companies. From a scientific viewpoint, an independent not-for-profit organization with the requisite testing experience and facilities is preferable. One such organization is the National Sanitation Foundation International or NSF International (not to be confused with the National *Science* Foundation). This is a nonprofit organization that began operation in 1944. Its focus was initially on water purity and then it began to branch out into public health. NSF International is used by the American Herbal Pharmacopoeia.

The USP also has a verification and testing program. In 2002, the USP launched an initiative entitled the Dietary Supplement Verification Program (DSVP) in which manufacturers voluntarily submit their products to USP testing. Any product passing USP testing will be awarded the DSVP verification mark. The goals of the DSVP are to ensure consumers and health care professionals that a dietary supplement product contains the ingredients listed on the label at the declared concentrations, that the product meets requirements (as listed in the USP-NF) on potential contaminants, and that the product has been manufactured in compliance with the GMPs proposed by the FDA and USP. Although manufacturer enrollment is voluntary, this program has examined and verified over 200 product lines to date. For pharmacists, the USP standard is perhaps the most trusted one in practice. Details of the verification program and an up-to-date list of verified companies can be found on the USP website (www.usp.org).

Potential Herbal-Drug Interactions

Just as with drug-drug interactions, the concomitant usage of herbal preparations with prescription drugs may lead to significant herbal-drug interactions with adverse outcomes. Herbals and orally administered drugs are absorbed across the GI tract, metabolized by the liver, and excreted by the kidneys. Therefore, it is not surprising that the presence of herbals may alter the absorption, metabolism, or excretion of drugs. For example, use of St. John's wort has been reported to decrease the absorption of digoxin and indinavir (an antiviral) and to increase the metabolism of warfarin, cyclosporine, and oral contraceptives. Each of these interactions would decrease the amount of prescription drug concentrations in patients, potentially resulting in subtherapeutic doses. In short, the patient might be undertreated even though he or she is receiving the correct dosage of prescription drug. The difficulty of predicting such interactions with herbals is greatly complicated because they are not single compounds. There is no evidence, for example, that the above-described effects of St. John's wort are due to a single constituent.

> ***Herb Contraindications & Drug Interactions*** a useful resource by Francis Brinker on herbal-drug interactions

A useful resource on herbal-drug interactions for the pharmacy is the text ***Herb Contraindications & Drug Interactions*** by Francis Brinker. Another recent publication that can be helpful is *Herbal Supplements: Efficacy, Toxicity, Interactions with Western Drugs, and Effects on Clinical Laboratory Tests*, edited by A. Dasgupta and C. A. Hammett-Stabler. This volume also deals with the potential interaction of herbals in a number of clinical lab tests.

Additional information can be found on the Natural Medicines Comprehensive Database website (www.naturaldatabase.com) under the "Natural Product/Drug Interaction Checker." In addition to being accessible via the Internet, this database may be downloaded to a mobile device making it handy during patient counseling and information review.

Therapeutic Value of Herbals

Most of the above discussion has focused on the issues of safety under the premise of "first do no harm." Of course, the real reason for using herbals is their potential therapeutic value. Unfortunately, there is no easy answer to the question "Do herbals have therapeutic effects?" While it is logical to expect some herbals to be very useful in treatment (after all, most of our early medications were derived from botanicals), clinical trials have been lackluster in demonstrating efficacy or in definitively ruling it out. There are a number of reasons for this state of affairs, including poor clinical trial design, poor execution, and clear bias. Moreover, the source of many herbals used in some trials has come under significant scrutiny. A well-designed clinical trial, that is well executed, is to no avail if the product tested does not actually contain the herbal compound under investigation. Thus, the source of the herbal (which has not been extensively considered or documented in most trials) is paramount to a sound study. For all these reasons, the effectiveness of herbals in treatment remains to be worked out on a case-by-case basis.

International Natural Medicines

Each region of the world has its own form of traditional medicine and natural product use. Some of these therapies have gained a large following in the United States such as traditional Chinese medicine (TCM), Japanese Kampo, and Indian Ayurvedic medicine. In addition, traditional African and South American medicines are becoming increasingly popular. The availability of the natural products for such traditional therapies has become greatly enhanced by the Internet and international online sales.

Although regional natural products are becoming increasingly accessible, the expert knowledge and skill needed for their use often is not. Furthermore, the details of a natural product's composition is often only available in the native language of the region. The dearth of such information makes it difficult for an American pharmacy to offer any informed decisions as to safety or potential herb-drug interactions.

Fortunately, some resources are becoming available that are filling that gap. There is an English language version of the Chinese pharmacopeia in a three-volume set published by the Chinese government (Chinese Pharmacopoeia Commission, 2011). Volume 1 deals with herbals and botanicals used in TCM. Another useful resource is the two-volume set entitled *Handbook of Chinese Medicinal Plants: Chemistry, Pharmacology and Toxicology* (Tang & Eisenbrand, 2010). This set of texts deals specifically and comprehensively with the herbals of TCM.

For Japanese traditional medicine (Kampo), the Japanese Society of Oriental Medicine has published an *Introduction to Kampo: Japanese Traditional Medicine* in English (Sato et al., 2005). This text not only describes the basics of Kampo and its approach to disease, but also provides brief descriptions of modern scientific investigations that have been performed to demonstrate the efficacy of a number of the traditional herbal compounds. Unfortunately, although a comprehensive pharmacopeia listing all the ingredients of Kampo medicines has been published by the Japanese Society of Oriental Medicine, it is currently only available in Japanese.

For Ayurvedic medicine, the Ministry of Health & Family Welfare of India has published several volumes detailing the composition of traditional Ayurvedic medicines. Some of these volumes are being made available in ebook format (usually PDF) free of charge on the Internet. One example can be found at www.ayurveda.hu/api/API-Vol-1.pdf It is recommended that the regional language package be activated on the computer or electronic reading device prior to downloading because some words (such as traditional names) are often in the original language. In the case of Ayurvedic herbals, the original name is often in Sanskrit.

It is probable that the American trend toward use of international or regional natural products will continue to increase. Therefore, every pharmacy needs to question its patients as to any natural product use and have reliable sources of information available and accessible in order to understand the natural product being used, its composition, and any potential interactions with other drugs or contraindications.

Where to Get More Information on Herbals

The concerns over safety and efficacy discussed in this chapter clearly underscore the need for information on herbals that is updated in a timely manner and made rapidly available to the pharmacy. Until recently, it has been hard to obtain such information in the United States. Now, however, some very useful sources are available:

1. The U.S. Pharmacopeia (USP) is a mainstay of pharmacy in the USA. The USP-NF publications essentially set the standard of practice in pharmacy. As such, USP monographs on particular herbals will be central to any pharmacy's information database. From 1995 to 2005, USP reinvigorated it efforts to publish up-to-date information on botanicals and herbals in its dietary supplements section. As of 2013, USP had more than 80 monographs on botanicals/herbals. Starting in 2008, all dietary supplements monographs began to be published in one volume. Furthermore, in November 2007, USP announced 11 new proposed monographs on dietary supplements with the following breakdown : 6 tumeric-related monographs, 3 soy isoflavones monographs, and 2 amino acid formulations (*Pharmacopeial Forum,* 33[6]). These monographs are in addition to ones announced in July 2007 on decaffeinated green tea extract and powdered bilberry extract. Updates as to the progress of these monographs can be found on the USP website at www.usp.org.
2. *The ABC Clinical Guide to Herbs* edited by Mark Blumenthal and published by the American Botanical Council (2003) (ISBN 1-58890-157-2) is a handy compendium of relevant facts on various herbals and summaries of published clinical trials. Although a number of similar publications are available, none has the range of information as well as the clinical data. Additionally, rapid updates on clinical information as well as a searchable database are available via the ABC website (www.herbalgram.org) for members of the American Botanical Council. As a single reference on herbals in the pharmacy, this text is a valuable resource. The ABC website also contains a wealth of information, but you must pay a fee to access some resources.
3. The Natural Medicines Comprehensive Database (www.naturaldatabase.com) is also a fee-based website. However, as noted earlier, it has many useful features including access to clinical trial information and updates.
4. The USP Dietary Supplement Verification Program (DSVP) sets a high standard for herbals in the United States and ensures the pharmacy of the safety of a product. Manufacturers voluntarily submit their products to USP testing. Updates and details about the DSVP can be found at the USP web site (www.usp.org). This program has verified over 200 product lines to date.
5. The NIH Office of Dietary Supplements website at http://ods.od.nih.gov is helpful. One of the provisions of the DSHEA of 1994 was the formation of an Office of Dietary Supplements (ODS) at the National Institutes of Health (NIH). The mission of the ODS is to "strengthen knowledge and understanding of dietary supplements by evaluating scientific information, stimulating and supporting research, disseminating research results, and educating the public. . . ." ODS has created and maintains two large databases on herbals: IBIDS (the International Bibliographic Information on Dietary Supplements) and CARDS (Computer Access to Research on Dietary Supplements). CARDS covers all federally funded

research projects such as those from the NIH from 1999 onward. IBIDS covers all "published, international, scientific literature on dietary supplements" and includes almost 700,000 entries. Both databases can be accessed free of charge at the ODS website.

6. Another very useful website is the National Center for Complementary and Alternative Medicine at http://nccam.nih.gov. This site contains information on current clinical trials and drug interactions between herbals and drugs.
7. Medwatch (www.fda.gov/medwatch) contains information from the FDA Safety Information and Adverse Event Reporting Program. This site is not focused exclusively on herbals or dietary supplements, but adverse events, drug interactions, and important safety announcements are reported here. This is a very useful site for the pharmacy.
8. The publication in English of the *German Commission E Monographs on Herbals* provides an excellent reference based on the accepted medicinal uses of herbals in Europe. The text is entitled *Herbal Medicine: Expanded Commission E Monographs*. It is edited by M. Blumenthal, A. Goldberg, and J. Brinckman, published by Integrative Medicine Communications (2000), and is available in hardback (ISBN 0967077214) and as a CD-ROM. This text gives a different perspective on the use of herbals in medicine that is quite useful in making clinical decisions.

Some Traditional Uses of Herbals

Listed next are some common herbal products and their traditional or common uses. Please note that this section is not an endorsement of the clinical efficacy of any particular herbal, nor is it meant to be an exhaustive list of all herbals used. Rather, these are merely examples of typical herbal products.

Common Name: Angelica
Botanical Name: *Angelica archangelica*
Typical Uses: To relieve symptoms of flatulence (i.e., GI gas), as a diuretic (i.e., to increase urine flow), and as a diaphoretic (i.e., sweat producer). Also used as a flavoring agent in several liqueurs and in gin (along with juniper berries).

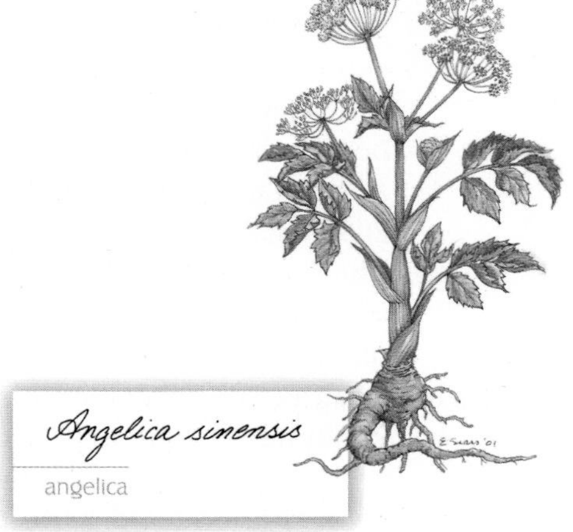

FIGURE 25-1 Angelica.

Common Name: Black cohosh (black snakeroot)
Botanical Name: *Cimicifuga racemosa*
Typical Uses: To relieve symptoms of menopause and various menstrual problems.

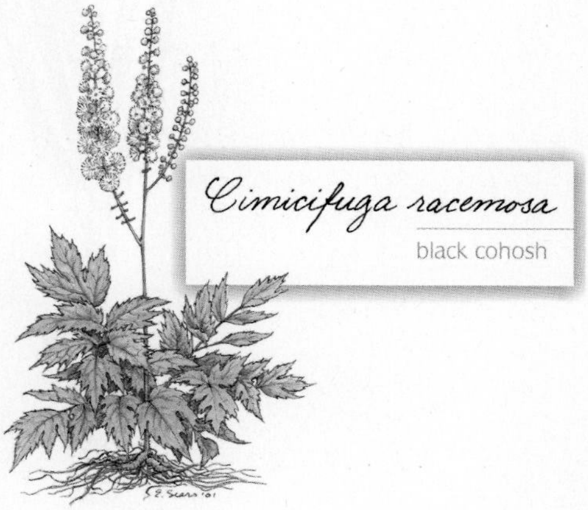

FIGURE 25-2 Black cohosh.

Common Name: Feverfew
Botanical Name: *Tanacetum parthenium*
Typical Uses: To relieve symptoms of migraine headaches, arthritis, and menstrual problems.

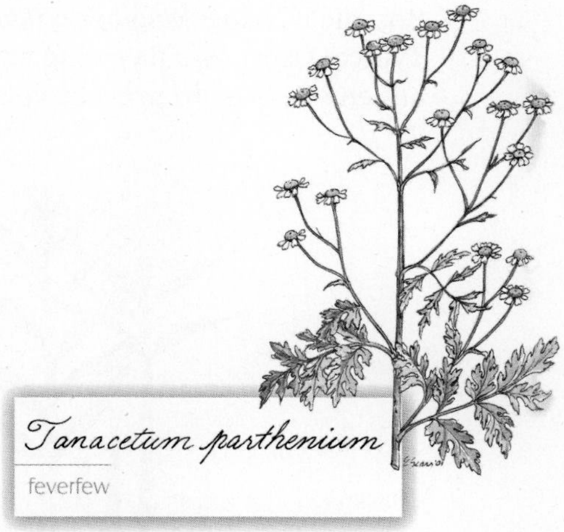

FIGURE 25-3 Feverfew.

Common Name: Garlic
Botanical Name: *Allium sativum*
Typical Uses: As a flavoring agent in salads, soups, and other foods; as a cholesterol-lowering agent.

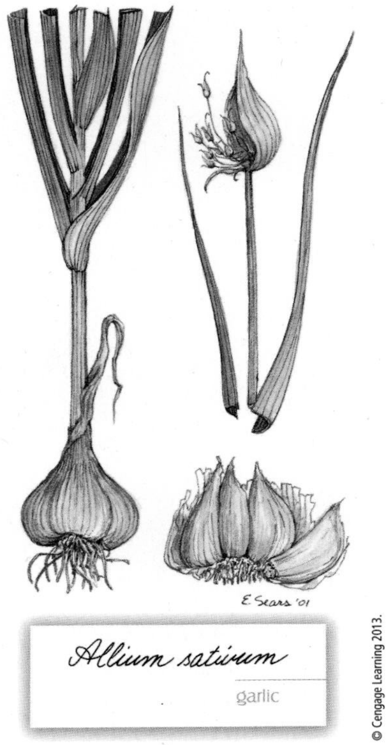

FIGURE 25-4 Garlic.

Common Name: Ginger
Botanical Name: *Zingiber officinale* Roscoe
Typical Uses: As a flavoring agent in foods, as a digestive aid, and as an antiemetic (i.e., to prevent vomiting).

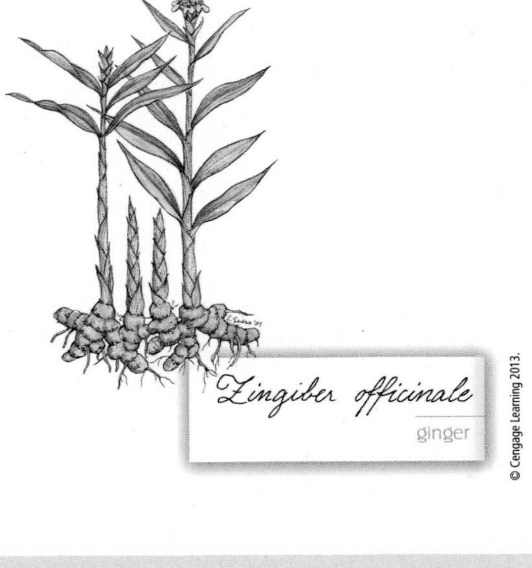

FIGURE 25-5 Ginger.

Common Name: Ginkgo
Botanical Name: *Ginkgo biloba*
Typical Uses: As an antiasthmatic, as a bronchodilator, and to treat memory loss or headache.

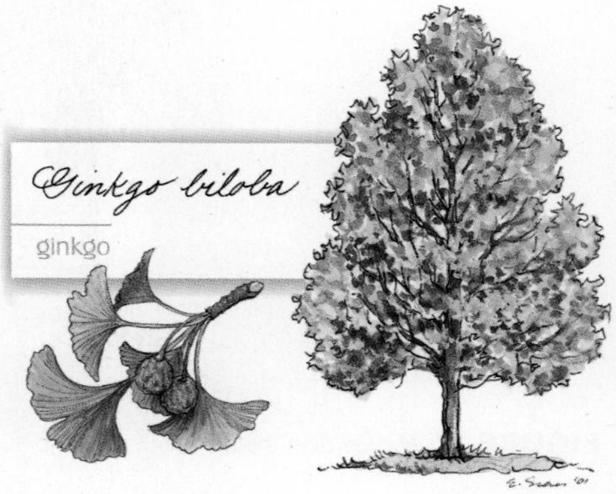

FIGURE 25-6 Ginkgo.

Common Name: Ginseng
Botanical Name: *Panax ginseng* (Asian ginseng) or *Panax quinquefolius* (American ginseng)
Typical Uses: As an "adaptogen" to increase resistance to environmental stress and to promote immune response.

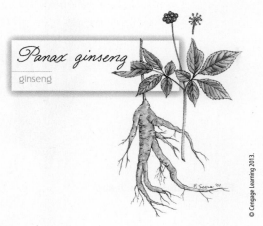

FIGURE 25-7 Ginseng.

Common Name: Golden Seal
Botanical Name: *Hydrastis canadensis*
Typical Uses: As a bitter tonic for gastric and urogenital disorders.

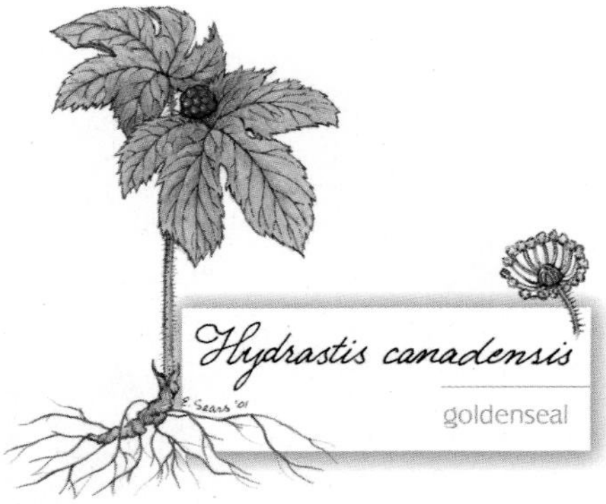

FIGURE 25-8 Golden seal.

Common Name: Milk thistle
Botanical Name: *Silybum marianum*
Typical Uses: As an antihepatotoxic agent (i.e., liver protectant) especially against poisoning from *Amanita* sp. mushrooms, which contain compounds such as phallotoxins.

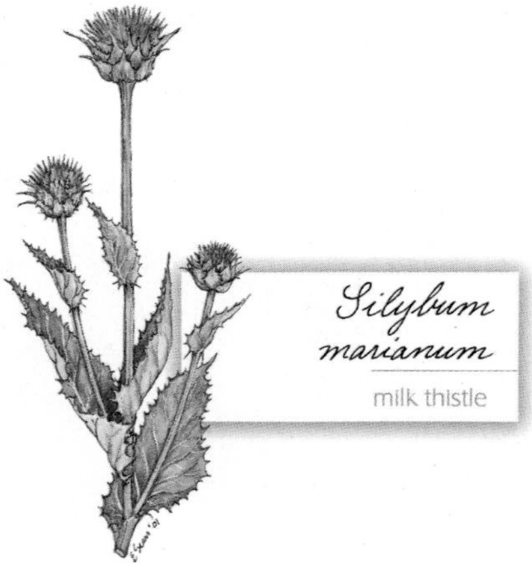

FIGURE 25-9 Milk thistle.

Common Name: Purple coneflower or echinacea
Botanical Name: *Echinacea purpurea*
Typical Uses: As an anti-infective, antiseptic, and immunostimulant agent.

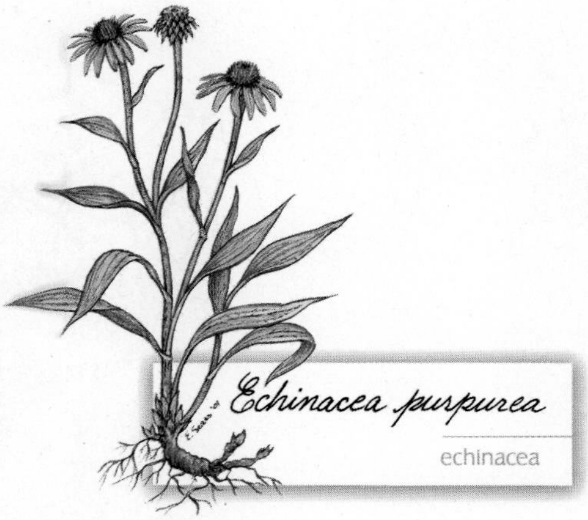

FIGURE 25-10 Purple coneflower (*Echinacea*).

Common Name: Saw palmetto
Botanical Name: *Serenoa repens*
Typical Uses: To relieve symptoms of benign prostatic hypertrophy (i.e., noncancerous enlarged prostate gland).

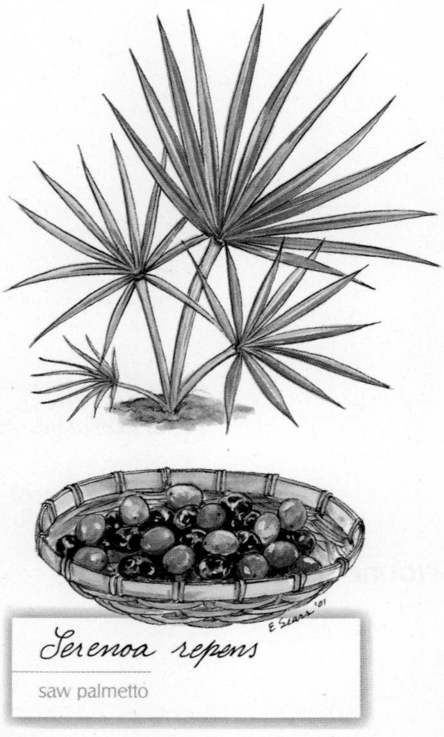

FIGURE 25-11 Saw palmetto.

Common Name: St. John's wort
Botanical Name: *Hypericum calycinum*
Typical Uses: To relieve symptoms of depression.

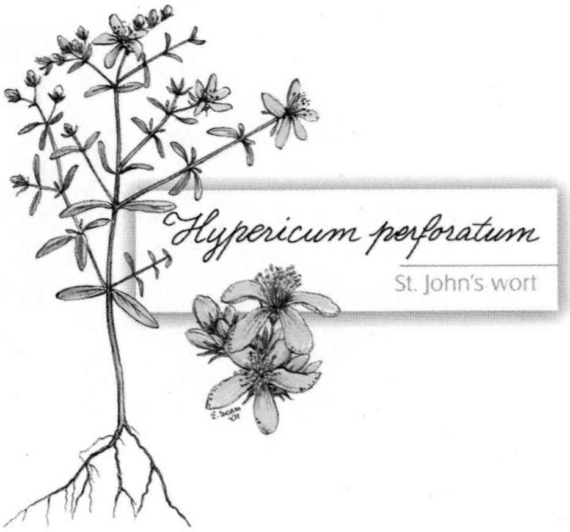

FIGURE 25-12 St. John's wort.

Common Name: Valerian
Botanical Name: *Valeriana officinalis*
Typical Uses: To relieve symptoms of restlessness, sleep disturbances, or nervousness.

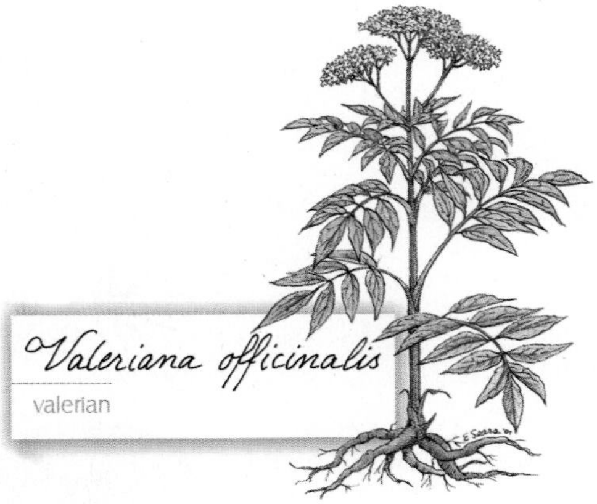

FIGURE 25-13 Valerian.

Summary

Historically, herbals, botanicals, and natural plant products have provided humans with a wealth of medicines. Herbals are currently regulated as dietary supplements and not as drugs under the 1994 Dietary Supplement Health and Education Act (DSHEA). According to the DSHEA, herbals may not claim to cure, mitigate, diagnose, or prevent disease. However, herbals have been and continue to be used by many consumers to prevent or self-treat disease. While some herbal preparations may be useful, the effectiveness (efficacy) and safety of many herbals has yet to be demonstrated. Fortunately, new regulatory initiatives and programs are beginning to address the safety concerns over herbals. Moreover, reliable, professional health care information is becoming increasingly available on the Internet, allowing rapid access for the pharmacy. This chapter reviews the regulatory history of herbal products in the United States, the major classes of secondary plant metabolites that make up most herbals, and the sites where professional herbal information is freely available.

TEST YOUR KNOWLEDGE

Multiple Choice

1. Which of the following is the best regulatory definition of an herbal?
   a. plant material that smells nice
   b. any substance or mixture of substances intended for the cure, mitigation, diagnosis, or prevention of disease
   c. a dietary supplement that contains an herb or other botanical for use to supplement the diet and to promote health
   d. all of the above

2. Which of the following prohibited misbranded or adulterated drugs, but did not require that a drug be safe or effective before being sold?
   a. 1906 Pure Food Act
   b. 1938 Federal Food, Drug, and Cosmetic Act
   c. 1962 Kefauver-Harris Drug Amendments
   d. 1994 Dietary Supplement Health and Education Act

3. Chemically most herbal products would described as
   a. proteins.
   b. primary metabolites.
   c. nucleic acids.
   d. secondary metabolites.

4. To be compliant with DSHEA, an herbal must be
   a. labeled as a dietary supplement.
   b. identify all ingredients by name and list the quantity of each ingredient.
   c. identify the plant by genus and species and the plant part from which the ingredient is derived.
   d. comply with any standards set forth by the USP-NF.
   e. all of the above.

5. Herbal remedies are never administered as
   a. tablets.
   b. lozenges.
   c. injections.
   d. topical ointments.
   e. tea.

6. Which of the following is *not* an important safety concern with the use of herbal products?
   a. the potential of a hypersensitivity (allergic) response to the herbal
   b. the potential that the product does not contain the herbal declared on the label
   c. the potential that the herbal product is contaminated with toxic material
   d. The potential that the herbal product does not taste very good
   e. The potential for an herbal-drug interaction when taking other medication

7. Which of the following is the website for the Dietary Supplement Verification Program and the updates on the U.S. Pharmacopeia–National Formulary monographs on herbals?
   a. http://ods.od.gov
   b. www.usp.org
   c. www.fda.gov/medwatch
   d. http://nccam.nih.gov
   e. none of the above

8. Which of the following is traditionally taken by individuals as an herbal treatment for depression?
   a. saw palmetto (*Serenoa repens*)
   b. milk thistle (*Silybum marianum*)
   c. St. John's wort (*Hypericum calycinum*)
   d. purple coneflower or echinacea (*Echinacea purpurea*)
   e. none of the above

9. Which of the following is traditionally taken by individuals to help prevent illness such as colds?
   a. saw palmetto (*Serenoa repens*)
   b. milk thistle (*Silybum marianum*)
   c. St. John's wort (*Hypericum calycinum*)
   d. purple coneflower or echinacea (*Echinacea purpurea*)
   e. none of the above

Matching

Match the use with the appropriate natural product.

1.	______ cholesterol-lowering agent	a.	ginger
2.	______ bronchodilator	b.	ginseng
3.	______ antiemetic	c.	garlic
4.	______ stimulates immune system	d.	valerian
5.	______ used for insomnia	e.	ginkgo

Suggested Readings

Applequist, W. (2006). *The identification of medicinal plants: A handbook of botanicals in commerce.* St. Louis, MO: Missouri Botanical Garden Press.

Blumenthal, M., et al. (Eds.). (2003). *The ABC clinical guide to herbs.* New York, NY: Thieme Publishers.

Blumenthal, M., Goldberg, A., & Brinckman, J. (Eds.). (2000). *Herbal medicine: Expanded commission E monographs.* Newton, MA: Integrative Medicine Communications.

Bowsher, C., Steer, M., & Tobin, A. (2008). *Plant biochemistry.* New York, NY: Garland Science, Taylor & Francis Group.

Brinker, F. (2010). *Herb contraindications & drug interactions* (4th ed.). Sandy, OR: Eclectic Press.

Buchanan, R.B., Gruissem, W., & Jones, R.L. (2000). *Biochemistry & molecular biology of plants.* Rockville, MD: American Society of Plant Physiologists.

Cavaliere, C., & Blumenthal, M. (2007). Review of the FDA's final GMPs for dietary supplements. *Herbalgram, 76*, 58–91.

Chinese Pharmacopoeia Commission. (2011). *Pharmacopoeia of the People's Republic of China* (English ed., 3 vols.). Beijing, China: Chemical Industry Press.

Dasgupta, A., & Hammett-Stabler, C.A. (Eds.). (2011). *Herbal supplements: Efficacy, toxicity, interactions with Western drugs, and effects on clinical laboratory tests.* New York, NY: John Wiley & Sons.

Dewick, P.M. (2009). *Medicinal natural products: A biosynthetic approach* (3rd ed.). New York, NY: John Wiley & Sons.

Dey, P.M., & Harborne, J.B. (Eds.). (1997). *Plant biochemistry.* San Diego, CA: Academic Press.

Gleason, F.K., & Chollet, R. (2012). *Plant biochemistry.* Sudbury, MA: Jones & Bartlett.

Goldman, P. (2001). Herbal medicines today and the roots of modern pharmacology. *Annals of Internal Medicine*, *135*, 594–600.

Grosse, Y., Baan, R., Straif, K., Secretan, B., El Ghissassi, F., Bouvard, E., et al. (2009). A review of human carcinogens. *Lancet Oncology, 10*(1), 13–14.

Harkey, M.R., Henderson, G.L., Gershwin, M.E., Stern, J.S., & Hackman, R.M. (2001). Variability in commercial ginseng products: An analysis of 25 preparations. *American Journal of Clinical Nutrition*, *73*, 1101–1106.

Israelsen, L.D. (1998, Fall). Botanicals and DHSEA: A health professional's guide. *Quarterly Review of Natural Medicine*, pp. 251–257.

Linde, K., Ramirez, G., Mulrow, C.D., Pauls, A., Weidenhammer, W., & Melchart, D. (1996). St. John's wort for depression—An overview and meta-analysis of randomized clinical trials. *British Medical Journal*, *313*, 253–258.

Nortier, J.L., Martinez, M-C.M., Schmeiser, H.H., Arlt, V.M., Bieler, C.A., Petein, M., et al. (2000). Urothelial carcinoma associated with the use of a Chinese herb (*Aristolochia fanchi*). *New England Journal of Medicine*, *342*, 1686–1692.

Nutrition Business Journal. (2002). U.S. nutrition industry. San Diego, CA.

Nutrition Business Journal. (2011). U.S. nutrition industry. San Diego, CA.

Robbers, J. E. , Speedie, M. K., & Tyler, V. E. (1996) *Pharmacognosy and pharmacobiotechnology.* Baltimore, MD: Williams & Wilkins.

Sato, Y., Hanawa, T., Arai, M., et al. (Eds.). (2005). *Introduction to Kampo: Japanese traditional medicine.* Tokyo, Japan: Elsevier.

Slifman, N. R., Obermeyer, W. R., Aloi, B. K., Mussler, S. M., Correll, W. A., Cichowicz, S. M., et al. (1998). Contamination of botanical dietary supplements by *Digitalis lanata*. *New England Journal of Medicine*, *339*, 806–811.

Srinivasan, V. S., & Kucera, P. (1998). Botanicals in the USP-NF. *Pharmacopeial Forum*, *24*, 6623–6626.

Tang, W., & Eisenbrand, G. (2010). *Handbook of Chinese medicinal plants: Chemistry, pharmacology and toxicology.* Germany: Wiley-VCH.

Temin, P. (1980). *Taking your medicine: Drug regulation in the United States.* Cambridge, MA: Harvard University Press.

U.S. National Toxicology Program. (2011). Aristolochic acids. In *Report on Carcinogens* (12th ed., pp. 45–49). Washington, DC: U.S. Department of Health and Human Services.

Websites

American Botanical Council www.herbalgram.org

Medwatch with information from the FDA Safety Information and Adverse Event Reporting Program www.fda.gov/medwatch

National Center for Complementary and Alternative Medicine http://nccam.nih.gov

National Institutes of Health Office of Dietary Supplements with the IBIDS (International Bibliographic Information on Dietary Supplements) and CARDS (Computer Access to Research on Dietary Supplements) databases http://ods.od.nih.gov

Natural Medicines Comprehensive Database www.naturaldatabase.com

U.S. Pharmacopeia (USP-NF) and the dietary supplement verification program (DSVP) www.usp.org

PART

V

Administrative Aspects of Pharmacy Technology

CHAPTER

26

The Policy and Procedure Manual

Competencies

Upon completion of this chapter, the reader should be able to:

1. Define and differentiate a *policy* from a *procedure*.
2. Give five reasons to justify the need for a policy and procedure manual.
3. Explain the rationale for inclusion of job descriptions in the policy and procedure manual.
4. Give examples of the sections that may be included in a pharmacy policy and procedure manual.
5. List five topics that could be included in each of the following pharmacy areas: administration, distribution, and clinical.
6. Describe the rationale for the use of a policy and procedure manual for new pharmacy employees.

Key Terms

policy **procedure**

Introduction

policy a defined course to guide and determine present and future decisions; established by an organization or employer who guides the employee to act in a manner consistent with management philosophy

In every organization rules or policies are developed to accomplish the objectives of the organization. There are also specific ways in which these policies are to be carried out. These ways of carrying out policies are called *procedures*.

A **policy** is an overall plan embracing general goals and objectives of what is to be done. A **procedure** is a particular way of accomplishing the objectives set forth in the policy—a series of steps and ways of doing things. In other words, a policy is a decision by an organization or a department to do something; a procedure is a step-by-step method used to accomplish that policy.

Need for Policies and Procedures

procedure guideline on the preferred way to perform a certain function; particular actions to be taken to carry out a policy

When new employees begin work in a pharmacy, they literally have hundreds of things to learn. Not only must the newcomers learn the work, but they must also learn about lunch hours, benefits, hours of operation, the chain of command, what scope of services is provided by the department, and so on. By reading a manual in which policies and procedures are described, new employees *will* be able to learn a considerable amount about their respective jobs. So the first reason for having a policy and procedure manual is to use it in the training of new employees.

If written policies and procedures did not exist, employees would have to be trained and instructed verbally by other employees. Because everyone may not be a good teacher or able to explain things fully or correctly, having information in writing ensures it is presented in a clear and consistent manner. Therefore, the second reason to have a written policy and procedure manual is to prevent *errors or misunderstandings when communicating verbally.*

People handle different situations in different ways. In a pharmacy, however, it is important to ensure that the same accurate and consistent results occur and that people and situations are treated the same way every time. Thus, a set way for doings things is established and set forth in a policy and procedure manual. Another reason for having a policy and procedure manual is consistency—to ensure that the same policy is followed in a particular situation at all times.

The pharmacy department uses a large number and variety of drugs and supplies. Although many drugs are expensive, labor and supplies used in compounding, packaging, and labeling in a pharmacy can also comprise a considerable component of the cost of getting drugs to patients. If procedures are performed in an efficient and economical manner, waste of both materials and manpower can be minimized, thus reducing the cost of providing services.

A good manager is responsible for ensuring that the work is *performed in a consistent manner* and that employers are aware of how well they are performing their jobs. One way this may be accomplished is through periodic evaluations of personnel job performance (i.e., how well an employee is following procedures). Effective evaluations can be accomplished only if there are written policies, procedures, and job descriptions against which job performance can be measured (**Figure 26-1**).

Because of potential harm to patients, pharmacy departments take considerable care to ensure that medications are purchased, stocked, packaged, compounded, labeled, dispensed, administered, and charted accurately. Despite this care, adverse outcomes do occur, *potentially* resulting in lawsuits. Unfortunately, these are not uncommon and it is sometimes necessary to determine how a specific procedure should have been performed. Policy and procedure manuals, therefore, often serve as legal documents in the event of a lawsuit to protect the individual and the institution or employer.

It must be recognized that pharmacies and hospitals are highly regulated establishments. They are governed by laws, rules, regulations, standards, and guidelines that must be followed. Many of these federal, state, and local regulating agencies require written policies and procedures.

MEDICAL CENTER
JOB DESCRIPTION – PERFORMANCE APPRAISAL

EMPLOYEE NAME:	EMPLOYEE NUMBER:

DATE OF HIRE:	DATE IN POSITION:
EVALUATION DATE:	EVALUATION PERIOD:

☐ INTRODUCTORY ☐ ANNUAL

JOB TITLE: Pharmacy Technician
DEPARTMENT: Pharmacy

JOB CODE: TECH04
REPORTS TO: Senior Pharmacist

JOB SUMMARY: Assist the pharmacist in the day to day activities of the hospital pharmacy with emphasis on cassette filling, label filling, and drug distribution. Adheres to the medical center/department policies and procedures and Joint Commission/regulatory agency requirements. Demonstrates and promotes service excellence at all times.

MINIMUM QUALIFICATIONS:

Education: High school diploma or equivalent

Experience/skills: Technician certification preferred.

Licensure:

Risk Exposure;
Hazard Assessment:
Physical Demands:
Mental Demands:

PERFORMANCE RATING SCALE:

Exceeds – Performance consistently exceeds performance standard. (Comments preferred.)
Meets – Performance consistently meets performance standards.
Needs Improvement – Performance inconsistently meets performance standards. **(Comments required.)**
Does Not Meet – Performance consistently does not meet performance standards. **(Comments required.)**
Not Applicable/Unable to Evaluate – Performance could not be evaluated to date for standard.

Validation methods used in evaluating performance are as follows, but not limited to, direct observation, written tests, skills checklist, attendance records, incident reports, patient comments/letters and medical record reviews.

Approval Signatures	
Department Head:	Date:
Human Resources:	Date:

(Continued)

FIGURE 26-1 Technician job description-performance apprasial form

PERFORMANCE	RATING SCALE					COMMENTS
STANDARD	EX	MTS	NI	DNM	UE	
***Standard #1. Demonstrates the ability to assist in inpatient drug distribution activities.**	☐	☐	☐	☐	☐	
A. Fills/exchanges patient's cassettes accurately and efficiently.	☐	☐	☐	☐	☐	
B. Fills prescription labels accurately and efficiently.	☐	☐	☐	☐	☐	
C. Delivers medications to patient care areas in a timely manner.	☐	☐	☐	☐	☐	
D. Assists pharmacists with phone/window in a courteous, professional manner.	☐	☐	☐	☐	☐	
***Standard #2. Demonstrates the ability to perform IV Room activities.**	☐	☐	☐	☐	☐	
A. Accurately prepares add-a-vial stock and adheres to logging procedures.	☐	☐	☐	☐	☐	
B. Sets up TPN pump/prepares TPN fluids.	☐	☐	☐	☐	☐	
C. Maintains inventory by ordering medications and restocking solutions.	☐	☐	☐	☐	☐	
D. Accurately labels premixed intravenous admixtures/piggybacks.	☐	☐	☐	☐	☐	
Standard #3. Able to assist in daily maintenance activities.	☐	☐	☐	☐	☐	
A. Generates and processes fill lists, transfer/discharge lists, reports, etc.	☐	☐	☐	☐	☐	
B. Maintains floor stock/Pyxis.	☐	☐	☐	☐	☐	
C. Pre-packs medications as per policy and procedure.	☐	☐	☐	☐	☐	
D. Files daily orders/controlled substance sheets.	☐	☐	☐	☐	☐	
Standard #4. Demonstrates the knowledge and skills necessary to provide care and/or services to patients/guests of specific age groups as designated.	☐	☐	☐	☐	☐	***Attach age specific competency, if applicable.***
A. Neonate/Infant (Birth–1 yr)	☐	☐	☐	☐	☐	
B. Child (1–11 yrs)	☐	☐	☐	☐	☐	
C. Adolescent (12–17 yrs)	☐	☐	☐	☐	☐	
D. Adult (18–65 yrs)	☐	☐	☐	☐	☐	
E. Older Adult (65+ yrs)	☐	☐	☐	☐	☐	
F. All Ages	☐	☐	☐	☐	☐	
Standard #5. Fosters change initiatives to ensure continued improvement of service quality and performance improvement.	☐	☐	☐	☐	☐	

* ADA Essential Functions

FIGURE 26-1 (Continued)

PERFORMANCE STANDARD	RATING SCALE					COMMENTS
	EX	MTS	NI	DNM	UE	
A. Facilitates change initiatives in a manner that promotes continued performance improvement.	☐	☐	☐	☐	☐	
B. Willingly contributes talents and skills to achieve individual, departmental, and hospital goals and objectives.	☐	☐	☐	☐	☐	
C. Attends meetings and participates on committees as directed.	☐	☐	☐	☐	☐	
D. Performs activities that foster a culture of safety within the department and organization.	☐	☐	☐	☐	☐	
E. Identifies safety/risk reduction strategies and communicates these to department director.	☐	☐	☐	☐	☐	
Standard #6. Incorporates Medical Center's service excellence standards by identifying patient/guest expectations and working to exceed them. Promotes positive "Guest Services" throughout the organization by demonstrating care, compassion, and respect to patients, physicians, guests, and staff.	☐	☐	☐	☐	☐	
A. Anticipates, understands, and meets the needs of the guest. Is supportive and gives help before asked. Is consistently courteous to all guests in all forms of communication including in person, on the telephone, and in writing.	☐	☐	☐	☐	☐	
B. Demonstrates compassion, empathy, concern, and a respectful behavior toward guests. Exhibits an "always caring" attitude.	☐	☐	☐	☐	☐	
C. Promotes positive co-worker, team building relationships, within the department and between departments. Works collaboratively and is respectful of others. Takes individual responsibility for living and energizing the Medical Center Service Excellence Standards.	☐	☐	☐	☐	☐	

(Continued)

FIGURE 26-1 (Continued)

PERFORMANCE	RATING SCALE					COMMENTS
STANDARD	EX	MTS	NI	DNM	UE	
Standard #7. Incorporates Hospital's Corporate Compliance Program into the work environment by adhering to the "Standards of Conduct" outlined in the Compliance Assurance Program Handbook.	☐	☐	☐	☐	☐	
A. Conducts himself/herself in a professional and ethical manner when acting on behalf of the Medical Center. Is honest and truthful in all of his/her dealings with other employees or organizations that do business with the Hospital.	☐	☐	☐	☐	☐	
B. Participates in Corporate Compliance Program by receiving formal in-service education, obtaining a copy of the Compliance Assurance Program Handbook, and attesting to abide by the Standards of Conduct outlined in the handbook.	☐	☐	☐	☐	☐	
C. Understands the disciplinary policies for violations of the Corporate Compliance Program.	☐	☐	☐	☐	☐	
D. Understands the manner in which a violation of the Corporate Compliance Program can be reported.	☐	☐	☐	☐	☐	
Standard #8. Complies with general policies and procedures of the organization/department including:	☐	☐	☐	☐	☐	
A. Is knowledgeable of and exemplifies the beliefs, mission, and vision of Health Services at the Medical Center.	☐	☐	☐	☐	☐	
B. Maintains confidentiality of patients, employees, department, and hospital information including computer passwords.	☐	☐	☐	☐	☐	
C. Follows emergency/disaster preparedness protocols.	☐	☐	☐	☐	☐	
D. Maintains safe work environment; follows fire/safety prevention protocols.	☐	☐	☐	☐	☐	

FIGURE 26-1 (Continued)

PERFORMANCE STANDARD	RATING SCALE					COMMENTS
	EX	MTS	NI	DNM	UE	
E. Complies with departmental and organizational in-service education program requirements.	☐	☐	☐	☐	☐	
F. Complies with dress, appearance, and uniform requirements.	☐	☐	☐	☐	☐	
G. Follows infection control practices and procedures.	☐	☐	☐	☐	☐	
H. Complies with Human Resources attendance/punctuality policy.	☐	☐	☐	☐	☐	
I. Adheres to Joint Commission and other regulatory requirements.	☐	☐	☐	☐	☐	
Standard #9. Provides support and leadership within the department.	☐	☐	☐	☐	☐	
A. Resolves problems regarding department operations and assists in resolving co-worker problems/issues.	☐	☐	☐	☐	☐	
B. Promotes and communicates commitment, values, and ethics within the department.	☐	☐	☐	☐	☐	
C. Provides assistance to co-workers in meeting the goals and objectives of the department.	☐	☐	☐	☐	☐	
D. Promotes continued development and morale among co-workers.	☐	☐	☐	☐	☐	
E. Fosters effective employee communications, teamwork, and participates in department staff meetings.	☐	☐	☐	☐	☐	
Standard #10. Works to enhance professional growth and development.	☐	☐	☐	☐	☐	
A. Participates in educational programs, in-service meetings, workshops, conferences, and committees.	☐	☐	☐	☐	☐	
B. Keeps abreast of current literature and professional trends.	☐	☐	☐	☐	☐	
C. Participates in professional organizations.	☐	☐	☐	☐	☐	
Standard #11. Performs related duties as necessary.	☐	☐	☐	☐	☐	
A. With appropriate training, accepts additional related duties as needed.	☐	☐	☐	☐	☐	

Responsibilities may be added, changed, or deleted at any time at the discretion of the Department Head or Administration formally or informally, either verbally or in writing.

FIGURE 26-1 (Continued).

In summarizing the need for policies and procedures, a policy and procedure manual exists for the following reasons:

- To train new employees or retrain existing employees.
- To prevent errors due to verbal communication.
- To ensure consistency of job performance.
- To minimize the waste of human resources and materials.
- To evaluate job performance.
- To serve as legal documents in the event of a lawsuit.
- To comply with regulatory and accreditation agencies' requirements.

Overview of a Policy and Procedure Manual

This section takes a look at the basic information contained in a pharmacy department's manual.

Format

To avoid confusion and for the sake of consistency, a similar format should be followed for all policies and procedures. Most institutions and employers, follow some kind of standard format that sets forth the basic information required. Let us examine some of the items that should be part of every policy and procedure manual.

Title

First, every policy and procedure should have a title. This tells the reader what subject is covered in the policy and procedure. This title is also used in a table of contents or an index.

Date

Every policy and procedure should be dated. Initially, a date of implementation indicates when the policy and procedure went into effect. Often, however, it is necessary to change, update, expand, or modify an existing policy or procedure. Therefore, additional dates indicate when the policy or procedure was revised. Many institutions use just the original and latest revision dates. For example:

Approved and Implemented: 9-19-13
Revised: 10-25-14

Design

It has been suggested that a useful policy and procedure manual must answer the following questions regarding a specific activity.

- What must be done?
- Who should do it?
- How should it be done?
- When should it be done?

The Approval Process

In most hospitals the Pharmacy and Therapeutics Committee serves as the liaison between the medical staff and the department of pharmacy services. The Joint Commission requires that the Pharmacy and Therapeutics Committee annually review

MEDICAL CENTER
DEPARTMENT OF PHARMACY

POLICY AND PROCEDURE MANUAL

THE POLICIES AND PROCEDURES OF THE DEPARTMENT OF PHARMACY
HAVE BEEN APPROVED BY THE MEDICAL STAFF OF THE HOSPITAL
THROUGH THE PHARMACY AND THERAPEUTICS COMMITTEE

Jack Royale
President & Chief Executive Officer

Elizabeth Prime
Director of Clinical Services

Alex Zimmerman, Chairman
Pharmacy & Therapeutics Committee

Alison Zaza
Pharmacy & Therapeutics Committee

FIGURE 26-2 Cover approval page for the policy and procedure manual.

and approve the policies and procedures of the pharmacy department. Pharmacy departments normally use a signature cover page at the beginning of the manual indicating the approval of the Pharmacy and Therapeutics Committee. **Figure 26-2** is an example of a cover page for approval of the policy and procedure manual.

Additionally, policies and procedures should also contain the signatures of those who wrote or approved the policy where the policy and procedure are most frequently carried out. These signature(s) are valuable because they indicate who is responsible for generating the policy and procedure and document the agreement of the administrative personnel on the highest level.

Format and Contents of a Policy and Procedure Manual

The format and contents of a policy and procedure manual vary from hospital to hospital. The most common methods for organizing policy and procedure manuals fall into two main groups. In the first method, policies and procedures are placed in a book in alphabetical order by title; for example, Abbreviations, Absenteeism, Adverse Drug Reactions, Ambulatory Care, and Aseptic Technique. A second common method of organizing a manual is to group policies and procedures into three or more categories with separate sections for each category. An example of this format follows:

- *Section I: Organization*—This section contains information on the hospital and pharmacy department itself, organizational charts for both the hospital and the department, services offered, pharmacy department participation on hospital committees (e.g., Pharmacy and Therapeutics Committee, the Infection Control Committee), security/confidentiality, and so forth.
- *Section II: Personnel*—This section may contain job descriptions/performance appraisals; orientation, staffing, and scheduling information; personnel policies; educational benefits, and so forth.
- *Section III: Administrative Policies*—This section contains policies and procedures on the department's hours of operation, purchasing policies and procedures, inventory control, interdepartmental requisitions, control and accountability of controlled drugs, performance improvement activities, safety data sheets, administrative reports, annual reports, in-service education, and so forth.
- *Section IV: Distribution Services*—These policies and procedures involve the compounding, labeling, packaging, dispensing of medications, and the control and accountability of controlled substances; formulary operation; automatic stop orders; intravenous admixture services, including parenteral nutrition and antineoplastic therapy; outpatient pharmacy services; nonsterile compounding and extemporaneous compounding manufacturing and so forth.
- *Section V: Clinical Pharmacy Services*—This section includes the clinical pharmacy services provided by the department: drug therapy monitoring, pharmacokinetic consultation services, drug information services, investigational drugs, in-service education, discharge counseling, and so forth.
- *Section VI: Facilities and Equipment*—These policies and procedures pertain to the use and maintenance of the department's physical facilities and equipment, their maintenance and repair, service contracts, and the like.

This format of grouping policies and procedures into categories with separate sections for each category requires a comprehensive table of contents or index for each section so that any policy and procedure can be easily and readily located. No matter which system a department uses to organize its policy and procedure manual, there is no one "right way." Some prefer not to include job descriptions in their manuals. Some have separate sections for inpatient and outpatient operations. The key factor of a good manual is that it meets the needs of the department or pharmacy practice and that it is a useful reference for the staff.

Distribution

A policy and procedure manual is a dynamic entity since it is constantly changing. Policies and procedures should be continually revised, added, or deleted on an ongoing basis. Copies of the policy and procedure manual should be readily available to every employee (and other departments in a hospital) so that it may be used as a reference. A number of pharmacy practices have hospital-wide computerized information systems, thus the policy and procedure manual is available for reference on the organization's computer network. This permits access to the policy and procedure manual from any terminal within the institution and makes updating the policy and procedure manual quick and easy since the network file can be easily modified. Individuals can also generate a printed of any policy and procedure as needed.

Summary

Each policy and procedure manual is unique for a particular pharmacy practice. It addresses the mission, goals, and objectives of the pharmacy; it incorporates the contemporary professional standards of practice as well as the current legal and quasi-legal regulations of the profession; and it provides the basis for a *cooperative* professional environment where there is a strong sense of direction for the pharmacy staff.

Comprehensive and current policy and procedure manuals are necessary, useful tools in the proper running of any well-managed organization. They should be viewed as meaningful, helpful guides in providing efficient and consistent service to the patients and staff served by the pharmacy department.

TEST YOUR KNOWLEDGE

Multiple Choice

1. A policy is
   a. a series of steps to follow.
   b. a memorandum to accomplish in a definite order.
   c. a statement of goals and objectives for a traditional way of doing a task.
   d. all of the above.

2. A procedure is
   a. a step-by-step method used to carry out a task.
   b. a verbal communication.
   c. a decision to do something.
   d. all of the above.

3. New employees must become familiar with
   a. their job description.
   b. the hours of work.
   c. policies and procedures.
   d. all of the above.

4. Policy and procedure manuals are used to
   a. train and inform new employees.
   b. prevent errors resulting from verbal communications.
   c. ensure that the same policies are followed in the same situations.
   d. all of the above.

5. Which of the following is not true regarding policy and procedure manuals?
   a. Many regulating agencies require written policies and procedures.
   b. Any change requires approval of the chief operating officer of the institution.

c. They minimize waste of manpower, time, and materials by providing direction in technical activities and tasks.
d. They provide a new employee with valuable information about his or her new job.

Matching

Match the term with its definition.

1. ______ job description
2. ______ policy
3. ______ memo
4. ______ policy and procedure manual
5. ______ procedure

a. overall statement of goals and what is to be done
b. specific job guidelines that outline an employee's responsibilities
c. a directive in message form
d. a reference for employees to follow to ensure consistency and accuracy in their daily pharmacy activities
e. steps in providing specific activities

Fill in the Blank

1. A definite course or method of action is a ______________.
2. An overall plan embracing general goals and objectives of what is to be done is a ______________.
3. Every policy and procedure should be ______________.
4. In most hospitals, the ______________ serves as the liaison between the medical staff and the department of pharmacy services and provides guidance in the development and approval of pharmacy policy and procedures.
5. Pharmacy policy and procedures provide guidelines for consistent ______________.

Suggested Reading

American Society of Health-System Pharmacists. (2010–2011). *Best practices for hospital and health-system pharmacy, 2010–2011*. Bethesda, MD: Author.

CHAPTER

27

Pharmaceutical Supply Chain

Competencies

Upon completion of this chapter, the reader should be able to:

1. List the functions involved in the drug procurement process in an institutional pharmacy.
2. Explain the methods used to manage major stock locations in a hospital.
3. Describe the roles and contracts of a group purchasing organization (GPO) and prime vendor.
4. List the seven basic principles essential for group purchasing.
5. Describe the procurement process for products obtained from vendors.
6. Describe acquisition alternatives when manufacturers' backorders or distributor shortages impose a supply dilemma.
7. State the information that must be included in a pharmacy purchase order.
8. Describe pharmacy's role in supplying medications to other areas in a hospital.
9. Describe what should be considered when storing medications.
10. Describe what should be considered in controlling inventory
11. Calculate an inventory turnover rate, and describe the implications of the result.
12. List the benefits associated with the use of a bar code medication administration program.

Key Terms

bioengineered therapies
contract
group purchasing organizations (GPOs)
just-in-time (JIT)
materials management
prime vendor
turnover rate

Introduction

Health care costs at both the federal and state levels have increased more rapidly than any other category of products or services used in our society. The cost has been driven by factors such as expensive state-of-the-art diagnostic procedures, sophisticated treatments, and newly developed therapies. Generally, the costs associated with medications continue to increase incredibly fast due to the constant flow of costly new bioengineered therapies such as epoetin alfa and various insulin preparations. The term **bioengineered therapies** (biotechnology) refers to the use of genetically modified living organisms in the production of pharmaceutical products.

bioengineered therapy the use of genetically modified living organisms in the production of pharmaceutical products

materials management the division of a hospital pharmacy responsible for the process of procurement, control, storage, and distribution of drugs and pharmaceutical products

Concurrent with the expansion in health care costs has been a decrease in the resources to pay. Additionally, in recent years the public awareness of safety issues related to health care has dramatically increased. The combination of these factors contributes to the pressures experienced by those in the pharmacy profession. In response to these pressures pharmacy must:

- Effectively manage the cost of medications through more effective contracting.
- Improve stock management processes for medications to reduce losses, streamline access, and minimize the value of inventory.
- Reduce the opportunities for medication errors, for example, the improper receipt and storage of temperature-sensitive medications.

The term **materials management** represents the collection of activities surrounding the purchase, storage, and control of stock for authorized requestors or customers. For a pharmacy department in a hospital, the term represents all elements in the medication supply chain from the manufacturer to the last stock site used to fill an individual patient medication order. Many medications are more expensive than diamonds and are subject to diversion and theft, resulting in a need for secure handling to prevent loss. Effective pharmacy materials management processes must help reduce the cost of acquiring the medications while minimizing the opportunities for loss.

This chapter addresses the components of pharmacy's materials management responsibilities:

- Contracting process
- Procurement processes
- Medication storage
- Inventory control
- Repackaging and relabeling
- Recapture and disposal.

In a hospital, the overall responsibility for the materials management of pharmaceuticals lies with the director of the pharmacy department. The Pharmacy and Therapeutics (P&T) Committee is responsible for approving all medications used in the institution. This committee is chaired by a physician appointed by the medical board, and the committee's secretary is generally the director of pharmacy services. The committee consists of representatives from the medical staff, pharmacy staff, nursing staff, dietary staff, quality assurance staff, and hospital administration. The clinical and technical knowledge of pharmacists, physicians, nurses, and other experts is essential when making decisions regarding which drug products should be included in the *hospital formulary*. The hospital formulary is the official list of medications available in the hospital (see Chapter 28 for more details).

Contracting Process

contract a written legal agreement between a vendor and a client that states the conditions and requirements that a client must fulfill to obtain a product or products for a cost less than the vendor's listed price

A **contract** is defined as a written legal agreement between a vendor and a client that states the conditions and requirements that a client must fulfill to obtain a product or products for a cost less than the vendor's listed price. The vendor might be a manufacturer or a third-party source for a product in the supply chain. Pharmacies have contracts for most of the medications they purchase. Contracts can be negotiated by pharmacy for some items and by the materials management department of the institution for others. Hospital policy usually determines who is allowed to negotiate a contract. Contracts are an essential part of managing the cost of required products in hospitals.

GPO Relationship

group purchasing organization (GPO) a group of hospitals or pharmacists that buys drugs directly from the manufacturer

Group purchasing organizations (GPOs) are an important source of contracting support for hospitals. Each GPO represents a cooperative of multiple hospitals in the contract negotiation process. Each member hospital provides the GPO with its individual hospital formulary. The GPO then uses its collective buying power to leverage or reduce the price of products. The negotiated price of a product generally decreases in relation to the volume of product the GPO can commit to buy during some period of time. A GPO negotiates contracts at two levels on behalf of its member hospitals:

- The GPO will negotiate with each manufacturer or supplier of a product(s) required by the member hospitals in the quantity their members estimate will be used for a specified period of time (e.g., 12 months). The process begins with the GPO issuing a request for a "bid" to the appropriate manufacturers or suppliers. The GPO assesses the responses to the bid for compliance with criteria established in conjunction with the member hospitals. The GPO awards a contract to a manufacturer or supplier for a product or products and records this action in its electronic approved contract file.
- The GPO will issue a request for prime vendor bids to the national drug wholesalers. The GPO assesses the wholesalers' responses to specific criteria established in conjunction with its membership. The GPO will award a prime vendor contract to the selected drug wholesaler and provide that prime vendor with an electronic version of their approved contract file for its member hospitals.

A GPO often provides other services to its member hospitals such as assisting members in establishing a drug utilization program. The following seven basic actions should be embraced by the member hospitals to maximize the effectiveness of the GPO's activities:

1. Member hospitals should have generic formularies to support the evaluation of all eligible vendors.
2. Member hospitals should be committed to buy from the GPO-awarded agreement.
3. The GPO should award each item to only one supplier with few exceptions.
4. A GPO pharmacy committee should be established to ensure thorough product quality and vendor review.
5. The management of member hospitals should support group programs, especially pharmacy purchasing.

6. The GPO should maintain open communication with contracted manufacturers and prime vendors through newsletters, active cooperation in dealing with compliance issues, and regular visits.
7. The GPO should be willing and able to consider the addition of new products to the bid (contract negotiations).

The technician's role with a GPO can include the review of GPO communications for product information requiring pharmacy actions such as a drug recall.

Prime Vendor Contract

prime vendor a drug wholesaler who contracts directly with hospital pharmacies for the purpose of providing their high-volume pharmaceuticals

The contracted **prime vendor** is responsible for stocking all of the GPO's contracted products for all of the GPO's member hospitals. The hospital pharmacy is encouraged to order the majority (90% to 95%) of all stock requirements from the prime vendor. Products provided by the prime vendor to a member hospital are sold to that hospital at the GPO's negotiated contract price. The prime vendor's negotiated agreement with the GPO describes the prime vendor fee for this service, which can range from 2% to −2% or lower. That's right; many prime vendor agreements have a fee of less than zero. When the fee is less than zero, then the value is deducted from the hospital's GPO contract price. The prime vendor cost can be even lower if the hospital pays its invoices sooner or even in advance of purchasing.

The prime vendor is required to stock all of the GPO-contracted products for the member hospitals in sufficient quantities to respond to the member orders. The prime vendor agreement also describes the number of deliveries it is required to make to the pharmacy each week. Generally the prime vendor will make one delivery every day, 6 days a week. A prime vendor enables the pharmacy to reduce the size of its inventory due to the ease of access to their required medications. They can order in the evening of one day and receive the product on the morning of the following day. This allows pharmacies to reduce the size of their inventory, thus reducing their inventory holding costs.

The pharmacy technician could be responsible for reviewing communications from the prime vendor for information requiring pharmacy action such as a drug recall or providing pharmacy management information on the prime vendor's performance.

Private Contracts

Private contracts are defined as those contracts directly negotiated between a hospital and a manufacturer or supplier. Private contracts are generally required to supplement contracts negotiated by the GPO for needed products that are not on the GPO contract file. Private contracts are also offered by manufacturers or suppliers when they are mounting special marketing efforts in a region that they do not want to offer to a larger population or when they just want to influence the purchasing decisions in a specific hospital. Note that a member hospital can damage a GPO's negotiation power by independently negotiating a contract for a lower price with a manufacturer or supplier. Most hospital pharmacies avoid private contracts unless they are required to use them because of special circumstances.

Procurement Processes

The procurement of medications is the responsibility of the pharmacy department. The diagram in **Figure 27-1** highlights the components of the generic procurement process. The description of the component parts of the procurement process is different depending on whether the process supports the acquisition of products from

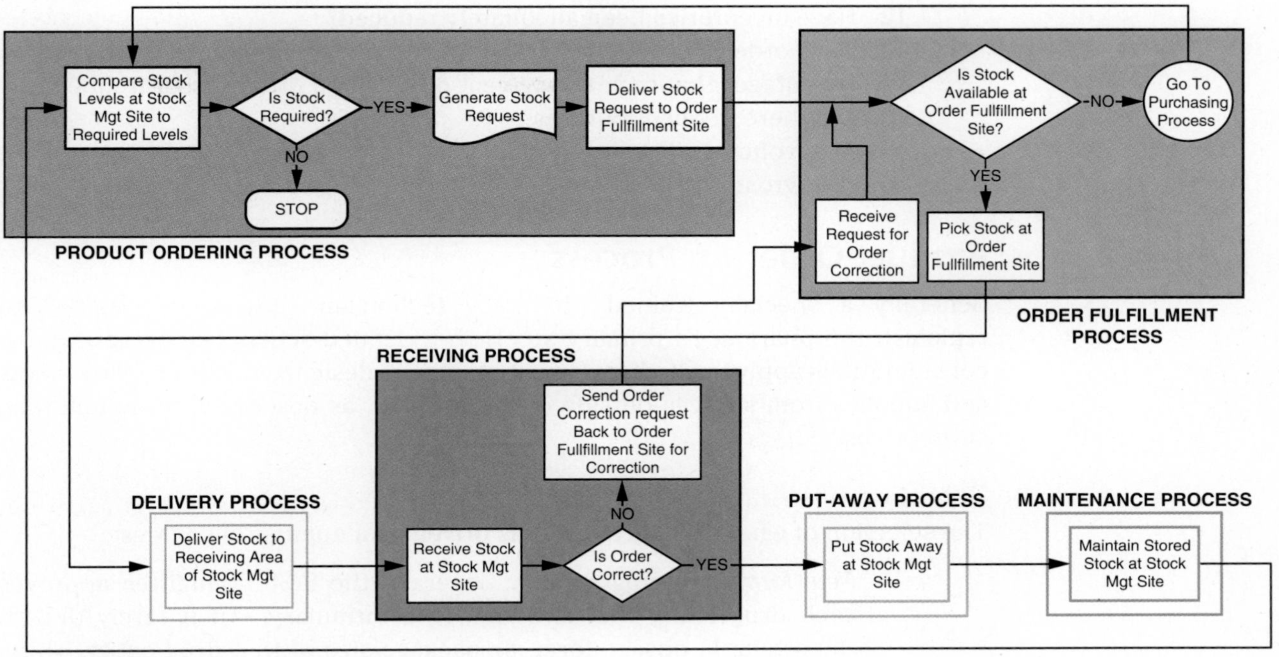

FIGURE 27-1 Flowchart of the procurement process.

sources outside of the hospital or whether the process supports the internal transfer of stock between stock sites. The descriptions that follow are divided along those lines.

Products Obtained from Vendors

Some products are obtained directly from sources outside of the hospital such as manufacturers, suppliers, or the prime vendor, and they may or may not be on the hospital's formulary. The answers to following questions will assist the pharmacy technician in a new hospital pharmacy to understand the hospital's procurement processes:

1. Is a single-brand purchasing policy in effect for the pharmacy department?
2. Has the P&T Committee approved a written therapeutic substitution policy?
3. Is competitive bidding used for high-cost items? For high-volume items?
4. Are either of these methods used to set prices: guarantee of bid prices or price ceiling set for the term of the contract?
5. Are the following considered when evaluating bids: prompt payment discount, terms of payment, nonperformance penalties, delivery time limitations, returned and damaged goods policy, and services?
6. Are contracts negotiated when appropriate?
7. Are contracts renegotiated on a regular basis (e.g., annually)?
8. Is a GPO used?
9. If a GPO is used, are prices guaranteed, and is there a mechanism for determining that GPO prices are competitive?
10. Is the prime vendor's contract used for specific drugs when appropriate?
11. Is the prime vendor's cost equal to or less than the cost of purchasing the same drug directly? Are factors such as increased investment revenues, decreased number of purchase orders, reduced inventory value, and receiving costs included in this assessment?

12. Have inventories been adequately reduced?
13. Have ordering and receiving costs been adequately reduced?
14. Do outages that require payment of premium prices occur frequently?
15. Are there frequent outages?
16. Are volume discounts evaluated for net savings before purchase (i.e., gross savings minus increased carrying costs)?

Product Ordering Process

Generally a specially trained pharmacy technician (buyer) is assigned to replenish the pharmacy's primary stock on a defined schedule. Several general considerations apply to all procurement processes designed to obtain medications and supplies from sources outside of the hospital, as described in the following subsections.

Selection of What Medication to Order

The selection of what drug(s) to order is driven by a number of sources:

- *New formulary drug request:* Generally the P&T Committee approves each drug entity that is added to a formulary, but it rarely defines the strength, dosage form, or package size of that drug entity. These decisions are left to the pharmacy to determine. Hospital pharmacies will have either an internal pharmacy committee that evaluates what to actually stock or someone designated to make those decisions.
- *Nonformulary drug request:* Most hospital pharmacies have a process in place for approving a prescriber's request for a nonformulary product for a specific patient.
- *Want-book requests:* Requests to replenish a specific medication are generally written on a spiral notebook or pad by a pharmacist or pharmacy technician.
- *Manual review of stock shelves:* This process is dependent on the knowledge of the individual scanning the shelves and that person's ability to remember what should be present on the shelf and in what quantity.
- *Computer-generated replenishment request:* The stock usage is managed by a computerized inventory management system that can electronically compare stock levels to required minimum or maximum inventory levels (par levels) to generate a suggested purchase request.

Source of Medication

The selection of the source for the majority of medications is made by the GPO through its bidding and negotiated contract process. The GPO generally selects one source for a product that is available from a number of manufacturers and/or suppliers. Such a product is called a *multisource product*. These multisource products are generally referred to as *generics*. All other products are known as *single-source products*. Source selection factors should include:

- Past performance of the manufacturer or supplier over the life of a contract to supply the product
- Quality assurance employed by the manufacturer or supplier in the production of the product
- Reputation of the manufacturer or supplier.

Occasionally, a contracted multisourced product is not available and an alternative must be selected. When this occurs the pharmacy buyer must exercise caution when making a source selection. Often the buyer will use the past performance of the manufacturer in supplying quality products as a guide. Comprehensive guidelines covering the sources of medications are available in the *ASHP Guidelines for Selecting Pharmaceutical Manufacturers and Suppliers* publication from the American Society of Health-System Pharmacists (ASHP).

Cost Analysis of What to Buy

The cost analysis of what to buy is generally incorporated into the GPO bidding and negotiation process. When an alternative product must be selected in the absence of a contract product, the buyer should compare prices to ensure the best value has been acquired. The prime vendor's ordering system generally electronically presents alternatives with current prices to the buyer when a requested product is not available. This action is intended to assist the buyer in his or her cost analysis decision for an alternative. In all procurement actions the buyer should consider the nonacquisition costs associated with the product such as storage, time required to prepare the product for patient use, and even the packaging. The cost of these additional considerations might override the differences in product cost.

Impact of Medication Shortages

The lack of availability of specific drugs has increased in frequency and severity during the past few years for many reasons. A major factor is the overwhelming economic pressure to decrease costs that affects all aspects of the health care industry. Hospitals generally receive less reimbursement from insurers. Prime vendors, manufacturers, and suppliers have to compete for lower-margin business that is driven by aggressive contracts from GPOs. Companies are continually reevaluating their product lines and dropping or adding items, packaging options, etc. When companies change their production schedules or lengthen the cycle between production runs of products, the availability of those products changes. When the frequency of litigation increases on a product or has the potential to increase, companies remove the product from their production lines. Drug shortages can also occur when the brand name drug's patent expires and the generic manufacturers are unable to expedite the manufacture of the generic equivalent.

Additional issues that can cause medication shortages include industry consolidation, complex manufacturing processes, underestimated demand, raw material shortages, U.S. Food and Drug Administration (FDA) certification problems, profitability, and obligation to shareholders. Last but certainly not the least important is the continuing shortage of certain raw materials needed in the manufacture of some drugs. All of these factors and more disrupt the supply chain availability of products.

Drug shortages can cause delays in patient treatments or even result in a patient having to use a less desirable alternative therapeutic approach. The pharmacy is generally responsible for identifying shortages or impending shortages, the causes of the shortage, and for notifying other members of the health care team.

In an ideal world, providers of health care would be able to anticipate and order the appropriate quantity of drugs in a timely manner. This would enable the manufacturers and suppliers to produce sufficient quantities of a medication so distributors could deliver the drugs just prior to the time they are needed. A **just-in-time (JIT)** inventory strategy minimizes the need to tie up large sums of money in inventory for long periods of time for both the manufacturer and the hospital pharmacy. Using a JIT strategy could enable manufacturers to accurately predict what would be needed in the future, distributors to manage their available stock to meet the needs of their clients, and clients to always have the drugs they

> **just-in-time (JIT)** an inventory strategy that minimizes inventory levels, thus minimizing the tying up of large sums of money

need for patient care in a timely and efficient manner. All elements of this supply chain would have lower inventories and less capital consumed by the process.

A pharmacy technician working as an inventory manager must constantly monitor the utilization trends of high-usage medications, critical medications, and expensive products. The technician needs to be able to generate reports for pharmacy management that communicate changes in a timely and accurate manner. The prime vendor needs to modify its stock levels based on demand in a timely manner and notify its clients as soon as shortages start to appear in the supply chain.

The impact that drug shortages have on the hospital pharmacy can be devastating and may include increases in drug expenditures as a result of purchasing noncontracted drugs, which may adversely affect bundled product contracts. Costs may be associated with getting manufacturers to drop-ship emergency allocations of product that are no longer available from the distributors. There is also a tendency to overstock an item when it has been backordered or difficult to obtain.

To be prepared, a hospital pharmacy buyer should take a proactive approach and establish contingency procedures. An excellent source of information on this topic can be found in the *ASHP Guidelines on Managing Drug Product Shortages* publication.

Prime Vendor Ordering Process

Each prime vendor provides each client with a very sophisticated computerized ordering system that connects electronically to the vendor's internal business systems. The ordering of medications from the prime vendor can occur in several ways:

- The buyer conducts a manual review of stock shelves and the information on those handwritten notes is manually entered into the prime vendor's ordering system.
- Products can be ordered using a handheld bar code scanning device provided by the prime vendor. The prime vendor provides bar-coded product shelf labels for all of the products purchased by the client. The client applies these to their stock shelves to aid in the ordering process. The buyer can scan these labels and enter a quantity to order directly into the handheld device. The scanned information is uploaded into the prime vendor computer ordering system for review by the buyer.
- Written requests or "want books," approved formulary requests, approved nonformulary request, and so forth, are manually transcribed into the prime vendor's ordering system by the buyer.
- If the pharmacy maintains a perpetual computerized inventory, then the inventory management system can generate a suggested order with suggested order quantities based on historical usage for review by the buyer. If the inventory management system is connected electronically to the prime vendor's ordering system, then the buyer's approved order can be transferred electronically to the prime vendor's distribution system.

Most hospital pharmacies use a combination of these ordering methods when placing their prime vendor orders. The prime vendor's ordering system generally provides a number of prompts during the ordering process. These prompts help ensure that the GPO contract product is chosen when possible or that the buyer is aware of the most cost-effective alternative generic products. The prime vendor's ordering system automatically queries the prime vendor's stock management system to determine if the product is available. If the product is available, then the prime vendor's stock management system reserves that item for the client. If the product is not available, then the prime vendor's ordering system notifies the buyer and suggests alternatives for the buyer to select. This process is iterative until the buyer is satisfied with the order and all of the requested products are confirmed as being in the prime vendor's inventory.

When the order is confirmed by the buyer, the vendor prints an order confirmation report at the client site. Most hospital pharmacies use this confirmation report as their purchase order. In some hospitals this confirmation report must be manually reentered into a materials management computer system to create a purchase order.

The pharmacy technician's role in the prime vendor ordering process can include functioning as the buyer and/or assisting the buyer in collecting and entering order information into the prime vendor's ordering system.

Manufacturer Direct Ordering Process

Hospital pharmacies try to avoid ordering products directly from a manufacturer unless that is the only source of the product or a significant savings can be obtained. When ordering directly from a manufacturer or supplier, the buyer generally places the order without any knowledge of whether the manufacturer has the product available to ship. Often the transport of the manufacturer or supplier order takes longer than a prime vendor order, which encourages the buyer to "stock up" rather than just buying what is needed today. If too much is purchased and needs to be returned, the process is much more complicated than returning a product through the prime vendor.

The buyer is restricted to a manual review process to identify when a product is required if the hospital pharmacy lacks a perpetual computerized pharmacy inventory system. When a direct product is needed, the buyer initiates the purchase by completing a purchase order (PO). The PO can be mailed, telephoned, or faxed to the manufacturer or supplier. Every attempt is made by the buyer to consolidate orders for each manufacturer or supplier to minimize the number of individual POs required.

The pharmacy technician's role in the manufacturer direct ordering process can include functioning as the buyer and/or assisting the buyer in collecting and entering order information into the prime vendor's ordering system.

Record Keeping

The hospital pharmacy must establish and maintain adequate records for the purchasing and distribution of the products purchased to meet the requirements of either government regulations, standards of practice requirements, accreditation standards, hospital policies, or management information requirements. Budget reports, productivity reports, workload reports, completed purchase orders, invoices, inventory reports, product receiving reports, and dispensing reports may be generated and maintained by a pharmacy technician. These reports are important to establish historical references to past performance and financial results.

Reports on controlled substances and alcohol purchases, invoices, completed receiving documents, inventory reports, and distribution reports can be maintained by a pharmacy technician. Records for the inventory management of controlled drugs must be maintained for 2 years. Some states may require these records to be maintained for 5 years.

The purchase order should be prepared prior to the time the order is placed by telephone, mail, computer, or fax. The information included on a PO typically includes the following:

- Name and address of the hospital
- Shipping address
- Date the order was placed
- Vendor's name and address
- Purchase order number
- Ordering department's name and location
- Expected date of delivery
- Shipping terms (e.g., FOB, Net 30)
- Account number or billing designation
- Description of items ordered
- Quantity of items ordered
- Unit price
- Extended price
- Total price of the order
- Buyer's name and phone number.

Order Fulfillment Process

The order fulfillment process for the prime vendor could be either automated or manual. Each prime vendor will have a distribution center designated to serving each client hospital pharmacy. The fulfillment process is often done overnight so that all of the ordering for each client is completed prior to starting the fulfillment process.

The order fulfillment process used by a manufacturer or supplier normally occurs as soon as the order has been received and the customer's creditworthiness has been confirmed.

Delivery Process

The prime vendor's delivery process is dictated by the negotiated contract. Delivery of completed orders generally occurs once each day, up to 6 days a week. In some cases the prime vendor may deliver orders twice a day. Most order delivery is accomplished by the prime vendor's own trucks as soon as the orders are ready at their distribution center. However, depending on the hospital's size and/or location in relation to the prime vendor's distribution center, completed orders may be shipped by third-party carriers.

Manufacturers ship completed orders by third-party carriers. If required, the order may be shipped via a carrier that uses an expedited process.

Receiving Process

All drugs should be delivered directly to the pharmacy department or a secured pharmacy receiving area to prevent diversion of the drug orders. Controlled substances and tax-free alcohol require special handling and must be closely supervised by a licensed pharmacist to minimize loss or adulteration. All controlled drugs and tax-free alcohol are accounted for in a perpetual inventory. Every individual dose of a controlled substance must be accounted for throughout the receiving process, storage, and distribution.

Note: A general rule promoted by auditors and security experts is to separate the ordering and receiving processes so that the same person is never be put in the position of doing both functions.

Managing the receiving process is an important role for the pharmacy technician. The following are important guidelines to ensure the successful management of that role:

- Verify the shipping address to ensure the package received was intended for delivery to the pharmacy department.
- Evaluate the outside of the package for visible signs of damage to the carton or the contents. Note any observed damage on the receiving document before you sign for the delivery.
- Look for any shipping documents attached to the outside of the package, and determine if special handling is required (e.g., store in freezer, controlled substance).
- Carefully open the package, and check each item for breakage.
- Check each item for expiration date, and make note of any short-dated material for immediate use or return.
- Verify the order received against a copy of the purchase order. Note any variations. Refer to the shipping document or packing slip to determine if items are backordered or out of stock.
- Refer any discrepancies to the supervising pharmacist.

Some prime vendors offer an automated receiving process that improves the accuracy and the timeliness of the process. An automated receiving process can be a free-standing computer application or it might be integrated into the vendor's ordering system. Products are marked as received when they are scanned into the prime vendor's receiving application by the client. The vendor's application compares what the product received to what was ordered and notifies the pharmacy technician of any discrepancies. The result of this receiving process can be electronically transferred to the client's accounts payable system.

Controlled substances and alcohol are normally received by pharmacy technicians or pharmacists familiar with the legal requirements associated with the receiving of these products. Often the outer shipping containers for these products are sent directly to the specialized area that handles these products where specified personnel conduct the receiving process. Under no circumstances should the person ordering controlled substances from a vendor receive those same controlled substances into the pharmacy. Separating these actions is imperative to limit the opportunities for diversion.

The PO, the receiving documents, and the order's invoice are provided to accounting for payment at the conclusion of the receiving process.

Put-Away Process

Received stock should be placed in the appropriate stock locations as soon as possible after the receiving process is complete. This helps ensure that duplicate product ordering does not occur. Any product requiring special storage such as refrigerated items should be put away immediately after receiving is complete. Care should be taken to ensure that all items are stored in the appropriate location. The pharmacy technician can support all of the activities associated with the put-away process.

Stock Maintenance Process

The maintenance of stock storage sites involves activities such as reviewing the stock for out-of-date products; maintaining the cleanliness of the stock storage area, shelves, and shelf labels; and keeping the stock straight and orderly. The pharmacy technician can support all of the activities associated with maintaining the stock holding areas.

Products Obtained from the Pharmacy

Medications are held in numerous stock sites throughout the hospital for a variety of reasons. Each stock site serves as a source of medications to support the delivery of patient care. All of these stock sites must be replenished routinely. The pharmacy is the only source of medications for these stock sites. The replenishment of these stock sites can represent a significant portion of the pharmacy's ongoing workload depending on the method of patient drug distribution used by the hospital. Some of the more common stock sites can include:

- Patient care area (nursing units, surgery, outpatient clinics, etc.) floor stock
- Emergency carts or code carts
- Specialty trays or boxes for surgery
- Automated dispensing cabinets (ADCs)
- Satellite pharmacies
- Specialty pharmacy order fulfillment areas.

The specific approach to replenishing these stock sites can vary from hospital to hospital. The following descriptions provide an example of how product could be ordered for some common stock sites.

Patient Care Area Floor Stock

Patient care area floor stock generally has a par level associated with the quantity of stock for each item held at each stock site. The type of stock and quantity for each item at each floor stock location are determined through agreement between the nursing and pharmacy departments generally with the approval of the P&T Committee. When a patient caregiver uses a floor stock item, the caregiver should provide documentation to pharmacy that indicates which patient received the floor stock. This documentation functions as the order to replace the stock. Periodically a pharmacy technician will reconcile the existing floor stock at each stock location to the approved par levels to identify any discrepancies. Nursing might be required to explain the discrepancies or the product may be charged to the nursing unit.

Orders for the patient care area floor stock are picked by a pharmacy technician from either the primary stock site in the central pharmacy or from a satellite pharmacy's stock. The picked items are packaged for each patient care area and set aside in a staging area for delivery or pickup. Patient care area floor stock is generally delivered by a pharmacy technician.

Patient care area floor stock maintenance is the responsibility of both nursing and pharmacy. A pharmacy technician is generally responsible for reconciling the actual floor stock levels with the par levels periodically to identify any discrepancies. The pharmacy technician is also responsible for reviewing the expiration dates and removing any expired products on a routine schedule. Nursing should assist in keeping the stock orderly and in its proper location as identified by labels applied by pharmacy to the stock sites.

Emergency or Code Carts

Emergency carts or code carts generally have a fixed number of medications in specific quantities suitable for treating patients under emergency conditions such as heart attacks. Generally, the types of items and quantity of each are fixed for all carts and approved by the P&T Committee. The return of the cart or tray to the pharmacy represents the order for replenishment.

The individual returning an emergency cart medication tray or code cart is provided a replacement by a pharmacy technician. A pharmacy technician replenishes the tray or cart to its par levels, replaces expired or nearly expired medications, generates appropriate charges for used items, and then reseals the tray or cart. The technician records the earliest expiration date on the outside of the tray or cart.

Emergency carts or code cart replacements are delivered to the patient care area by either a caregiver or a pharmacy technician depending on the hospital's policies. The cart is replaced as soon as possible in case it is needed again.

The expiration dates of medications stocked in emergency carts or code carts should be reviewed routinely during patient care area inspections conducted either by a pharmacist or trained pharmacy technician. Carts with expired medications should be replaced immediately by the pharmacy technician.

Specialty Trays/Boxes

Specialty trays or boxes for surgery are generally treated as a single product. A caregiver will request a tray or box prior to the start of a surgical procedure or at the beginning of a day depending on hospital policies. Each tray or box contains a fixed number of items in a specific quantity. The content is determined jointly between pharmacy and the area using the tray or box.

The items in the used specialty trays or boxes for surgery are compared by a pharmacy technician to the par levels for that tray or box to determine what needs to be replenished. The technician reviews the expiration date of all items and notes the earliest expiration date on the outside of the tray or box.

Specialty trays or boxes for surgery are picked up by a caregiver from the pharmacy when they are needed. In some hospitals, anesthesia trays and surgery boxes are delivered by pharmacy to a cabinet or storage locker that is only accessible by authorized personnel. In these cases the caregiver could obtain a tray or box from that storage location using a sign-out process.

The expiration dates for products in stored specialty trays or boxes should be reviewed routinely by a pharmacy technician. Expired products in trays or boxes should be removed and updated as described earlier.

Automated Dispensing Cabinets

Automated dispensing cabinets (ADCs) can contain 300 or more different stock items. par levels are generally set for the inventory in the ADC. An ADC's master computer controller, located in the pharmacy, can either generate a stock replenishment list automatically or on request by a pharmacy technician to bring the ADC's inventory back to the par level.

The ADC's computer-generated replenishment lists are filled by a pharmacy technician for each ADC location. The majority of hospitals use an area similar to a unit-dose cassette filling area to support the processing of ADC replenishment orders. Some hospitals have connected the ADC's replenishment lists electronically to automated stock carousels and packaging equipment to streamline the picking process. In either case, the completed replenishment order is set aside in the pharmacy staging area for delivery.

The pharmacy technician delivers the ADC stock directly to the cabinet. The technician uses the cabinet's automation features to ensure that each item is placed in the appropriate location. In some hospitals a caregiver may be required to verify what is loaded, especially for controlled substances.

Stock added to an ADC must be recorded in the ADC's computer records. Generally, the ADC guides the pharmacy technician through the restocking process by prompting the technician on what product to load next. The ADC organizes the loading process to minimize the time required to execute the process. The technician must acknowledge each item on the ADC with the quantity being loaded. Some ADCs require the technician to scan the bar code on the item being loaded and the bar code on the location where the item is being placed for a match to ensure accurate restocking.

An ADC's content should be routinely reviewed electronically to identify items that are not being used anymore and can be removed to make space for other items. The par levels set for each item should be reviewed routinely to identify any need for adjustment. This helps ensure that sufficient product is available to serve changing patient care needs. The items in each ADC storage compartment should be review routinely to remove items that have expired or will expire soon. The ADC's storage compartments should be cleaned periodically. The manufacturer's routine maintenance guidelines should be observed for each ACD.

Pharmacy Satellite

A satellite pharmacy technician might either order replenishment products from the central pharmacy or place his or her order directly with the prime vendor in conjunction with the buyer as described earlier. Par levels for the inventory are often used to determine the quantity of an item to order.

A satellite pharmacy's replenishment order might be picked from existing pharmacy stock by a pharmacy technician and set aside in the pharmacy staging area for delivery or pickup. Alternately, the replenishment order might be incorporated into the prime vendor order. If so, then those items ordered for the satellite pharmacy would be set aside by a pharmacy technician in the pharmacy staging area for delivery or pickup during the receiving process.

Replenishment orders for satellite pharmacies or specialty pharmacy order fulfillment areas may be delivered by a pharmacy technician or picked up by the area's pharmacy technician. The controlled substance vault's replenishment order is delivered by the prime vendor to the pharmacy and moved immediately to the vault for completion of the receiving process.

Satellite pharmacy locations and specialty pharmacy order fulfillment areas should be routinely reviewed by a pharmacy technician to identify expired or damaged items for removal. Storage areas should be kept clean and free of dust. Stock storage locations should be labeled according to the requirements of regulatory agencies such as the Joint Commission.

Specialty Pharmacy Order

The pharmacy technician for a specialty pharmacy order fulfillment area might either order replenishment items from the pharmacy's primary stock site or add his or her order requirements to the prime vendor order process described earlier. Specialty order fulfillment sites can include the unit-dose cassette filling area, the sterile compounding area, the specialty tray replenishment area, and so forth. The replenishment order for the controlled substance vault is incorporated into the prime vendor order process described earlier.

Orders for the specialty pharmacy are generally processed by a pharmacy technician from the main pharmacy stock area. However, the controlled substance vault order fulfillment process is done by the prime vendor.

Medication Storage Considerations

Stock Organization

Many different methods are used by hospital pharmacies to organize their drug inventories.

The inventory may be divided into an active drug inventory and a backup storeroom inventory for large, bulky items that require more space. The inventory may also be divided by how the drugs will be used. For example, parenteral medication for intravenous (IV) administration may be stored in the IV admixture room only.

Stock may be shelved alphabetically by the generic name of the active ingredient(s) or by the trade name of the product. Stock may be divided by the route of administration (e.g., oral solids, oral liquids, ear, eye, nasal, injectable) and then stocked by each item's generic name. Some pharmacies assign a bin location to each product, allowing for a random storage pattern. If this system is used, then all orders requiring selection of a product must reflect that bin location on the picking document to locate the stock. Retail pharmacies will often arrange their stock alphabetically by trade name.

A newer method of stocking involves the installation of automated carousels that can store large numbers and quantities of items. A vertical carousel is a device that brings the stock to the pharmacy technician. This eliminates the need for the technician to find the stock in the pharmacy. These devices are controlled by a software program. Such a device can be electronically integrated with other devices such as ADCs to automate the ADC replenishment process. Vertical carousels contain multiple shelves (up to 12 feet long) that rotate to the specific shelf where a product is stored and then provide direction with lights to the specific stock location for the pharmacy technician. Most of these devices have integrated bar code scanning to aid the pharmacy technician in verifying that she or he picked the right medication for the order.

Storage Environment

Certain environmental factors must be considered when storing medications such as temperature, ventilation, humidity, light, and sanitation. National standards have been developed for these factors and can be found in the U.S. Pharmacopeia (USP) and National Formulary (NF). The storage standards were designed to ensure that the strength, quality, purity, packaging, and labeling of drugs and related articles are maintained until the items are needed by patients.

Manufacturers are required to print specific storage conditions on drug packaging and drug labels to ensure proper storage and product integrity. The following terms are nationally recognized definitions for storage temperature:

- *Cold*—any temperature not exceeding 8°C (45°F). A refrigerator is a cold place in which the temperature is maintained thermostatically between 2°C (36°F) and 8°C (46°F). A freezer is a cold place in which the temperature is maintained thermostatically between −20°C (−4°F) and −10°C (−14°F).
- *Protection from freezing*—When freezing causes an item to lose strength or potency or to destructively alter the item's characteristics, then the container label must bear an appropriate instruction to prevent the item from freezing.

- *Cool*—any temperature between 8°C (46°F) and 15°C (59°F). An item for which storage in a cool place is required may be stored in a refrigerator, unless otherwise specified in the individual monograph.
- *Room temperature*—the temperature prevailing in a working area. Controlled room temperature is a temperature maintained thermostatically between 15°C (59°) and 30°C (86°F).
- *Warm*—any temperature between 30°C (86°F) and 40°C (104°F).
- *Excessive heat*—any temperature above 40°C (104°F).

When specific storage directions or limitations are not provided in the package insert, it is understood that the storage conditions include protection from moisture, freezing, and excessive heat. In many hospitals, the pharmacy technician may be required to check and record the temperatures in refrigerators and freezers used to store drugs throughout the facility. Recording devices are also used to monitor the temperature continuously and alert the pharmacy of significant variations so appropriate actions can be taken when the temperature is outside an acceptable range.

Additional standards regarding the preservation, packaging, storage, and labeling of drugs are described in the "General Notices and Requirements" section of the USP-NF. Those involved in any aspect of materials management of pharmaceuticals must be familiar with the official standards and definitions as they relate to the proper storage and handling of drugs. The pharmacy technician shares this obligation with all other members of the health care team involved in medication-related activities.

Hospital pharmacies will have some form of an automatic temperature recording device on all pharmacy refrigeration and freezer storage areas with suitable alarms when the refrigerator's or freezer's temperature varies outside of the national standards. The pharmacy is also responsible for monitoring the refrigerator and freezer temperatures for any medication storage location outside of the pharmacy. Electronic temperature monitoring devices are now available to install in all refrigeration units and freezers where medications are stored throughout a hospital. These devices enable the pharmacy to monitor all of these devices remotely and maintain the required records. The devices can alert the pharmacy technician when any monitored refrigerator or freezer fails to maintain the appropriate temperature.

Security

All medications must be maintained in locations that restrict access to only the professional and technical staff members who are authorized to receive, store, prepare, dispense, distribute, or administer medications.

Legend drugs (i.e., federal law prohibits dispensing without a prescription) must be dispensed by a licensed pharmacist. However, a pharmacy technician under the direct supervision of a pharmacist can receive and fill stock orders as described earlier. Medications stored in the patient care areas must also be secured and restricted to authorized personnel only. Even the medication carts used to support medication administration must be kept locked at all times when they are not being used by a caregiver.

Controlled substances and tax-free alcohol require additional security restrictions. Only a licensed pharmacist can order, receive, prepare, and dispense these drugs. However, a qualified pharmacy technician under the direct supervision of a pharmacist can assist in storing and delivering these products. Special security procedures, such as daily physical counts of pharmacy and nursing unit inventories, are essential to limit the opportunities for the diversion or misuse of controlled substances. ADCs are commonly used in hospitals to manage the record-keeping requirements for controlled substance use with patients and to provide security for the products. Similar devices are used in the main pharmacy as a controlled substance vault in some hospital pharmacies. Software applications are available to support audits of these products and detect diversion.

It is important for the pharmacist or technician involved in the ordering, receiving, or other management of controlled substances to avoid any discussion of their roles in these activities outside of the pharmacy. Unfortunately we live in a violent world in which certain individuals will often do anything to acquire these drugs, including committing violent acts. It is far better not to bring attention to yourself by discussion of the purchase and storage of these products anywhere except in the pharmacy.

Tax-free alcohol is generally used only by the hospital's pathology department. Security of tax-free alcohol is generally accomplished through a periodic audit of dispensing records and physical inventories.

Hazardous Substances

Safety precautions must also be considered when handling materials that have a high potential for danger. Pharmacy technicians should be aware of the following important guidelines for handling hazardous substances:

- *Volatile or flammable substances* should be stored in a cool, properly ventilated location that has been specially designed to reduce fire and explosion potential.
- *Caustic substances*, such as acids, should be stored in a location that would reduce any potential for dropping or breaking the container such as a locked cabinet instead of an open shelf.
- *Oncology drugs* used to treat cancer are often toxic themselves and therefore must be handled with extreme care. These drugs should be received in a sealed protective outer bag that restricts leakage of the drug in the event the container leaks or is broken. These drugs should also be stored in a secure area that has limited access and a restricted traffic flow. When the potential exists for exposure to chemotherapy drugs (i.e., a breakage or spill), all personnel involved must wear protective clothing and equipment while following a hazardous materials cleanup procedure. All exposed materials must be properly disposed of in chemo-hazardous waste containers.

Inventory Control Considerations

The overall management of the inventory is important for a number of reasons. Well-managed inventory requires less storage space, which is often at a premium in a hospital pharmacy. Additionally, well-managed inventory consumes less capital. The following sections provide some details about what a pharmacy technician should consider when managing a pharmacy's inventory.

Stock Rotation and Segregation

The rotation of stock is critical to minimizing losses because it helps prevent medications from becoming outdated. Stock rotation ensures that stock received first is dispensed first. This is accomplished by always placing new stock behind the existing stock of the same item. This type of inventory management is called FIFO (first in-first out) stocking. Rotation allows the pharmacy technician to look at the existing stock and be sure that it is in the right place and still in-date for use in order filling. These actions contribute to the overall safety checks made by a pharmacy.

The segregation of the inventory into internal medications and external medications is mandated by a number of regulatory and accrediting bodies such as the Joint Commission. Some drugs have names that sound alike and/or look alike that can lead to errors in picking and dispensing. It is important for these drugs to be physically separated to reduce the opportunity for a picking error. Stickers for "STOP" or "LOOK" can be placed on the storage bins for these types of drugs to further call attention to the potential hazard.

Computerized Inventory Control

Many of the inventory management functions can be better controlled with the use of computer programs dedicated to monitor the purchasing, receiving, and dispensing functions. Perpetual inventory systems are now being utilized to indicate when predetermined reorder points have been reached. The automated stock management programs can be integrated with ADCs, carousels, and automated packaging equipment to facilitate enhanced stock management at all remote locations.

Most dedicated pharmacy systems can generate management reports that allow pharmacy management and the buyer to review drug use. For example, the monthly usage rate of each drug can be monitored and utilization tracked to determine which clinical department or patient population is using specific drugs. Computers also enable the pharmacy manager to closely monitor budget trends and year-to-date purchases by drug category. The pharmacy technician must remember that computer systems are only as effective as the accuracy of the information entered. Therefore, the pharmacy technician must have a basic understanding of how the pharmacy computer works and must be properly trained to maximize the potential benefits of inventory control programs. More detail on pharmacy computerization is given in Chapter 29.

Turnover Rate

turnover rate the rate of drug inventory; calculated by dividing the total dollars spent to purchase drugs in 1 year by the actual pharmacy inventory dollars

Determining a pharmacy's inventory **turnover rate** is a good method of measuring the overall effectiveness of the pharmacy's purchasing and inventory control programs. The inventory turnover rate does not mean that all medications in the pharmacy are turned over (i.e., used up and replaced). The inventory turnover rate refers to how many times the inventory value is recycled during a year. The inventory turnover rate is calculated by dividing the total dollars spent to purchase drugs for 1 year by the actual value of the pharmacy inventory at the end of the year. The number produced by this calculation defines how many times the value of the inventory was completely replaced during a year. The larger the number of inventory value turns, the stronger the financial indicator that the inventory control program is efficient. This approach encourages the pharmacy to focus on keeping only the bare minimum quantity of high-cost products in stock at any one time.

The definition of inventory is very important to this calculation. Some pharmacies that appear to have a high turnover rate may have defined their inventory as only that stock in their central pharmacy storage area. For the turnover rate to truly reflect the efficiency of the purchasing and inventory control program, all inventory from all pharmacy stock locations must be included in addition to the central pharmacy stocks. The floor stock locations, stock in the ADCs, outpatient clinics, and so forth, should be included in the valuation of the inventory.

In the 1980s, a turnover rate of 6 to 7 was considered acceptable. In the 2000s, turnover rates of 12 to 15 were easily achievable because of more efficient methods of purchasing, such as prime vendor programs and computerized order-entry systems. Even higher turnover rates might be achieved in the twenty-first century due to improved materials management techniques and business strategies such as consignment of inventory programs. Note, however, that a measure of effective inventory management and reasonable turnover rates is often reflected in how many products were not available when needed.

The following questions may further assist the pharmacy manager in his or her attempt to maintain adequate controls on a very large and complex inventory:

1. Has an inventory turnover rate been calculated for your hospital?
2. Is this rate optimal for the facility?
3. Is the storeroom checked at regular intervals to verify that appropriate purchasing and inventory methods are being followed?
   a. Are reorder points adjusted as needed?
   b. Is this rate optimal for the facility?
4. Are inventories controlled in dispensing areas?
   a. Are minimum and maximum inventories maintained?
   b. Is the space allotted for each product restricted?
   c. Is there a routine check for outdated drugs and excesses?
   d. Are exchange systems used when appropriate (e.g., carts, self-units, boxes)?
5. Are nursing-unit drug inventories controlled?
   a. Is an approved floor stock list used for drug items?
   b. Have maximum allowable quantities been established for each item?
   c. Are inventory dollar limits set for each nursing unit?
   d. Are units checked monthly for excesses and outdated drugs?
6. Are inventories controlled in the emergency, operating, and recovery departments?

Drug Recall Process

Drug recalls are generally issued by manufacturers when they become aware of a defect in their manufacturing process or labeling processes that would affect the use of their product in the marketplace. Notices of a drug recall are distributed by manufacturers to hospitals electronically and by mail; however, the most important route is through the hospital's prime vendor. The prime vendor reviews its records of a hospital's purchases and notifies the hospital if they have shipped the recalled product to the hospital. Drug recalls can range from minor labeling errors to catastrophic formulation problems that can lead to patient deaths.

Hospital pharmacies are required by both regulatory and accrediting bodies to have a clearly defined process in place for managing drug recalls. Drug recalls are generally related to a specific lot of the affected product. The drug recall notice includes at least the drug name, strength, dosage form, and the affected lot number(s) with an indication of the nature of the recall. Pharmacy technicians generally review all stock sites and remove the appropriate items. The technician completes the drug recall records and disposes of the recall product as directed by the manufacturer. Often the manufacturer requests the pharmacy to inventory the recalled product and provide the results of that inventory for the manufacturer to use in crediting the hospital. The actual recalled product is often sent back through a reverse distributor who will return it to the manufacturer for credit or for disposal of the product.

Out-of-Date Medications

Medications that are expired may have unpredictable results if used in patient care. At the very least the product may have lost its labeled potency. Regulatory and accrediting bodies require hospital pharmacies to have established guidelines for the routine review of all stored stock to identify and remove expired medications. This task is often coupled with the cleaning efforts for shelves and storage areas. Each hospital pharmacy defines its own procedures and who is responsible for this activity. Generally it is the responsibility of the pharmacy technician.

Repackaging and Labeling

In-house packaging and labeling are sometimes necessary when required dosage forms are not available commercially. Hospitals that have adopted the bar code medication administration program may have a substantial secondary labeling activity. Robotic automation to support the unit-dose drug distribution system may require specialized packaging. The pharmacy technician must be adequately trained for each of these repackaging, labeling, and relabeling activities to ensure compliance with regulatory requirements and the stability of the final product.

There are many different types of containers to choose from depending on the product, the desired route of administration, and the method of dispensing—for example, unit-dose packaging for solid oral forms (e.g., tray-fill blister packaging, cadet foil packaging) and oral liquids (e.g., cups, oral syringes). In addition, some of the new automated dispensing technologies require packaging unique to their dispensing design (e.g., robot-ready cards, Pyxis CUBIES).

Regardless of what type of packaging container is used, it should be clean. Special precautions and cleaning procedures may be necessary to ensure that extraneous material is not introduced into or onto the drugs being packaged. It is also essential to be sure that the container does not interact physically or chemically with the drug being placed in it. Any interaction might alter the strength, quality, or purity of the article beyond the official requirements.

Some drugs may have special packaging requirements as described in the manufacturer's literature and in official monographs published in the USP-NF. The following requirements for use of specified containers may apply when in-house packaging is required:

- *Light-resistant containers* protect the contents from the effects of light through the use of the special properties of their composition or an applied coating. Even a clear and colorless (translucent) container may be made light resistant by covering it in an opaque covering. If an opaque covering is used, the container should bear a statement that the covering is needed until either the contents are used or administered to a patient. If the pharmacist is directed to "protect from light" in an individual monograph, preservation in a light-resistant container is required.

- *Tamper-resistant packaging* is required for a sterile product intended for ophthalmic or otic use, unless it has been extemporaneously compounded for immediate dispensing on prescription. The contents are sealed so that they cannot be opened without obvious destruction of the seal.
- *Tight containers* protect the contents from contamination by extraneous liquids, solids, or vapors, from loss of the item, and from efflorescence, deliquescence, or evaporation under ordinary or customary conditions of handling, shipment, storage, and distribution.
- *Hermetic containers* are impervious to air or any other gas under ordinary or customary conditions of handling, shipping, storage, and distribution.
- *Single-unit containers* are designed to hold a quantity of drug product intended for administration as a single dose, or a single finished device intended for one-time use promptly after the container is opened. Each single-unit container should be labeled to indicate the identity, quantity, strength, name of manufacturer, lot number, and expiration date of the drug or item.
- *Single-dose containers* are single-use containers for articles intended for parenteral administration only. Examples of single-dose containers include prefilled syringes, cartridges, fusion-sealed containers, and closure-sealed containers when so labeled.
- *Unit-dose containers* are single-unit containers for articles intended for administration by routes other than the parenteral route as a single dose, direct from the container.

Each label must include at least the following information:

- Generic name of the product (brand name optional)
- Strength in units (e.g., mg, mL, oz)
- Drug form (e.g., tablet, capsule, suppository)
- Lot number and manufacturer's name
- Expiration date for repackaged drug.

The expiration date used on repackaged drugs should be based on the prevailing community standard of practice or on an evaluation of scientific information. In all cases the maximum expiration date should be compliant with applicable laws and regulations. The USP states, "In the absence of stability data to the contrary, such date should not exceed

1. 25 percent of the remaining time between the date of repackaging and the expiration date on the original manufacturer's bulk container, or
2. A six-month period of time from the date the drug is repackaged, whichever is earlier."

All repackaged drugs must be carefully checked by a licensed pharmacist, and approvals must be documented in writing before repackaged drugs are put into active inventory. Documentation of the repackaging process should include the following information:

- Date of repackaging
- Name and strength of drug

- Quantity of drug repackaged
- Manufacturer's name
- Manufacturer's lot number
- Manufacturer's expiration date
- In-house code number
- In-house expiration date
- Initials of packaging technician
- Initials of pharmacist.

Record-Keeping Recommendations

Repackaging, relabeling, or the application of a secondary label all require detailed record keeping of what was processed. Any time a product's labeling is altered by a pharmacy, extreme caution must be exercised to prevent errors. The pharmacy technician should be aware of these guidelines for repackaging, relabeling, or adding secondary labels to medications:

- Quantities of an item to repackage, relabel, or add a secondary label to should be of sufficient size to last for a reasonable period of time.
- Complete the batch production record reflecting the item's name, lot number, strength, dosage form, quantity to be processed, and the batch number prior to starting the activity.
- Print only the number of labels that will be required for the quantity of product to be processed.
- Account for all printed labels at the end of the process.

Record-keeping requirements may vary by hospital. Most of the needed information could be kept in a log book or a computer spreadsheet. Records for the repackaging, relabeling, and application of secondary labeling must be available for review during regulatory visits.

Bar Code Usage

In March 2003, the FDA announced that it would require bar codes on all medications in an effort to reduce the high rate of medical errors. This was an important step in automating the medication use process and reducing the amount of human interpretation in the ordering, dispensing, and administration of drugs. During a study of more than 88 million doses from April 2002 to June 2003, it was estimated that only 36% of the drugs down to the dose level had bar codes. The FDA estimated that it would cost pharmaceutical companies $50 million to add bar codes to all drugs manufactured and used in the United States, and hospitals would spend over $7 billion on scanners and computer systems to support the initiative. However, the FDA fell short of requiring manufacturers to place bar codes on the actual unit-of-use package. They required that the manufacturer place a bar code on the commercial sale unit, which may be a package of 100 or more unit-of-use packages. The FDA did not mandate what information should be contained in the bar code, leaving that decision to each manufacturer.

The Institute of the National Academy of Sciences estimated that more than 98,000 people were killed by medical errors each year with about 7,000 of those deaths directly attributable to medication errors. According to Michael R. Cohen, president of the Institute for Safe Medication Practices, early studies indicate that bar coding should reduce the number of medications errors by over 50%.

The use of bar codes to identify a product is a critical component of the new medication administration computer programs and is rapidly being adopted by many hospitals (**Figure 27-2**). Hospital pharmacy will be challenged to ensure that every product provided for use with patients in their institution has a "machine-readable" bar code. Until all manufacturers are able to overcome the issues associated with placing bar codes on their unit-of-use packaging, the hospital pharmacy will be required to apply secondary labeling.

Caregivers will probably rely more on the product's bar code than the printed label where bar code medication administration (BCMA) programs are present. This probability further increases the importance of pharmacy having "bullet-proof" processes equivalent to those of manufacturers for applying the secondary labeling. The pharmacy technician will need to:

- Understand how to use different types of packaging and scanning equipment.
- Understand the limitations and compatibility of the bar code system used at their hospital.
- Understand the associated changes in the medication use process driven by the use of BCMA.
- Understand the content in the bar code used by the hospital.

The information contained in the bar code varies depending on the type of bar code used and the landscape or label area available for the bar code. The bar code placed on products by the manufacturers varies from their company's list number to the product's National Drug Code (NDC) number. Unlike the grocery industry,

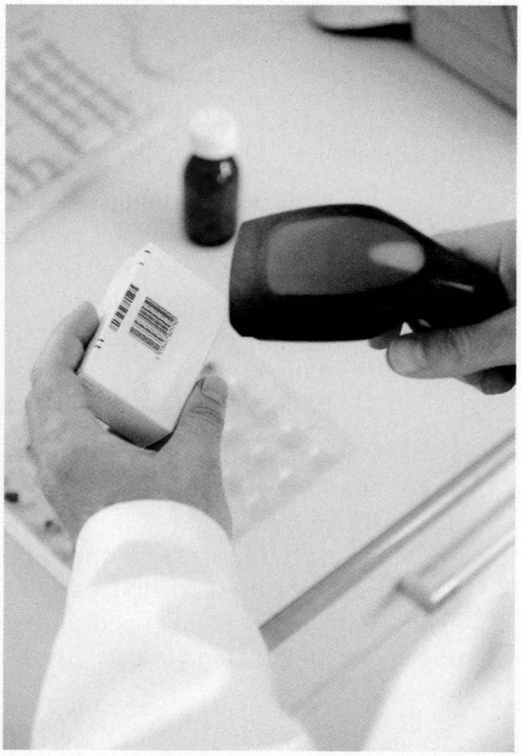

FIGURE 27-2 Bar code scanning is becoming an advantageous investment toward decreasing medication errors.

health care lacks a clearinghouse for the assignment of a universal product code (UPC). This leads to highly customized solutions that are often hospital specific. Hospital pharmacies try to use the NDC number where possible but often they have a multitude of exceptions. For that reason it is very important for the pharmacy technician to have a clear understanding of what drug identifier is used by their hospital and how exceptions are handled.

Hospital pharmacies can use bar codes to support the transfer of products between their stock sites and stock sites located in patient care areas. The use of bar codes to validate accurate replenishment of ADCs is critical to the integrity of that system. Hospital pharmacies will continue to develop new applications that use bar codes to manage their stock responsibilities.

Bar codes may ultimately be replaced by the use of a different technology called radio-frequency identification device (RFID) coding. This technology does not need to appear on a label's surface. It can be imbedded in the labeling material. RFIDs communicate with computerized listening devices to indicate when a product changes location. Retailers have become the early adopters of RFID technology to manage their inventories and minimize theft. Just try to walk out of a Walmart with an expensive item that has not been through the checkers. The future use of RFID technology will substantially change the management of products inside of health care organizations.

Recapture and Disposal Considerations

The recapture or retrieval of unused medications and the removal of expired or damaged medications is an important part of a pharmacy's responsibilities. The effective removal of these types of products contributes to the overall safety of patient care.

Returned Medications

Most approaches to drug distribution described in Chapter 20 can result in the return of medication originally intended for a patient. The return might be a result of:

- A failure to administer the medication
- The discontinuance of the medication by the prescriber
- The transfer of a patient within the hospital without moving the medications with the patient
- Damage to the medication during preparation for administration to a patient
- Patient refusal of the medication after it was prepared for administration.

The unit-dose drug distribution approach to drug distribution normally generates the largest volume of returned medications due to a combination of the reasons listed above.

Some hospitals require that all returned medications issued to a specific patient are credited to that patient unless the medication has been partially used. Returned partially used patient-specific medications are set aside by the pharmacy technician in a secure and isolated location to await the disposal process.

If the returned medication is packaged as a unit-dose, then the pharmacy technician checks the return medication packaging for integrity and proper dating. If the medication was dispensed for a specific patient, then hospital policy might require the dose to be credited to that patient. If the product is expired or damaged, the pharmacy technician will set the item aside in a secure and isolated location to await the disposal process. Usable medications are restocked by the pharmacy technician.

If the returned medication is packaged as a multidose item and has not been used, then the pharmacy technician will check the expiration date on the container and evaluate the container for damage. Expired or damaged multidose items are set aside by the pharmacy technician in a secure and isolated location to await disposal. Usable multidose items are restocked by the technician.

Expired Medications

All medications have an expiration date identified on their labeling. The expiration date indicates that the medication is no longer suitable for use. The expiration date can be designated in one of two ways:

- Month and year (e.g., June 20XX), which means that the packaged material, if properly stored, is good until the last day of the month, or
- Month, day, and year (e.g., June 15, 20XX).

Every hospital pharmacy must have a process for checking the expiration date on all drugs stocked on a regular basis. This process guarantees that only properly dated drugs are available for use. Expired drugs must be set aside in a secure and isolated location to await disposal. This action is designed to prevent an expired drug from being dispensed.

Disposal of Medications

Both regulatory and accrediting bodies for pharmacy require that a formal process be defined for the disposition of medications that are expired, damaged, or partially used. The Environmental Protection Agency (EPA) and the Occupational Safety and Health Administration (OSHA) both have rules on how to dispose of medications. EPA's rules apply to all medications and OSHA's rules apply only to "hazardous substances." In 1976, the Resource Conservation and Recovery Act (RCRA) was enacted to provide a mechanism for tracking hazardous waste from generation of medications to their disposal. These regulations are enforced by EPA. Several drugs (e.g., epinephrine) require handling, containment, and disposal as RCRA hazardous waste. Today, many pharmacy departments contract with a "reverse" distribution company. These companies provide pharmacy support for all of the required tracking and documentation that the drugs have been properly destroyed. The inventory personnel will keep a manifest of those medications destroyed on file.

The reverse distribution company often is responsible for sorting the items stored in the pharmacy's secure and isolated storage area that is designated for damaged, partially used, and expired medications. The reverse distributor may sort the products on site or may package the product and ship it to its facility for sorting. The reverse distributor identifies those items that could be returned to the manufacturer for credit. Those items are submitted to the appropriate manufacturer for credit. A complete listing of these items with their value is generated for the hospital's records. Many pharmaceutical companies will give full credit for expired medication.

The remaining items are sorted into their appropriate disposal groups according to existing rules and regulations. The items are inventoried and a list is generated for the hospital pharmacy's records recording how the products were destroyed with appropriate descriptive information.

All controlled drugs returned through or destroyed by a reverse distributor must be removed from perpetual inventory. Records pertaining to returned or destroyed controlled drugs must be kept for 5 years.

If the hospital pharmacy elects to manage the disposition of all of these items, then the pharmacy would be responsible for sorting, applying for credit, and arranging for destruction of all noncreditable products awaiting the disposal process. For patients and consumers in the community, the EPA suggests that tablets and capsules be crushed and mixed with water. The resultant slurry can be put in coffee grounds or kitty litter and disposed of in the regular trash. Liquids can be poured directly into the kitty litter and the kitty litter placed in the trash.

Summary

Pharmacy technicians have many different opportunities to contribute to pharmacy materials management. The integration of automation into pharmacy materials management has created additional opportunities that are still being defined. As drugs become more expensive, more complex to manage, and more desirable to the criminal element in our society, the role of pharmacy materials management will intensify. The pharmacy technician must work closely with pharmacy management to minimize the cost of drugs, assist in designing better ways to manage the complexity of drug distribution, and protect the pharmacy's drug supply from the ever-present criminal activities to divert drugs.

TEST YOUR KNOWLEDGE

Multiple Choice

1. An institutional pharmacy materials management program includes
   a. procurement.
   b. drug storage.
   c. inventory control.
   d. all of the above.

2. In a hospital, overall responsibility for the materials management of pharmaceuticals lies with the
   a. chairperson of the Pharmacy and Therapeutics Committee.
   b. director of pharmacy services.
   c. hospital administration.
   d. chief pharmacy technician.

3. Environmental considerations in the storage of pharmaceuticals include
   a. proper ventilation.
   b. proper humidity.
   c. proper temperature.
   d. all of the above.

4. The pharmacy department is responsible for
   a. preparing purchase orders.
   b. receiving and securing shipments of pharmaceuticals.
   c. monitoring the inventory of controlled substances and tax-free alcohol.
   d. all of the above.

5. Inventory control may include
   a. maintaining minimum and maximum reorder points.
   b. return of outdated stock.
   c. drug usage reports.
   d. all of the above.

6. The Food and Drug Administration's bar-coding rules are estimated to reduce the number of medication errors by which of the following percentages?
   a. 36%
   b. 50%
   c. 70%
   d. 90%

Matching

Match the description to the appropriate temperature range.

1. ______ cold temperature	a.	-20°C (-4°F) to -10°C (14°F)
2. ______ freezer	b.	15°C (59°F) to 30°C (86°F)
3. ______ room temperature	c.	not exceeding 8°C (46°F)
4. ______ refrigerator	d.	30°C (86°F) to 40°C (104°F)
5. ______ excessive heat	e.	2°C (36°F) to 8°C (46°F)
6. ______ warm	f.	above 40°C (104°F)

Match the task with the correct person's responsibility. Answers are used more than once.

1. ______ Select the drug source.	a.	pharmacist's responsibility
2. ______ Prepare the drug order.	b.	technician's responsibility
3. ______ Check the incoming drug products.		
4. ______ Maintain a proper drug storage environment.		
5. ______ Prepare formulary revision.		

Suggested Readings

ASHP guidelines for drug distribution and control: Preparation and handling. (2006). *American Journal of Health-System Pharmacy, 63*, 1172–1193.

ASHP guidelines for selecting pharmaceutical manufacturers and suppliers. (1991). *American Journal of Health-System Pharmacy, 48*, 523–524.

ASHP guidelines on formulary system management. (1992). *American Journal of Health-System Pharmacy, 49*, 648–652.

ASHP guidelines on managing drug product shortages. (2001). *American Journal of Health-System Pharmacy, 58*, 1445–1450.

Joint Commission. Pharmacy services. (2007). In *Comprehensive accreditation manual for hospitals*. Oak Brook Terrace, IL: Author.

Okeke, C.C., Bailey, L., Medwick, T., & Grady, L. T. (2000). Revised USP standards for product dating, packaging, and temperature monitoring. *American Journal of Health-System Pharmacy, 57*(15), 1441–1445.

U.S. Pharmacopeial Convention. (2007). General notices and requirements: Preservation, packaging, storage, and labeling. *In U.S. Pharmacopeia, 30th ed./National Formulary, 25th ed.*, pp. 10–13. Rockville, MD: Author.

CHAPTER

28

The Pharmacy Formulary System

Competencies

Upon completion of this chapter, the reader should be able to:

1. Outline the five core attributes of the formulary system.
2. Explain the impact of a formulary in pharmacy practice in relation to managed care organizations such as pharmacy benefit managers and health plans.
3. List the steps in the process for adding a new drug to the formulary.
4. List three surveillance activities fostered by the formulary system.
5. Describe how using new technologies will improve formulary compliance.
6. Illustrate why it is important to revise the formulary regularly.

Key Terms

dossier
monograph
National Formulary

Introduction

Throughout much of the history of pharmacy, the term *formulary* has referred to a listing of drugs. The spectrum of sophistication of a formulary can range from a simple list for use in a small institution to an elaborate compendium of detailed standards, which may carry some official weight as a legally recognized standard. In some cases, an institution's formulary is actually a complete reference manual of policies and procedures, guidelines for use, and criteria for evaluation of medications approved for use at that particular institution. Formularies can be used for many purposes.

Perhaps the most historically significant of the ancient formularies is the Ebers Papyrus (c. 1500 B.C.), a listing of complex prescriptions and cures from ancient Egypt. Formularies have documented the state-of-the-art therapeutic knowledge of the cultures that compiled them. Not all formularies are from the Old World, however. Some very complete ones, usually described as *codices*, are attributed to Central American native civilizations. In fact, some of the drugs, such as digitalis and cocaine, appeared in these formularies many years before they were "discovered" by Western or Oriental medicine.

National Formulary
a database of drugs of established usefulness not found in the U.S. Pharmacopeia

The most revered formulary in the United States is the **National Formulary**, which was first published in 1888 and includes standards for excipients, botanicals, and other similar products. Many pharmacists are familiar with the initials *NF* following drug names. The National Formulary has since been incorporated into the U.S. Pharmacopeia (USP) as the official compendium of drug standards in the United States. Formularies, then, are a continuation of a worldwide, centuries-old pharmacy tradition.

In their modern form, formularies are usually associated with hospitals or other organized medical care settings, but increasingly managed care organizations (MCOs), such as health plans and pharmacy benefit managers (PBMs), and other payer-based entities have established their own formularies for their beneficiaries or member populations. In some instances, formularies are identified as preferred drug lists or PDLs. Managed care organizations and Medicare Part D brought formularies to the forefront of the general public's attention.

According to the Academy of Managed Care Pharmacy's (AMCP's) Concept Series paper on formulary management, a formulary is one component of health care management. It enhances other existing medication management practices designed to optimize patient care, including:

- Sound medical treatment and prescribing guidelines or protocols
- Drug utilization reviews and drug use evaluation programs
- Physician, pharmacist, and patient drug education programs.

The federal Veterans Affairs system has adopted a "national" formulary (not to be confused with the official compendium, the National Formulary) and uses it to optimize therapy and as a tool to negotiate price savings. The Centers for Medicare and Medicaid Services (CMS) developed specific guidelines and requirements for all prescription drug plans (PDPs) when developing formularies for the Medicare Part D prescription drug program. Formularies are tools, and like any tool, how it is used determines the overall judgment of its value. As part of this tradition, certain attributes come to mind when using the term *formulary*. It is interesting that some ancient concepts embodied in formularies are now being used to expand the role of the pharmacy profession for technician practitioners as well as for pharmacists.

The Formulary System

The formulary system describes how formularies are derived and how the drug use process can be guided, controlled, and accounted for when a particular formulary is in effect. The core attributes of a formulary and formulary system include the following:

- Formularies represent a selective list of the drugs available for beneficiaries.
- Formularies are either considered open or closed. An open formulary provides coverage for all drugs; however, some drug classes, such as those for cosmetic use or over-the-counter drugs, may be excluded from coverage. A closed formulary provides coverage for only those drugs listed on the formulary. Formulary exception policies allow patients and physician reimbursement and access to nonformulary medications when medically necessary.
- A formulary is developed through the consensus of the Pharmacy and Therapeutics (P&T) Committee. The committee reviews drugs in each therapeutic class, looking for any superiority within a class, placing emphasis on the most cost-effective therapeutic agents to be used in the practice.
- Formularies can contain additional information about covered drugs and their use, such as dosing guidelines, tables comparing similar drugs within a class, common drug interactions, suggestions for patient information, and so forth.
- The formulary system defines policies and procedures along with coverage criteria concerning drug use, and it defines the scope of the formulary.
- Formularies must be continuously reviewed and revised.

Consensus is important for the formulary to be effective. The members of the P&T Committee should be selected with this in mind and should represent a cross section of disciplines from the medical and pharmacy community.

Today, MCOs utilize the clinical pharmacy department in a lead role in formulary development. The clinical pharmacy department develops monographs that provide detailed information about drugs under consideration by a P&T Committee. Several strategies are used to gain consensus:

1. Additions to the formulary should be requested in a formal fashion through the use of a request form. This form can channel the thoughts of the requester by including some questions such as "Are there similar drugs on the formulary?" or "What are the advantages of this drug?"
2. Requests to add drugs to the formulary are generally forwarded to the chairman or secretary (usually the director of pharmacy) of the P&T Committee.
3. The pharmacy department should prepare a monograph for each drug being considered for addition to the formulary that includes its advantages, disadvantages, and therapeutic impact. Some monographs also include information about the financial impact of a medication, but not all P&T Committees request this data when reviewing products. When researching and comparing drugs, it helps to have all the information about those drugs in a standardized format. The *AMCP Format for Formulary Submissions* has become

the accepted standard used by most MCOs and pharmaceutical manufacturers. The *Format* is a set of guidelines that pharmaceutical manufacturers can use to prepare submissions of new (and existing) pharmaceuticals for a health system's P&T Committee. This information set is referred to as a **dossier**. Manufacturers submit the dossier to the plan, and the pharmacy department uses the information in the development of its **monograph**. Further information about the *Format* may be found on the AMCP website (http://www.amcp.org). A fully electronic version of the *Format*, the eDossier System, has also been developed; information about this electronic version may be found at https://amcp.edossiers.com.

dossier a set of guidelines that pharmaceutical manufacturers can use to prepare submissions of new (and existing) pharmaceuticals for a health system's P&T Committee

monograph a compilation of information about a specific drug product; contains a list of and amounts of ingredients, instructions on usage, the circumstances under which it may be used, and any contraindications for use of the product

4. The actions of the P&T Committee and their reasons for including or rejecting a drug should be published as soon as possible after the meeting. If the voted action was to reject a drug, it is particularly important to specify the reasons for its rejection.

A drug monograph is a compilation of information about a specific drug product; it contains a list of and amounts of ingredients, instructions on usage, the circumstances under which it may be used, and any contraindications for use of the product. Drug monographs are found in the USP-NF and spell out the requirements for each drug product, excipient, or other product, such as chemical formula and physical description of the compound (e.g., $C_6H_{12}O_6$, white crystalline powder), purity requirements, melting point, and solubility.

MCOs prepare monographs for review by their P&T Committees. These monographs typically contain much information about the clinical usefulness of the drug, its indications, side effect profile, normal dosing range, drug interactions, and more. The MCO uses this information when making formulary coverage decisions.

The formulary should be selective and represent the most cost-effective drugs available for the population covered by the formulary. The factors contributing to cost-effective drugs vary, but include the following: approved indications, adverse event profile, factors affecting patient compliance, ease of administration, special storage or security requirements, the inherent safety profile, and cost of the medication.

There are many reasons to support a selective formulary; the elimination of unnecessary and potentially confusing duplications is one. A second reason deals with economics. Carefully watching how money is spent is very important for all institutions, hospitals, and health insurance companies. The advent of biotechnology drugs (also referred to as *specialty drugs*) such as colony-stimulating factors, monoclonal antibodies, drugs produced by recombinant technology, and genetically engineered drugs can precipitate a financial crisis for a hospital or MCO if the economic impacts of the use of these agents are not monitored. The pharmacy budget as a percentage of total medical spending has increased dramatically in the past few years. All indications are that this trend will continue in part because of the many new, high-tech, and innovative agents in the pipeline. Note, however, that many new drugs coming to the market are in fact very similar to drugs already available. These drugs may contribute little added therapeutic value, but may increase the cost of therapy for a particular disease state. A formulary is a tool that allows MCOs and hospitals to provide optimal drug coverage to its members/patients while offering some economic containment.

Application of Formulary in the Community

Formularies are used in many settings. They are important components in hospital systems and are now extremely prevalent in the community setting. A majority of health insurance plans and PBMs use formularies in the administration of prescription drug coverage for their subscribers/members. This includes the Medicare Part D prescription drug benefit. The predominant formulary seen in the marketplace today is an open formulary. An open formulary, sometimes referred to as a *preferred drug list*, provides subscribers with access to quality, appropriate, clinical drug therapy at various cost-share levels.

Many managed care organizations use a "tiered" pharmacy benefit design. All medications and related products subject to clinical review are assigned to a formulary "tier." The tier represents the level of coverage the health plan will provide. The most cost-effective agents (often generics) are usually assigned to the most preferred tier and have the lowest patient out-of-pocket costs. The least cost-effective agents are usually assigned to the least preferred tier and have the highest patient out-of-pocket costs or the plan offers no coverage. The preferred tier(s) are commonly referred to as *formulary* and nonpreferred tier(s) as *nonformulary*. In other cases, nonformulary drugs are not assigned a tier and are not listed on the formulary. A formulary may be published in a variety of ways including by tier status, by therapeutic class, or alphabetically. The goal is for physicians to prescribe cost-effective medications for their members, because studies show patient compliance is generally better when their cost share is less.

Prior authorization (PA) is another way health plans encourage appropriate use of medications. Prior authorization is an administrative tool normally used by a health plan or PBM that requires a prescriber to receive preapproval for prescribing a drug in order for the drug to qualify for coverage under the terms of the pharmacy benefit plan. Guidelines and administrative policies for prior authorization are developed by pharmacists and/or other qualified health professionals who are employed by or under contract with a health plan or PBM. Each plan develops its own guidelines and makes its own decisions about how they are implemented and used.

Additional methods to encourage appropriate use of medications include *step therapy* and *quantity limits*. Step therapy is the practice of beginning drug therapy for a medical condition with the most cost-effective and safest drug, and stepping up through a sequence of alternative drug therapies if the preceding treatment option fails. Step therapy programs apply coverage rules at the point of service when a claim is adjudicated (e.g., a first-line drug must be tried before a second-line drug can be used). If a claim is submitted for a second-line drug and the step therapy rule was not met, the claim is rejected, and a message is transmitted to the pharmacy indicating that the patient should be treated with the first-line drug before coverage of the second-line drug can be authorized. When quantity limits are instituted, the amount of medication a member may obtain in a given time period is capped. Limits are typically based on dosage or length of therapy guidelines.

The Medicare Part D prescription drug program is of major importance due to the growing number of senior citizens in the United States. Many Part D beneficiaries have difficulty choosing a prescription drug plan due to the large number of programs and the different options (i.e., formularies and cost share) available within each plan. Many MCOs offer one or more Medicare Part D plans, and each plan may have its own formulary with each formulary offering different deductibles, copayment tiers, and varying tier placements of medications. In addition, the same medications may not be covered by all formularies and different plans may have different prior authorization, step therapy, and quantity limits for the same medication. Disruption of patient therapy may occur if patients are forced to change medications due to their Medicare Part D plan. Prescription drug plan formulary information is available to beneficiaries, pharmacists, and pharmacy technicians on the CMS website; however, patients may still be confused.

The CMS website provides the following Medicare Part D drug definitions:

- Covered drugs are those that are included in a Part D plan's formulary, or treated as being included in a Part D plan's formulary, as a result of a covered determination or appeal.
- Noncovered drugs are those that are categorized as "less than effective" (LTE). Such drugs are identified by having a DESI (Drug Efficacy Study Implementation) indicator code of either 5 or 6.

Excluded drugs are listed below:

- Agents used for anorexia, weight loss, or weight gain
- Agents used to promote fertility
- Agents used for cosmetic purposes or hair growth
- Agents used for the symptomatic relief of coughs and colds
- Prescription vitamins and mineral products, *except* prenatal vitamins and fluoride preparations
- Nonprescription drugs
- Barbiturates
- Benzodiazepines
- Agents used for the treatment of sexual or erectile dysfunction.

Like hospital-based formularies, community-based formularies may include clinical programs that require certain trials and failures of preferred drugs prior to coverage of nonpreferred drugs. It is important to understand the procedures for requesting coverage for nonpreferred drugs.

Complications can arise when trying to be selective and trying to reach a consensus at the same time. Little doubt remains that as pressure increases to become more selective, consensus will also become important and possibly more difficult to achieve.

The information a formulary contains, aside from the listing of the available drugs, can often be a decisive factor in determining its effectiveness and quality over another formulary. Reviewing formularies from different PBMs reveals a remarkable similarity in the drugs contained in them. Although the additional information they convey may be different, even in this aspect, uniformity seems to be more common. For example, many formularies list policies about drug use in a separate chapter. Sample protocols for drug use can be listed. (Think of a protocol as a recipe for how to use a specific drug.) Often, charts comparing the features or costs of an important drug class are included.

The formulary system defines the policies of drug use and can be effective in several aspects. For example, the system not only has the responsibility to select drugs and to foster rational drug therapy, but can also function in an educational role as a means of quality assurance. The educational role of the P&T Committee is carried out through the formulary system. Traditionally, education was in the form of written communications. Today's education involves more direct in-service programs as well as podcasts, web-based videos, and so on, sponsored or conducted by the P&T Committee.

Some surveillance activities fostered by the system have an educational and quality assurance aspect. For example, monitoring the use of both formulary and nonformulary drugs can provide staff members with information about drug utilization trends that would otherwise go unnoticed. Many monitoring activities or drug use evaluations (DUEs) that fall into this category are discussed elsewhere.

An exciting outgrowth of the formulary system linked to computer technology is the ability to track adverse drug reactions (ADRs). Sophisticated database management programs often allow for rapid identification of trends that might not otherwise be obvious and thus result in interventions to avoid such reactions. Recent literature provided data that quantify the cost of ADRs—and the number is remarkable! For example, in a *JAMA* study published in 1997, an overall average of the additional cost involved with ADRs was $2,000 per incident, but the range varied from $6,700 per case for "bleeding" to $9,000 for "induced fever." A study in Germany, published in *Pharmacoepidemiology & Drug Safety* in June 2011, estimated the average treatment cost for a single ADR at €2,250 (approximately $2,950). These observations support the view that there is more to the relationship of formulary management, drug therapy, and cost than may be at first apparent.

The traditional application of the formulary system could be described as occurring in two dimensions: (1) mostly in writing and (2) often after the fact. However, the growing trend is to apply sophisticated computer techniques to information use. As a result, many of the formulary system's procedures and protocols can move away from the "scripture-like" status of written documents to a prospective and often interactive status. For example, in some computer applications, the program can alert the pharmacist to a drug's formulary status and to any restrictions that apply and document special criteria for use—all while the order is being entered. Pharmacists are encouraged to discuss available formulary alternatives with prescribing physicians.

The use of electronic prescribing (e-prescribing) systems in physicians' offices has brought formulary information to the point of prescribing. A prescriber using an e-prescribing system is able to view the formulary information, including prior authorization and step therapy requirements, for a patient as he or she is writing a prescription. E-prescribing increases the efficiency and safety of the medication use process because prescriptions are no longer handwritten (resulting in no misreading due to handwriting), the medications ordered are covered by the patient's prescription drug plan (coverage is checked before prescribing), and phone calls between the pharmacy and physician are significantly reduced or eliminated.

Other methods to improve the medication use process are also the focus of medical safety efforts. *Computerized physician order entry (CPOE)* or, more precisely, *computer-assisted provider order entry (CAPOE)* systems are routinely being installed in hospitals and health systems. While such technologies are promoted as the ultimate answer to medical safety, they are not an easy or inexpensive answer. The principles of the formulary system design discussed in this chapter will continue to play an important role in the success or failure of CAPOE system development and implementation.

Electronic health records (EHRs) are also being installed in many prescribers' offices. This allows the physician's office to keep a complete patient medical record on a computer. EHR systems typically contain an e-prescribing component, allowing the physician to electronically submit prescriptions directly to the pharmacy.

The e-prescribing system checks for possible drug interactions, correct dosing, available generic medication, duplications, and formulary tier substitutions before the prescription is transmitted. It will also alert the physician if a prior authorization, step therapy requirement, or quantity limit for the prescribed drug has been implemented by the patient's insurance company, saving a telephone call later from the pharmacy or patient when the pharmacy claim is rejected. In cases where the pharmacy is unable to receive electronic prescriptions, the system allows for the prescription to be faxed directly to the pharmacy.

As stated previously, these electronic systems are complicated and expensive, so movement away from paper-based records and prescriptions is slow, but advances are occurring. The federal government has instituted incentive programs to bolster the uptake of both e-prescribing and EHR systems. Ultimately, EHRs, connected through the national health information network (NHIN), will make a patient's medical information portable, allowing medical professionals access to a patient's medical data even when that patient is in a different area of the country.

Revisions to a formulary are important because its effectiveness depends on how current the information contained in the formulary is. Keeping a formulary current is a difficult task. Currently, new drugs are being introduced at a faster rate than in previous years, making formulary revision a constant activity.

Formularies are usually published once a year, even though they may be revised after each P&T Committee action. Changes that occur between official revisions can be communicated in several ways. Communication may be done via newsletters sent to physicians and pharmacy providers, or the P&T Committee may release a special publication when changes are made. The information contained in classic formularies is printed and published in book form. Formularies are revised continuously, and the logistics of ensuring that all previous copies are updated can be overwhelming. Typically, new editions of the formulary are published on a regular basis, and this too can get extremely expensive. More recently, the trend has been to use electronic means to disseminate formularies, and a vast array of drug information has revolutionized health care practice. Thousands of articles on the use of web-based (Internet and Intranet) media and mobile versions of formulary information have been published, and commercial information services are competing for attention in this dynamic market. The use of the Internet and mobile communications makes it even more imperative that information in a formulary is updated on a regular basis, and in some areas, immediately.

As you have learned in this chapter, formularies are used in almost all health care delivery situations. Formularies are used to promote rational, cost-effective drug therapy, and are developed for specific populations of patients. As drug therapy has become more sophisticated, formularies have adapted and grown, and their use by hospitals, MCOs, and other health care delivery systems will continue into the foreseeable future.

Summary

Formularies and the formulary system are ancient concepts that have been adapted to the dynamic environment of modern medical care. When sound therapeutic management principles are applied in a practical, scientific manner, they can also become very effective tools for clinical safety and quality of care.

TEST YOUR KNOWLEDGE

Multiple Choice

1. An institution's ______________ is actually a complete reference manual for the policies and procedures, guidelines for use, and criteria for evaluation of the medications approved for use at that particular institution.
a. policy and procedures manual
b. formulary
c. compendium
d. risk management plan

2. A formulary consisting of tiered benefits is considered
a. regulated.
b. closed.
c. open.
d. static.

3. The committee that develops the formulary is the
a. Pharmacy and Therapeutics Committee.
b. U.S. Pharmacopeia.
c. Veterans Affairs system.
d. pharmacy benefits managers.

4. The specific information that the Pharmacy and Therapeutics Committee reviews when considering a drug for addition to the formulary is contained in a
a. monograph.
b. white paper.
c. business plan.
d. research journal.

5. Health insurance companies may utilize ______________ to administer prescription drug coverage for their subscribers.
a. private pharmacists
b. a board of directors
c. Medicare and Medicaid officers
d. pharmacy benefit managers

6. The portion of the Medicare plan that specifies how prescription coverage is handled is
a. Medicare Part A.
b. Medicare Part B.
c. Medicare Part C
d. Medicare Part D.

7. How many times in a year are formularies typically published?
a. once
b. twice
c. four times (quarterly)
d. twelve times (monthly)

Fill in the Blank

1. The most revered formulary in the United States is the ______________ Formulary.
2. A ______________ formulary excludes drugs from various therapeutic classes.
3. Insurance companies may try to control costs through ______________.
4. The use of computer technology for formularies has led to the ability to better track ______________.
5. ______________ is an important function.

Suggested Readings

Academy of Managed Care Pharmacy. (2005, May). *Principles in practice*. Alexandria, VA: Author.

Academy of Managed Care Pharmacy. (2005, November). *Concepts in managed care pharmacy: Prior authorization and the formulary exception process*. Alexandria, VA: Author.

Academy of Managed Care Pharmacy. (2009, November). *Concept series in managed care pharmacy: Formulary management*. Alexandria, VA: Author.

Academy of Managed Care Pharmacy (2013). *Glossary of managed care pharmacy terms*. Retrieved from http://www.amcp.org/ManagedCareTerms

American Society of Health-System Pharmacists. (1996–1997). ASHP technical assistance bulletin on assessing cost-containment strategies for pharmacies in organized health-care settings. In *Practice standards of ASHP, 1996–1997* (p. 147). Bethesda, MD: Author.

American Society of Health-System Pharmacists. (1997). ASHP statement of the pharmacy and therapeutics committee. In *Practice standards of ASHP, 1997*. Bethesda, MD: Author.

American Society of Health-System Pharmacists. (2003). ASHP guidelines on formulary management. *Practice standards of ASHP formulary management, 2003*. Bethesda, MD: Author.

American Society of Health-System Pharmacists. (2004–2006). ASHP hospital drug distribution and control. *Practice standards of ASHP, 2004–2006* (update). Bethesda, MD: Author.

Centers for Medicare and Medicaid Services. *CMS Medicare Part D manual. Chapter 6: Part D drugs and formulary requirements.* Baltimore, MD: Author.

Joint Commission. (2013). *Accreditation manual for hospitals*. Oak Brook Terrace, IL: Author.

MacKinnon, N. J., & Kumar, R. (2001). Prior authorization programs: A critical review of the literature. *Journal of Managed Care Pharmacy, 7*, 297.

Rottenkolber, D., et al. (2011). Adverse drug reactions in Germany: Direct costs of internal medicine hospitalizations. *Pharmacoepidemiology & Drug Safety, 20*(6), 626–634.

CHAPTER 29

Computer Applications in Drug Use Control

Competencies

Upon completion of this chapter, the reader should be able to:

1. List various pharmacy activities that automation and computerization have improved.
2. Describe how computer systems interact within the pharmacy and with other systems in the health care delivery process.
3. Describe how computerization within the health care system can provide better patient care.
4. Explain the concept of project management relating to the implementation of a computer system.
5. Describe the role of the pharmacist and the pharmacy technician in the management of a pharmacy information system.
6. Describe the general terms used in reference to information systems and automation.

Key Terms

admission, discharge, and transfer system (ADT)
charge capture system
computerized physician order entry (CPOE)
electronic data interchange (EDI)
hospital information system (HIS)
patient accounting system

Introduction

The management of medication administration plays a critical role in the patient care process. The data stored in the pharmacy information system is not only vital to the operation of the pharmacy, but it is also extremely important to other health care professionals in the management of the patient's care. Many extremely important decisions are made each day concerning drug therapy and the adjustment of drug therapy based on information that is retrieved from the pharmacy information system.

Pharmacy information systems have been used successfully in hospital and retail pharmacies for many years. In recent times, automation has become more and more prevalent in pharmacy practice. These automated systems not only improve productivity, but also help in reducing errors. Today it would be hard to find a pharmacy that does not have a pharmacy information system and some level of automation. As a matter of fact, without the use of a pharmacy information system, it would be nearly impossible to comply with all state, federal, and third-party insurance companies' demands.

As medical care becomes more and more complex, both clinically and administratively, pharmacy information systems have also become more and more complex. In the past, pharmacy information systems did nothing more than retrieve prescription data in order to generate a label for a prescription or drug order. Now pharmacy information systems screen for drug allergies and drug interactions, perform drug reviews, perform billing functions, automatically transmit information to insurance companies, allow the user to do sophisticated database searches or queries, interface with other information systems such as laboratory computer systems, and link themselves to other devices in the pharmacy that are involved in automation.

Note also that as more and more hospitals and pharmacies merge, the need for these information systems to communicate with each other (networking) becomes extremely important. Chain drugstores can now look up prescription data from any of the stores in their network or chain. The same holds true for hospitals. The sharing of information between hospitals not only helps with the efficiency of the member institutions, but it also helps disseminate vital information to members of the health care team.

This chapter reviews the evolution of information systems within the hospital pharmacy and the role that pharmacists and technicians have played in their use. Some of the basic terminology that information technology specialists use when speaking of these integrated pharmacy information systems is also discussed. Finally, a look toward what the future may hold is addressed.

Computer Terminology

Computer systems have a language all their own. Understanding of computer technologies hinges on understanding the language used. **Table 29-1** summarizes computer terminology.

TABLE 29-1 Computer Terminology

Abort	The abnormal termination of a program or process through user input or program failure.
Access speed	The average amount of time it takes for a storage device (flash drive) to find a particular piece of data.
ADT	Admission, discharge, and transfer.
Algorithm	A detailed sequence of actions performed to accomplish a task of some kind.
Alias	A name, usually short and easy to remember, that is translated into another name, usually long and difficult to remember.
Application	Software that one uses to perform a specific task (e.g., word processors, spreadsheets, database programs).
Backbone	Carries data to smaller lines of transmission, just as the human backbone carries signals to many smaller nerves in the body. A local backbone refers to the main network lines that connect several local-area networks together. The result is a wide-area network (WAN) linked by a backbone connection.
Backup	The action of copying important data to a second location to protect against data loss through equipment failure and unforeseen events.
Bandwidth	Refers to how much data can be sent through a network or modem connection. It is usually measured in bits per second (bps).
Batch file	A type of script that contains a list of commands. These commands are executed in sequence and can be used to automate processes.
Beta software	A version of an application or software made just prior to its accepted completion. Beta testing is carried out after alpha testing and involves ironing out any of the last few bugs or issues.
Bluetooth	Wireless technology that enables communication between Bluetooth-compatible devices. It is used for short-range connections between desktop and laptop computers, PDAs (like the Palm Pilot or Handspring Visor), digital cameras, scanners, cellular phones, and printers.
Booting	The act of starting up a computer and loading the system software into memory.
Cache	A section of memory used to temporarily store files.
Client	A computer that is able to access the resources of other computers on the network.
Cookie	Data sent to a computer by a Web server that records the user's actions on a certain website.
CPU (central processing unit)	The brain of the computer where almost all information processing is carried out.
Crash	A sudden, unexpected system failure.
Data	Any information stored in an electronic fashion.
Driver	A piece of software that tells the computer how to operate an external or added device, such as a printer or hard disk.
Ethernet	A common method of networking computers.
File attributes	Markers assigned to files that describe properties of the file and limit access to the file. File attributes include archive, compress, hidden, read-only, and system.
File server	A computer that controls access to its storage media by other computers.
File transfer	Transferring files electronically from one computer to another, whether the computer is in the same room or miles away.
File transfer protocol (FTP)	Protocol used to move files between two computers linked via a network.
Firewall	A combination of hardware and software that acts as a gatekeeper. Firewalls restrict other computers from gaining access to data.
Firewire	High-speed interface used to connect peripherals.
Firmware	A software program or set of instructions programmed on a hardware device.
Gateway	Hardware or software that acts as a bridge between two networks so that data can be transferred between several computers.

(Continued)

TABLE 29-1 (Continued)

Gigabyte	1,024 megabytes (MB) or 1,073,741,824 bytes.
Graphical user interface (GUI)	Allows users to click on buttons with a mouse, light pen, or touch screen.
Hard drive	The main storage device in a computer's hardware.
HIS	Hospital information system.
Hyperlink	A word, phrase, or image that the user can click on to jump to a new document or a new section within the current document.
IP (Internet Protocol)	A standard set of rules for sending and receiving data through the Internet.
IP address	A code, also known as an "IP number" or simply an "IP," made up of numbers separated by three dots, that identifies a particular computer on the Internet. Every computer, whether it is a Web server or a personal computer, requires an IP address to connect to the Internet. IP addresses consist of four sets of numbers from 0 to 255, separated by three dots. For example "66.72.98.236" or "216.239.115.148."
Kilobyte	1,024 bytes.
Local-area network (LAN)	A computer network limited to the immediate area, usually the same building or floor of a building.
MAC address (Media Access Control address)	A hardware identification number that uniquely identifies each device on a network.
Megabyte	1,024 kilobytes or 1,048,576 bytes.
MIPS	Millions of instructions per second.
Motherboard	The main circuit board of a computer. The motherboard is the part of the computer where all other components are attached.
Network	A group of computers set up to communicate with one another. A network can be as small as two computers linked together or millions of computers linked together.
Operating system	The software on the computer that allows all other software to run. It is also the software that tells the computer how to run and execute commands.
Peripheral	A piece of hardware that is located outside of the main computer. Examples include printers and monitors.
Print queue	A list of print jobs waiting to be sent to a printer.
Print server	A software program that manages print jobs and print devices.
Protocol	A specific set of communication rules. When computers communicate with each other, each computer follows a common set of rules and instructions.
Query	The process by which a user can ask for specific information from a database.
Queue	A set of instructions waiting to be executed.
Random-access memory (RAM)	The physical memory installed in a computer.
Read-only memory (ROM)	Computer memory that can be read, but not erased.
Router	A network device that channels information from one computer to another across a network.
SATA (Serial Advanced Technology Attachment)	An interface used to connect ATA hard drives to a computer's motherboard.
Uninterruptible power supply (UPS)	A device that has an internal power source (battery) that enables a computer to continue operations for a short period of time during a power outage.
Upload	To send a file to another computer.
URL (Uniform Resource Locator)	The address of a specific website or file on the Internet.
Wide-area network (WAN)	Any Internet or network that covers an area larger than a single building or campus.

TABLE 29-1 (Continued)

Wildcard	A character (usually *) that can stand for one or more unknown characters during a search.
Workstation	Any computer that is attached to a network.
WYSIWYG (what you see is what you get)	What is seen on the screen will be pretty close to what the finished product looks like.
Zip	A zip file (.zip) is a "zipped" or compressed file.

Components of a Pharmacy Information System

Pharmacy information systems have four basic components: (1) computer hardware, (2) application software, (3) system network, and (4) information server.

Computer Hardware

A computer's hardware consists of the physical components of the computer systems and related devices. Computer hardware can be classified as internal and external. Internal computer hardware includes things like memory chips, hard drives, and the motherboard, while external computer hardware consists of components such as monitors, keyboards, mice, printers, and so on. Computer hardware is the part of the computer system that can be physically handled.

Storage of Data

All information or data that resides in the computer system is stored on the system's hardware. This information can be stored locally (i.e., on the user's desktop computer) or on a server. Storing the information on a server is the more common configuration, since doing so will make it accessible to all others on the network and will prevent the end user from entering the same data more than once. When thinking about the information commonly stored, it is easy to understand why network storage makes sense. The user wouldn't want to have to enter demographic information on every patient on every machine. It makes a lot more sense to have this type of information stored in one place so that all other users can obtain this information when necessary.

The two main categories of storage devices are (1) disk devices (e.g., hard drives, CD-ROM drives, flash drives) and (2) memory. Memory on a computer usually refers to random-access memory (RAM) chips. The main difference between these two types of storage devices is that disk drives can store information, and this information will only be erased if the user directs the computer to do so. All information stored on RAM chips, however, will be lost when the computer is turned off or when it is rebooted.

The speed at which computers can access the information on disk drives and RAM memory differs greatly. It takes the computer much longer to access information on disk drives than it does to access information on RAM. Typically, when a particular program is run, some of the information needed to run the program is copied to the RAM chips inside the computer. The computer now runs the program from the RAM and not the disk drives. This speeds up information processing. When the user is finished working on a particular program, information is transferred back to the disk drive for safety intermittently, at specified times determined by the application. Remember that if at any time power is lost to the RAM chips, all information on these chips will be lost.

Some devices serve more than one purpose. For example, memory sticks may also be used as input devices if they contain information to be used and processed by the computer user. In addition, they can be used as output devices if the user wants to store information for archival purposes.

Application Software

Application software is nothing more than the programs one uses. Application software is the software that is running on any computer system in use. It could be the pharmacy software package used to enter physician orders and prescriptions into the computer, or it could be the software used by the laboratory department or software used by the payroll department to pay the employees within the company or institution. Application software used in pharmacies is usually leased from companies that supply the same software to many different pharmacies or hospitals. Usually, the organization will pay an initial fee for the installation of the software in the pharmacy or on the hospital's network and then pay monthly maintenance fees to the software company, which ensures that the software is kept current. These monthly maintenance fees also pay for any technical support that the end user might need.

System Network

The system network, simplistically, is a collection of wiring, hardware, and software that allows all computers linked to the network the ability to share information. Network management (i.e., client–server technology) controls the security of the network as well as the transfer of all data passing through the network. Client–server technology determines what information is passed back and forth from computer to computer. It also determines where information will be processed and on what machine the data will be stored. An example of this would be the calculation of a drug dosage. A pharmacist using a local computer in the pharmacy would obtain the age, weight, height, sex, and all other patient information needed to calculate the correct dosage from demographic information that most likely is stored on the hospital's main information server. Once all of the necessary information or data is obtained, the process of calculating the dosage can be done on the local pharmacy computer. The results of this calculation can then either be stored on the server or on the pharmacy system, depending on the way the network is set up. Normally, information is stored locally only when that information is specific for that one department.

The important thing to remember here is that, in most cases, specific data is never stored in more than one place. It would be foolish to store everything about every patient on every computer in the network. Modern networking applications allow the local computer to run local applications that obtain specific data only when needed. Storing data on multiple computers or storage devices could lead to individual users having different data sets. Storing the data on one computer or storage device ensures that everyone in the network has access to the exact same data.

Until recently, all computers on a network were physically linked together by high-capacity copper or fiber cable. More recently, wireless networks have become the standard. Wireless networks have many advantages. Probably the biggest one is that buildings no longer have to be "wired." One must remember that wiring a large building with high-speed networking cable can be very expensive, and adding new computers to the network after the building is already wired is an ongoing and expensive chore. With a wireless network, any new computer can very easily be added to the network. At the present time, these wireless networks are used in most institutions and one can easily predict that within the near future, copper or fiber networks will be a thing of the past. While wireless technology is much easier and possibly less expensive to set up, there are many security issues surrounding this technology that sometimes outweigh its benefits.

Information Server

The information server is usually a large-capacity computer that serves as an online repository of information resources. Demographic information such as patient names, addresses, phone numbers, ages, and sex are all types of information that would be stored on an information server. Other computers on the network access this information according to the software running on the computer and the privileges that the operator of the computer has.

Management

Computer systems throughout most hospitals are administered or controlled by the institution's information technology (IT) department. The IT department is broken down into many divisions, but typically most IT departments will have people assigned to the following divisions:

- *Integration*—The role of this department is to make sure that the applications the institution is running integrate with the other applications on the network.
- *Help desk*—This is a support group that helps the client use applications. It is analogous to a technical support number that the user might call with software or hardware questions at home.
- *Medical informatics*—This is a group of people that make sure state-of-the-art clinical information is available for use. This could include anything from drug information applications to video conferencing with other hospitals.
- *Networking services*—This group of people maintains the institution's network.
- *Patient information services*—These are the people who ensure proper patient information (e.g., demographic information, previous admission information, drug history information) is available to all end users.
- *Technical services*—These are support personnel who maintain the information system.

Individual departments might have someone designated as the liaison between his or her department and the IT department. This person could be anyone in the department who has more than the usual computer skills. This person works with the IT department to make sure the systems in the department are running correctly and also makes sure training is available to all staff members who use applications on the system. The liaison would also be involved in the decision-making process if and when new hardware or software is deemed necessary.

Changing primary system applications or, for that matter, making major hardware revisions usually involves a team effort and is not an easy undertaking. Data on the old system must be able to be integrated into the new application, and any new hardware must be able to perform its given tasks.

Because of the complexity of such changes, a team effort is usually needed to make these major changes in operation run smoothly. The team participates in the tasks necessary to implement the system project in accordance with a well-defined work plan. The implementation of the system follows a well-defined project management methodology. A systems administrator will handle the ongoing management of the system once it is put into production.

When large revisions in hardware or system applications are necessary, the end user's responsibility is to justify and obtain funding for the procurement and ongoing enhancements for a particular system. This individual also defends departmental initiatives for the system.

Generally, when these types of large projects are initiated, someone within the department is named the project manager. The project manager is the field boss during the implementation or upgrade of the computer system. In the pharmacy, a pharmacist or pharmacy technician best fills this job. That person should have an intimate knowledge of the operation to be automated and must understand the goals and objectives of the project. In addition, this individual should possess sufficient skills to manage the pharmacy staff, participating staff from other departments, vendors, and assigned technical personnel. The project manager develops the work plan and uses it to manage the project through to its completion.

One job of the project manager is to manage the expectations of all who are involved in the project. The project manager must manage the expectations of the department, the members of the project team, and the other members of the hospital community who will be relying on the system when it goes into production. The work plan developed by the project manager must be realistic. Project milestones and other deliverables should take into consideration all steps necessary to complete the assigned tasks in a professional manner.

The project manager becomes the principal architect in designing how the system will be used in the pharmacy and how it will interact with other systems and departments throughout the hospital. The project manager also will coordinate how the work flow of the area(s) being automated will interact with the system.

A computer system can serve as a change agent to facilitate improvements of the processes being automated. If a system project automates a manual process without materially improving that process, the benefits of the system investment may be subject to question. Through the work flow design process and the development of policies, procedures, and forms, the project team has a real opportunity to effect positive change.

A well-managed system project is supported by a team working under the direction of the project manager. The project team should consist of people containing the right mix of skills, experience, and knowledge to build the desired system. The team should consist of representatives of the areas being automated. They should be intimately familiar with the work flow in their areas of responsibility and all relevant policies and procedures of the area. Subject to the components of the system being implemented, the project team should include information systems staff with hardware, network, or programming expertise. Additional participants should be considered from areas with which the pharmacy interfaces on a regular basis (e.g., nursing, admitting, medical staff). These additional team members can assist in incorporating into the system those features and functions that will promote increased customer satisfaction through the use of the system.

Hospital Information System Application Relationships

To begin the discussion about pharmacy computer applications, an understanding of how these applications fit within the framework of the hospital's other critical applications is important.

hospital information system (HIS) a system that integrates information from many parts of the hospital

The basic **hospital information system (HIS)** manages the processes of patient admission, charge capture, and billing. Although this is an oversimplification, it is, in essence, the set of features and functions performed within the HIS.

Admission, Discharge, and Transfer System

admission, discharge, and transfer system (ADT) a computer program for admission, discharge, and transfer of patients that provides significant demographic and clinical information for each patient

The admission process is, of course, a more complex process often referred to as the **admission, discharge, and transfer system (ADT)**. The ADT is the system that first acknowledges a patient's existence in the hospital to every other system. The pharmacy system depends on the ADT system to know that a patient is a current patient of the hospital. It also distinguishes whether or not the patient is an outpatient or an inpatient. The ADT provides the pharmacy system with basic demographics on each patient (e.g., name, address, telephone numbers of the patient and next of kin, medical record number, bill/account number, date of birth, sex). The ADT keeps the pharmacy system informed as to each patient's location in the hospital. It also constantly updates the pharmacy system when patients are transferred or discharged. With this information, the pharmacy will know the room and bed location of each patient, where to send medication orders, where to send reports concerning patients, and if the patient has been discharged and is no longer entitled to filled orders.

In addition, the ADT provides other systems with critical information necessary to manage other processes within the hospital. Insurance information is collected here to facilitate the billing process. The ADT can also be used to help the hospital collect other valuable information such as whether the patient has a living will or durable power of attorney, who referred the patient to the hospital, and the name of the patient's physician.

The Charge Capture System

charge capture system a component of a hospital information system whereby every time an order is entered on a patient, a charge is captured for billing purposes, and a statistic is captured for management monitoring purposes

The next component of the HIS is the **charge capture system**. A modern HIS system is referred to as an *order entry system*. Every time an order is entered on a patient, a charge is captured for billing purposes, and a statistic is captured for management monitoring purposes. Depending on the nature of an order, some charges are not computed until a test's results are delivered or the order is completed. In the case of physical therapy, an order for such a service is typically not finalized until after the physical therapist can assess the patient's condition and determine the amount of therapy required.

Medical records own a piece of the HIS. At discharge, the medical records department codes the chart with procedure and diagnostic information. This information is required for regulatory and billing purposes. A link between this coded information, charge information, and admitting information forms the basis of the billing and accounting functions performed relative to the services rendered to each patient.

Patient Accounting System

patient accounting system a component of a hospital information system that allows the hospital to bill and collect for its services

The **patient accounting system** forms the last piece of the HIS, which is the final piece into which all previously collected information flows. This system allows the hospital to bill and collect for its services. Components of this system include charge capture, accounts receivable, a collection system, and a cash receipts system. This system, and its relationship to the other components of the patient flow cycle, forms the basis for compliance with the regulatory reporting standards of state, federal, and other accrediting organizations.

Ancillary Systems

The pharmacy system is one of many ancillary departmental systems. Other departments have specialized systems that support their operations, such as radiology, clinical pathology, surgical pathology, food and nutritional services, the operating room, and other procedure areas and specialty labs. These systems relate to the HIS system in the same manner as the pharmacy system.

The relationships of systems in many hospitals allow ancillary systems to communicate with one another to support patient care needs. For example, if a lab result indicates the need for a patient's medication to be adjusted, then such a result can be triggered to automatically place a notification in the pharmacy system for a pharmacist to review. Because a dietitian may have a similar need to manage patients' nutritional intake, certain lab values can also be automatically sent to the food and nutritional services system.

Services provided by the ancillary departments are captured within the ancillary systems. Each order entered is processed to interact with the inventory that the department manages. Issuing an item results in a reduction of the inventory on hand. The item that has been ordered and issued to the patient, with the patient's identifying information, is communicated back to the hospital's billing system so that the hospital can bill correctly for the item. To the extent that test results would accompany this communication from the ancillary system (in the case of radiology or laboratory systems), the result would be placed in a portion of the hospital's information system where it can be retrieved by caregivers who need to access such information. Many HIS environments support order entry via the HIS. These orders can be transmitted directly to each ancillary system via an automated interface. Order entry interfaces and their implications in the pharmacy are addressed later in this chapter.

Business Systems

Several other systems support the day-to-day activities of a hospital. For the purposes of this chapter, they are classified as *business systems*.

The finance department requires a number of systems to support its operations: payroll systems, accounts payable systems, general ledger and budgeting systems, and cost-accounting systems. For the most part, the functions performed by these systems are self-evident from their names. It is also important to understand that the pharmacy interacts with each of these systems on paper or, in an automated sense, as it relates to the business processes of the pharmacy.

The hospital's payroll system is the vehicle used to pay the employees of the pharmacy as well as other employees within the institution. Hours have to be collected for input at the end of each pay period. Adjustments in vacation time, sick time, and staffing shift differential pay (for evening and night shift staff) need to be collected and submitted by the pharmacy's management in a timely manner so that payroll can pay all employees.

The accounts payable system processes the pharmacy's bills for payment, as it does for every other department of the hospital. This system requires that the pharmacy verify all purchases of supplies, products, or services on invoices prior to processing payment. Accounts payable systems are often linked to materials management systems to facilitate the link between purchasing and receiving and accounting for the payment of purchases.

The general ledger and budget systems allow the pharmacy to submit its budget for the coming year and track its actual expenditures against the approved budget.

Although only one system may reside in the pharmacy, it must interact with the vast majority of other computer systems in the hospital to conduct its day-to-day business.

The Hospital Pharmacy Application

Pharmacy information systems are designed to support the specific needs of pharmacy operations. These systems support activities that fall into several broad categories: inventory management, purchasing, and clinical support.

Inventory Management

A good place to start is with the maintenance of the pharmacy's inventory. The level or quantity of an item in inventory triggers the need to order more product. What this means is that when the quantity on hand of a particular item reaches a certain predefined level or quantity (sometimes called the PAR level), some sort of notification must be sent out so that the materials management people or the purchasing component of the system knows that the item needs to be reordered.

When shipments are received, they must be checked against the purchasing documentation and then logged into inventory. Many pharmacy systems employ bar code scanners, which speed up the process of item identification and input into the system. When an order received is incomplete, the pharmacy system will track open order or back order situations. When the inventory level dips to a critical low, it will notify the purchasing component of the system and the key system user that follow-up is necessary.

As patient medication orders are filled, stock levels are automatically reduced in the inventory system. As stock items are taken to create new products (e.g., IV admixtures), the inventory system also reduces the inventory by the quantity of the item used. The term *perpetual inventory* is best understood as the quantity count of items in stock, based on the computer's calculations of purchases, less medications dispensed, plus the inventory item count at the last physical inventory. Its accuracy is dependent on several variables, including compatibility of the unit of issue with the unit of purchase, the accurate reporting of inventory shrinkage (e.g., items removed from stock due to expiration), and the accuracy of reporting of every item added to and removed from stock. It is up to the pharmacist or pharmacy technician to maintain the definitions in the inventory system in a manner so that the system can correctly perform the necessary calculations. Periodic physical counts of the inventory in stock must be performed and the results compared with the system inventory. This procedure will ensure the integrity of the information in the system and will alert the pharmacy as to any shrinkage of inventory that requires follow-up.

Purchasing/Receiving

When drugs, supplies, or other items in inventory require restocking, or new items must be purchased, the purchasing system is the vehicle that serves to facilitate the process. The purchasing system enables the management of orders placed, tracks open orders and backorders, and possesses the capability to electronically communicate new purchases to suppliers.

Whether the order for restocking is computed electronically (i.e., calculated by the system) or an item is manually entered for purchasing, most modern systems will be able to create a purchase requisition. Subject to the nature of the item(s) to be purchased, the system provides analysis tools to assist in analyzing supplier pricing. Once the supplier for each item is identified, requisitions are converted into purchase orders. Each purchase order contains those items to be acquired from one supplier and contains all agreed terms and conditions of the purchase.

When a purchase order is generated by the system and signed by an authorized signatory, it becomes a legally binding agreement when accepted by the supplier. Most suppliers will ship an order based only on receiving a purchase order number. Pharmacy computer systems are usually capable of generating purchase orders and transmitting them to suppliers electronically. In these instances, both the pharmacy (hospital) and the supplier are usually bound by certain terms and conditions as if a purchase order was duly signed by the purchaser and accepted by the supplier.

electronic data interchange (EDI) technology commonly used to order merchandise, transfer funds, and facilitate billing

An electronically transmitted purchase order employs a technology referred to as **electronic data interchange (EDI)**. EDI technology is commonly used for ordering merchandise, transferring funds (e.g., electronic payroll deposits), and billing. Upon receipt of merchandise ordered, pharmacy personnel must count the items received and compare them with the items, quantities, and pricing ordered. Although the process can occur directly online on a computer terminal, it typically is more expeditious to check the order against the vendor's packing list and then check the packing list against the order and the invoice. If there is any discrepancy in the shipment against the order, the system will facilitate correcting the error. It is important to understand that the system will not correct the error, but merely provide the pharmacist or technician with sufficient information to follow up on the discrepancy. When ordered merchandise is acknowledged to the system as received, the inventory on hand is updated.

Clinical Support

The production side of pharmacy operation relates to the receipt of medication orders for patient care, the processing of the orders, and the tracking of patients' medication histories. The features and functions of pharmacy information systems and the relationship they bear to a hospital's order entry system vary widely.

Most physicians generate medication orders in their own handwriting. The issues surrounding physicians entering orders directly into a system are complex and will be discussed briefly later in this chapter. In most hospitals today, physician orders are keyed into systems in the pharmacy. Fax machines, pneumatic tubes, and couriers or transporters are all being used to transmit orders from nursing units to the pharmacy. In some instances, physicians are entering orders directly into the HIS, which is interfaced to the pharmacy system or order entry.

Upon entry of the medication order, some systems will immediately identify existing medication orders, laboratory test results, or allergies that may be incompatible with the order just placed. Other systems have a functionality that will suggest to the user that certain laboratory tests should be ordered with the medication order and other open orders should be discontinued based on the current literature. Still other features include suggesting more cost-effective medications than the one ordered. In such instances, the system is not designed to terminate the order, but merely to suggest to the pharmacist that the physician who wrote the order should be contacted to verify that the order is as intended.

The pharmacy system will generally receive relevant information on every patient from the HIS to facilitate the processing of appropriate doses. Date of birth, sex, height, weight, medical record number, and admitting (or billing) number of the patient are critical pieces of information. These data, coupled with the history of medications already ordered and dispensed to the patient, laboratory results, vital signs, diet orders and restrictions, and knowledge of procedures that have been ordered or scheduled, provide the system and the pharmacist with critical information to assist in managing the patient toward a speedy recovery.

When orders are entered, the system queues them for a regular production cycle. Pharmacists and technicians prepare medication doses in accordance with schedules prepared by the system. The system also generates the appropriate labels for the medication to be administered. When robotics are being utilized, pharmacy information systems can electronically pass the order to the robot.

As the orders are packaged for shipping to the patient units, the inventory system is automatically adjusted to reflect a reduction in stock. In addition, each patient's medication administration record is updated to reflect the order and the medications dispensed. Medication lot numbers are also tracked to facilitate patient identification in the event of a manufacturer's recall.

Orders issued are communicated to other systems such as the hospital patient accounting (or billing) system, cost-accounting system, utilization review system, or other systems with authorized access.

For a pharmacist to fill a patient's medication order, the pharmacist must determine that the order was written by a physician and that the medication, dosage, and frequency of its administration are in accordance with the physician's order. The accepted mechanisms for accomplishing this process are as follows: (1) The pharmacist visually inspects the physician's written order and then enters it into the system, or (2) the physician enters the order directly into the system and uses a secret password that only he or she would know. Medication orders transcribed by a unit secretary or other personnel may result in errors and should not be considered reliable. Most of the HIS implementations to date have not been successful in inducing the medical staff to enter medication or other orders directly into the computer without transcription, but in the near future this will change.

computerized physician order entry (CPOE) a drug order entered into a hospital-wide computer system and transmitted to a pharmacy

Soon most hospitals will incorporate some sort of **computerized physician order entry (CPOE)** process. CPOE is the process of electronic entry of physician orders for the treatment of their patients. These orders are communicated over a computer network to the medical staff (nurses, therapists, or other physicians) or to the departments (pharmacy, laboratory, or radiology) responsible for fulfilling the order. Use of a CPOE system decreases delays in order completion, reduces errors related to handwriting or transcription, allows order entry at point-of-care or off-site locations, provides error-checking for duplicate or incorrect doses or tests, and simplifies inventory and posting of charges.

Most available clinical pharmacy information comes from third-party vendors that link their products with pharmacy software. The vendors' core business is the maintenance of current information concerning medications, general pharmacology, drug-drug and drug-food interactions, and other related health care information in the form of numerous computerized database products.

The Health Information Technology for Economic and Clinical Health Act

On February 17, 2009, the federal government signed into law the Health Information Technology for Economic and Clinical Health (HITECH) Act. This legislation was created to stimulate the use of electronic health records (EHRs) in the United States. This law earmarked $18 billion as incentives to help hospitals and physicians offices use EHRs in their practices and institutions. These incentives will be offered until 2015, after which time penalties may be levied for failing to demonstrate such use. The act also established grants for training centers for the personnel required to support a health IT infrastructure.

The Future of Pharmacy Information Systems

The future of pharmacy information systems appears to be heading in two distinct directions. The first is the integration of the data and information-driven systems with robotics for drug dispensing. The second is the improvement of voice recognition technology to attract more physicians to enter their own orders directly into a system.

In a truly integrated environment, the management of patient medications is closely tied to laboratory results and diet. Abnormal laboratory test results can trigger alerts to clinical decision makers, which can result in a change to the patient's medications or diet. As physician order entry occurs, integrated systems can provide educational reminders or a series of cost-effective options for physicians and other clinical decision makers to consider. When orders inconsistent with the patient's treatment plan are about to be entered, the system can also alert the system user to the potential problem.

An order system linked to a robotics system can then complete the automation loop by processing and filling the orders without human involvement from the moment the order is entered. Pharmacy personnel must manage these robotic systems. Inventory levels within the robot must be periodically checked. The restocking of the robot's inventory levels also must be manually supervised.

True integration allows the hospital to operate as a whole. Information concerning all services provided to a patient can interact against a common data repository, which will form the true source for all patient information. These repositories will not only hold patient data, but also diagnostic images such as x-rays and lab slides. Clinical data repositories will form the basis of online, computerized patient records. A patient record contains information concerning the most recent patient encounter and all information concerning a patient's medical history throughout a patient's life.

Voice recognition is a vehicle that holds much promise for bringing more physicians into the world of automated order entry. Consider the fact that the effort required to write an order is much easier than the effort involved in signing onto a system, flipping through order entry screens, identifying medications from the formulary, and validating the entry. Many physicians are reluctant to undertake this responsibility. Once perfected, voice recognition will provide a vehicle that will require little training and actually ease the effort for physicians.

Although the technologies described in this section do exist today, they are not widely used or are in early stages of development or release. By looking at what they are being designed to accomplish, they create a clear vision of what the near future will look like.

Summary

Early forms of automation dealt with speeding the processing of information so that productivity gains could be reached. As computers and technology have become more sophisticated, speeding the ability to access information has allowed decision makers to make more intelligent decisions. This is true for the pharmacy, as well.

This chapter was written with the goal of letting the reader understand that the role of the pharmacist and pharmacy technician is a critical one in the implementation and management of systems in a hospital pharmacy operation. A systems consultant can certainly play a role in managing a system, but the consultant ultimately leaves the project when it is completed. The pharmacists and pharmacy technicians are the individuals who will be responsible for the care and feeding of the system after the consultants leave, and they are the ones responsible for linking the features and functions of a system with the operational needs of the workplace. Lastly, it will be the pharmacists and the pharmacy technicians who will play a major role in the evolution of these systems.

Society has grown more dependent on automation over the years. Successful pharmacy professionals will be those who understand what automation can contribute, are able to harness its power, and are able to align its power with the tactical and strategic requirements of the business of pharmacy and hospital management.

TEST YOUR KNOWLEDGE

Multiple Choice

1. The software that provides desirable features and functions is the
 a. operating system software.
 b. files.
 c. application software.
 d. data.

2. Under a software lease, a user
 a. pays an installation fee.
 b. pays a monthly maintenance fee.
 c. receives technical support.
 d. all of the above.

3. A benefit of using a server for file storage is *not*
 a. to facilitate sharing common files.
 b. to store computer programs.
 c. to facilitate communication between different computer systems.
 d. to provide improved access security.

4. Which of the following describes inventory management software?
 a. It can automatically order inventory when needed from a wholesaler.
 b. It can incorporate bar code technology to aid in inventory control.
 c. It is very costly and not actually used in many hospitals.
 d. a and b.

5. The information server
 a. is no longer used in most pharmacies because smaller PC-type terminals are now used.
 b. is always housed a far distance from the hospital or pharmacy.
 c. takes up too much room to be housed in a normal hospital setting.
 d. can be used by other computers to obtain information such as patient demographics.

6. The system network is
 a. a collection of wiring, hardware, and software that allows all computers that are linked to the network to share information.
 b. a place where the IT department is usually housed.
 c. a technical instruction manual.
 d. a tool used to communicate with other people in the organization.

Matching

Match the computer term with its definition.

1. ______ ADT
2. ______ Bluetooth
3. ______ CPU
4. ______ DOS
5. ______ firewall
6. ______ HIS
7. ______ MIPS
8. ______ query
9. ______ RAM
10. ______ UPS

a. wireless technology that enables communication between compatible devices
b. hospital information system
c. a combination of hardware and software that acts as a gatekeeper that restricts other computers from gaining access to data
d. millions of instructions per second
e. an electronic pathway
f. the process by which a user can ask for specific information from a database
g. admission, discharge, and transfer
h. the physical memory installed in a computer
i. a device that has an internal power source (battery) that enables a computer to continue operations for a short period of time during a power outage
j. central processing unit

Suggested Readings

Austin, C.J., & Boxerman, S.B. (2003). *Information systems for healthcare management* (6th ed.). Ann Arbor, MI: Health Administration Press.

Campbell-Kelly, M., & Aspray, W. (2005). *Computer: A history of the information machine* (2nd ed.). New York, NY: Basic Books.

Drazen, E.L., Ritter, J.L., Schneider, M.K., & Metzger, J. (1996). *Patient care information systems: Successful design and implementation (Computers in health care)*. New York, NY: Springer Verlag.

Dudeck, J., Blobel, B., Lordieck, W., & Burkle, T. (Eds.). (2000). *Studies in health technology and informatics* (Vol. 45). Amsterdam, The Netherlands: IOS Press.

Englander, I. (2003). *The architecture of computer hardware and systems software: An information technology approach*. New York, NY: John Wiley.

Haux, R. (Ed.). (2004). *Strategic information management in hospitals: An introduction to hospital information systems (health informatics)*. New York, NY: Springer Verlag.

Kreider, N.A., & Haselton, B.J. (1997). *The systems challenge: Getting the clinical information support you need to improve patient care*. San Francisco, CA: Jossey-Bass.

Long, L., & Long, N. (2003). *Computers: Information technology in perspective* (11th ed.). Upper Saddle River, NJ: Prentice-Hall.

Reis, R.A. (1996). *Understanding electronic and computer technology* (3rd ed.). Chico, CA: Technical Education Press.

Turban, E., Kelly Rainer, R., & Potter, R.E. (2002). *Introduction to information technology*. New York: John Wiley.

CHAPTER

30

Preventing and Managing Medication Errors: The Technician's Role

Competencies

Upon completion of this chapter, the reader should be able to:

1. Discuss the role of the pharmacy technician in preventing medication errors.
2. Determine and state the cause of system breakdowns that result in medication errors.
3. Define the types of medication errors that occur during the ordering and dispensing process.
4. State the 11 steps necessary for proper dispensing of medications.
5. List some commonly used drugs that result in medication error–related deaths.
6. Define confirmation bias.
7. List the steps that should be taken to minimize errors when taking verbal orders.

Key Terms

confirmation bias

Introduction

The Institute of Medicine (IOM) released a report in 2006 entitled *Preventing Medication Errors.* The report indicated that medication errors are among the most common medical errors, harming at least 1.5 million people every year. The report concluded that studies indicated 400,000 preventable drug-related injuries occur each year in hospitals. Another 800,000 occur in long-term care settings, and roughly 530,000 occur just among Medicare recipients in outpatient clinics. The committee noted that these are likely underestimates.

With increasing attention to medical and medication errors by the lay media, concern has intensified in both the public and health care sectors. Health professionals acknowledge that medication errors are a growing concern because of the increased numbers of critically ill patients, the development of more potent and potentially dangerous drugs and methods of administration, and more emphasis on fiscal constraints that affect hospital staffing and workloads in all sectors. Protecting patients from inappropriate administration of medications has become an important focus for pharmacists and technicians, including those in community and institutional settings.

Technicians play a major role in modern pharmacy practice. A large-scale study (conducted by the American Pharmaceutical Association) of both new prescriptions and prescription refills found an error rate of 1.7%. This dispensing error rate translates into approximately 4 errors per 250 prescriptions per pharmacy per day, or an estimated 51.5 million errors during the filling of 3 billion prescriptions each year. While most of these errors probably have minimal clinical relevance and do not adversely affect patients, many experts believe that the medication error rate in less controlled environments—such as in the ambulatory setting where a patient purchases nonprescription medications or picks up prescription medicines from a community pharmacy—is probably higher.

This chapter focuses on system enhancements and the checks and balances needed to provide the maximum degree of safety as pharmacists and technicians prepare, dispense, and control medications in both community and institutional pharmacy settings. In addition, focus is placed on the importance of determining latent failures that contribute to medication errors by developing effective medication error reporting programs to discover how latent failures occur and how they can be prevented.

Background

Currently, many organizations take an ineffective approach to preventing medication errors. Investigations tend to focus on the front end or active end of the error (e.g., the front-line practitioner, such as the pharmacy technician picking the wrong medication from stock). When an error occurs, human nature needs to assign blame. In addition, health care practitioners work in an environment where they strive for perfection. Individuals involved in the commission of an error may be considered inattentive, incompetent, lazy, and uncaring. They are often subject to punitive action such as public or private reprimands, remedial education, disciplinary action, suspensions, or termination.

On the other hand, effective approaches to remedying medication errors consider factors that contribute to medication errors that occur at the organizational level, known as the latent end or blunt end of an error. Latent failures are weaknesses in organizational structure or processes, such as faulty information management or ineffective personnel training, that may have resulted from decisions made by upper management (Reason, 1990). Latent failures can also stem from having incomplete information for a patient, such as missing allergy or diagnosis information, unclear communication of a drug order, lack of an independent double-check, lack of computer warnings, ambiguous drug references, drug storage issues, and look-alike/sound-alike medications. These latent failures are properties of the medication use system. To prevent medications errors, we must change and improve the system and not rely on changing people. By themselves, latent failures often are subtle and may not cause problems directly. The potential consequences are often hidden, becoming apparent only when they occur in a certain sequence and combine with the active failures of an individual.

Medication use is a complex process that consists of subprocesses that include the work of a pharmacy technician such as the ordering, preparing, and dispensing.

Ordering Medications

Physicians or their designees (i.e., nurse practitioners, physician assistants) initiate the drug-dispensing and administration process through the medication order or prescribing process. While computerized prescriber order entry (CPOE) and electronic prescribing (e-prescribing) systems, each with clinical decision-support tools, are being implemented in more settings, as of 2011, still many pharmacies are dispensing from handwritten medication orders. These prescribing systems may help reduce certain types of errors, such as illegible handwriting errors. (Note, however, that they may introduce new types of errors, such as prescribers selecting the wrong medication from a list.) Illegible, ambiguous, or incomplete handwritten prescriptions or medication orders can contribute to many errors made by nurses, pharmacists, pharmacy technicians, and other health care workers.

Illegible Handwriting

To minimize the chance of misinterpretation due to illegibly handwritten orders, physicians should be encouraged to print prescriptions and medication orders in block letters. In the institutional setting, physicians can review orders with the nursing staff before leaving the patient care area. In addition, including the purpose of the medication as part of the prescription or medication order can help readers distinguish the drug names when legibility of handwriting is less than ideal. Many medications have similar names, but very few name pairs that are spelled similarly are used for similar purposes. Preprinted orders, dictation, and direct order entry into the computer by physicians are other solutions for poor handwriting and improper orders.

Because even skilled individuals can misread good handwriting, a system of order/prescription transcription should be in place in which several individuals interpret and transcribe an order. In many hospitals each order is read by a unit secretary and reviewed by a nurse. At the same time, an exact copy of the order is sent to the pharmacy either directly, electronically, by fax machine, or with scanning technology. In the pharmacy, pharmacists and technicians have a number of opportunities to check the order, including a double-check against labels, printouts, and the drug containers. A technician often screens the order and sometimes enters it into the computer. After data entry, a label is printed and a pharmacist should interpret the original order/prescription and verify the technician's computer entry by comparing it to the label. Later, the order and label again will be read by technicians and pharmacists as doses are prepared and dispensed. In the outpatient

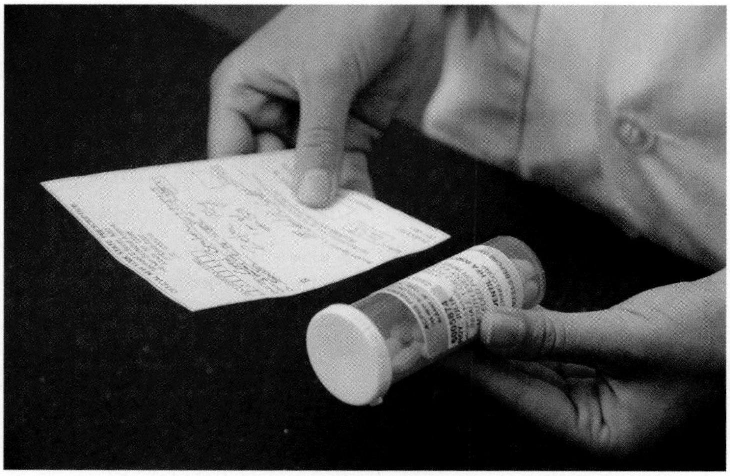

FIGURE 30-1 The pharmacist is responsible for ensuring that the final product is properly labeled and matches the prescription the physician wrote.

setting, this system should include a final check when providing counseling to the patient. In no case should pharmacy technicians interpret orders on their own, since this process does not offer enough checks in the event an error is made. In addition, orders must not be filled only from computer-generated labels; rather, the original order should accompany the label to serve as another check (**Figure 30-1**).

Look-Alike Drug Names

Medications with similarly spelled names can easily be misread for one another. In fact, from January 2000 to March 2004, close to 32,000 reports were submitted to the USP's MedMarx Reporting System that linked errors to look-alike or sound-alike drug names. Technicians must be alert to this problem and should never guess about the prescriber's intent.

Study the handwriting in **Figures 30-2 through 30-8**. Would you have had difficulty reading these medication orders correctly? These are actual examples of handwritten orders in both the inpatient and outpatient setting, and each led to medication errors. The problem was not uncertainty. On the contrary, each order

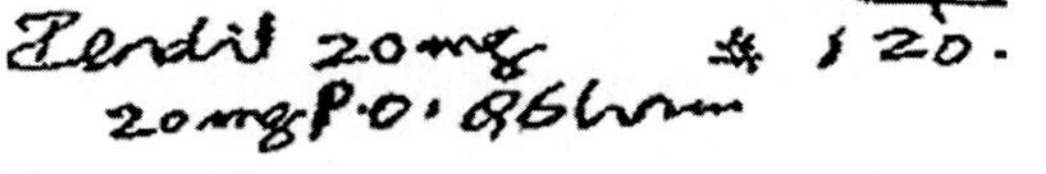

FIGURE 30-2 Prescription order for Isordil 20 mg, misread as Plendil 20 mg.

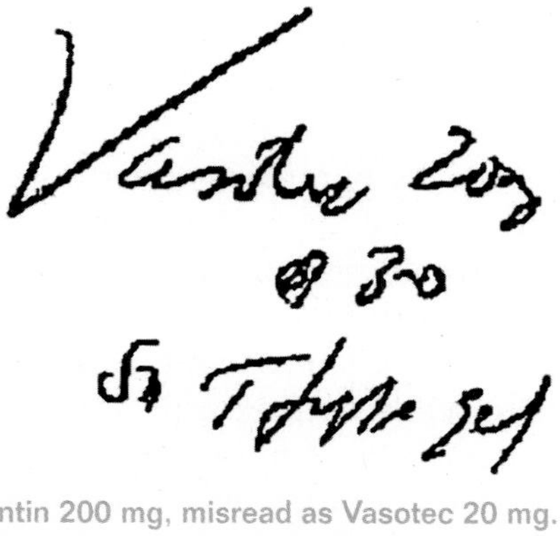

FIGURE 30-3 Order for Vantin 200 mg, misread as Vasotec 20 mg.

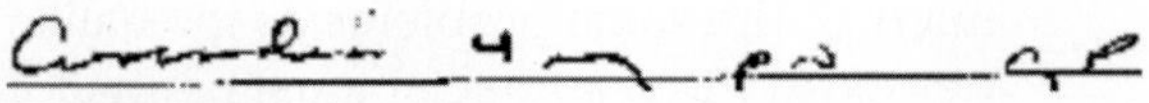

FIGURE 30-4 Order for Avandia 4 mg, misread as Coumadin 4 mg.

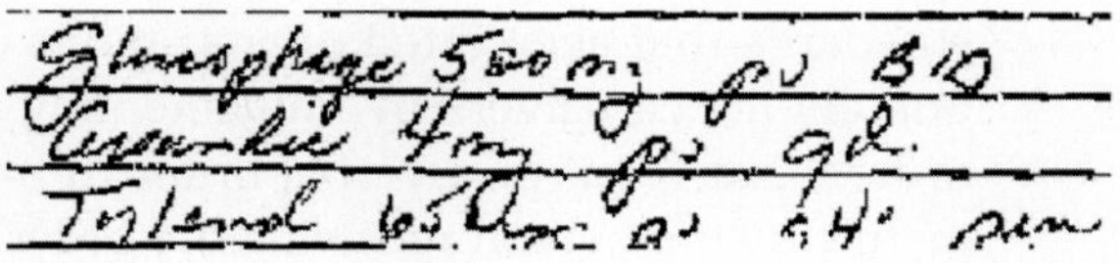

FIGURE 30-5 Order for Avandia 4 mg, misread as Coumadin 4 mg (second order).

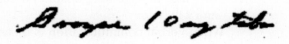

FIGURE 30-6 Order for BuSpar 10 mg, misread as Prozac 10 mg.

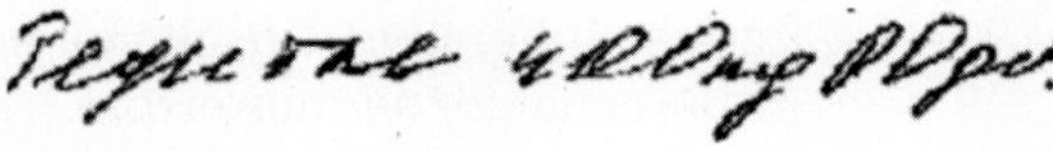

FIGURE 30-7 Order for Tequin 400 mg (misspelled with an "e"), misread as Tegretol 400 mg.

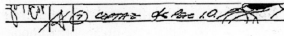

FIGURE 30-8 Ceftazidime "OK" per I.D., misread as ceftazidime "d/c" per I.D.

was misread from the start; no consideration was ever given to the alternative drug, because in each case the pharmacy staff members thought they were reading the order correctly.

When pharmacists and technicians interpret prescriptions and medication orders, new drugs are a particular problem. Pharmacy technicians may not be as familiar with the names of newly marketed drugs and, hence, may misinterpret them as older drugs. This is a good reason for health care facilities to establish policies that prohibit oral requests for medication without the pharmacy reviewing a copy of the order. Facsimile machines and scanners on nursing units make the process of having a pharmacist review the order easier. In the community, physicians can write both the generic and trade names legibly on the prescription, and they can add the intended purpose of the medication to further alert the pharmacy staff to the correct medication name. As mentioned earlier, many medications have look-alike names, but very few name pairs that are spelled similarly are used for similar purposes.

Sound-Alike Drug Names

Drug orders communicated orally often are misheard, misunderstood, misinterpreted, or transcribed incorrectly. Celebrex and Cerebyx sound alike, as do alprazolam and lorazepam, Sarafem and Serophene, Lopid and Slo-bid, and many other name pairs. All of these have been confused at one time or another, resulting in patients receiving incorrect medications. In many cases, serious injuries have occurred because of misinterpreted verbal orders. Sound-alike drug names present many of the same problems as look-alike drug names. Obviously, when uncertainties exist, the pharmacist must contact the prescriber for clarification.

To decrease the opportunity for misunderstanding, health care facilities and community pharmacies should discourage telephone orders. The Joint Commission, a national accrediting agency for health care organizations, requires in its standards that accredited organizations improve the effectiveness of communication among caregivers by implementing a process for taking verbal or telephone orders that requires a verbal order to be transcribed and then "read back" completely by the person receiving the order (Joint Commission, 2011).

To decrease the opportunity for misunderstanding, health care facilities and community pharmacies should seriously discourage verbal orders. Greater use of facsimile machines among hospital areas, medical offices, pharmacies, and nursing units will help.

When verbal communication is unavoidable, strict adherence to these procedures for verbal orders can minimize errors:

- Verbal orders should be taken by a pharmacist whenever possible.
- Prohibit spoken orders for selected high-alert medications (e.g., chemotherapy, IV insulin for neonates) because of their complexity and potential for serious errors.
- If possible, a second person should listen while the prescription is being given.
- The order should be transcribed and read back, repeating exactly what has been understood, sometimes spelling the drug name and strength for verification (e.g., "one, five milligrams" for 15 mg).
- Obtain the prescriber's phone number in case follow-up questions arise.
- The prescribed agent must make sense for the patient's clinical situation.

To prevent sound-alike and look-alike errors, physicians must be encouraged to include complete directions, strengths, route of administration, and indication (purpose) for use. All of these elements can serve as identifiers. It cannot be stressed enough that even if such information is lacking on orders, by knowing a drug's purpose as well as the patient's problems, skilled health care professionals can judge whether the drug ordered makes sense for the patient in the context in which the order is written. For example, knowing that the patient has a diagnosis of diabetes would be an important clue in determining that Avandia is intended by the orders in Figures 30-4 and 30-5. Diagnostic procedures along with orders also could provide important information. This is why it is important for pharmacists to verify all orders processed by technicians. When in doubt, check with the pharmacist, who can call the physician for clarification if the intent is not completely clear. A list of sound-alike drug names can be found in Appendix C.

Certain abbreviations are easily misinterpreted. Avoiding dangerous abbreviations can reduce communication errors. Although many health care facilities have lists of abbreviations that are approved for use by the professional staff, it would be far safer if each hospital also developed a list of abbreviations that should *never* be used. In fact, such a negative list is easier to maintain and enforce. In addition, The Joint Commission has recommended that accredited organizations standardize abbreviations, acronyms, and symbols used throughout an organization, including a list of abbreviations, acronyms, and symbols not to use.

The Institute for Safe Medication Practices (ISMP) has developed a list that contains several easily misinterpreted abbreviations from actual medication errors reported to ISMP, some of which resulted in patient harm (ISMP, 2010). **Table 30-1** contains several easily misinterpreted abbreviations from that list.

TABLE 30-1 Misinterpretation of Abbreviations and Associated Errors

ABBREVIATION/ DOSE EXPRESSION	INTENDED MEANING	MISINTERPRETATION	CORRECTION
ʒ	Dram	Misunderstood or misread as "3"	Use the metric system
m	Minim	Misunderstood or misread as "mL"	Use the metric system
AU	Aurio uterque (each ear)	Mistaken for OU (oculu uterque—each eye)	Do not use this abbreviation
D/C	Discharge or discontinue	Premature discontinuation of medications when D/C (intended to mean "discharge") has been misinterpreted as "discontinued" when followed by a list of drugs.	Spell out "discharge" and "discontinue"
μg	Microgram	Mistaken for "mg" when handwritten	Use "mcg"
o.d. or OD	Once daily	Misinterpreted as "right eye" (OD—oculus dexter) and results in administration of medications in the eye	Use "daily"
TIW or tiw	Three times a week	Mistaken for "three times a day"	Do not use this abbreviation
q.d. or QD	Every day	Mistaken as "q.i.d.," especially if the period after the "q" or the tail of the "q" is misunderstood as an "i"	Use "daily" or "every day"
qn	Nightly or at bedtime	Misinterpreted as "qh" (every hour)	Use "nightly"
qhs	Nightly at bedtime	Misread as every hour	Use "nightly"
q6PM, etc.	Every evening at 6 p.m.	Misread as every six hours	Use "6 p.m. nightly"
q.o.d. or QOD	Every other day	Misinterpreted as "q.d." (daily) or "q.i.d." (four times daily) if the "o" is poorly written	Use "every other day"
sub q	Subcutaneous	The "q" has been mistaken for "every" (e.g., one heparin dose ordered "sub q 2 hours before surgery" misunderstood as every 2 hours before surgery)	Use "subcut" or write "subcutaneous"
SC	Subcutaneous	Mistaken for SL (sublingual)	Use "subcut" or write "subcutaneous"
U or u	Unit	Read as a zero or a four, causing a 10-fold overdose or greater ("4u" seen as "40" or "4u" seen as "44")	Unit has no acceptable abbreviation; use "unit"
IU	International Unit	Misread as IV (intravenous)	Use "units"
cc	Cubic centimeters	Misread as "u" (units)	Use "mL"
X3d	For three days	Mistaken for "three doses"	Use "for three days"
BT	Bedtime	Mistaken for "BID" (twice daily)	Use "bedtime"
ss	Sliding scale (insulin) or 1/2 ss	Mistaken for "55"	Spell out "sliding scale"; use "one-half" or use "1/2 ss"
> and <	Greater than and less than	Mistakenly used or interpreted as the opposite symbol	Spell out "greater than" or "less than"

(Continued)

TABLE 30-1 (Continued)

ABBREVIATION/ DOSE EXPRESSION	INTENDED MEANING	MISINTERPRETATION	CORRECTION
/ (slash mark)	Separates two doses or indicates "per"	Misunderstood as the number 1 ("25 units/10 units" read as "110 units")	Do not use a slash mark to separate doses; spell out "per" when that is intended
Name letters and dose numbers run together (e.g., Inderal 40 mg)	Inderal 40 mg	Misread as Inderal 140 mg	Always use a space between drug name, dose, and unit of measure
Zero after decimal point (e.g., 1.0)	1 mg	Misread as 10 mg if the decimal point is not seen	Do not use terminal zeros for doses expressed in whole numbers
No zero before decimal point (e.g., .5 mg)	0.5 mg	Misread as 5 mg	Always use zero a before a decimal when the dose is less than 1
per os	Orally	The "os" can be mistaken for "left eye"	Use "PO," "by mouth," or "orally"
Drug Names			
ARA-A	Vidarabine	Cytarabine (ARA-C)	Use the complete spelling for drug names
AZT	Zidovudine	Azathioprine	
CPZ	Compazine (prochlorperazine)	Chlorpromazine	
HCl	Hydrochloride salt	Potassium chloride (the "h" can be interpreted as "k")	
HCT	Hydrocortisone	Hydrochlorothiazide	
HCTZ 50	Hydrochlorothiazide 50 mg	Hydrocortisone (seen as hct250 mg)	
$MgSO_4$	Magnesium sulfate	Morphine sulfate	
MSO_4	Morphine sulfate	Magnesium sulfate	
MTX	Methotrexate	Mitoxantrone	
TAC	Triamcinolone	Tetracaine, Adrenalin, cocaine	
$ZnSO_4$	Zinc sulfate	Morphine sulfate	
Stemmed Names			
Nitro drip	Nitroglycerin infusion	Sodium nitroprusside infusion	Use the complete spelling for drug names
Norflox	Norfloxacin	Norflex (orphenadrine)	

These should never be used in medication orders, on pharmacy labels, in newsletters or other communications that originate in the pharmacy, or in pharmacy computer systems because they may find their way to medication orders, labels, and reports.

Here are examples of some of the most problematic abbreviations used to communicate orders:

- The abbreviation "U" for units is an example of what can go wrong; it should be on every organization's list of unacceptable abbreviations. Errors have occurred when the letter "U" was mistaken for the numerals 0, 4, 6, and 7, and even "cc," resulting in disastrous drug

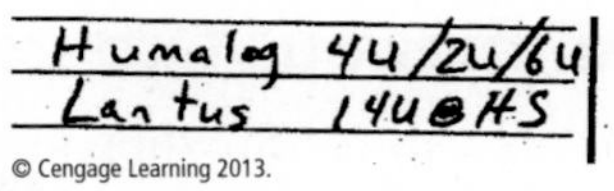

FIGURE 30-9 Erroneous order for insulin due to the use of the letter "U" for units.

overdoses with insulin, heparin, other medications whose doses are sometimes expressed in units. For example, orders written as "6U Regular Insulin" have been misinterpreted as "60 Regular Insulin," with patients receiving 60 units rather than the intended 6 units. A report sent to ISMP stated that a nurse, who was taking a patient's history, recorded his insulin dose using the letter "u" instead of the word "unit" (see **Figure 30-9**). The physician misread the "u" as a "4" and wrote orders for doses of 44 units, 24 units, and 64 units, which is dramatically different from what the patient had been taking.

- Q for "every," as well as other abbreviations with this letter (QD, QID, and QOD; or qd, qid, and qod), is often involved in medication errors. QD for "daily" can result in fourfold overdosages if seen as QID (q.i.d.) for "four times daily," or subtherapeutic doses if seen as QOD for "every other day." In one case, an order for Zithromax (azithromycin) 500 mg written as QD was misinterpreted as QID. The patient was not harmed, despite receiving the medication four times daily. In another report, an order was written for digoxin 0.125 mg po QOD (every other day), but the medication was given QD (every day). The patient received two extra doses before the error was discovered.
- D/C is another example of an abbreviation that should not be used. It has been written to mean either discontinue or discharge, sometimes resulting in premature stoppage of patient's medications. In Figure 30-8, the "d/c" order was incorrectly interpreted as discontinuation of an antibiotic that the patient had never even received. In reality, the "d/c" is really "OK," meaning that the drug was approved for use by the infectious diseases physician.
- Do not abbreviate drug names. For example,
    - "MTX" means "methotrexate" to some health professionals, but others understand it as "mitoxantrone."
    - "AZT" has been misunderstood as "azathioprine" (Imuran) when "zidovudine" (Retrovir) was intended. In one case, this misinterpretation led to a patient with AIDS receiving azathioprine, an immunosuppressant, instead of the intended antiretroviral agent. The patient's immune system worsened, and he developed an overwhelming infection.
    - One problematic example includes using abbreviations for magnesium sulfate ($MgSO_4$ or simply Mg) and morphine sulfate (MSO_4 or simply MS). In one example reported in Pennsylvania, a prescriber used an abbreviation for magnesium sulfate and wrote "$MgSo_4$ 2g IV x 1 dose" for a 45-year-old female patient. However, the unit clerk and nurse misinterpreted the order as morphine sulfate (MSO_4) 2 mg IV x 1 dose, and the patient received a 2-mg dose of morphine sulfate. Contributing to this error was the fact that the patient was having pain, so morphine seemed reasonable. The prescriber was notified, and magnesium was administered to the patient (Pennsylvania Patient Safety Authority, 2005).

Ambiguous Orders

Errors can result when ambiguous orders are interpreted in a manner other than what the prescriber intended. Proper expression of doses is vital in a drug order. Technicians should be able to recognize improper expressions of doses—and the potential for error—when they see them, and they should bring them to the pharmacist's attention. When the prescriber's clarification is needed, the pharmacist must contact the prescriber. Pharmacists and technicians should avoid using improper expressions of doses as they process orders, type labels, and communicate with others. Several improperly expressed orders are analyzed and corrected in the following examples.

- *Zeros and decimal points*—When listing drug doses on labels or in other communications, never follow a whole number with a decimal plus a zero (i.e., a "trailing zero"). For example, "Coumadin 1.0 mg" is a very dangerous way to express this dose. If the decimal point is not seen, the dose would be misinterpreted as "10 mg" and a 10-fold overdose would result. The same could happen if "Dilaudid 1.0 mg" is written. The proper way to express these orders would be "Coumadin 1 mg" and "Dilaudid 1 mg," respectively. On the other hand, always place a zero *before* a decimal point when the dose is smaller than 1 (i.e., a "leading" zero"). For example, "Synthroid .1 mg" may be seen as "Synthroid 1 mg," especially when a poor impression of the decimal is written, such as on faxes or carbon or no-carbon-required copies. Avoid using decimal expressions at all where recognizable alternatives exist because whole numbers are easier to work with. In the above example, "Synthroid 0.1 mg" would be good, but "Synthroid 100 mcg" would be better. Use "Digoxin 125 mcg" rather than "Digoxin 0.125 mg." Use "500 mg" instead of "0.5 grams."
- *Spacing*—Potentially serious medication errors have been reported to the ISMP because a lowercase "L" was the last letter in a drug name and was misread as the number 1. For example, a prescription for 300 mg of TEGRETOL (carbamazepine) BID was misinterpreted as 1,300 mg BID (**Figure 30-10**). The letter "L" at the end of Tegretol had been written very close to the numerical dose of 300 mg on a prescription for the patient (e.g., Tegretol300 mg). The pharmacist was unfamiliar with the medication, and the pharmacy computer did not alert him that the dose exceeded safe limits. A similar error occurred with a prescription written for AMARYL (glimepiride) 2 mg. The "2" was written close to the "L," which led the pharmacist to misinterpret the order as Amaryl 12 mg. Luckily, this error did not reach the patient (**Figure 30-11**).
- *Apothecary system*—Use the metric system exclusively. You may have learned about the apothecary systems and its grains, drams, minims, and ounces, but this form of measure can be easily mistaken. For example, symbols for dram have been misread as "3" and minim misread as "55." Orders for phenobarbital 0.5 gr. (30 mg) have been mistaken for 0.5 grams (500 mg). The use of the apothecary system is no longer officially recognized by the U.S. Pharmacopeia.
- *Label preparation*—When typing labels, always place a space after the drug name, the dose, and the unit of measurement. It is difficult to read labels when everything runs together. Do not type "Tegretol300mg," because this can be misinterpreted as "Tegretol 1,300 mg." Instead, type "Tegretol 300 mg."

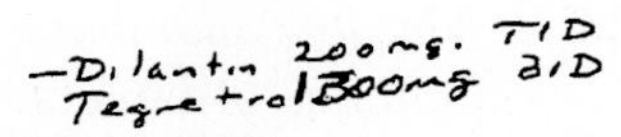

FIGURE 30-10 Order for 300 mg of Tegretol (carbamazepine) BID, misinterpreted as 1,300 mg BID.

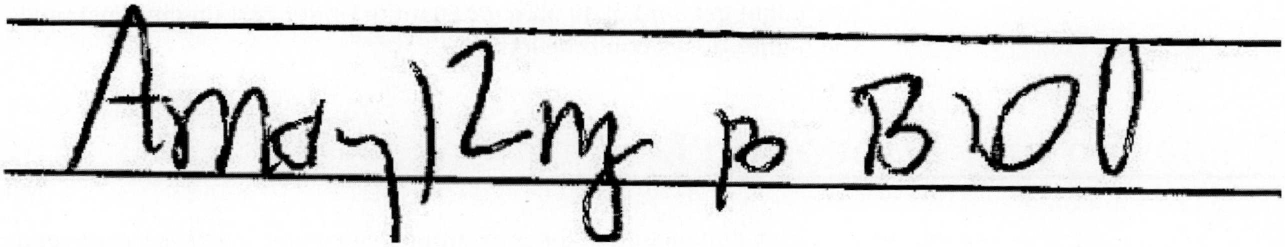

FIGURE 30-11 Is this order for Amaryl 12 mg or 2 mg?

- *Tablet strengths*—Orders specifying both strength and number of tablets are confusing when more than one tablet strength exists. For example, "Atenolol 1/2 tablet 50 mg once daily" appears clear enough; however, when you realize this product is available in both 50-mg and 100-mg tablets, it becomes clear that this order is ambiguous. What is the intended dose, 50 mg or 25 mg? Orders are clearer if the dose is specified regardless of the strengths available: "Atenolol 50 mg once daily." For doses that require several tablets or capsules, the pharmacy label should note the exact number of dosage units needed. For example, the label on a 400-mg dose of Tegretol (carbamazepine), which is available in 200-mg tablets, should read "2 × 200 mg tablets = 400 mg." For a 25-mg dose of prednisone, which is available in 50-mg tablets, the label should read "1/2 tablet 25 mg." If your pharmacy prepares a computer-generated medication administration record (MAR) for the nurses, this same type of notation should be used.
- *Liquid dosage forms*—Expressing the dose only in milliliters (or teaspoonfuls) for liquid dosage forms is confusing. For example, acetaminophen elixir is available in many strengths including 80 mg per 5 mL, 120 mg per 5 mL, and 160 mg per 5 mL. If the prescriber wrote "5 mL," the intended number of milligrams would be unclear, but "80 mg" is clear. The amount of drug by metric weight as well as the volume always should be included on the pharmacy label: "Acetaminophen elixir 80 mg/5 mL." Further, the patient dose should also be included. For a 320-mg dose the label should read "320 mg = 20 mL." The same holds true for unit-dose labels and bulk labels.
- *Injectable medications*—For injectable drugs, the same rule applies. List the metric weight or the metric weight and volume—never the volume alone—because solution concentrations are variable. This problem at a hospital where hepatitis B vaccines were being administered and resulted in an error. A preprinted physician's order form was used to prescribe the vaccine, listing only the volume to be given. When the clinic switched to another brand of vaccine, containing a different concentration of vaccine, the same preprinted forms continued to be used, underdosing hundreds of children until the error was discovered. This could have been avoided had the amount of vaccine been prescribed in micrograms, rather than just the volume in milliliters.

- *Variable amounts*—A drug dose should never be ordered solely by number of tablets, capsules, ampoules, or vials because the amounts contained in these dosage forms are variable. Drug doses should be ordered with proper unit expression; for example, 20 mEq of magnesium sulfate. A patient whose physician orders "an amp" of magnesium sulfate might get 8 mEq, 40 mEq, or 60 mEq. Under certain circumstances, the higher doses could be lethal.

Preparing and Dispensing Medications

An important safety enhancement for preventing dispensing errors is the development of a system of redundant checks from the time a prescription order is first written in the physician's office or on the nursing unit, to receipt in the pharmacy, through dispensing and administration. Such a system is suggested in this section. Obviously, the more "looks" an order receives (while efficient work flow is maintained), the better. Health professionals can review orders at several checkpoints and thereby maximize the chances of errors being discovered.

Steps in Prescription Filling

The following list describes the steps a prescription goes through in the filling process:

1. The physician sees the patient; performs an assessment; determines appropriate medication, dose, and frequency; and writes the order or communicates the order verbally to nursing personnel or the pharmacy.
2. In the institution, a unit secretary reads and transcribes the order onto the medication administration record. This step is unnecessary in hospitals where computers generate the MAR or where physicians can enter orders by computer, although the nurse and the pharmacist still must verify the order.
3. In the institution, a nurse checks the unit secretary's transcription for accuracy.
4. In both community and institutional settings, a direct copy of the order is carried, scanned, or faxed to the pharmacy, or the physician's computer entry reaches the pharmacy via electronic means. The pharmacy technician reads the order and enters it in the pharmacy computer system. If the technician finds a duplicate order, an incorrect dose, an allergy, or the like, the discrepancy should be documented and called to the attention of the pharmacist during the clinical screening in step 5.
5. A pharmacist reviews the technician's computer entry, compares it with the original prescription (handwritten or electronic), and performs a clinical screening of the prescription with respect to the need for the drug, allergies or other contraindications, proper dose, and proper route of administration.
6. A label or a medication profile is printed. A copy of the original prescription or medication order continues to accompany the label or medication profile while the order is filled. No orders should be filled solely on the basis of what appears on the label or medication profile, because the computer entry may have been in error.

7. To choose an item for dispensing, a technician reviews both the label and the medication order for possible discrepancies. If no discrepancies are identified, the technician fills the order.
8. A pharmacist checks the technician's work, reviewing the label against the medication order copy and the dose that has been prepared. The drug is dispensed. In the community setting, the pharmacist uses the patient counseling session to further assess that the correct medication is being dispensed and that the patient has a condition treatable with the product being provided.
9. Pharmacists should *not* simply ask patients if they have any questions about their medication, but confirm their understanding of the medication and its proper use. For refills and medications patients have taken in the past, they should be informed about any changes in the appearance of the product. Patients should be counseled about the common adverse effects of medications they are taking, and they should be instructed on any clinical signs to watch for and report to health professionals. In addition to providing patients with appropriate devices for measuring doses, such as oral syringes for administering oral solutions or suspensions, practitioners must ensure that the patient or caregiver understands how to properly use them with the medication. Demonstrate for patients how to use the device, and follow up with a return demonstration by the user.
10. In the institution, the nurse receives the drug and compares the medication and pharmacy label against the copy of the physician's order as well as the handwritten transcription made earlier in the MAR. The nurse administers the dose, explaining the drug's purpose and potential adverse effects, and answers questions and concerns raised by the patient.
11. The final step in the process is the assurance of adherence to medication therapy. If the patient is taking too much medication or is not taking the drug as frequently as prescribed, the pharmacist should speak with the patient to determine the reasons and address the variation. In addition, patients should be asked about common adverse effects and about signs of serious drug toxicities.

Selecting Medications

The importance of reading the product label while selecting medications and filling prescriptions cannot be overemphasized. Too often the wrong drug or wrong strength is dispensed, and such errors usually stem from failure to read the label. During drug preparation and dispensing, the label should be read three times: when the product is selected, when the medication is prepared, and when either the partially used medication is disposed of (or restocked) or product preparation is complete.

Selecting the correct item from the shelf, drawer, or bin can be complicated by many factors. Similar labeling and packaging as well as look-alike names are a common trap that leads to medication errors. Restocking errors are quite common and can lead to repeated medication errors before being detected.

Automated dispensing machines have become more common on the nursing units of many hospitals. The nurse must punch a security code and a password into the dispensing device, along with the name of the patient and the name of the medication, before the machine will allow access to the medication. This system allows more control of items kept on the nursing unit and serves as a check for the nurse who retrieves the medication, more so than for regularly stocked floor stock items. In some cases, online communication with the hospital computer information system or pharmacy system allows a pharmacist to review medication orders before nursing access to the medication is allowed.

Automated dispensing devices create several situations that can result in errors. The machines are routinely restocked, and the incorrect restocking of items (i.e., placing the wrong drug into the wrong bin) can occur. Devices that have multiple medications in each drawer and that do not require pharmacist review of orders before access have drawbacks that are identical to flaws in the old floor stock systems, in that the nurse can retrieve either the wrong item or additional items to use for other patients, and lack of pharmacist double-checking and screening of orders allows prescribing errors, wrong dosages, incorrect routes of administration, and other clinical errors to occur.

confirmation bias a term used to describe errors that occur in selection of medication by either pharmacy or nursing staff; when choosing an item, people see what they are looking for, and once they think they have found it, they stop looking any further

When errors occur in selection of medication by either pharmacy or nursing staff, the term **confirmation bias** is used to describe the phenomenon. When choosing an item, people see what they are looking for, and once they think they have found it, they stop looking any further. Often the health professional chooses a medication container based on a mental picture of the item. Staff members may be looking for some characteristic of the drug label, the shape and size or color of the container, or the location of the item on a shelf, in a drawer, or in a storage bin instead of reading the name of the drug itself. Consequently, they may fail to realize that they have the wrong item in hand.

A number of approaches can be used to minimize the possibility of such errors in the pharmacy and in automated dispensing machines. One strategy would be to change the appearance of look-alike product names on computer screens, pharmacy shelf labels and bins, and pharmacy product labels by highlighting, through boldface, color, or by the use of "tall man" letters, the parts of the names that are different (e.g., hydrOXYzine, hydrALAzine). In fact, the U.S. Food and Drug Administration (FDA) Office of Generic Drugs requested manufacturers of 16 look-alike name pairs to voluntarily revise the appearance of their established names in order to minimize medication errors resulting from look-alike confusion. Manufacturers were encouraged to visually differentiate their established names with the use of "tall man" letters. Examples of established names involved include chlorproMAZINE and chlorproPAMIDE, vinBLAStine and vinCRIStine, and niCARdipine and NIFEdipine.

Physically separating drugs with look-alike labels and packaging reduces the potential for error. Some pharmacy technicians also separate drugs with similar names and overlapping strengths, especially those labeled and packaged by the same manufacturer. For example, metformin 500-mg tablets and metronidazole 500-mg tablets, both from the same unit-dose packager, might pose a problem. So might chlorproMAZINE 200 mg and chlorproPAMIDE 200 mg, traMADol 50 mg and traZODone 50 mg, and injectable morphine 1 mg/mL and HYDROmorphone 1 mg/mL.

In institutional and community pharmacies with several staff members, everyone should have input in deciding how and where drugs are available, how doses are prepared, who is responsible for preparing them, the appearance of the storage containers, and how they are labeled. In addition, staff members should be encouraged to use a technique known as failure mode and effects analysis (FMEA) to examine the use of new products to determine points of potential failures and their effects before any error actually happens. In this regard, FMEA differs from root-cause analysis (RCA). RCA is a reactive process, employed after an error occurs, to identify its underlying causes. In contrast, FMEA is a proactive process used to carefully and systematically evaluate vulnerable areas or processes. FMEA can be employed before the purchase and implementation of new products to identify potential failure modes so that steps can be taken to avoid errors before they occur (ISMP, 2010). Procedures to ensure safe medication use must be written, and the importance of adhering to the guidelines must be shared by all involved pharmacy, medical, and nursing personnel. Pharmaceutical companies are aware of labeling and packaging problems, and many have responded to suggestions made by technicians and pharmacists. Health professionals can alert manufacturers about errors caused by commercial packaging and labeling problems by using the ISMP's national Medication Error Reporting Program (MERP). Reports are forwarded to the individual pharmaceutical company and the FDA and the ISMP provide follow-up when appropriate. Call 1-800-FAIL-SAF(E) or go to www.ismp.org to complete a ISMP MERP report. All reports are confidential.

Selecting Auxiliary Labels

To help prevent errors, pharmacists and technicians should apply auxiliary labels in as appropriate, especially in the community setting. For example, amoxicillin oral suspension is available in dropper bottles for pediatric use. When the suspension is used for an ear infection, some parents have been known to place the suspension in the child's ear rather than give it properly, that is, orally. An auxiliary label, "For Oral Use Only," would help prevent this error. Other such labels are "For the Ear," "For the Eye," and "For External Use Only."

However, this practice can be unsafe if the patient is unable to understand the warning, and the application of an auxiliary label should not be done in lieu of speaking with the patient. A study that appeared in the *American Journal of Health-System Pharmacy* showed that there is a high level of misunderstanding of auxiliary labels among adults with low literacy, a reading level at or below the sixth-grade level. The rate of correct interpretation of these labels ranged from 0% to 78.7%. With the exception of the label "Take with Food," less than half of all patients were able to provide adequate interpretations of the warning labels' messages. In fact, none were able to correctly interpret the label "Do not take dairy products, antacids, or iron preparations within one hour of this medication." Studies have also shown that a combination of a verbal description of a warning along with visual symbols improves the overall comprehension of the warning.

Sterile Admixture Preparation

In preparing fluids for injectable administration, the potential for grave error is increased for several reasons. First, patients who are sicker often need intravenous drugs, so the medications used have more dramatic effects on the body's function and physiology. Further, most injectable solutions are simply clear, colorless, water-based fluids, so they may look alike, regardless of what drug and how much of it is actually in the fluid.

Errors during pharmacy preparation of parenteral products and admixtures may happen more often than you think. A five-hospital observational study on the accuracy of preparing small- and large-volume injectables, chemotherapy solutions, and parenteral nutrition showed a mean error rate of 9%, meaning almost 1 in 10 products was prepared incorrectly and then dispensed (Flynn, Pearson, & Barker, 1997). Error rates for complex solutions such as parenteral nutrition were especially high—37% for manual preparation and 22% for preparations that were partly automated. More recently, a 2009 State of Pharmacy Compounding Survey showed that 30% of hospitals have experienced a patient event involving a compounding error in the past 5 years (Pharmacy Purchasing & Products, 2009). In 2006, an infant received a lethal dose of zinc stemming from an error that occurred during the order entry and compounding of a total parenteral nutrition (TPN) solution. TPN was prescribed for a preterm infant born at 26 weeks' gestation. On the day of the event, the physician's TPN order included directions to add zinc in a concentration of 330 mcg/100 mL. Because the automated compounder used for TPN required entry of zinc in a mcg/kg dose, the pharmacist converted the mcg/mL dose to a mcg/kg dose. She performed this calculation correctly, but accidentally entered the zinc dose in the pharmacy computer in mg, not mcg. This resulted in a final concentration of 330 mg/100 mL—a 1,000-fold overdose (ISMP, 2007).

Thus, in the sterile admixture preparation setting, the chance of dosage miscalculation or measurement error must be minimized by systems designed with procedures that require independent double-checks by two staff members. The independent double-check in some pharmacies might be required for all calculations or measurements, while others require it only for calculations falling into special categories, such as dosage calculations for admixture compounding for any child under 12, critical care drug infusions requiring a dose in micrograms per kilogram per minute, insulin infusions, chemotherapy, and patient-controlled analgesia. Calculators and computer programs may improve accuracy, but they do not eliminate the need for a second person to review the calculations and solution concentrations used. Another important way to minimize calculation errors is to *avoid* the need for performing calculations. This can be accomplished by using the unit-dose system exclusively through the following methods:

- Use commercially available unit-dose systems, such as premixed critical care parenteral products.
- Standardize doses and concentrations, especially of critical care drugs such as heparin, DOBUTamine, DOPamine, or morphine.

Similar steps can be taken in community pharmacies that provide sterile admixtures to physician's offices, home care programs and patients, long-term care facilities, and other clients.

The use of standard dosage charts on the floors and standard formulations in the pharmacy minimizes the possibility of error and makes calculations much easier for everyone. For example, in critical care units, physicians need order only the amount of drug they want infused and list any titration parameters. No one has to perform any calculations because dosage charts are readily available for choosing appropriate flow rates by patient weight and dose ordered.

Standard concentrations for frequently prepared formulations should be recorded and be readily accessible for reference in the admixture preparation area in the pharmacy. Of course, all calculations must be double-checked and documented by the pharmacist. Diluents as well as active drugs must be checked *before* they are added to the base solution. The stock container of each additive with its accompanying syringe should be lined up in the order in which it appears on the container label to facilitate the checking procedure. When compounding TPN solutions, at least three verification processes should occur in the pharmacy: after initial order entry of TPN, before manually injecting additives into the TPN, and once the TPN has been compounded. Each verification should require a pharmacist to compare the actual prescriber's order to the printed labels, and the printed labels to the additives and final product, as appropriate. Verification of manual additives should include inspection of the actual vials and syringes that contain the additives. The final verification of the compounded TPN should include a comprehensive review of the TPN order, the label on the product, and the work label.

In many hospitals, automated compounders are being used for admixing both large- and small-volume parenterals. Automated equipment has been known to fail occasionally. Also, some accidents have occurred in which solutions were placed on the wrong additive channel. In either case, the result could be a serious medication error. Therefore, pharmacies must have an ongoing quality assurance program for the use of automated compounding equipment. This program should include double-checks and documentation of solution placement within the compounder, final weighing or refractometer testing of the solution to ensure that proper concentrations have been compounded, and ongoing sampling of electrolyte concentrations. Pharmacists that prepare special parenteral solutions in batches (e.g., total parenteral nutrition base solutions, cardioplegic solutions) should have additional quality assurance procedures in place, including sterility testing and quarantine until confirmation.

Effective Medication Error Prevention and Monitoring Systems

All drug-dispensing procedures should be examined regularly, and the cause of system breakdowns must be discovered so that prevention measures can be designed. Pharmacy technicians need to communicate clearly to their pharmacist supervisors what it takes to do the job correctly in terms of personnel, training programs, facilities design, equipment, drug procedures and supplies, computer systems, and quality assurance programs.

Multidisciplinary educational programs should be developed for health care personnel that address medication error prevention. Because many errors happen when procedures are not followed, this is one area on which to focus through newsletters and in-service training. It also is important for pharmacy staff members to focus not just on their own internal errors, but to look at other pharmacies' errors and methods of prevention and to learn from these. The ISMP provides ongoing features to facilitate these reviews in publications such as *Pharmacy Today, Hospital Pharmacy*, and *Pharmacy & Therapeutics*. The ISMP also publishes its own biweekly *ISMP Medication Safety Alert!* for hospitals and a monthly newsletter for community/ambulatory care practices that reports on current medication safety issues and offers recommendations for changes.

Medication Error Reporting Programs

All pharmacy procedures should be examined regularly, both proactively and retrospectively, in an effort to discover the potential problems as well as causes of system breakdowns so that prevention measures can be designed. Pharmacy technicians need to communicate clearly to managers what it takes to do the job correctly in terms of personnel, training programs, facilities design, equipment, drug procedures and supplies, computer systems, and quality assurance programs. In addition, reducing medication errors requires using a number of effective risk identification methods, including a nonpunitive environment and a voluntary medication error reporting system.

Currently, many pharmacies approaches to error reduction are ineffective. An organization's primary means of identifying risk involves investigations that occur during the error reporting process that tend to focus their attention on the front end or active end of the error such as the front-line practitioner. While these actions may not seem outwardly punitive, these forms of reprimand lead to underreporting of errors. In fact, punishing individuals for errors actually can be dangerous to an organization. It inhibits open discussion about errors, creates a defensive and reactive environment, and hinders careful and unbiased consideration of the system-based root causes of errors. Pharmacies are weakened further by punitive actions, especially if the sole responsibility for safe medication practices rests on individuals rather than on strong systems that make it difficult for practitioners to make errors.

The goal of patient safety is best served within a nonpunitive environment that places more value on a variety of risk identification methods, in addition to reporting problems so that they can be remedied rather than on pursuing the unprofitable path of disciplining employees for errors.

A retrospective, voluntary, confidential reporting program provides pharmacy technicians with the opportunity to tell the complete story without fear of retribution. The depth of information contained in these stories is critical to understanding the error. This information is critical to identification of system deficiencies that can be corrected to prevent future errors. However, successful and sustained improvement of error-prone processes cannot occur if little information is available about factors that contribute to an error.

Many organizational factors inhibit the reporting of medication errors. Examples include inconsistent definitions of a medication error, a punitive approach to medication errors, failure to improve the medication system or address reported problems reported by staff, lack of feedback to staff, overconcern with medication error rates, complex reporting processes, and the perception that reporting is a low priority. A voluntary program encourages practitioners to report hazardous situations and errors that have the potential to cause serious patient harm. A confidential reporting system where everyone understands that errors will not be linked to performance appraisals is critical. Many organizations have regular meetings where medication errors are addressed. The results of these meetings often are not shared with the front-line staff, therefore giving the impression that "nothing is being done" when errors are reported. In addition, busy practitioners tend to avoid reporting errors owing to the cumbersome nature of their organizations' reporting forms and processes. It is important to make error reporting easy, reward error reporting, and provide timely feedback to show what is being done to address problems.

Consistently applying a nonpunitive approach to errors is important. If even one person is disciplined for an error, mistakes will be hidden. Employees should not be evaluated based on errors or lack of making mistakes but on positive measures that evaluate an employee's overall contribution to the organization. Armed with these tools, pharmacy technicians can become aware of the deficiencies in their organizations and make performance improvement changes. Without them, we are only addressing errors at the surface rather than at the root cause.

To be successful, medication error-reduction efforts must result in system improvements that are identified through a four-pronged analysis of errors. The first two prongs, both reactive in nature, include analysis of organization-specific errors that have caused some degree of patient harm and analysis of aggregate medication error data (e.g., trends by drugs or location of drugs involved in errors). Equally important, the other two prongs, both proactive in nature, include analysis of "close calls" (errors that have the potential to cause patient harm) and analysis of errors that have occurred in other organizations. Each prong contains valuable information about weaknesses in the system that, collectively, can lead to effective error-reduction strategies. Yet many organizations focus primarily on the first two prongs of error analysis and action. Most often proactive efforts are not given high priority. As a result, organizations may be busy "fighting fires" rather than preventing them. A near miss should be clear evidence that a tragic event could occur. Unfortunately, too often this wakeup call is not heard. Little attention is focused on thorough analysis of errors that, fortunately, do not cause actual patient harm, especially if organizations identify errors that require analysis by a severity rating that is based on actual patient outcome. For example, a serious overdose detected before administration may not be given the same priority and analysis as a similar error that actually reached and possibly harmed the patient. Worse, some organizations fail to use errors that have occurred elsewhere as a road map for improvement in their own organization. Staff members will be more comfortable discussing a serious external error than one that has occurred within their own organization. Because blame is not an issue, defensive posturing and other obstacles to effective discussion will not be present. Staff can identify possible system-based causes of the error more easily and the likelihood of a similar error occurring in their facility and make suggestions for improvement. As improvements are made, enthusiasm builds for identifying, reporting, and analyzing errors that are actually occurring within the organization. In the end, discussion about external errors leads to more effective analysis of internal errors.

Summary

In institutions, the pharmacy department is responsible for the drug use process throughout the facility. Pharmacists and other members of the pharmacy department should lead a multidisciplinary effort in examining where errors arise in this process. Pharmacists and pharmacy technicians should work together when designing quality assurance programs to obtain information that helps establish priorities and make changes. For example, joint reviews of the accuracy of unit-dose cart fills are of great help in detecting reasons for missing or inaccurate doses and changing the drug-dispensing system accordingly. Programs can be established to monitor the accuracy of order entry into computers in the pharmacy. Quality assurance efforts that include a review of medication error reports help to develop a better understanding of the kinds of system or behavioral defects being experienced so that necessary corrections can be identified. The medication error problem will never be completely eliminated, but pharmacists and pharmacy technicians, working together, can use their expertise to address issues of safety and thus ensure the safest environment possible.

TEST YOUR KNOWLEDGE

Multiple Choice

1. Medication errors are a growing concern in hospitals because of
   a. increased numbers of critically ill patients.
   b. development of more potent medications.
   c. increased media awareness.
   d. all of the above.

2. Medication errors are estimated to occur at a rate of
   a. one per patient per day.
   b. one per hospital per day.
   c. one per health care personnel per day.
   d. one per nursing unit per day.

3. The five "rights" of medication prescribing, dispensing, and administration for medications include all but
   a. patient
   b. route.
   c. dose.
   d. prescriber.

4. Which of the following changes in process could minimize the chance of misinterpretation of handwritten orders?
   a. prescribers printing prescriptions and medication orders in block letters
   b. physicians reviewing orders with the nursing staff before leaving the patient care area
   c. including the purpose of the medication as part of the prescription
   d. all of the above

5. An order for a drug whose strength is a whole number should never be followed by a zero (e.g., 10.0 mg) because
   a. the patient could be underdosed 10-fold.
   b. the patient could be overdosed 10-fold.
   c. the patient could be underdosed 100-fold.
   d. the patient could be overdosed 100-fold.

6. Which order below is the most clearly written and least ambiguous?
   a. "Synthroid 100 mcg daily"
   b. "Synthroid 1 tablet daily"
   c. "Synthroid 0.1 mg daily"
   d. "Synthroid 100 mcg daily"

7. Which order below is the most clearly written and least ambiguous?
   a. "Phenobarbital elixir 15 mg/5 mL: Give 15 mg 5 mL at bedtime."
   b. "Phenobarbital elixir: Give 5 mL at bedtime."
   c. "Phenobarbital elixir 15 mg/5 mL: Give 5.0 mL at bedtime."
   d. "Phenobarbital elixir: Give one teaspoonful at bedtime."

8. When you see an order for "AZT" written, it could stand for
   a. azidothymidine.
   b. azathioprine.
   c. aztreonam.
   d. all of the above—check with prescriber before filling.

9. Computerized order entry enhances routine drug-dispensing activities by
   a. serving as a double-check of the patient's medication for physicians, nurses, and pharmacists.
   b. eliminating the pharmacist from having to check the technician's filled bins.
   c. eliminating the technician from having to restock floor stock items.
   d. none of the above.

10. Confirmation bias occurs when
    a. a physician orders medication for the wrong patient.
    b. an item is chosen once you confirm what you think you are looking for on the label.
    c. a nurse confirms the identity of a patient before administering medication.
    d. a pharmacist does a clinical screening of a patient's medication profile.

11. Medication errors can be reported to the ISMP MERP by
    a. pharmacists.
    b. pharmacy technicians.
    c. the public.
    d. all of the above.

Suggested Readings

Cohen, M.R. (Ed.). (2007). *Medication errors* (2nd ed.). Washington, DC: American Pharmaceutical Association.

Flynn, E.A., Barker, K.N., & Carnahan, B.J. (2003). National observational study of prescription dispensing accuracy and safety in 50 pharmacies. *Journal of the American Pharmaceutical Association, 43*(2), 191–200.

Flynn, E.A., Pearson, R.E., & Barker, K.N. (1997). Observational study of accuracy in compounding IV admixtures at five hospitals. *American Journal of Health-System Pharmacy, 54*, 904–912.

Institute for Safe Medication Practices (ISMP). (2003, January). Misidentification of alphanumeric characters. *ISMP medication safety alert! Community/ambulatory edition* (p. 3). Horsham, PA: Author.

Institute for Safe Medication Practices (ISMP). (2004). Stop U be 4 errors. *ISMP Medication Safety Alert!, 9*(21), 1.

Institute for Safe Medication Practices (ISMP). (2007). Fatal 1,000-fold overdoses can occur, particularly to neonates, by transposing mcg and mg. *ISMP Medication Safety Alert!, 12*(18), 1–2.

Institute for Safe Medication Practices (ISMP). (2010). *ISMP's list of error-prone abbreviations, symbols, and dose designations.* Retrieved from http://www.ismp.org/Tools/errorproneabbreviations.pdf

Joint Commission, 2011

Lesch, M.F. (2003). Comprehension and memory for warning symbols: Age-related differences and impact of training. *Journal of Safety Research, 34*(5), 495–505.

Pennsylvania Patient Safety Authority. (2006). Improving the safety of verbal orders. *Patient Safety Advisory, 3*(2), 1–7.

Reason, J. (1990). The contribution of latent human failures to the breakdown of complex systems. *Philosophical Transactions of the Royal Society B: Biological Sciences,* 327.

Santell, J.O., & Camp, S. (2004). Similarity of drug names, labels, or packaging creates safety issues. *U.S. Pharmacist, 29*(7), 89–91.

State of pharmacy compounding 2009: Survey findings. (2009). *Pharmacy Purchasing & Products, 6*(4), 4–20.

Wolf, M.S., Davis, T.C., et al. (2006). Misunderstanding of prescription drug warning labels among patients with low literacy. *American Journal of Health-System Pharmacy, 63*(1), 1048–1055.

CHAPTER

31

Communication Skills

Competencies

Upon completion of this chapter, the reader should be able to:

1. Define the three major types of communication skills.
2. Avoid common communication mistakes.
3. Understand how communication skills are linked to excellent customer service.
4. Communicate successfully on a job interview.

Key Terms

communication skills **phonetic alphabet** **read-back verification**

Introduction

Clear, concise, and complete communication is essential in today's health care arena. As practitioners from all disciplines work together to improve the well-being of patients, communicating timely and accurate patient information is crucial. Thus, an essential skill that employers consistently search for in potential employees is the ability to communicate effectively.

communication skills skills that are used to effectively convey a message, either verbally or in writing

Why is developing **communication skills** important for pharmacy technicians? Pharmacy technicians are the lifeblood of most pharmacies. They interact every day with patients, nurses, physicians, pharmacists, and other health care professionals and communicate key pieces of patient information that are needed to help all members of the patient's medical team take care of the patient. In many settings, pharmacy technicians are often the face of the pharmacy, directly interacting with patients or customers on the front lines, while pharmacists may be behind the scenes. High-quality customer service is the foundation of pharmacy services and technicians are at the forefront of delivering the patient's needs and expectations. Thus, the professionalism and communication skills possessed by a pharmacy technician have the potential to directly impact the reputation of the entire pharmacy. Communication skills, then, should not be taken lightly. Communication skills are an art, and like any art form, mastering them takes training, practice, and refinement.

Often, the term *communications skills* is used to refer to oral or verbal communication skills—but that definition is incomplete. Several other essential types of communication exist, including written and nonverbal. Mastering all three types is necessary to developing skills as a high-performing communicator.

Oral Communication Skills

Oral communication skills come in many varieties. They can be the formal type, such as those skills used when performing an in-service or giving a presentation, or the more informal, yet equally important, communication that occurs daily among peers, colleagues, coworkers, and patients. In either setting, formal or informal, basic principles of communication apply. These basic principles are at the core of any good presentation or conversation.

First, attention should be given to speaking clearly and fluently. While this might seem intuitive, health care professionals from different backgrounds with unique dialects and accents often interact on behalf of patients. Because important information is being conveyed, perhaps patient information that cannot afford to be misinterpreted, speakers should avoid using slang or rushing through their message. Slang should be viewed as unprofessional and has no place in professional patient communications. Rushing through a message makes it difficult to follow and may also lessen the value of the message to the listener. Instead, clearly articulating each word and idea with proper diction is essential. Also, speakers should focus on volume. In a formal presentation setting with a microphone, volume can be adjusted. However, in most settings, appropriate volume is essential when conveying a message. After all, no matter how important the message is, if the recipient cannot hear it, its value may be lost.

One manner in which pharmacy technicians communicate daily with colleagues and customers is via the telephone. Telephones should be answered with a warm greeting that is welcoming to the caller and let's them know with whom they are speaking. The best communicators can transmit their positive, enthusiastic demeanor and smile across the telephone line, by the warm manner in which the telephone is answered. Answering the phone by saying "Watson's Pharmacy, Jennifer," leaves a lot to be desired. However, with a smiling face, using the greeting "Good morning! You've reached Watson's Pharmacy. This is Jennifer speaking. How may I help you today?" sends a message that is powerful and welcoming.

Telephone communication is, however, a common channel for misinterpretation. Technicians receiving patient information via telephone should take care to use **read-back verification**. When an important message is delivered on the telephone, the best communicators will read the message back and ensure that it was clearly understood. As an example, when a pharmacy technician is receiving a prescription or transfer via telephone (laws vary by state), the pharmacy technician should repeat the information about the medication being ordered and, if needed, spell out the letters in words as necessary. Note, however, that letters may be hard to hear due to poor connections, static, or heavy accents. The critical nature of medical messages should prompt the technician to spell out the word using a **phonetic alphabet** ("That's *A* as in alpha, *B* as in bravo," and so on). Numbers should also be clarified when necessary. The numbers *50* and *15* look different, as do the words *fifty* and *fifteen*. However, when spoken, these numbers can easily be mistaken. Thus, a skilled communicator will break the number down into its individual numbers for read-back verification. For a dose of 50 milligrams, the confirmation would be stated as "five-zero" to confirm the strength as fifty milligrams.

> **read-back verification** a process in which the recipient of a message speaks the message back to the sender of the message to confirm the message was received correctly
>
> **phonetic alphabet** an alphabet that is used to prevent miscommunication by spelling a word out by the way it sounds; for example, "A is for alpha, B is for bravo," etc.

Finally, take care to ensure that you have good documentation regarding the communication, including the name and return telephone number of the individual with whom you spoke, in case additional information later becomes necessary. Incomplete communication is just as dangerous as inaccurate communication. Thus, if a technician routinely finds he is leaving out important information, he might consider developing a brief script that can be kept in a lab coat pocket and referred to during a conversation to ensure all information is conveyed.

Terminology

Pharmacy terminology can be likened to learning a new language. Pharmacy technicians should work hard to immerse themselves in the pharmacy vocabulary and to master it. This may not happen overnight, but with practice and attention, the vocabulary can be learned. Mispronouncing or misspelling medication names can be interpreted by others as the technician being disinterested or uneducated. Because each medication has two names (brand and generic), a skilled technician will take the time to practice going back and forth between both names, using flash cards as necessary, or working with a pharmacist who can help.

Customer Service

A good communicator will take time to acknowledge the patient. Often, a technician might be tempted to treat people as numbers. When the first words of a greeting to a patient are "Who's next?" "Number 87," or "Date of birth?" it can be difficult to build a relationship of trust and respect. Instead, greet a customer with a simple "Hello, how are you today? I'm Chalyse. How may I help you?" When you have time, let the customer know a little bit more about yourself and find out more about them, as individuals.

Take a moment to reflect on the following two encounters, from both the perspective of a technician and a customer.

EXAMPLE

Technician: Who's next?

Patient: Hi, I'd like to pick up my prescription.

Technician: Name and date of birth.

Patient: Virginia Smith. November 24, 1983.

Technician: I have two prescriptions for Smith. That'll be twenty dollars. Sign here. Got any questions?

Patient: No.

Technician: Next!

EXAMPLE

Technician: Hello, how are you today? I'm Tameka, one of the pharmacy technicians here. How may I help you?

Patient: Hi. I'm Virginia Smith. I'd like to drop off these two prescriptions.

Technician: No problem, Ms. Smith. I'd be happy to help. Can you please confirm your date of birth, current address, and medication allergies?

Patient: November 24, 1983. 100 Elm Drive. No allergies that I know of.

Technician: Excellent! Well, it looks like I have all of your insurance information on file. I see you visited Dr. Jones. Isn't he fantastic!

Patient: Yes. He is great.

Technician: Well you picked the right pharmacy. We take care of his patients here all the time. I've been working here as a pharmacy technician for about ten years and most of our pharmacy team has worked here for even longer than that. You're in great hands. How are you feeling today?

Patient: I'm okay. Feeling a little tired. I've been at the doctor's office all day long and can't wait to get home.

Technician: I understand. I know that feeling. Please have a seat in our waiting room and relax. We should have these prescriptions filled for you in 30 minutes. If there is any change, I'll be sure to let you know.

Certainly, time may not always lend itself to such a lengthy conversation. However the basic principles apply. Take time to introduce yourself and to put the patient at ease. Remember to find out how the patient is feeling. Take time to celebrate the fantastic team that you work with. Doing so will help the customer to have a positive experience. Also, make sure to set the expectation with regards to wait time, communicating often when the promised time cannot be met. Most importantly when communicating with patients and setting expectations, you should underpromise and overdeliver. If you tell a patient that a prescription will only take 5 minutes and then the phone rings and there is a problem with the insurance claim, the patient will undoubtedly be upset, even when the circumstances were out of the technician's control. However, if a patient expects 20 minutes and the prescription is ready in 15, the customer will leave with a positive experience, feeling that she received a small gift of time back in her already busy day.

The bottom line is that patients will react poorly when treated as a number. They react well when treated with respect and when communicated with effectively. When any communication with a patient is complete, be sure to thank them. A good communicator uses "Thank you" generously.

Written Communication Skills

Written communication skills paint a picture of an individual without them being present. Discretion, then, is needed as is careful attention to detail. Concise writing is often warranted in health care. Make messages short, clear, and accurate.

Consult online templates for assistance with formal correspondence. Generally speaking, written communication needs to be at least as formal, if not more formal, than oral communications. Many times, written communications leave a lasting impression about the level of professionalism and education of the writer. Thus, take time to read and reread the printed words. Do not rely on an automatic spell-checker as the sole check for correct spelling. When in doubt, consult a dictionary. Above all, avoid typos. An obvious typo in a paper may stand out far more than the actual content of the message.

Electronic Communication

As electronic communication continues to become the accepted norm, be very cautious when sending e-mails in a professional environment. Separate your work and personal e-mails—it is not professional to mix personal business with your work. Be wary of the "Reply to All" feature, because unintended messages can easily reach a large audience with a simple click of a button. Pay careful attention to whom messages are addressed to before pressing "send." Remember, it is next to impossible to retrieve a message once it has been sent. Writing an e-mail when angry or emotionally stirred up can result in regret or be a career-limiting move. Take the time to cool down and reread a message carefully prior to pressing "Send." Use caution when sharing patient information over electronic communications and be sure to consult your institution's policy for this type of information exchange. Protecting patient confidentiality should be a priority; thus be very careful about what printed information is shared. Be sure to destroy all patient information as soon as it is no longer necessary. Failing to do so can lead to a breach in confidentiality and can put the pharmacy technician, pharmacist, and pharmacy at risk for substantial penalties.

Additionally, social media is an excellent tool to quickly disseminate information to a large population and to connect people in new and varied ways. For all of its benefits, however, social media can have potentially negative or unintended consequences with respect to health care. Care should be taken to avoid disparaging talk about patients or employers on social media. Additionally, no protected health information should be shared.

Nonverbal Communication Skills

Body language may be the most important thing never said. It communicates a message in a manner that words may not adequately describe. It allows patients to understand that pharmacy technicians care about them as people, and while they are in the pharmacy, they are the top priority. Appropriate body language can be used to display kindness, humility, and empathy. A gentle touch on the arm or shoulder, when appropriate, or kindly expression can be consoling to a patient experiencing grief. Folding arms can portray arrogance. A facial grimace and rolling eyes can show disinterest or disrespect. Avoid slouching or body language that portrays a lack of poise. Instead keep a balanced posture with shoulders square toward the individual or audience. A brief glance at a watch or clock may indicate boredom or the need to conclude a conversation. Holding one's head up with a hand may make an individual appear lazy or tired. A speaker with poor eye contact comes across as uninterested and unconfident. Looking a customer or colleague in the eye, without staring, allows a connection that sends a powerful message. A firm handshake and a bright smile are appropriate and appealing during an initial greeting, and can often soften a disgruntled customer. These basic examples all demonstrate the power of body language. The best communicators use nonverbal communication to engage their audience and to show respect.

The Job Interview

The job interview is the ultimate test of oral, written, and nonverbal communication skills. An employer assesses a candidate's communication skills as much as his knowledge and abilities. Employers are interested in building a team that communicates well, has a positive spirit, and treats customers and patients with respect. Because many candidates have similar skills on paper, the job interview is where candidates can show true differentiation.

When interviewing, a candidate should use the potential employer's formal title when addressing the person, until given permission otherwise. A candidate should speak with confidence regarding past and current experiences. Ensure that answers to questions are well thought out and complete. Employers are looking for more than one-word answers, so elaborate on answers in a clear and concise manner. Avoid the frequent use of word whiskers (um, uh, etc.).

Many employers will ask an interviewee to tell them about an experience at her past place of employment that illustrates a particular skill. One suggestion is to have mentally prepared a collection of stories that can be easily adapted to any question. These might be stories about a time when the candidate went above and beyond for a patient or completed a project that led to cost savings or improved efficiency within the pharmacy. A skilled communicator will practice sample questions with a friend or respected colleague prior to the interview. Having practiced concise responses to several sample questions will allow communication skills to shine.

To effectively communicate on a job interview, a candidate needs to fine tune her listening skills. Be sure to understand exactly what is being asked, clarifying if necessary, and responding in turn. Finally, when an employer asks a candidate whether she has any questions, a skilled communicator will ask an educated question that shows interest and that she has been listening to the conversation.

As far as written communication skills are concerned on a job interview, a current curriculum vitae or resume should be provided. This document should be carefully prepared. Interviewees should consider asking a trusted friend, colleague, or career mentor to provide a review and feedback. Employers often require a cover letter. Rather than use a standard cover letter for many positions, prepare a customized cover letter for each employer. Within the cover letter, be specific and include why you are interested in the specific job with the particular employer/company, and what skills you possess that make you an ideal candidate for the position.

Finally, to be successful on a job interview, a candidate will want to maintain good eye contact with the potential employer, have a firm handshake at the beginning and end of the interview, and maintain a smile and positive demeanor.

Communication Barriers

Several barriers exist to good communication between colleagues. Avoiding or overcoming these barriers can transform a work environment.

Time

One common barrier to good communication is time. We may not feel that we have enough time to make every patient feel like a priority. Several telephones ringing at the same time or requests for information coming from several directions simultaneously could cause poor communication. However, a simple prevailing principle should apply. Patients' lives are at stake. Thus, a good communicator will make time for each patient, asking a supervisor or peers for help when patient care is in jeopardy.

Listening

Good communication starts with good listening skills. In a busy pharmacy, it can be very easy to spend more time talking than listening. A high-performing communicator, however, will spend time listening to ensure he understands the complete set of facts. Asking specifically targeted questions to help obtain appropriate information is essential. Often, pharmacists rely on information obtained by technicians in order to provide the highest level of patient care. Failing to listen effectively can result in incomplete or inaccurate information that can adversely impact the patient.

Gossip

Next, working in a pharmacy may mean interacting with only a few people per day, or may mean working with dozens of different people during each shift. A positive and enthusiastic personality and a can-do attitude are critical. Certain types of communication, such as gossip or half-truths, can be toxic to the workplace. It can make the workplace environment unpleasant and uncomfortable. When exposed to such an environment, some individuals may look for alternative employment, not because they dislike their job, but because the communication has reached an unacceptable level. Avoid participating in such negative communication and set the example by encouraging others to focus on the patients.

Stereotyping

Also, pharmacy technicians should avoid stereotyping other health care professionals. If a particular physician is difficult to work with at times, a skilled communicator will not take out her frustration on others and will recognize that, although being negative is not appropriate, it may be a part of a bigger picture for which she may not have all of the facts. Keeping in mind that there is often more to a situation than meets the eye is important. For instance, a particularly grumpy patient may have just received some bad news about his health. An angry physician may have just come from the hospital after having to tell someone's family members that their loved one has died. A demanding nurse may be taking care of a patient who desperately needs a medication from the pharmacy to take care of an emergency situation. Skilled communicators will always respond positively and professionally, even when the recipient does not respond in kind.

Cultural Competency

One final barrier to the effective use of communication skills that must be considered is cultural and background differences. Living in an increasingly multicultural population and working in a customer service industry, pharmacy technicians must be sensitive to the needs of a wide range of patients. Heavy accents or unique dialects, religious customs or observances, language differences, and sexual orientation are just a few of the cultural and lifestyle differences that must be considered when communicating with patients. Failure to do so could result in a poor patient experience or, worse yet, a poor patient health outcome. Pharmacy technicians must remain nonjudgmental regarding the choices and decisions of patients and work hard to provide consistent services regardless of one's personal preferences. Additionally, techs may find it helpful to have a good working understanding of the backgrounds, values, and customs that affect health care decisions for the common patient populations encountered in their particular area. Being informed about different customs and lifestyles is a key step to gaining cultural competence and, thus, providing consistent, high-quality care. Try to keep resources handy that might be helpful when working with patients from different backgrounds and be familiar with organizational references specifically designed for reaching out to individuals who have unique communication needs.

Summary

As the profession of pharmacy advances, pharmacy technicians will be increasingly called on to advance and expand their skills. To meet that challenge, the development of comprehensive oral, written, and nonverbal communication skills is essential. Pharmacy technicians are often the face of the pharmacy and, thus, the reputation of the pharmacy team and the overall patient or customer experience may very likely be dependent on positive communications.

TEST YOUR KNOWLEDGE

Multiple Choice

1. Which of the following represents an example of communication skills?
   a. an in-service on a newly approved medication
   b. a compassionate response to someone who just received bad news
   c. an e-mail to a manager about a performance improvement idea
   d. all of the above
2. Which of the following is an example of nonverbal communication?
   a. handshake
   b. telephone call
   c. typos
   d. none of the above
3. Which of the following is a common barrier to communication skills?
   a. a perceived lack of time
   b. stereotyping
   c. rumors
   d. all of the above

4. Eye contact is an example of what type of communication?
   a. oral
   b. nonverbal
   c. written
   d. none of the above

True/False

1. Sharing patient information on social media is permissible as long as the patient cannot view it.
2. Electronic spelling correction programs are sufficient for proofreading written communications.
3. Read-back verification should not be used in retail pharmacies because it takes too long.
4. Job interviews are an excellent way to showcase all three types of communications skills.

References

DeCoske, M. A., & White, S. J. (2010). Public speaking revisited: Delivery, structure, and style. *American Journal of Health-System Pharmacy, 67*(15), 1225–1227.

Kallos, J. (2007). *Email etiquette, made easy.* Retrieved from http://www.emailetiquettemadeeasy.com

Reinders, T. P. (2011). *The pharmacy professional's guide to resumes, CVs and interviewing* (3rd ed.). Washington, DC: American Pharmacists Association.

CHAPTER

32

Reimbursement for Pharmacy Services

Competencies

Upon completion of this chapter, the reader should be able to:

1. Describe the trends in the costs of pharmaceuticals since 1990.
2. Compare the roles of private versus publicly funded prescription drug plans.
3. Explain the different measures that pharmacy benefit managers use in reimbursement formulas.
4. Differentiate between the three methods of patient cost sharing for prescription drugs.
5. Discuss the various strategies employed by pharmacy benefit managers to reduce drug costs.
6. Describe the different billing methods employed in long-term care, home health care, and institutional pharmacy settings.

Key Terms

coinsurance
copayments
deductibles
dispensing fee
formulary
medication therapy management (MTM)
National Drug Code (NDC)
pharmacy benefit manager (PBM)
prior authorization
step therapy
tiered copayment schedules

Introduction

Prescription drug expenditures have been one of the fastest rising health care costs during the past 20 years. The majority of prescription drug expenditures are paid for by some form of health insurance, be it a private form of health insurance or a government-sponsored program such as Medicare or Medicaid. Medicare is funded by the federal government and provides coverage for hospitalization and medical expenses to those who are 65 years of age or older and for certain people under the age of 65 who have disabilities. Medicaid is also a federal program that is financed by federal and state funds. Medicaid provides coverage for hospitalization and medical expenses for persons of all ages within certain income limits. As costs have risen, insurance companies have modified prescription drug insurance plans to reduce the costs of prescription drug coverage. These modifications have served to curtail the growth of spending for prescription drugs. However, some of the changes to prescription drugs plans have left consumers confused at pharmacies about what is covered by their prescription drug plan and how much they will have to contribute for the payment of prescription drugs.

This chapter first provides an overview of prescription drug plans and then offers an historical perspective on rising drug costs and the various types of prescription drugs plans. Next, we describe the methodologies used for the payment of prescription drugs in the following health care settings: community pharmacies, long-term care facilities, home care pharmacies, and institutional or hospital pharmacies.

Overview of Prescription Drug Plans

The rate of spending for prescription drugs in the United States has risen from $40.3 billion in 1990 to $234.1 billion in 2008. For a period of time since 2000, prescription drug spending declined, only to increase again with the implementation of Medicare Part D in January 2006. **Figure 32-1** illustrates the annual percentage of spending for prescription drugs from 1996 to 2008, compared to two other components of health care spending: hospital care and physician services.

As drug spending rose, so did the payment of prescription drug expenses by health insurance plans. Most health insurance companies have chosen to

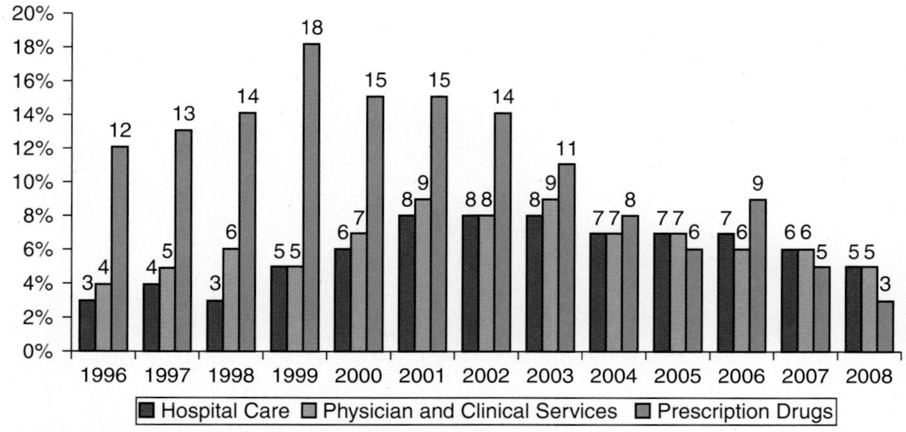

Historical data from *National Health Expenditure* report of the Centers for Medicare and Medicaid Services, http://www.cms.hhs.gov/NationalHealthExpendData.

FIGURE 32-1 Average annual percentage change in selected national health expenditures, 1996–2008.

pharmacy benefit manager (PBM) a provider of prescription drug programs; can be a third-party administrator or part of an integrated healthcare system

separate, or "carve out," coverage for prescription drug benefits from health insurance plans. Health insurance companies and employers have contracted with **pharmacy benefit managers (PBMs)**, also known as *third-party plans*, for the administration of prescription drug insurance plans. Pharmacy benefit management companies specialize in the administration of prescription drug plans. They typically manage prescription drug benefits for millions of individuals, known as *members* of a prescription drug plan. They have become very efficient at providing all of the management functions associated with prescription drug plans, including contracting with pharmacies to supply pharmacy services, payment of claims to pharmacies for prescriptions, and managing the utilization of prescription drugs by plan members. Payments by prescription drug plans have increased dramatically since 1990. **Figure 32-2** illustrates the increase in payments for prescription drugs by private or public insurance plans and the significant decrease in consumer spending for prescription drugs.

As illustrated in Figure 32-2, public and private health insurance programs increased their coverage and payment for prescription drugs, resulting in consumers paying less out of their own funds for prescription drugs. Private health insurance plans, most of which are employer sponsored, provided coverage for 58% of Americans in 2008. Nearly all of the workers covered by employer-sponsored plans have a prescription drug benefit. Employers are often referred to as *plan sponsors*.

Publicly funded programs also pay a significant portion of the national expenditures for prescription drugs. Publicly funded expenditures increased significantly in 2006 with the implementation of the Medicare Part D program. This program was created by the Medicare Prescription Drug, Improvement, and Modernization Act of 2003. This act provided for prescription drug coverage for those eligible for the Medicare program through the establishment of the Medicare Part D program. Medicare Part D plan members are referred to as *beneficiaries*. As of 2010, 41.8 million of the 46.6 million eligible Medicare beneficiaries had drug coverage. This enrollment was distributed as follows:

- Medicare Part D: 27.7 million
- Employer, union retiree, TRICARE, or Veteran's Administration plans: 14.2 million
- No drug coverage: 4.7 million.

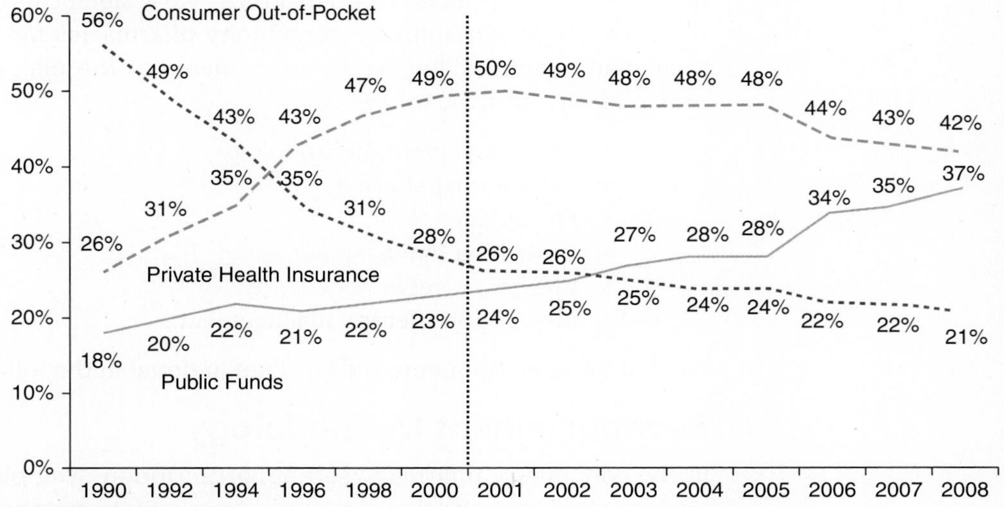

Historical data from *National Health Expenditure* report of the Centers for Medicare and Medicaid Services, http://www.cms.hhs.gov/NationalHealthExpendData.

FIGURE 32-2 Distribution of total national prescription drug expenditures by type of payer, 1990–2008.

Private insurance and Medicare Part D plans operate on a contract year basis. This means that every year, plans establish what they will cover and how they will reimburse for covered products and services for the upcoming contract year.

Medicaid is another public insurance program. It is a joint federal-state program that provides coverage for medical care to approximately 60 million Americans. The Centers for Medicare and Medicaid Services (CMS) is a federal agency that regulates the Medicare and the Medicaid programs. CMS has established a list of health care services that must be covered by Medicaid and a list of optional services that states may include in their Medicaid programs. Although prescription drug coverage is considered an optional service by CMS, all states include prescription drug coverage in their Medicaid programs. Coverage terms vary significantly, however, from state to state.

Reimbursement Methodologies of Prescription Drug Plans

Prescription drug plans vary in their coverage of and payment for prescription drugs. Differences in plan design exist across various pharmacy practice settings (community, home health care, etc.) and within pharmacy practice settings. One of the major reasons for this difference in plan design is the fact that employers are the primary source of health insurance coverage. Employers typically provide health insurance coverage as a benefit to full-time employees, and they typically are looking for the ways to provide their employees and their dependents (such as a spouse or child) with the most coverage at the most reasonable cost. The differences in plan design include differences in how much the consumer pays for drugs, how prescription drugs are billed to insurance plans, how PBMs reimburse pharmacies for the drugs they dispense, and how plans contract with pharmacies who participate in the drug plan.

The balance of this chapter examines prescription drug benefit design for community practice, home health care pharmacy services, long-term care pharmacy, and institutional (or hospital) pharmacy.

Community Pharmacy

Prescription drug plans, through PBMs, vary significantly from plan to plan in terms of how they reimburse community pharmacies for the drugs dispensed to their plan members. Important components of the plan design for prescription drug plans include the following:

- Reimbursement methodology
- Patient cost sharing
- Formulary
- Utilization management
- Pharmacy networks
- Medication therapy management

Each of these components is described in detail in the following sections.

Reimbursement Methodology

In the community pharmacy setting, prescription drug plans reimburse pharmacies for every prescription dispensed to one of its members or their dependents. Typically, PBMs set reimbursement as the lower of the following: the usual and customary price or the price calculated through a reimbursement formula. The usual and customary price is also known as the cash price and is the price charged to cash customers, or those individuals who do not have prescription drug coverage. Typically, reimbursement is based on a reimbursement formula. Reimbursement formulas use three components:

Payment to pharmacies = (ingredient cost + dispensing free) − patient cost sharing
(reimbursement) (drug cost)

These three components—ingredient cost, dispensing fee, and patient cost sharing—are part of every prescription drug claim that is submitted to a PBM for reimbursement. Each of the three components of this reimbursement equation is examined in the following subsections.

Ingredient Cost

The ingredient cost component of the reimbursement formula represents the cost of the drug dispensed to the patient. Pharmacies bill for the cost of the drug by submitting a **National Drug Code (NDC)** on the claim sent to the plan for payment. NDC numbers are 11 digits long and unique to each drug product, strength, and package size:

National Drug Code (NDC) a unique 11-digit identifier for a drug's product, strength, and package size

11111	–	2222	–	33
(drug)		(drug strength)		(package size)

When entering NDC number information into a computer system to bill a drug claim, you must do so accurately so that the PBM can pay the correct amount for the ingredient cost component of each claim.

Typically, PBMs reimburse the ingredient cost of a claim on the basis of the average wholesale price (AWP). The AWP is a price published by drug manufacturers in a number of drug pricing publications and electronic reference files. The AWP is higher than the actual cost paid by pharmacies to purchase the drug. Pharmacies typically receive discounts off of the AWP from manufacturers and wholesalers, which lower a pharmacy's actual acquisition cost of the drug. Actual acquisition costs vary from pharmacy to pharmacy so that information is not published in any reference. PBMs attempt to manage drug costs for plan sponsors by reimbursing pharmacies at a rate as close to the actual acquisition cost as possible. They approximate the actual acquisition cost (AAC) through an estimate. This estimate is calculated by subtracting a set percentage from the AWP. This results in a new reimbursement formula:

Payment to pharmacies = [(AWP − x%) + dispensing free] − patient cost sharing
(reimbursement) (drug cost)

This revised reimbursement formula represents the methodology most widely used in practice.

As drug prices have risen during recent years, PBMs have tried to use other methods to estimate the actual acquisition costs paid by pharmacies for drugs. One other method worth consideration is one based on the wholesale acquisition cost (WAC). The WAC is defined by the federal government's guidelines as the manufacturer's published price to wholesalers and other purchasers in the United States. As is the case with AWP, the WAC does not take into account any discounts received by the wholesalers from manufacturers. PBMs use the WAC measure to estimate what a pharmacy has paid a wholesaler for a drug based on what the wholesaler paid to acquire the drug. Since wholesalers will charge pharmacies a higher price for a drug than what they paid to acquire it, PBMs often add a set percentage to the WAC to estimate a pharmacy's AAC. A reimbursement formula that utilizes the WAC to estimate acquisition cost would be:

Payment to pharmacies = [(WAC − x%) + dispensing free] − patient cost sharing
(reimbursement) (drug cost)

PBMs often reimburse pharmacies for generic drugs using other measures of cost. Brand name drug products may have more than one generic equivalent. When a brand name drug has generic equivalents, PBMs often limit the reimbursement of a generic drug to the price of the generic equivalent most commonly used. That price is then referred to as the maximum allowable cost (MAC) for the generic product. Each prescription drug plan establishes MAC prices for each generic drug. In addition, the federal government publishes a list of MAC prices for selected generic drugs. For all generic versions of a drug, a PBM will pay the MAC price, regardless of the drug's actual cost. MAC prices are also calculated for all multisource drugs, which are brand name drugs and at least one generic equivalent. As a result, the calculated MAC price may be used for reimbursement for the brand name drug and the generic equivalent(s). In cases where a patient requests that a brand nam drug be dispensed and MAC pricing is used for reimbursement, pharmacies are often required to collect the difference between the MAC price and the cost of the brand name drug from the patient.

The Medicaid program also establishes limits on what it will pay for generic equivalents and for reimbursement of multisource drugs. The federal government uses the term *federal upper limit* (FUL) instead of maximum allowable cost (MAC). In the past, Medicaid has used established MACs for each product as a basis for reimbursement.

Federal legislation passed in 2005 specified that reimbursement for generic drugs in the Medicaid program should be based on the average manufacturer price (AMP). The AMP for a drug is the average price received by a manufacturer from a wholesaler for drugs that are distributed by the wholesalers to pharmacies classified by the federal government as a *retail class of trade*. Retail class of trade pharmacies sell drugs to the general public and include chain pharmacies, independent pharmacies, and mail-order pharmacies. The AMP level of reimbursement for generic drugs is significantly less than previously established rates (FUL or MAC) for reimbursement. Pharmacy associations representing retail pharmacies were successful in blocking the implementation of AMP for reimbursement of generic drugs. In 2010, the Patient Protection and Affordable Care Act redefined the calculation of AMP prices. The result of this modification is that AMP prices will not reduce reimbursement to pharmacies to the extent originally planned. As a result of this modification, it remains to be seen if CMS, which sets the regulations and reimbursement formulas for Medicare and Medicaid, will ever adopt AMP pricing for multisource drugs paid by the Medicaid program.

Table 32-1 provides a review of the different pricing methods used for the reimbursement of generic drugs.

Dispensing Fee

dispensing fee the fee charged by a pharmacy for the cost of dispensing a prescription

The **dispensing fee** component of the reimbursement formula is intended to reimburse pharmacies for the cost of dispensing a prescription. In addition to the cost of the drug dispensed, many other costs are associated with filling a prescription such as labor costs, the cost of utilities, rent expense for the pharmacies, and insurance premiums. One way to understand the costs associated with filling a prescription is to categorize them as *fixed, semifixed,* or *variable.*

TABLE 32-1 Pricing Methods Used for Reimbursement of Generic Drugs

METHODOLOGY	DEFINITION
Actual acquisition cost (AAC)	• Price that a pharmacy actually pays to purchase a drug • Price that PBMs want to use to reimburse pharmacies for a drug • Not published
Average wholesale price (AWP)	• Price published by the drug manufacturer • Higher than the price actually paid by the pharmacy for the drug • Often reduced by a percentage to estimate actual acquisition cost
Wholesale acquisition cost (WAC)	• Published manufacturer's price to wholesalers • Does not reflect any rebates or discounts • Percentage usually added to WAC to estimate pharmacy's actual cost
Maximum allowable cost (MAC)	• Used for reimbursement of multisource drugs (brand name drugs with at least one generic equivalent) • Some plans limit reimbursement of multisource drugs to the price of the most commonly dispensed generic equivalent
Average manufacturer price (AMP)	• Price paid by wholesalers to manufacturers for drugs distributed to pharmacies classified as retail class of trade • Lower rates that other established rates; would significantly reduce reimbursement to pharmacies • Rates recently revised to higher rates of reimbursement than originally planned

TABLE 32-2 Examples of Dispensing Costs

TYPE OF COST	EXAMPLE
Fixed	• Property insurance • Property taxes • Rent
Semifixed	• Hours available to schedule pharmacists • Hours available to schedule technicians
Variable	• Prescription vials • Prescription labels

Fixed costs, as the term implies, are costs that do not change with changes in prescription volume (the number of prescriptions). *Semifixed* costs are costs that change only with significant changes in prescription volume. *Variable* costs change in proportion to any change in prescription volume. Examples of fixed, semifixed, and variable costs are provided in **Table 32-2**.

The dispensing fees paid by plans are meant to cover all of the fixed, semifixed, and variable costs associated with filing a prescription. This has been disputed by pharmacy organizations, which have studied the costs associated with filling a prescription and maintain that dispensing fees only partially cover dispensing costs.

Patient Cost Sharing

The third component of the reimbursement formula is patient cost sharing. Patients are required to pay some portion of the cost of prescriptions. Patient cost sharing reduces the amount paid by the PBM for prescriptions on behalf of the plan sponsor. PBMs typically link patient cost sharing to the type of drug dispensed. For example, cost sharing for a generic drug is lower than that for a brand name drug. (This concept of linking patient cost sharing to the type of drug dispensed is discussed later in this chapter.) Three different types of patient cost sharing modules used in prescription drug plans: deductibles, copayments, and coinsurance.

deductible a set dollar amount that must be paid by the patient before an insurance plan will begin to cover prescription costs

A **deductible** is a set dollar amount that must be paid by the patient before an insurance plan will begin to cover prescription costs. If a prescription plan requires patients to pay a deductible, patients will be required to pay for the entire cost of their prescriptions (ingredient cost plus dispensing fee) until they have paid an amount equal to the total deductible. For example, if a drug plan has a $500 deductible, each plan member has to pay the total price for each prescription until they have paid an amount equal to $500. Once the $500 has been paid by a patient, the plan will begin to cover some or all of the costs for prescriptions obtained by the patient. Deductibles are set for and begin with each contract year. Therefore, plan members have to satisfy a deductible every year.

copayment a set dollar amount that a patient must pay every time he or she obtains a prescription

coinsurance a set percentage of the cost of a prescription that the patient must pay

Copayments are the most widely used method of patient cost sharing. Copayments are a set dollar amount that a patient must pay every time he or she obtains a prescription. The plan will reimburse the pharmacy for the remaining dollar amount of the claim.

Coinsurance is a set percentage of the cost of a prescription that must be paid by the patient. For example, if a plan has a coinsurance rate of 20%, then patients will pay 20% of the price for each prescription they obtain. The plan will reimburse the pharmacy for the remaining dollar amount of the claim.

As the price of prescriptions has increased, plan sponsors have worked with PBMs to find ways to reduce or control drug costs. Copayments have increased steadily since 2000. Also, coinsurance has become more popular because as drug prices increase, the patient's share will also increase because the coinsurance rate applies to the entire cost of the claim.

Formularies

formulary a listing of drugs approved by the medical staff of a hospital or a health care system for use within their institution or by health care insurers as determined by the safety, efficacy, effectiveness, and cost of the drugs

PBMs use drug formularies to control drug costs for their plan sponsors. **Formularies** are listings of drugs that are covered by an insurance plan. When designing a formulary, PBMs examine the benefits and costs of drugs. PBMs typically establish a Pharmacy and Therapeutics (P&T) Committee, which is comprised of physicians and pharmacists who evaluate the scientific literature and make decisions as to whether a drug should be covered by a plan. These decisions are made after a thorough evaluation of the literature. Formularies are explained in detail in Chapter 28.

Formularies list drugs as:

- Generics
- Preferred brand name drugs
- Nonpreferred brand name drugs
- Specialty or lifestyle drugs.

tiered copayment schedule a prescription drug payment schedule that aligns the amount of a copayment to the formulary tier of the drug dispensed

Preferred brand name drugs are brand name drugs that are deemed to be cost effective by the P&T committee and the PBM. In an effort to control drug costs, PBMs encourage patients to use generic drugs and preferred brand name drugs. To achieve this goal, copayment schedules have been coordinated with the formulary categories to form a **tiered copayment schedule**. With this type of schedule, the lowest copayment category is for generic drugs (tier 1), followed by preferred brand name drugs (tier 2), and nonpreferred brand name drugs (tier 3).

Some plans have a three-tier system, while other plans have adopted a four-tier schedule, which includes a fourth tier for specialty or lifestyle drugs, which are typically very expensive.

Formularies may be classified as *open*, *incented*, or *closed*. With an open formulary, a plan will pay for all drugs. With an incented formulary, patients are encouraged through lower copayments to use generics and preferred brand name drugs. With a closed formulary, only drugs listed on the formulary are covered. As prescription drug costs have risen, tiered formulary systems have replaced the open and closed formulary models.

Utilization Management

In addition to patient cost sharing, plans also employ other strategies to reduce costs. A description of commonly used methods is provided next.

Quantity Limits

Plans may dictate a limit on the amount of medication dispensed per prescription. These limits are in place to reduce waste in the event that a drug is discontinued by a physician or fraud. Usually, a patient may not receive more than a 30-day supply of a medication at a time from a community pharmacy. A patient may not receive more than a 90-day supply from a mail-order pharmacy.

Prior Authorization

prior authorization a request to a pharmacy benefit manager to cover the cost of a drug that is outside the formulary

Prior authorization programs are designed to allow physicians to prescribe noncovered or nonpreferred drugs for their patients. A physician must contact the PBM to request permission to prescribe a noncovered prescription for a patient or to request that a patient be allowed to obtain a nonpreferred drug for a lower, preferred drug copayment.

Step Therapy

step therapy a system designed to allow physicians to first try the least expensive drug alternative before progressing to more expensive alternatives to treat diagnosed conditions

Step therapy programs have been used to encourage physicians and their patients to first try less expensive drugs before using a more expensive drug used to treat the same condition. If the patient tries the less expensive drug and the drug does not adequately treat the condition, the plan will authorize payment for the more expensive drug. Step therapy models are often used for certain drug classes that include new expensive drugs and less expensive alternatives such as generic drugs or over-the-counter (OTC) drugs. Examples of such drug classes are drugs used to treat insomnia, gastroesophageal reflux disease (GERD), and intranasal steroids to treat allergies. Using GERD as an example, step therapy would be employed as shown in **Figure 32-3**.

Step therapy requires that meticulous records be kept of the patient's history in each phase of this process. These notes may be maintained in the pharmacy's computer system and/or in a database that is maintained by the third-party plan. In addition, notes can be maintained by the physician in the patient's chart and submitted to the third-party plan.

If a physician wants a patient to take a particular prescription drug and does not want his or her patient to go through the step therapy process, the physician must write to the third-party plan to request an override of the step therapy requirement. If the override is granted, the patient may receive the prescription drug requested by the physician for the copayment amount established for the drug.

Technicians play a key role in step therapy. Technicians assist in this process by first explaining step therapy to patients and answering questions. It is important to stress to patients that step therapy is instituted as a means to reduce health

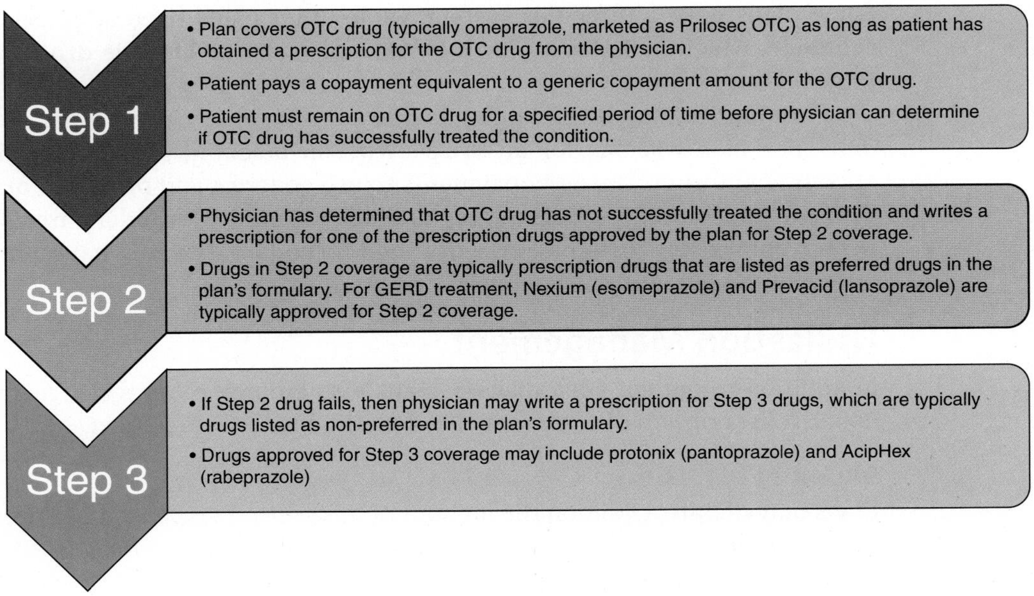

FIGURE 32-3 Step therapy using GERD as an example.

care costs and that step therapy protocols are designed by physicians and pharmacists with patients' well-being in mind. Technicians also play an important role in documenting each step of the process in the patient's history in the pharmacy computer system.

Pharmacy Networks

As previously stated, health insurance plans, including prescription drug plans, operate on a contract year basis. PBMs contract with pharmacies for their services. Contracts specify how pharmacies will be reimbursed, how often they will be paid, which drugs will be covered by the plan, and who will be covered by the plan. Pharmacies that agree to the terms of the contract are part of a pharmacy network. Plan members must patronize a pharmacy in the network in order to receive the benefits of their drug plan.

Medication Therapy Management

medication therapy management (MTM) a distinct service or group of services that optimize therapeutic outcomes for individual patients; these services are independent of, but can occur in conjunction with, the provision of a medication product

Medication therapy management (MTM) is a comprehensive approach to patient care that is proactive in nature. The goal of MTM is to manage drug therapy so that patients can benefit from the best possible outcome. This is accomplished through a variety of ways, including educating patients about their drug therapy, talking to them about the importance of compliance with their therapy, offering wellness programs that often provide screening services, and assisting with the management of diseases.

MTM is the latest step in the evolution of the pharmacist's role from being primarily a dispenser of medication to a provider of pharmacy products and services. Pharmacists may bill and receive reimbursement for their MTM services. Payment for MTM services has accelerated greatly since the implementation of the Medicare Part D program in 2006. The regulations that created this program required each plan to provide and reimburse for MTM services. Each plan can design its MTM program as it wishes.

Although pharmacists are playing a major role in the provision of MTM services, some plans have opted to provide services using nurses and other health professionals. Some MTM services take place in a face-to-face setting, such as a consultation in a pharmacy. Other plans use call centers staffed by health professionals to conduct interviews with patients. Although plans have some latitude in the design of their MTM programs, the criteria used to determine eligibility for MTM services is standard and required for all plans. MTM services must be provided for beneficiaries who have multiple chronic conditions, are using multiple medications for chronic conditions, and have annual drug costs that exceed a predetermined threshold. The threshold is established annually by the CMS. For 2012, this eligibility threshold was $3,000 or greater.

MTM services are billed using the Current Procedural Terminology (CPT) codes. These codes were originally established by the American Medical Association so that physicians would have a standard method of billing for services. The CPT codes are widely used by physicians, laboratories, radiology centers, and other health care providers to bill for procedures performed. In recent years, a series of CPT codes have been established for pharmacists to use when billing for MTM services.

In addition to providing a CPT code, the pharmacist may also provide a National Provider Identifier (NPI) number. The NPI number is 10 digits in length and specific to the pharmacy provider. If a pharmacy is the billing unit, then the pharmacy's NPI number must be used in billing. If a pharmacist is the billing unit, then the pharmacist must use his or her NPI number when billing. The Medicare Part D program has spurred the growth of the payment of MTM services provided by pharmacists. Other health insurance programs have begun to follow suit by paying pharmacists for MTM services.

Long-Term Care Pharmacies

Long-term care (LTC) is defined as a "set of health, personal care, and social services delivered over a sustained period of time to persons who have lost or never acquired some degree of functional capacity." Long-term care services may be provided in the home, adult day care centers, retirement homes, and nursing homes in additional to other settings. Individuals who required LTC services are primarily the elderly. Approximately 70% of those over 65 years of age will require LTC at some point in their lifetime (U.S. Department of Health and Human Services, 2009).

Reimbursement for LTC services, including pharmacy services, may be paid by Medicare, Medicaid, private insurance, or by the patient. For those covered by Medicare, the type of service provided or the setting in which services are delivered will determine the payer of prescription drugs. If a patient receives prescription drugs in a nursing facility, the time when the patient received the drugs will also determine the payer. Medicare Part A (which covers care provided in an institutional setting) will pay for nursing home care if a beneficiary has spent at least 3 days in a hospital and then immediately goes from the hospital to a nursing home. Medicare will pay 100% of the cost for the first 20 days of long-term care in a nursing home, then the patient will have to pay a copayment for days 21 to 100. Medicare payments during this period also include payments for medications. Medicare will not pay any services delivered after the first 100 days of nursing home care. After this time period, Medicare Part D will pay for any prescription drugs administered to patients.

Medicaid will pay for LTC services for those who financially qualify for Medicaid benefits. Frequently, nursing home residents qualify for Medicaid coverage of LTC services after they have exhausted their own personal finances. Typically, patients covered by Medicaid for nursing home services have prescription drug coverage through a Medicare Part D plan. In other words, Medicaid pays for all services with the exception of prescription drugs, which are covered by Medicare Part D.

As is the case in the community pharmacy setting, formularies play a role in the management of drug costs. Patients in a LTC setting may require a nonformulary drug or a drug that is not on the approved list of drugs covered by the Medicare Part D plan. Each Medicare Part D plan has an appeals process for physicians and their patients to use to obtain coverage for noncovered drugs. Approval of reimbursement for noncovered drugs must be obtained before the drug may be dispensed to the patient. Accuracy when billing the Part D plan for nonformulary drugs is important so that the claim may be properly processed and reimbursed. Please refer to Chapter 4 for more information on long-term care.

Home Health Care Pharmacy

Home health services are typically provided by home health agencies. These services include nursing care, physical therapy, speech therapy, and rehabilitation services. Home health care services allow a patient to recover from illness in a familiar setting: the home. Many insurance plans reimburse home health providers for their services. Each plan, whether public or private, has specified what it will cover, its billing procedures, and the reimbursement rates. Generally speaking, private insurance plans cover more home health care services than public plans.

Billing for home health care products and services is done through the use of the billing codes shown in **Table 32-3**.

Different plans have different requirements for the billing of home health care services. Reimbursement rates also vary from plan to plan. Due to the significant variation in billing practices, pharmacy technicians must understand what is covered by each plan and the billing guidelines specific to each plan. Please refer to Chapter 3 for more information on home health care.

TABLE 32-3 Home Health Care Billing Codes

CODE TYPE	MEANING
J codes	• Used to bill drugs to Medicare • Used for drugs that cannot be self-administered • *Example:* J0120 is the code for "injection, tetracycline, up to 250 mg"
K codes	• Used to bill for certain noncompounded services • Used to bill or devices needed for drug therapy • *Example:* K0552 is the code used for "external drug infusion pump, syringe type cartridge, sterile"
S codes	• Used to bill drugs to Blue Cross/Blue Shield and other commercial (non-Medicare) carriers • Also used for drugs that cannot be self-administered • *Example:* S0093 is the code used for "injection, morphine sulfate 500 mg (loading dose for infusion pump)

Hospital or Institutional Setting

The most common method of reimbursement for inpatient care (care delivered while a patient is in a hospital) is a form of prospective reimbursement. Prospective reimbursement systems specify what a plan will pay for care in advance of a contract year. By doing so, the plans establish a limit on the maximum amount of money they will pay for an inpatient visit. As a result of prospective reimbursement systems, hospitals know in advance what each plan will pay for each type of care or case.

The goal for hospitals is to provide care for each case in an efficient way so that the costs of services during a visit do not exceed the predetermined rate of reimbursement. Some prospective systems use capitated rates (per person) based on a per diem charge (per day). Others use a case-based rate, which establishes payment based on the patient's diagnoses. Diagnosis-related groups (DRGs) are an example of a case-based method of prospective reimbursement. DRG codes are specific to disease of organ systems. For example, DRG codes with values of 326 to 395 cover disease and disorders of the digestive system.

Prospective reimbursement rates are established at the beginning of a contract year. The rates are fixed, meaning that hospitals will receive only the published rate as payment for a visit of care, even if the total cost to provide care of a patient exceeds the published rate. Therefore, hospitals strive to keep the cost of care for patients to an amount that is in alignment with the reimbursement rate for that particular type of care. Hospital pharmacies play a major role in helping hospitals to achieve this goal. The cost of pharmaceuticals typically used in an inpatient setting have escalated, as have all drugs. To keep costs under control in the institutional setting, hospitals establish formularies. Adherence to the formulary when dispensing medication to patients helps to control costs. In addition to formularies, hospital pharmacies often utilize dispensing protocols, which specify which drugs should be tried before an expensive product is dispensed. When hospital pharmacies purchase drugs, they often solicit bids for manufacturers to obtain the best possible pricing. This enables the pharmacy to provide drugs to the patients in a cost-efficient manner.

Summary

During the past 20 years, prescription drug costs have grown significantly. Prescription drug plans, which pay for prescription drugs dispensed in the community setting, have established reimbursement formulas and utilization management practices to contain these costs. In other settings, such as home health care, long-term care, and institutional settings, specific procedures must be followed in order to obtain reimbursement from prescription or health insurance plans. Accuracy in billing for prescription drugs is key to securing adequate reimbursement for insurance plans.

TEST YOUR KNOWLEDGE

Multiple Choice

1. Prescription drug prices increased in 2006 due to
   a. manufacturer price increases.
   b. wholesaler price increases.
   c. implementation of the Medicare Part D plans.
   d. a spike in illnesses in 2006.

2. In 2008, private prescription drug coverage provided coverage for which of the following percentage of Americans ?
   a. 62%
   b. 58%
   c. 44%
   d. 71%

3. Typically, pharmacy benefit managers reimburse pharmacies on the basis of
   a. wholesale acquisition cost.
   b. maximum allowable cost.
   c. federal upper limit.
   d. average wholesale price.

4. The average wholesale price is typically
   a. lower than the price paid by pharmacies to acquire drugs from a wholesaler.
   b. higher than the price paid by pharmacies to acquire drugs from a wholesaler.
   c. higher than the price wholesalers pay to acquire drugs from a manufacturer.
   d. lower than the price wholesalers pay to acquire the drugs from a manufacturer.

5. Consider the following scenario: You are filling a prescription for a patient who has prescription drug insurance. This patient's third-party plan will reimburse you fully for the drug cost of $101.93 and will pay you $3.50 for dispensing the prescription. The patient is responsible for paying you a copay of $40.00. What is the amount of the reimbursement that the pharmacy expects to receive from the third-party plan?
   a. $62.93
   b. $64.93
   c. $104.93
   d. $65.43

6. In the scenario in Question 5, what would be the total amount of the payment (from the third-party plan and the patient) that the pharmacy would receive if the third-party plan discounted the ingredient cost by 15% ?
   a. $86.64
   b. $90.14
   c. $105.43
   d. $98.43

7. An example of a fixed cost is
   a. rent expense.
   b. prescription vials.
   c. technician hours.
   d. prescription labels.

8. The most widely used method of patient cost sharing is
   a. deductibles.
   b. coinsurance.
   c. copayments.
   d. none of the above.

9. You are filling a prescription for 60 antibiotic capsules. The prescription is covered by the patient's third-party insurance coverage. The wholesaler average cost for 100 capsules of the antibiotic is $226.00. The third-party plan will reimburse you for the wholesale cost plus 15%. In addition, the plan will pay you $3.25 for dispensing the prescription. After you collect a $20.00 copayment from the patient, what is the reimbursement you expect to receive from the third-party plan ?
a. $159.19
b. $139.19
c. $118.85
d. $135.94

10. In a tiered copayment schedule, the tier with the most expensive copayment is
a. tier 1.
b. tier 2.
c. tier 3.
d. tier 4.

11. In Medicare Part D plans, medication therapy management programs must be provided to beneficiaries who satisfy all of the following requirements *except*
a. be enrolled in a Medicare Part D plan for at least 5 years.
b. have multiple chronic conditions.
c. be using multiple medications for chronic conditions.
d. have annual drug expenses of at least $3,000 in 2012.

12. In the home health care setting, which of the following codes are used to bill drugs to the commercial health insurance plans?
a. S codes
b. A codes
c. J codes
d. K codes

13. In the institutional setting, which of the following codes are used part of a prospective payment system?
a. National Drug Codes
b. diagnostic-related group codes
c. K codes
d. S codes

Matching

Match the drug reimbursement method with the description that best describes the method.

1.	______ average wholesale price	a.	limit of payment for generic drugs
2.	______ maximum allowable cost	b.	published price of a drug
3.	______ average manufacturer price retail class of pharmacies	c.	federally established price for drugs sold to
4.	______ actual acquisition cost	d.	price paid by a pharmacy for a drug
5.	______ wholesale acquisition cost		
		e.	price charged by manufacturers to wholesalers for drugs

Suggested Readings

Desselle, S.P., & Zgarrick, D. (2009). *Pharmacy management* (2nd ed.). New York, NY: McGraw-Hill.

Kaiser Family Foundation. (May 2010). *Prescription drug trends*. Retrieved from www.kff.org/rxdrugs/3057.cfm

Kane, R.A., & Kane, R.L. (1987). *Long-term care: Principles, program, and policies.* New York: Springer.

McCarthy, R.L., Schafermeyer, K.W., & Plake, K.S. (2011). *Introduction to Health Care Delivery* (5th ed.). Sudbury, MA: Jones and Bartlett.

ReimbursementCodes.com. Assessed July 3, 2011, at www.reimbursementcodes.com.

U.S. Department of Health and Human Services. (2009). *Understanding long-term care.* Available at www.longtermcare.gov

Vogenberg, F.R. (2006). *Understanding pharmacy reimbursement.* Bethesda, MD: American Society of Health-System Pharmacists.

CHAPTER

33

Accreditation of Technician Training Programs

Competencies

Upon completion of this chapter, the reader should be able to:

1. State four objectives of the accreditation process for pharmacy technician training programs.
2. Articulate the primary reason for a well trained workforce in the pharmacy profession.
3. Explain the ASHP's involvement in accrediting pharmacy technician training programs rather than in evaluating the competency achievement of individual pharmacy technicians.
4. List the eight areas that comprise the Accreditation Standard for Pharmacy Technician Training Programs.
5. Outline the objectives that form the basis for pharmacy technician training programs.

Key Terms

accreditation
Commission on Credentialing
outcome competencies
site survey

Introduction

The process of accreditation (recognition of a particular set of standards) for pharmacy technician training programs includes the following main objectives: (1) to protect the public; (2) to upgrade and standardize the formal training that pharmacy technicians receive; (3) to guide, assist, and recognize those health care facilities and academic institutions that wish to support the profession by operating such programs; (4) to provide criteria for the prospective technician trainee in the selection of a program by identifying those institutions conducting accredited pharmacy technician training programs; (5) to provide prospective employees a basis for determining the level of competency of pharmacy technicians by identifying those technicians who have successfully completed accredited technician training programs; (6) to serve as a guide for pharmacy technician education and training program development; and (7) to encourage improvement of established programs.

The Need for a Standardized Pharmacy Technician Training

During the past decade, many of the American Society of Health-System Pharmacists' (ASHP's) initiatives have centered on pharmacy's movement toward becoming a full-fledged clinical profession. The ASHP has long recognized that as we continue to move in this *clinical* direction, other health care professions and the public will increasingly look to pharmacy for answers to complex questions in drug therapy. More recently, since 2008, ASHP has been working toward a more futuristic model pharmacy practice that includes the advancement of the health and well-being of patients by developing and disseminating a practice model that supports the most effective use of pharmacists as direct patient care providers. This effort, the Pharmacy Practice Model Initiative (PPMI), included a summit of many key leaders in pharmacy practice in November 2010 who worked extensively to provide a think tank to provide the roots of the new model for pharmacy practice. Much discussion surrounded the importance of the involvement of the pharmacy technician as a member of the health care team to support the pharmacist is providing direct patient care. Many new opportunities for pharmacy technicians, including the management of new technologies and pharmacy informatics, are extremely important elements for the success of the model. ASHP and the ASHP Research and Education Foundation are supporting the efforts. More information regarding PPMI can be found at www.ashp.org.

ASHP also supports the triad needed for standardized training of the pharmacy technician: completion of an ASHP-accredited pharmacy technician training program, successful passing of the Pharmacy Technician Certification Board (PTCB) national exam, and registration. An advocacy group within the organization has operated an initiative entitled the Pharmacy Technician Initiative (PTI). This group (www.ashp.org) was established to work with state affiliates and their boards of pharmacy to require the aforementioned triad to standardize work as a pharmacy technician. As of 2013, 26 states had signed on and committed to endorse the initiative.

The purpose of the PTI initiative is to enhance the safety and welfare of patients served by pharmacy technicians who have been appropriately trained as certified technicians and to encourage involvement in database management, management of automated drug distribution devices, pharmacy billing, telepharmacy, and many more innovative positions that are not offered to those without advanced pharmacy technician training.

Historical Perspective

> **outcome competency** the measurable desired ability, knowledge, and skill achieved upon completion of a program

For over three decades the ASHP, in response to an obvious void, has promulgated documents that specifically address **outcome competencies** (standardized training goals) for pharmacy technicians. However, to date, these have not been uniformly recognized and accepted throughout pharmacy. Although these documents are gaining a greater degree of acceptance among pharmacists, it remains clear that the job category of technician continues to be interpreted differently because no two technicians are necessarily measured by the same yardstick.

The ASHP has remained steadfast in its belief that an absolute prerequisite for the orderly development of pharmacy support personnel is uniform recognition and acceptance of a competency or performance standard. Moreover, it has agreed that such a standard provides the basic objective for supportive personnel training programs.

Early on, the ASHP recognized that a competency standard alone could not suffice for development of pharmacy technician training programs. In fact, the ASHP considered as part of its early deliberations such programs and whether competency-based training would be acceptable. The realization that the structure and process of these training programs would be of secondary importance was key to these deliberations; competency outcomes would be the primary concern. Further, it was agreed that the feasibility of developing competency-based training programs, which depend largely on the ability to evaluate competency achievement, would not be difficult.

Despite these considerations, and due in large measure to the advice of its members, the ASHP expressed uneasiness about promoting establishment of competency-based technician training programs. As a consequence, the ASHP decided to follow the more traditional pattern of evaluating each training program through the process of accreditation. It is easy to understand how the ASHP chose this avenue, since it has had a well-established accreditation process for postgraduate pharmacy residency training programs in place since 1963.

> **accreditation** the process by which an agency or organization evaluates and recognizes a program of study or an institution as meeting predetermined qualifications or standards

Accreditation is defined as the process by which an agency or organization evaluates and recognizes a program of study or an institution as meeting certain predetermined qualifications or standards. It applies only to institutions and their programs of study or their services.

Obviously, to establish an accreditation program, the ASHP knew firsthand that it would be necessary to develop an accreditation standard that would delineate specific facilities and process requirements in addition to competency outcome criteria. Therefore, in November 1980, the ASHP Board of Directors requested that an accreditation standard for technician training programs be developed. They also authorized implementation of an accreditation process for such programs at the earliest possible time.

An accreditation standard for pharmacy technician training programs was approved by the ASHP board in April 1982. The first program was accredited in September 1983. Now, more than 250 programs are ASHP accredited in 40 states. Only 120 programs were ASHP accredited when the previous edition of this book was published.

Accreditation Program

Commission on Credentialing the ASHP body appointed to formulate and recommend standards and administer programs for accreditation of pharmacy personnel training programs

site survey a visit by representatives of the ASHP to review training programs and ascertain compliance with standards

As noted in the ASHP regulations on accreditation of pharmacy technician training programs, the accreditation service is conducted by authority of the ASHP Board of Directors under the direction of the **Commission on Credentialing**. The commission reviews and evaluates applications and survey reports and, as delegated by the board, takes final action on all applications set forth in the regulations.

All pharmacy technician training programs applying for accreditation by the ASHP are evaluated by **site survey** against the ASHP Accreditation Standard for Pharmacy Technician Training Programs. The standard outlines specific requirements for administrative responsibility for the training program, qualifications of the training site, qualification of the pharmacy service that is used to provide trainees with practical experience, qualifications of the pharmacy director and preceptors, qualifications and selection of the applicant, the overall structure of the pharmacy technician training program, experimentation and innovative approaches to training, and issuance of the certificate of completion. More information regarding ASHP accreditation can be found at www.ashp.org. A tool called *RU Ready* is available for those contemplating applying for ASHP accreditation. This tool is used to determine if a program is at the point where pursuing the process makes sense. In addition, sample forms, frequently asked questions, and other useful tips are available on the ASHP accreditation website.

With respect to the competency-based objectives that must be developed as a fundamental component of any ASHP-accredited technician training program, individuals are encouraged to use the ASHP publication *Model Curriculum for Pharmacy Technician Training*, third edition. This is the updated version of the manual that was developed as a nationwide project to provide technician educators with a prototype for training technicians in all practice settings and geographic locations. Specifically, it provides a guide for structuring the curriculum of a technician training program, a checklist of quality components of existing training programs, suggestions for strengthening technicians' skills in specific areas, a list of job responsibilities and tasks that technicians can assume to allow pharmacists time to provide direct patient care, and a descriptive list of tasks to assist technicians when writing job descriptions. A user's guide is included with the curriculum to help pare down the training menu to suit individual training needs. The curriculum consists of four components: (1) goal statements, objectives, and instructional objectives; (2) a curriculum map with suggested sequencing of the modules for instruction; (3) descriptors for each of the instruction modules; and (4) a tracking document that identifies where each objective and instructional objective are taught. The technician's role in enhancing safe medication use, use of the tech–check–tech method, and how to assist with immunizations are included in the curriculum. The model curriculum was a collaborative project undertaken by the American Association of Pharmacy Technicians, the American Pharmacists Association, the American Society of Health-System Pharmacists, the National Association of Chain Drug Stores, and the Pharmacy Technician Educators Council. The project was under the leadership of the American Society of Health-System Pharmacists.

The ASHP accreditation standards accommodate training programs offered by hospital and health system pharmacy departments, managed care facilities, community colleges, vocational/technical institutes, proprietary agencies, chain pharmacies, and military facilities. A directory of these programs is located at www.ashp.org under the technician section.

Pharmacy technicians completing ASHP-accredited programs are provided with a wealth of opportunities to learn didactic information, hands-on laboratory training, and experiential rotations in a variety of pharmacy settings. Each program must be at least 600 hours in duration to be considered for accreditation and must include didactic, laboratory, and experiential elements. Graduates completing such programs gain perspective on all aspects of pharmacy technician training practice, a substantial added value that cannot be acquired from undertaking just on-the-job training. Instructors and preceptors provide one-on-one instruction and guidance for the students to ensure that each trainee is appropriately trained to succeed as a pharmacy technician. Many of the students undertaking ASHP-accredited pharmacy technician training programs are offered job opportunities upon completion of their experiential training rotations at the specific site.

Many of the employers in areas where pharmacy technician training programs are available only hire graduates from ASHP-accredited training programs. Some employers provide higher entry-level salaries to those who are graduates from ASHP-accredited pharmacy technician training programs. ASHP accreditation is a nationally recognized accreditation. An employer in any state can review the ASHP standards for accreditation and review the different areas of practice in which a graduate has training. Employers reap the benefits of employing someone who is already familiar and trained in many areas of pharmacy technician practice.

Summary

ASHP accreditation of pharmacy technician training programs is becoming more widely required and important in the health care area to substantiate compliance with national standards and provide evidence of standardization in pharmacy technician education. Employers respect and prefer to hire pharmacy technicians graduating from ASHP-accredited pharmacy technician training programs. New national initiatives such as the PPMI and PTI support the need for appropriately trained, accredited pharmacy technicians who have passed the PTCB exam and state registration to undertake the management of the parts of the drug distribution process that do not need to be relegated to the pharmacist. Pharmacists' involvement in providing more direct patient care services will more widely occur as pharmacy technicians begin to manage supportive roles in practice.

TEST YOUR KNOWLEDGE

Multiple Choice

1. The ASHP has accredited pharmacy technician training programs in
   a. colleges of pharmacy.
   b. vocational/technical schools.
   c. military institutions.
   d. all of the above.

2. Continuing accreditation of a pharmacy technician training program depends on
   a. a site visit.
   b. adherence to accreditation standards.
   c. an increased number of graduates over previous years.
   d. all of the above.

3. A pharmacy technician may engage in which of the following activities?
   a. packaging and labeling of medication doses
   b. maintaining patient records
   c. preparing intravenous admixtures
   d. all of the above

4. A well trained workforce is needed in pharmacy because
   a. pharmacists provide direct patient care services.
   b. technicians answer complex questions in drug therapy.
   c. pharmacists must perform many technical functions.
   d. the personnel best suited for the role perform specialized functions.

Suggested Readings

American Society of Health-System Pharmacists. (1980). ASHP position on long-range pharmacy manpower needs and residency training. *American Journal of Health-System Pharmacy, 37*, 1220.

American Society of Health-System Pharmacists. (1998). ASHP accreditation standard for pharmacy technician training programs. *Practice Standards of ASHP, 1998–1999.* Bethesda, MD: Author.

American Society of Health-System Pharmacists. (1998). ASHP regulations on accreditation of pharmacy technician training programs. *Practice Standards of ASHP, 1998–1999*. Bethesda, MD: Author.

American Society of Health-System Pharmacists. (2001). *Model curriculum for pharmacy technician training* (2nd ed.). Bethesda, MD: Author.

Cobaugh, D. J. (2011). Advancing pharmacy practice models: Achieving consensus. *American Journal of Health-System Pharmacy, 68*(12), e40–e41.

CHAPTER 34

Pharmacy Technician Certification

Competencies

Upon completion of this chapter, the reader should be able to:

1. Describe pharmacy technicians' evolving roles in pharmacy practice.
2. Explain the importance of the Pharmacy Technician Certification Exam (PTCE) in the protection of public health and safety.
3. Discuss the nature of pharmacy technician regulatory oversight by state boards of pharmacy.
4. Differentiate between the processes of PTCB certification and recertification.
5. Describe the value of National Commission for Certifying Agencies (NCCA) accreditation to a national certification program.
6. Describe the goals and outcomes of the PTCB C.R.E.S.T. Initiative.

Key Terms

certification **certified pharmacy technician (CPhT)** **recertification**

Introduction

The role of pharmacy practice in modern health care continues to evolve. Today, in addition to the oversight of traditional medication dispensing and product fulfillment activities, the responsibilities of pharmacists include direct patient care services such as medication therapy management (MTM) and the delivery of immunizations. As medication regimens become more complex and cost-conscious insurers rely on pharmacists to provide increased direct patient care, the certified pharmacy technician (CPhT) will continue to be relied on to keep pharmacy operations running smoothly.

The Joint Commission of Pharmacy Practitioners (JCPP) Future Vision of Pharmacy Practice in 2015 calls for qualified support personnel who will enable pharmacists to provide patient-centered care where they have the authority and autonomy to manage medication therapy while working cooperatively with practitioners of other health disciplines to care for patients. For this reason, pharmacy technicians must be well qualified to meet the challenges and fulfill their supporting roles in drug preparation and distribution.

Pharmacy technicians have been certified in all pharmacy practice settings, including community pharmacy, hospitals and health systems, and long-term care pharmacy. Pharmacists and the public require assurance that pharmacy technicians are qualified to handle the responsibilities delegated to them. CPhTs provide pharmacists with logistical support; they also perform additional functions to keep operations running smoothly and allow pharmacists more time to work directly with patients. A prime example is the critical roles CPhTs play in immunization campaigns in pharmacies across the nation that allow pharmacists to vaccinate millions of patients during flu season each year.

Background

The first pharmacy technician certification exam was created in 1981 by the Michigan Pharmacists Association (MPA). In 1988, the Illinois Council of Health-System Pharmacists (ICHP) created a certification exam for pharmacy technicians. Although designed to specifically address pharmacy practice in their own states, both the MPA and ICHP certification exams were being used under contract by other states to assess the knowledge of pharmacy technician candidates across the United States.

Review of the results of a profession-wide Scope of Pharmacy Practice survey in 1993 determined that there should be one national certification exam for pharmacy technicians. Therefore, working with the American Pharmacists Association (APhA) and the American Society of Health-System Pharmacists (ASHP), leaders from MPA and ICHP joined to create the Pharmacy Technician Certification Board (PTCB) in 1995, a nonprofit organization. In 2001, the National Association of Boards of Pharmacy (NABP) joined the PTCB Board of Governors.

PTCB develops, maintains, promotes, and administers a nationally accredited certification and recertification program for pharmacy technicians to enable the most effective support of pharmacists to advance patient safety. Since 1995, over 450,000 pharmacy technicians nationwide have earned the PTCB CPhT credential.

PTCB promotes patient safety by serving as the national standard for the certification of pharmacy technicians. The methods used to develop and administer the Pharmacy Technician Certification Exam (PTCE) promote the validity, measurement precision, and integrity of the program. The PTCE offers pharmacy technicians an opportunity to demonstrate that they have mastered knowledge across pharmacy practice settings.

In 2005, a second national certification exam was founded in the United States. The Exam for the Certification of Pharmacy Technicians (ExCPT) was originally established by the Institute for the Certification of Pharmacy Technicians (ICPT) and is now a part of the National Healthcareer Association (NHA).

Regulation of Pharmacy Technicians

Pharmacy technicians are accountable to their supervising pharmacist, who is legally responsible through state licensure for the care and safety of patients served by the pharmacy. State rules and regulations, as well as employer policies and procedures, may require and specifically define the functions and responsibilities of pharmacy technicians.

State boards of pharmacy provide regulatory oversight of the profession, most often through their state pharmacy practice acts. State boards of pharmacy continually revise their practice acts to align with their mission to protect public safety. As of 2012, 44 states boards of pharmacy regulated pharmacy technicians, with 18 requiring national certification for registration, 16 requiring an official background check, and 18 requiring continuing education (CE) to maintain registration. Of these states, many require pharmacy technicians to register with the state prior to working as a pharmacy technician and may require PTCB certification as a component of registration. It is common for states to tie specific responsibilities, pharmacist-to-technician ratios, supervision, or other requirements to pharmacy technicians' certification status.

The Model State Pharmacy Act and Model Rules of the National Association of Boards of Pharmacy (the *Model Act)* provide state boards of pharmacy with model language that may be used when developing state laws or board rules. The Model Act includes sections on the state boards of pharmacy, licensing (pharmacists, pharmacy technicians, and facilities), and discipline. The Model Act recommends that states that certify pharmacy technicians recognize PTCB certification and that all pharmacy technicians become PTCB certified by 2015.

Certification

certification a process by which a nongovernmental association or agency grants recognition to an individual who has met certain predetermined qualifications specified by that association or agency

certified pharmacy technician (CPhT) a pharmacy technician who has successfully passed the national Pharmacy Technician Certificate Examination

Certification is the process by which a nongovernmental association or agency grants recognition to an individual who has met certain predetermined qualifications specified by that association or agency. PTCB develops and implements practices related to national certification for pharmacy technicians. Pharmacy technicians who want to work more effectively with pharmacists to offer greater patient care and service should consider taking the PTCE to become a CPhT. Professional development, such as PTCB certification, enables many pharmacy technicians to progress through career ladders, satisfy employer requirements, and develop skills in specialty areas of practice.

To become a PTCB **certified pharmacy technician (CPhT)**, candidates must pass the PTCE. The PTCE contains 90 multiple-choice questions. The exam samples pharmacy technician knowledge of activities performed in settings throughout pharmacy practice. Each question is carefully written, referenced, and validated to determine its accuracy and correctness. Once a pharmacy technician passes the exam, he or she may use the designation of CPhT.

CPhTs who have become certified through the PTCB report higher earnings and increased promotion opportunities. Benefits to becoming a CPhT include enhanced self-worth, improved job satisfaction, increased knowledge, and the ability to make a positive impact on patient care. Employers trust that with PTCB certification, the CPhTs they work with have met predetermined qualifications by passing the PTCE.

PTCB's certification is valid nationwide and is recognized across states and practice settings. Specific regulations to work as a pharmacy technician vary from state to state. For more information regarding specific state requirements, pharmacy technicians should contact the state board of pharmacy for the state in which they wish to work.

Testing Process

The PTCE is available at more than 225 Pearson Professional Centers (the same centers used by the NABP), which administer the North American Pharmacist Licensure Examination (NAPLEX) and are located throughout the United States and its territories. The exam is administered in all locations in a computer-based format. Candidates have 2 hours to complete the exam tutorial, the PTCE, and the exit survey. Pearson Professional Centers are carefully controlled testing environments, dedicated to both test security and candidate comfort. A complete list of test center locations is available at www.ptcb.org.

Additional PTCE testing benefits include:

- Immediate pass/fail results at the test center
- Online application and test scheduling
- Daily test center hours
- Scheduling flexibility to allow candidates to schedule or reschedule their exams up to 48 hours prior to the testing time
- State-of-the-art testing facilities
- Increased exam security.

Job Analysis Study

The PTCE samples pharmacy technician knowledge of activities performed in settings throughout pharmacy practice. To ensure that the exam is psychometrically sound and legally defensible, the content framework of the exam is supported by a nationwide study, called a Job Analysis Study.

PTCB conducts a Job Analysis Study approximately every 5 years to gather firsthand information on the current roles and tasks performed by pharmacy technicians in every state and practice setting. The results of the survey are then used to construct a new blueprint, or content outline, for the PTCE.

PTCB's most recent Job Analysis Study was completed in 2012, with over 25,000 pharmacy technicians from across the United States participating in the survey. PTCB's Certification Council and Board of Governors reviewed the 2012 Job Analysis Study and approved a new blueprint for the PTCE, which served as the content outline for a revised PTCE in 2013.

Recertification

recertification
a renewal of an individual's certification

Recertification is the renewal of an individual's certification. All CPhTs must complete the recertification process in order to maintain their status as a CPhT. Recertification involves the completion of CE credits and submission of the appropriate application on the PTCB website. Failure to successfully complete the recertification requirements will result in the loss of PTCB certification.

Maintaining certification demonstrates pharmacy technicians' commitment to the profession, allowing them to keep up with the latest advances in the field through CE. Various state boards of pharmacy and employers have requirements for pharmacy technicians to maintain their PTCB certification in order to retain their state registration and/or employment.

To recertify, CPhTs are required to fulfill recertification requirements every 2 years. Visit the PTCB website, www.ptcb.org, to access current recertification requirements.

Reinstatement

CPhTs are required to renew their PTCB certification every 2 years. If a pharmacy technician does not recertify by the deadline, they are no longer recognized as a CPhT. PTCB offers pharmacy technicians the opportunity to reinstate their certification status for up to 1 year after their most recent recertification deadline. This allows pharmacy technicians whose certification has lapsed to reinstate their certification without having to reapply for certification. If a pharmacy technician does not reinstate within 1 year, however, she or he will be required to retake the PTCE in order to become an active CPhT again.

NCCA Accreditation

In 2006, PTCB joined the elite group of organizations that have received and maintained National Commission for Certifying Agencies (NCCA) accreditation. NCCA is the accrediting body of the Institute for Credentialing Excellence (ICE), which accredits certification programs based on the highest quality standards in professional certification. The accreditation process ensures that programs adhere to current standards of practice in the certification industry. NCCA has developed criteria used to ensure that accredited programs provide fair, valid, and reliable assessment tools; defined levels of accountability and decision making; and continuing competency.

PTCB's initial accreditation in 2006 and renewal in 2011 entailed a lengthy review of PTCB's procedures, protocols, and operations. NCCA standards address the structure and governance of PTCB; the characteristics of PTCB's certification program; the information that must be available to exam candidates, certificants, and the public; and the recertification initiatives of PTCB. PTCB's test development and administration procedures, psychometric analyses, and policies and procedures all meet NCCA's stringent standards. These methods follow certification exam testing procedures recommended in the Standards for Educational and Psychological Testing and testing guidelines published by ICE and the Council on Licensure, Enforcement and Regulation. NCCA's accreditation of PTCB's certification program verifies its adherence to the industry's highest standards.

Practice Test

PTCB has developed a series of online practice exams using the same rigorous processes and standards as the PTCE. These practice exams provide candidates with an opportunity to experience question content, formats, and a test structure similar to what they may experience when sitting for the PTCE. The sole function of these practice exams is to provide familiarity with content, format, and structure. Other study materials do exist, however, PTCB does not endorse, recommend, or sponsor any review courses, manuals, or books for the PTCE. Any resources listed at www.ptcb.org are provided for informational purposes only.

Future for Pharmacy Technicians

The Bureau of Labor Statistics reports that employment of pharmacy technicians is expected to increase by 31% from 2008 to 2018, which is faster than the average for other occupations. The increased number of middle-aged and elderly people—who use more prescription drugs than younger people—will spur demand for pharmacy workers throughout the projection period. In addition, as scientific advances lead to new drugs, and as more people obtain prescription drug coverage, pharmacy workers will be needed in growing numbers.

As cost-conscious insurers begin to use pharmacies as patient care centers, and as pharmacists become more involved in patient care, pharmacy technicians will continue to see an expansion of their role in the pharmacy. Job opportunities for pharmacy technicians are expected to be good, especially for those with previous experience, formal training, or certification. Job openings will result from employment growth, as well as the need to replace workers who transfer to other occupations or leave the labor force.

C.R.E.S.T. Initiative

PTCB launched the Consumer Awareness, Resources, Education, State Policy, and Testing (C.R.E.S.T.) Initiative in 2011 by hosting a summit focused on the C.R.E.S.T. areas as they relate to pharmacy technicians. Attendees included pharmacists, CPhTs, educators, major employers, state board of pharmacy representatives, as well as representatives from state and national pharmacy organizations.

During the summit, participants expressed the need for the profession to move beyond philosophical discussion and make decisions on the future of pharmacy practice and the role of pharmacy technicians. Recommendations from the summit include eligibility requirements for the PTCB certification program, requirements for recertification, and the creation of new specialty certification programs (**Figure 34-1**).

In response to the recommendations made during the summit, more than 17,000 pharmacists and pharmacy technicians participated in the C.R.E.S.T. Initiative

Certification Program Recommendations

- Require a minimum period of practical experience
- Require criminal background checks
- Require candidates to complete an accredited education program

Recertification Recommendations

- Accept only pharmacy technician targeted designated CE credits
- Change the number of CE credits allowed to be provided through practical/employer-based in-service training opportunities from ten to five
- Require one of the 20 required CE credits to be in medication/patient safety

New Certification Programs

Develop certification programs in the areas of sterile compounding, technology, medication safety, regulatory compliance, medication therapy management, inventory management, and/or medication reconciliation

- Establish an advanced CPhT credential

FIGURE 34-1 Recommendations from the C.R.E.S.T. Initiative.

Survey in early 2012. Results from the survey provided the PTCB Board of Governors and Certification Council with important input from the profession on advancing the work of pharmacy technicians and the future of the PTCB certification program.

C.R.E.S.T. Initiative Survey Findings

The majority of respondents, 90%, were pharmacy technicians. The two primary work environments of pharmacy technicians were retail pharmacies, 39% (chain and independent combined), and health system pharmacies, 27%. In contrast, of the 7% of respondents that identified themselves as pharmacists, 48% worked in a health system pharmacy, compared to 19% who worked in a retail pharmacy (chain and independent combined). Pharmacy technicians working in every state and several territories responded to the survey, and pharmacists from every state except Vermont responded.

Findings Related to C.R.E.S.T. Initiative Recommendations

Key survey findings related to C.R.E.S.T. Initiative recommendations are provided in **Table 34-1**.

TABLE 34-1 C.R.E.S.T. Survey Findings

		PHARMACY TECHNICIAN	PHARMACIST
Require background checks?	Yes	88%	92%
	No	12%	8%
Require accredited education?	Yes	53%	62%
	No	47%	38%
Is 2020 reasonable?	Yes	78%	79%
	No	22%	21%
Barriers to accredited education?	#1	Cost	Cost
	#2	State Regs	State Regs
	#3	Employers	# of Programs
Require practical experience?	Yes	72%	83%
	No	28%	17%
Accept only technician CE credits?	Yes	15%	24%
	No	85%	76%
Require a med safety CE credit?	Yes	89%	88%
	No	11%	12%
Support specialty certifications?	Yes	83%	74%
	No	17%	26%
Support advanced designations?	Yes	73%	70%
	No	6%	14%
	Unsure	21%	16%
Separate or comprehensive?	Sep	55%	74%
	Comp	33%	18%
	Unsure	12%	9%

Summary

There are numerous benefits to becoming a CPhT. CPhTs enhance the pharmacy team, bring higher quality care to patients, and add value to the pharmacy. PTCB certification also provides the public with basic protections for public health and the knowledge that those who they trust to handle their medications in a variety of settings are appropriately, consistently, and adequately tested across practice settings.

The success of the PTCB certification program has not gone unnoticed in the credentialing and association management fields. PTCB works diligently to meet the needs of the pharmacy profession and its stakeholders. With more than 450,000 CPhTs since 1995, PTCB has proven that CPhTs are an integral part of the pharmacy team.

TEST YOUR KNOWLEDGE

Multiple Choice

1. Pharmacy technician roles have grown to now support pharmacists in which of the following areas?
   a. medication therapy management (MTM)
   b. delivery of immunizations
   c. medication supply ordering and inventory
   d. pharmacy logistical support

2. Pharmacy practice acts may require which of the following as a prerequisite for pharmacy technicians to work within the state?
   a. registration with the board of pharmacy
   b. national certification exam
   c. background check
   d. continuing education credits

3. To maintain national certification, certified pharmacy technicians (CPhTs) need to recertify with the PTCB
   a. every year.
   b. every 2 years.
   c. every 5 years.
   d. never.

4. The C.R.E.S.T. Initiative addresses which of the following regarding pharmacy technicians?
   a. checking programs
   b. reimbursement
   c. error rates
   d. state policy
   e. temporary solutions

5. How many pharmacy technicians have been certified by PTCB since 1995?
   a. 10,000
   b. 150,000
   c. 300,000
   d. 450,000

True/False

1. _______ The Pharmacy Technician Certification Exam (PTCE) offers pharmacy technicians an opportunity to demonstrate that they have mastered knowledge in only the community pharmacy practice setting.
2. _______ State boards of pharmacy provide regulatory oversight of the profession, most often through their state pharmacy practice acts.
3. _______ All states have adopted the same requirements for pharmacy technicians to work within their state.
4. _______ The Pharmacy Technician Certification Exam (PTCE) has 120 questions.
5. _______ PTCB is accredited by the National Commission for Certifying Agencies (NCCA).

References

Bureau of Labor Statistics. (2011). *Pharmacy technicians and pharmacy aides*. Retrieved from http://www.bls.gov/oco/ocos325.htm

Gans, J.A., & Manasse, Jr., H.R. (2008). Certification of pharmacy technicians. *American Journal of Health-System Pharmacy, 48*(5), 568–572.

Manasse, H.R., Jr., & Menighan, T.E. (2010). Single standard for education, training, and certification of pharmacy technicians. *Journal of the American Pharmacists Association*, *50*, 116.

APPENDIX

A Long-Term Care

A–1: Examples of Guidelines for Automatic Stop-Order Policy in a Skilled Nursing Facility (Unless Otherwise Specified by Physician)

Drug Type

Analgesics .... 30 days
Darvon, Darvocet

Antianemia drugs .... 30 days
iron

Antibiotics .... 7 days
Keflex, tetracycline

Antiemetics .... 4 days
Compazine, Tigan

Anticoagulants .... 30 days
Coumadin

Antihistamines .... 7 days
Chlor-Trimeton, Seldane, Sudafed

Antineoplastics .... 30 days
Nolvadex, Hydrea

Barbiturates .... 30 days
phenobarbital

Cardiovascular .... 30 days
digoxin, Vasotec, quinidine

Cathartics .... 30 days
Peri-Colace, Colace, Senokot

Cold preparations .... 5 days
Phenergan Expectorant, Robitussin

Dermatologicals .... 30 days
Lidex, hydrocortisone, Synalar

Diuretics .... 30 days
HCTZ, Dyazide, Aldactazide, Lasix

A–2: Medication Order Entry Flow Chart

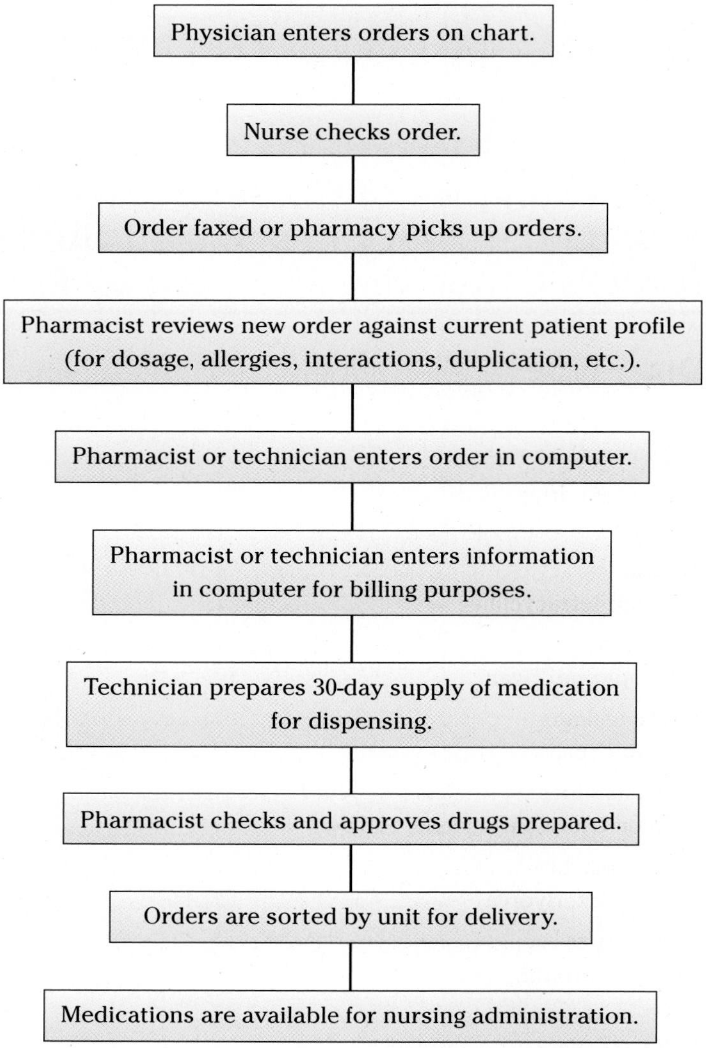
Physician enters orders on chart.
Nurse checks order.
Order faxed or pharmacy picks up orders.
Pharmacist reviews new order against current patient profile (for dosage, allergies, interactions, duplication, etc.).
Pharmacist or technician enters order in computer.
Pharmacist or technician enters information in computer for billing purposes.
Technician prepares 30-day supply of medication for dispensing.
Pharmacist checks and approves drugs prepared.
Orders are sorted by unit for delivery.
Medications are available for nursing administration.

APPENDIX

B The Hospital Formulary System

B–1: The Pharmacy and Therapeutics Committee

The Pharmacy and Therapeutics (P&T) Committee is a policy-recommending body to the medical staff and the administration of a healthcare organization on matters related to the therapeutic use of drugs. It develops policies for managing drug use and drug administration, and manages the formulary system. This committee is selected so as to represent different medical departments or divisions. The P&T Committee should be composed of at least the following voting members: physicians, pharmacists, nurses, administrators, quality assurance coordinators, and others as appropriate. A chairperson from among the physician representatives should be appointed. A pharmacist should be designated as secretary.

The committee functions in both an advisory and an educational capacity.

1. It deals with contemporary problems in therapeutics.
2. It selects for routine use within the institution (and its ambulatory services and clinics) therapeutic agents that represent the best available for the prophylaxis or management of disease.
3. It recommends the deletion of drugs from the formulary that no longer meet the needs of the hospital patients.

The department of pharmacy services recommends to the P&T Committee quality control specifications, methods of distribution and control, and drug utilization reviews.

Function

1. To serve as an advisory group to the medical staff, to the hospital administration, and to the department of pharmacy services on matters pertaining to drug utilization, drug use control, and standards of practice concerning the use of drugs.
2. To evaluate clinical and scientific data regarding new drugs or agents proposed for formulary addition.
3. To establish a formulary of accepted drugs for use in the hospital and to provide for its constant revision.
4. To establish policies regarding the surveillance of investigational drugs.
5. To serve as a focal point for collecting data obtained from drug utilization reviews throughout the hospital.

B–2: Definitions and Categories of Drugs to Be Stocked in the Pharmacy

Formulary Drugs

A formulary drug is a therapeutic agent whose place in therapy is well established. It is selected by the P&T Committee as essential for the best patient care.

Clinical Evaluation Drugs

A clinical evaluation drug is a commercially available, nonformulary agent that is temporarily made available to a particular physician or physicians for the purpose of evaluation for formulary inclusion. The P&T Committee will review these requests and, if approved, the requesting physician completes a Clinical Evaluation Drug Request Form that contains the following information:

- Objectives of the clinical evaluation
- Criteria for selection of patients who will receive the drug
- Parameters to be assessed
- Estimated number of patients to be studied
- Duration of study.

The requesting physician submits the results of the evaluation after an interim period of time (usually 6 months) to the P&T Committee.

The final report contains conclusions and recommendations to the P&T Committee concerning the drug's role relative to formulary alternatives.

Restricted Drug Guidelines

A restricted drug is a therapeutic agent, admitted to the formulary, the use of which is authorized to either specific physicians or under specific guidelines for use. The following procedures apply:

- Drugs in the category can be dispensed only if prescribed with the approval of specific physicians, and/or if they meet specific indications for use, and/or are prescribed on specific order forms (e.g., antibiotic order form, TPN Order Sheet).

Investigational Drugs

An investigational drug is a therapeutic agent undergoing clinical investigation that is not approved by the Food and Drug Administration.

The pharmacy is responsible for the storage, dispensing, recordkeeping, and disposition of investigational drugs. In addition, the pharmacy is charged with the responsibility for providing written drug information to the respective nursing units using these drugs.

The chief investigator must do the following:

- Get approval for the use of the investigational drugs from the Institutional Review Board.
- Provide the pharmacy with a copy of the signed patient consent form.
- Provide the pharmacy with all available pharmacologic data from the manufacturer.
- Arrange for transfer of the drug to the pharmacy.
- Indicate if the pharmacy is to have responsibility for ongoing ordering and storage of the investigational drug.

Nonformulary Drugs

A nonformulary drug is any drug other than one classified as a formulary drug, evaluation drug, restricted drug, or investigational drug. Nonformulary medications may only be prescribed by chiefs of service or attending physicians. These medications will not be dispensed without the prior submission of a Nonformulary Drug Request Form.

Upon receipt of a medication order, the pharmacist notifies the prescriber if the prescribed medication is nonformulary and suggests alternative formulary medications in the same therapeutic class. If the prescriber still wishes to use the nonformulary medication, he or she must complete a Nonformulary Drug Request Form.

B–3: Additions to the Formulary

Requests for the addition of drugs to the formulary may be initiated by an attending physician of the medical staff. The requesting physician completes and signs a Request for Formulary Addition form and submits it to the secretary of the P&T Committee.

The Drug Information Service is responsible for preparing all drug evaluation reports. These reports review the pertinent literature concerning the requested drug and make recommendations to the committee with regard to addition of the drug based on other formulary medications, its comparable cost, adverse effects, etc.

The formulary status of a new drug may be reviewed and evaluated by the committee after a specific period of time, usually 6 months.

B–4: Deletions from the Formulary

Drugs may be deleted from the formulary as a result of the addition of more efficacious or safer agents, duplication of drugs in the same therapeutic category, or upon review of the annual usage.

Additions and deletions are published in a pharmacy newsletter, which is distributed to the medical staff.

APPENDIX

C Common Sound-Alike Drug Names

The following is a list of common sound-alike drug names; trade names are capitalized. In parentheses next to each drug name is the pharmacologic classification/use for the drug. (Reprinted from *PDR Nurse's Drug Handbook* by G. R. Spratto and A. L. Woods. Clifton Park, NY: Thomson Delmar Learning, 2004.)

Accupril (ACE inhibitor)	Accutane (antiacne drug)
acetazolamide (antiglaucoma drug)	acetohexamide (oral antidiabetic drug)
AcipHex (proton pump inhibitor)	Accupril (ACE inhibitor)
Actos (oral hypoglycemic)	Actonel (diphosphonate—bone growth regulator)
Adriamycin (antineoplastic)	Aredia (bone growth regulator)
albuterol (sympathomimetic)	atenolol (beta blocker)
Aldomet (antihypertensive)	Aldoril (antihypertensive)
Alkeran (antineoplastic)	Leukeran (antineoplastic)
allopurinol (antigout drug)	Apresoline (antihypertensive)
alprazolam (antianxiety agent)	lorazepam (antianxiety agent)
Amaryl (oral hypoglycemic)	Reminyl (anti-Alzheimer's drug)
Ambien (sedative-hypnotic)	Amen (progestin)
Amiloride (diuretic)	amlodipine (calcium channel blocker)
amiodarone (antiarrhythmic)	amrinone (inotropic agent)
amitriptyline (antidepressant)	nortriptyline (antidepressant)
Apresazide (antihypertensive)	Apresoline (antihypertensive)
Aripiprazole (antipsychotic)	lansoprazole (proton pump inhibitor)
Arlidin (peripheral vasodilator)	Aralen (antimalarial)
Artane (cholinergic blocking agent)	Altace (ACE inhibitor)
Asacol (anti-inflammatory drug)	Avelox (fluoroquinolone antibiotic)
asparaginase (antineoplastic agent)	pegaspargase (antineoplastic agent)
Atarax (antianxiety agent)	Ativan (antianxiety agent)
atenolol (beta blocker)	timolol (beta blocker)
Atrovent (cholinergic blocking agent)	Alupent (sympathomimetic)
Avandia (oral hypoglycemic)	Coumadin (anticoagulant)
Bacitracin (antibacterial)	Bactroban (anti-infective, topical)
Benylin (expectorant)	Ventolin (sympathomimetic)
Brevital (barbiturate)	Brevibloc (beta-adrenergic blocker)
Bumex (diuretic)	Buprenex (narcotic analgesic)
bupropion (antidepressant; smoking deterrent)	buspirone (antianxiety agent)
Cafergot (analgesic)	Carafate (antiulcer drug)
calciferol (vitamin D)	calcitriol (vitamin D)
carboplatin (antineoplastic agent)	cisplatin (antineoplastic agent)
Cardene (calcium channel blocker)	Cardizem (calcium channel blocker)
Cardura (antihypertensive)	Ridaura (gold-containing anti-inflammatory)
Cataflam (NSAID)	Catapres (antihypertensive)
Catapres (antihypertensive)	Combipres (antihypertensive)
cefotaxime (cephalosporin)	cefoxitin (cephalosporin)
cefuroxime (cephalosporin)	deferoxamine (iron chelator)

Celebrex (NSAID)	Cerebyx (anticonvulsant)
Celebrex (NSAID)	Celera (antidepressant)
chlorpromazine (antipsychotic)	chlorpropamide (oral antidiabetic)
chlorpromazine (antipsychotic)	prochlorperazine (antipsychotic)
chlorpromazine (antipsychotic)	promethazine (antihistamine)
Clinoril (NSAID)	Clozaril (antipsychotic)
clomipramine (antidepressant)	clomiphene (ovarian stimulant)
clonidine (antihypertensive)	Klonopin (anticonvulsant)
Combivir (AIDS drug combination)	Combivent (combination for COPD)
Cozaar (antihypertensive)	Zocor (antihyperlipidemic)
cyclobenzaprine (skeletal muscle relaxant)	cyproheptadine (antihistamine)
Cyclophosphamide (antineoplastic)	cyclosporine (immunosuppressant)
cyclosporine (immunosuppressant)	cycloserine (antineoplastic)
Cytovene (antiviral drug)	Cytosar (antineoplastic)
Cytoxan (antineoplastic)	Cytotec (prostaglandin derivative)
Dantrium (skeletal muscle relaxant)	danazol (gonadotropin inhibitor)
Darvocet-N (analgesic)	Darvon-N (analgesic)
daunorubicin (antineoplastic)	doxorubicin (antineoplastic)
desipramine (antidepressant)	diphenhydramine (antihistamine)
DiaBeta (oral hypoglycemic)	Zebeta (beta-adrenergic blocker)
digitoxin (cardiac glycoside)	digoxin (cardiac glycoside)
diphenhydramine (antihistamine)	dimenhydrinate (antihistamine)
dopamine (sympathomimetic)	dobutamine (sympathomimetic)
Edecrin (diuretic)	Eulexin (antineoplastic)
enalapril (ACE inhibitor)	Anafranil (antidepressant)
enalapril (ACE inhibitor)	Eldepryl (antiparkinson agent)
Eryc (erythromycin base)	Ery-Tab (erythromycin base)
etidronate (bone growth regulator)	etretinate (antipsoriatic)
etomidate (general anesthetic)	etidronate (bone growth regulator)
E-Vista (antihistamine)	Evista (estrogen receptor modulator)
Femara (antineoplastic)	FemHRT (estrogen-progestin combination)
Fioricet (analgesic)	Fiorinal (analgesic)
Flomax (alpha-adrenergic blocker)	Volmax (sympathomimetic)
flurbiprofen (NSAID)	fenoprofen (NSAID)
folinic acid (leucovorin calcium)	folic acid (vitamin B)
Gantrisin (sulfonamide)	Gantanol (sulfonamide)
glipizide (oral hypoglycemic)	glyburide (oral hypoglycemic)
glyburide (oral hypoglycemic)	Glucotrol (oral hypoglycemic)
Hycodan (cough preparation)	Hycomine (cough preparation)
hydrocodone (narcotic analgesic)	hydrocortisone (corticosteroid)
Hydrogesic (analgesic combination)	hydroxyzine (antihistamine)
hydromorphone (narcotic analgesic)	morphine (narcotic analgesic)
Hydropres (antihypertensive)	Diupres (antihypertensive)
Hytone (topical corticosteroid)	Vytone (topical corticosteroid)
imipramine (antidepressant)	Norpramin (antidepressant)
Inderal (beta-adrenergic blocker)	Inderide (antihypertensive)
Indocin (NSAID)	Minocin (antibiotic)
Lamictal (anticonvulsant)	Lamisil (antifungal)
Lanoxin (cardiac glycoside)	Lasix (diuretic)
Lantus (insulin glargine)	Lente insulin (insulin zinc suspension)
Lioresal (muscle relaxant)	lisinopril (ACE inhibitor)
Lithostat (lithium carbonate)	Lithobid (lithium carbonate)
Lodine (NSAID)	codeine (narcotic analgesic)
Lopid (antihyperlipidemic)	Lorabid (beta-lactam antibiotic)

lovastatin (antihyperlipidemic)	Lotensin (ACE inhibitor)
Ludiomil (alpha and beta-adrenergic blocker)	Lomotil (antidiarrheal)
Medrol (corticosteroid)	Haldol (antipsychotic)
metolazone (thiazide diuretic) methotrexate	misoprostol (prostaglandin derivative)
(antineoplastic)	minoxidil (antihypertensive)
metoprolol (beta-adrenergic blocker)	nevirapine (antiviral)
Monopril (ACE inhibitor)	nifedipine (calcium channel blocker)
nelfinavir (antiviral)	Norlutin (progestin)
nicardipine (calcium channel blocker)	Neurontin (anticonvulsant)
Norlutate (progestin)	Navane (antipsychotic)
Noroxin (fluoroquinolone antibiotic)	Retrovir (antiviral)
Norvasc (calcium channel blocker)	Ocuflox (fluoroquinolone antibiotic)
Norvir (antiviral)	Ornade (upper respiratory product)
Ocufen (NSAID)	Percodan (narcotic analgesic)
Orinase (oral hypoglycemic)	paclitaxel (antineoplastic)
Percocet (narcotic analgesic)	penicillin (antibiotic)
paroxetine (antidepressant)	Parlodel (inhibitor of prolactin
penicillamine (heavy metal antagonist)	secretion)
pindolol (beta-adrenergic blocker)	Paraplatin (antineoplastic)
Platinol (antineoplastic)	Plavix (antiplatelet drug)
Pletal (antiplatelet drug)	Prevacid (GI drug)
Pravachol (antihyperlipidemic)	propranolol (beta-adrenergic blocker)
Pravachol (antihyperlipidemic)	prednisone (corticosteroid)
prednisolone (corticosteroid)	Procan SR (antiarrhythmic)
Procanbid (antiarrhythmic)	Propulsid (GI drug)
propranolol (beta-adrenergic blocker)	Premarin (estrogen)
Provera (progestin)	Proscar (androgen hormone inhibitor)
Prozac (antidepressant)	clonidine (antihypertensive)
quinidine (antiarrhythmic)	quinidine (antiarrhythmic)
quinine (antimalarial)	Hygroton (diuretic)
Regroton (antihypertensive)	Robinul (muscle relaxant)
Reminyl (anti-Alzheimer's drug)	Ritonavir (antiviral)
Retrovir (antiviral)	rifampin (antituberculous drug)
Rifamate (antituberculous drug)	flutamide (antineoplastic)
rimantadine (antiviral)	Roxicet (oxycodone/acetaminophen
Roxicodone (oxycodone alone—analgesic)	analgesic)
Sarafem (for PMS)	Serophene (ovulation stimulator)
Seroquel (antipsychotic)	Serzone (antidepressant)
Serzone (antidepressant)	Seroquel (antipsychotic)
Soriatane (antipsoriasis)	Loxitane (antipsychotic)
Stadol (narcotic analgesic)	Haldol (antipsychotic)
sulfadiazine (sulfonamide)	sulfasalazine (sulfonamide)
Tegretol (anticonvulsant)	Tequin (antibacterial)
terazosin (antihypertensive)	temazepam (sedative-hypnotic)
terbinafine (antifungal agent)	terfenadine (antihistamine)
terbutaline (sympathomimetic)	tolbutamide (oral hypoglycemic)
Ticlid (antiplatelet drug)	Tequin (fluoroquinolone antibiotic)
tolazamide (oral hypoglycemic)	tolbutamide (oral hypoglycemic)
torsemide (loop diuretic)	furosemide (loop diuretic)
trifluoperazine (antipsychotic)	trihexyphenidyl (antiparkinson drug)
Trimox (amoxicillin product)	Diamox (carbonic anhydrase inhibitor)
Ultram (analgesic)	Ultrase (pancreatic enzymes)
Vancenase (corticosteroid)	Vanceril (corticosteroid)
Vasosulf (sulfonamide/decongestant)	Velosef (cephalosporin)
Versed (benzodiazepine sedative)	Vistaril (antianxiety agent)

Versed (benzodiazepine sedative)	VePesid (antineoplastic)
Xanax (antianxiety agent)	Zantac (H_2 histamine blocker)
Xenical (antiobesity)	Xeloda (antineoplastic)
Xydis*	
Zebeta (beta blocker)	DiaBeta (oral hypoglycemic)
Zinacef (cephalosporin)	Zithromax (macrolide antibiotic)
Zocor (antihyperlipidemic)	Zoloft (antidepressant)
Zofran (antiemetic)	Zantac (H_2 histamine blocker)
Zosyn (penicillin antibiotic)	Zofran (antiemetic)
Zovirax (antiviral)	Zyvox (antibiotic)

****Note:*** Xydis is a technology consisting of a freeze-dried wafer that dissolves almost instantly on the tongue or in contact with saliva. The name of the technology has been confused because it is written on prescriptions as if it were a drug name.

GLOSSARY

Abbess Hildegard—writer of *Causae et Curae*

abbreviated new drug application (ANDA)—a request to create a generic version of a drug or product with an expired patent

absorption—a process by which drugs move from the site of administration into the body's systemic circulation

Academy of Managed Care Pharmacy (AMCP)—a professional association of pharmacists and associates who serve patients in the managed health care system environment

Accreditation Council for Pharmacy Education (ACPE)—the accrediting body for colleges of pharmacy by which high educational standards are established and monitored; formerly known as the American Council of Pharmacy Education

accreditation—the process by which an agency or organization evaluates and recognizes a program of study or an institution as meeting predetermined qualifications or standards

additive—an active ingredient added to a solution that is intended for intravenous administration or irrigation

adherence—the act of complying with prescribed directions

admission, discharge, and transfer system (ADT)—a computer program for admission, discharge, and transfer of patients that provides significant demographic and clinical information for each patient

adult day care facility—an institution for adults that provides long-term care that supplements the care an individual may be receiving at home by providing opportunities for socialization and care while the primary caregiver is at work

adverse drug reaction (ADR)—any unexpected, obvious change in a patient's condition that the physician suspects may be due to a drug

aerosol—a finely nebulized medication for inhalation therapy

agent—disease causing; may be biological, such as a bacteria or virus; chemical, such as medications or pesticides; or physical, such as radiation or heat

Agreement State—state to which the NRC delegates part of its governing authority in the regulation and safe use and handling of radioactive materials

airborne droplet nuclei—small-particle residue (5 microns or smaller in size) of evaporated droplets, containing microorganisms that remain suspended in the air for long periods of time

airborne transmission—infection by contact with airborne particles that contain infectious organisms

alkaloid—a nitrogenous basic substance found in plants or in synthetic substances with structures similar to plant structures (e.g., atropine, caffeine, morphine)

allergy—a disorder in which the body becomes hypersensitive to a particular antigen (called an allergen).

alligation—the relative amounts of solutions of different percentages from a mixture of a given strength

allopathy—a method of treating a disease by administering an agent that has the opposite characteristics of the disease (e.g., antipyretics to reduce fever)

almshouse—a home for the sick poor and indigent

alternative medicine—herbal supplements, megavitamins, and other nontraditional remedies

ambulatory care—care provided to individuals who do not require either an acute care (hospital) or chronic care (skilled nursing facility) setting; patients come in for treatment and go home the same day; they are not hospitalized

American Association of Colleges of Pharmacy (AACP)—an organization of pharmacy colleges primarily concerned with education issues, such as curricula and teaching methodologies

American Association of Pharmacy Technicians (AAPT)—professional organization that provides leadership and education to pharmacy technicians; recognizes pharmacy technicians as part of the health care team

American College of Apothecaries (ACA)—a small, selective association of community-based practitioners whose membership is granted only if the pharmacy and practitioners comply with specified pharmacy professional standards

American Society of Consultant Pharmacists (ASCP)—an organization of pharmacists who provide drug therapy management services in long-term care

American Society of Health-System Pharmacists (ASHP)—a national organization established in 1942; its current membership of 35,000 includes pharmacists in various institutional health care settings and contains a section for pharmacy technicians

American College of Clinical Pharmacy (ACCP)—organization with a membership that consists primarily of PharmD clinical practitioners and faculty members of colleges of pharmacy; its mission is to transmit the application of new knowledge in the science of pharmacotherapy

American Pharmacists Association (APhA)—founded in 1852, this is the largest association in pharmacy with more than 60,000 members; formerly known as the American Pharmaceutical Association

analgesic—an agent that relieves pain without causing loss of consciousness (e.g., codeine)

anhydrous—containing no water

anionic—carrying a negative charge

antacid—an agent that neutralizes gastric acid

antianginal—a drug used to relieve heart-related chest pain

antiarrhythmic—an agent that restores normal heart rhythm

antidote—a remedy for counteracting a poison

antihistamine—a drug used to reduce runny nose and sneezing

antihypertensive—an agent that reduces blood pressure

antitussive—a drug used for relief of a cough

apothecary system—an early English system of weights and liquid measures

area under the plasma concentration–time curve (AUC)—the plasma drug concentration can be determined by calculating the rate and extent of systemic absorption, as visualized by the plasma concentration–time curve

as low as reasonably achievable (ALARA)—principle used when working with radioactive materials to reduce an individual's exposure to them

asepsis—free from germs; sterile

assisted living facility—a community-like institution that provides care (such as meal service) for individuals who can no longer remain in their homes, but who do not need the level of care provided in nursing homes

asylum—an institution for the relief or care of orphans and those with mental illnesses, especially those who were insane

authorized nuclear pharmacist (ANP)—licensed pharmacist who has undergone NRC required classroom training (200 hours) and hands-on training (500 hours) and completed certification to become classified as an authorized user in the handling of RAM

automatic stop order—a requirement for particular drugs that ensures the proper monitoring of drug usage; mandates that a patient's drug response be reevaluated after specific time intervals; a medical decision is then made to continue the drug, change the dosage, or discontinue the drug

automatic substitution—a policy that allows a pharmacist to substitute a formulary drug for the drug ordered without any additional approvals

autonomy—the ability to act independently

bacteria—small, one-celled microorganisms that need a nourishing environment to survive

bar code medication administration (BCMA)—is a barcode system designed to prevent medication errors in healthcare settings and improve the quality and safety of medication administration. The overall goals of BCMA are to improve accuracy, prevent errors, and generate online records of medication administration.

beneficence—the practice of doing good; a kindly action

beta blocker—a drug that selectively blocks beta receptors in the autonomic nervous system

beta particle—a negatively or positively charged electron originating from the nucleus of a neutron-rich (negaton) or proton-rich (positron) radionuclide

bile—a fluid secreted by the liver

bioavailability—the fraction of an administered dose that ultimately reaches the systemic circulation

bioengineered therapy—the use of genetically modified living organisms in the production of pharmaceutical products

bioequivalence—the comparison of the bioavailability of different drug products with the same active ingredient

biologicals—medicinal preparations made from living organisms or their products; include serums, vaccines, antigens, and antitoxins

bloodborne pathogen—a microorganism that is transmitted through exposure to contaminated blood products

board of trustees/directors—the body responsible for governing the hospital in the community's best interest

body surface area (BSA)—the measurement of the height and weight of a patient to establish an estimate of his or her body surface

buffer system—used to maintain the pH of a drug solution within the range of optimum stability; when the pH of blood and body fluids is maintained virtually constant although acid metabolites are continually being formed in the tissues or lost in the lungs

Bureau of Alcohol, Tobacco, Firearms and Explosives (ATF)—a department of the U.S. Treasury that establishes regulatory standards for procuring, storing, dispensing, and using tax-free alcohol for specific clinical uses

capsule—a soluble container enclosing a drug

carminative—a medicine that relieves stomach/intestinal gas

cationic—carrying a positive charge

Center for Devices and Radiological Health (CDRH)—a federal department that is responsible for the premarket approval of all medical devices; also oversees the manufacture, performance, and safety of these devices and the radiation safety performance of nonmedical devices that emit certain types of electromagnetic radiation, such as cellular phones and microwave ovens

Center for Drug Evaluation and Research (CDER)—a federal department that regulates over-the-counter and prescription drugs, including biological therapeutics and generic drugs

Centers for Medicare and Medicaid Services (CMS)—a federal agency that administers the Medicare program and works in partnership with state governments to administer Medicaid, the Children's Health Insurance Program, and health insurance portability standards

certification—a process by which a nongovernmental association or agency grants recognition to an individual who has met certain predetermined qualifications specified by that association or agency

certified pharmacy technician (CPhT)—a pharmacy technician who has successfully passed the national Pharmacy Technician Certificate Examination

chain of infection—the elements needed in order for an infection to occur

chain pharmacy—a retail pharmacy owned by a corporation that consists of many stores in a particular region or across the nation

charge capture system—a component of a hospital information system whereby every time an order is entered on a patient, a charge is captured for billing purposes, and a statistic is captured for management monitoring purposes

chemical sterilization—the process of completely removing or destroying all microorganisms by exposure to a chemical

Class A prescription balance—balance scale that has a sensitive balance range of 6 mg with a maximum capacity of 120 g

code of ethics—a set of standards and beliefs maintained by a specific group of people

cohorting—infection control process in which a patient is placed in a room with another patient who has an active infection or colonization with the same microorganism but with no other infection

coinsurance—a set percentage of the cost of a prescription that the patient must pay

cold—a self-limiting viral infection of the respiratory tract

collaborative drug therapy agreement—an agreement between a physician and a pharmacist that gives the pharmacist expanded prescription authorization regarding management of drug therapy

colonized—term used to describe the result when a group of microorganisms has grown from a single infectious microorganism within a particular part of the body, causing an infection

combining form—a word type that facilitates the attachment of a prefix or suffix; formed when a word root is incorporated into a medical term

Commission on Credentialing—the ASHP body appointed to formulate and recommend standards and administer programs for accreditation of pharmacy personnel training programs

communication skills—skills that are used to effectively convey a message, either verbally or in writing

compounded sterile preparation (CSP)—relates to the compounding of preparations, such as intravenous admixtures, ophthalmics, and intrathecals, prepared in a controlled sterile environment

computerized physician/prescriber order entry (CPOE)—a drug order entered into a hospital-wide computer system and transmitted to a pharmacy

confirmation bias—a term used to describe errors that occur in selection of medication by either pharmacy or nursing staff; when choosing an item, people see what they are looking for, and once they think they have found it, they stop looking any further

constipation—difficult, incomplete, or infrequent bowel evacuation

consultant pharmacist—individual responsible for monitoring drug usage and drug therapy of residents in skilled nursing facilities

Consumer Product Safety Commission (CPSC)—an independent agency that does not report to, nor is it part of, any other department or agency in the federal government; created to protect the public "against unreasonable risks of injuries associated with consumer products"

contact transmission—a mode of transmission for microorganisms; divided into two subgroups: direct-contact transmission and indirect-contact transmission

contract—a written legal agreement between a vendor and a client that states the conditions and requirements that a client must fulfill to obtain a product or products for a cost less than the vendor's listed price

Controlled Substances Act (CSA)—federal law regulating the manufacture, distribution, and sale of drugs that have the potential for abuse

copayment—a set dollar amount that a patient must pay every time he or she obtains a prescription

counter balance—a double-pan balance capable of weighing relatively large quantities; they have a sensitivity of 100 mg and a weight limit of about 5 kg

covered entities—something to which HIPAA regulations apply; namely, health plans that provide or pay the costs of medical care, health care clearinghouses that facilitate the processing of health information from another entity, and health care providers of medical or health services

credentialing—a process in which a formal, organized agency recognizes and documents the competencies and abilities performed by an individual or an organization

C_{max}—the maximum plasma concentration of a drug

deductible—a set dollar amount that must be paid by the patient before an insurance plan will begin to cover prescription costs

deinstitutionalization—the discharge of people with a history of long-term mental health care in a hospital back to the community

delayed-release dosage form—specifically formulated pharmaceutical dosage form in which the active ingredient is released at a constant rate over a specific time period

density—weight per unit volume

Department of Justice (DOJ)—the federal executive department responsible for the enforcement of the law and administration of justice, equivalent to the justice or interior ministries of other countries

diagnosis—the determination of the nature of a disease or symptom through physical examination and clinical tests

diarrhea—increased frequency of stool that is loose and watery

dietary supplement—any product containing a vitamin, mineral, amino acid, or herb that is intended to supplement the diet by increasing overall intake of a particular substance

diluent—an agent that dilutes or reconstitutes a solution or mixture; also called *bulking agent*

direct-contact transmission—infection through body surface–to–body surface contact with an infected person

dispensatory—a treatise on the quality and composition of medicine

dispense as written (DAW)—notation on a prescription that means the medication indicated on the prescription may not be substituted with a generic or other brand drug without the authorization of the prescriber

dispensing fee—the fee charged by a pharmacy for the cost of dispensing a prescription

dissolution—breakdown of a drug so that it can be absorbed into the body

distribution—the movement of a drug from the bloodstream to other body tissues

dosage form—a system or device designed to deliver a drug or other medicinal agent to the biological system at the site of absorption or the site of therapeutic action; dosage forms include capsules, patches, injections, etc.

dosage schedule—the frequency, interval, and length of time a medicine is to be given

dose calibrator—used for compounding and dispensing patient doses; an ionization chamber allowing for the measurement of the amount of radiation present in a source in millicuries or curies

dossier—a set of guidelines that pharmaceutical manufacturers can use to prepare submissions of new (and existing) pharmaceuticals for a health system's P&T Committee

droplet transmission—infection through contract with microscopic liquid particles coming from an infected person

Drug Enforcement Administration (DEA)—a federal agency established to enforce the rules and regulations of the Controlled Substances Act (CSA), which was designed to combat controlled substance abuse

drug information center (DIC)—a center directed by a drug information specialist, most commonly funded by or located in a hospital, academic institution, or pharmaceutical company; it provides information and education on drugs, develops policies or guidelines for appropriate use of medications, and coordinates medication error programs

drug manufacturer—a company responsible for developing, producing, and distributing pharmaceutical products

drug wholesaler—a company responsible for delivering medication, medical devices, appliances, and so forth, to pharmacies and retailers

drug information—information about drugs and the effects of drugs on people, the provision of which is part of each pharmacist's practice

drug—the active ingredient in a medication or pharmaceutical substance intended to cure, prevent, or diagnose a disease or disease process

dumbwaiter—an in-house elevator used to transport medications and supplies

durable medical equipment (DME)—health-related equipment that is used for long periods of time, is not disposable, and is rented or sold to patients for home care, such as wheelchairs, hospital beds, walkers, canes, and crutches

durable medical equipment, prosthetics, orthotics, and supplies (DMEPOS)—durable medical equipment is any medical equipment used in the home to aid in a better quality of living; prosthetics are artificial devices that replace a missing body part lost through trauma, disease, or congenital conditions; orthotics are externally applied devices used to modify the structural and functional characteristics of the neuromuscular and skeletal system; and supplies include medical instruments, apparatus, implants, in vitro reagents, and similar or related articles that are used to diagnose, prevent, or treat diseases or other conditions and that do not achieve their purpose through chemical action within or on the body (which would make it a drug)

Durham-Humphrey Amendment—an amendment that established two classes of drugs, over-the-counter and prescription, and mandated that labels of prescription drugs include the legend "Caution: Federal law prohibits dispensing without a prescription"

e-prescribing—the ability to digitally send a prescription to the pharmacy

elastomeric devices—a device used to administer therapeutics (e.g., analgesics, antimicrobials, chemotherapy)
electronic balance—a digital weighing balance scale that varies based on its purpose; can be used to weigh bulk quantities greater than 1 g. Standard prescription balances are accurate up to 1 mg or smaller quantities down to 0.001 mg
electronic data interchange (EDI)—technology commonly used to order merchandise, transfer funds, and facilitate billing
elimination half-life—the amount of time it takes to eliminate one-half of the total amount of a drug in the blood
elimination—the removal of waste material from the body
emulsifying agent—a substance used in preparing an emulsion
emulsion—a heterogeneous system of at least one immiscible liquid intimately dispersed in another in the form of droplets, stabilized by the presence of an emulsifying agent
Environmental Protection Agency (EPA)—a federal agency tasked with protecting human health and the environment by writing and enforcing regulations based on laws passed by Congress
ethical code—a set of standards and responsibilities among members a group that governs interactions with other organizations, patients, colleagues, and society
ethical dilemma—a difficult moral problem involving two or more mutually exclusive and morally equal courses of action
ethics—the study of precepts or principles used to assist us in making the correct choice when faced with alternative possibilities in a moral situation
evidence-based medicine (EBM)—the use of information about health practices and drugs that has been validated as useful and accurate by appropriate reference sources
excipient—an inert substance that is added to a drug to give the drug form or consistency
expectorant—a substance that promotes the ejection of mucus or an exudate from the lungs, bronchi, and trachea
exposure control plan—guidelines to follow in the event of an exposure to an infectious disease; includes infection control training
extemporaneous compounding—the act of preparing a drug product at the time it is required with materials on hand
extended-release dosage form—specifically formulated pharmaceutical dosage form in which the active ingredient is gradually released over a predetermined time period
extravascular—outside of the blood vessels or lymphatic vascular channel
False Claims Act (FCA)—a law that makes it a crime to file a false claim for monetary reimbursement from the government, to withhold overpayments, or to induce someone else to file a false claim
false statement—deliberate communication of information that is misleading or incorrect
Family Smoking Prevention and Tobacco Control Act—a federal statute that gives the U.S. Food and Drug Administration the power to regulate the tobacco industry
fast-dissolving tablet—a tablet that disintegrates rapidly when contact with saliva is made without the need for water; also known as orally dissolving
FDA Adverse Event Reporting System (FAERS)—a computerized information database designed to support the FDA's postmarketing safety surveillance program for all approved drug and therapeutic biological products
Federal Anti-Kickback Statute—42 USC 1320a-7b illegal payments/bribes that are offered, requested or paid or accepted by any party to influence the sale of a drug, device or other product that is reimbursed under a federal or state program is a felony. Penalties include prison time and monetary fines
Federal Hazardous Substances Act (FHSA)—act that requires hazardous household products to bear cautionary labels to alert consumers of potential dangers and to inform them of measures to take to protect themselves
Federal Register—a publication announcing a new rule or regulation and requesting a public comment period on it
Federal Trade Commission (FTC)—a federal agency that promotes consumer protection and the elimination and prevention of anticompetitive business practices, such as coercive monopolies
fidelity—remaining true to a promise; promise keeping
filtration—the process of passing a liquid through a porous substance that arrests suspended solid particles
first-pass metabolism—occurs when a drug is rapidly metabolized in the liver after oral administration with minimum bioavailability
floor stock system—system in which medications are provided to the nursing unit for administration to the patient by a nurse, who is responsible for preparation and administration
Food and Drug Administration (FDA)—prómulgates rules, regulations, and standards; inspects drug and food facilities to ensure public safety regarding drug products
Food and Drug Administration Modernization Act of 1997 (FDAMA)—legislation that streamlined regulatory procedures and encouraged manufacturers to conduct research for new uses of drugs and perform pediatric studies of drugs
Food, Drug, and Cosmetic Act of 1938 (FDCA)—federal law through which the Food and Drug Administration enforces its rules and regulations
formulary—a listing of drugs approved by the pharmacy and therapeutics committee of a hospital or a health care system for use within their institution or by health care insurers as determined by the safety, efficacy, effectiveness, and cost of the drugs
fungi—yeasts or molds that obtain food from living organisms
galenical—a standard preparation containing one or several organic ingredients (e.g., elixirs, tinctures)
gamma camera—camera used in nuclear medicine, along with scintillation detectors, to image patients who ingested, inhaled, or were injected with a radiopharmaceutical
gastroesophageal reflux disease (GERD)—disease in which excess stomach acid causes a burning sensation in the esophagus due to eructation of small amounts of acid into the esophagus
geometric dilution—the addition of approximately equal amounts of prescribed drugs when mixing in a mortar
graduate—a marked (or graduated) conical or cylindrical vessel used for measuring liquids
grain—a base unit of weight in the apothecary system
gram—a base unit of weight in the metric system
granule—a very small pill, usually gelatin or sugar coated, containing a drug to be given in a small dose
GRAS list—a list of food additives generally recognized as safe by the Food and Drug Administration
group purchasing organization (GPO)—a group of hospitals or health systems whose collective buying power allows the group to obtain favorable pricing, such as discounts, when making large, ongoing purchases. Pharmaceutical

companies ship large quantities of drugs to the warehouses of these hospital buying groups

group purchasing organization (GPO)—a group of hospitals or pharmacists that buys drugs directly from the manufacturer

guidance documents—included under the umbrella title of FDA Information Sheets, these documents represent the Food and Drug Administration's current thinking on protection of human subjects in research

half-life ($t_{1/2}$)—the time an isotope requires to decay by 50% of measured activity

Hazard Communication Standard (HCS)—a regulation to ensure that information about hazardous chemicals is communicated to the workers handling them

Health Insurance Portability and Accountability Act (HIPAA)—an important law that requires the adoption of security and privacy standards in order to protect personal health care information

Herb Contraindications & Drug Interactions—a useful resource by Francis Brinker on herbal-drug interactions

herbal—a plant with therapeutic properties that can be used for nutritional or medicinal purposes

herb—a leafy plant used as a healing remedy or flavoring agent

heterogeneous—composed of parts having various and dissimilar characteristics or properties

Hippocrates—a Greek physician; considered the "father of medicine"

home care—care given to patients in their own homes

home equipment management services—the selection, delivery, setup, and maintenance of equipment and the education of the patient in the use of the equipment, all performed in the home or patient's place of residence

home health care—provision of health care services to patients at their place of residence

home health agencies—public (governmental) agencies, nonprofit agencies, proprietary agencies, and hospital-based agencies that provide health services in the home

home health services—the provision of health care services by a health care professional in the patient's place of residence on a per-visit basis

home infusion therapy (HIT)—intravenous drug therapy provided in the patient's place of residence

home medical services—physician services provided in the home

Homeopathic Pharmacopoeia of the United States—one of the three official drug compendia specified in the Federal Food, Drug, and Cosmetic Act

homeopathy—a method of treating or preventing disease by administering very dilute substances that cause the same effect as the symptom (e.g., giving a minute quantity of a fever-producing substance to reinforce the body's defense system)

homeostasis—a tendency toward stability in the internal body environment; a state of equilibrium

home medical equipment (HME)—health-related equipment used at home (e.g., hospital beds, crutches)

homogeneous—of uniform composition throughout

hospice—an institution that provides a program of palliative and support services to patients with terminal illnesses and their families in the form of physical, psychological, social, and spiritual care

hospital information system (HIS)—a system that integrates information from many parts of the hospital

hospital-acquired infection—an infection or illness that occurs as a result of a patient's stay in a hospital or health facility

Humanitarian Use Device (HUD)—a device that is intended to benefit patients by treating or diagnosing a disease or condition that affects or is manifested in fewer than 4,000 individuals in the United States per year

hydro-alcoholic—a mixture of water and alcohol

hydrophilic—water loving

hydrous—combined with water; forming a compound with one or more molecules of water

hygroscopic—moisture absorbing

hypersensitivity reaction—a reaction that occurs after a person is exposed to a compound and has generated antibodies against the compound

hypoglycemic—a drug that lowers the level of glucose in the blood; used primarily by people with diabetes

immunity—the condition of being resistant to a particular disease (e.g., polio)

immunomodulator—an agent that adjusts the immune system to a desired level

independent pharmacy—a retail pharmacy owned and operated by an individual pharmacist or group of individuals, in contrast to chain drug stores

indirect-contact transmission—infection through contact with a contaminated object

individual prescription system—a system in which a multiple-day supply of each medication is dispensed for a patient upon receipt of prescriptions or medication orders

infection—the state or condition in which the body (or part of it) is invaded by an agent that multiplies and produces an injurious effect

informed consent—giving permission for a specific treatment or action to take place

infusion—the introduction of a solution into a vein by gravity or by an infusion control device or pump

intended use—the stated manner in which a product was created to act and be used

intermittent infusion—the administration of an IV infusion over a period of time followed by a period of no administration. The same cycle is usually repeated at scheduled times, hence the name *intermittent*

International System of Units (SI)—internationally used system of weights and measures; commonly known as the metric system

interstate commerce—exchange of goods between states

intra-arterial—into an artery

intra-articular—into a joint, such as the elbow or knee

intracardia—into the heart

intradermal (ID)—situated or applied within the skin

intramuscular (IM)—within the muscle

intranasal—within the nose

intraocular—within the eye

intraperitoneal—into the peritoneal or abdominal cavity

intrapleural—into the sac surrounding the lungs

intrathecal—within the subdural space of the spinal cord

intravascular—injection into a blood vessel

intravenous (IV)—within a vein; administering drugs or fluids directly into the vein to obtain a rapid or complete effect from the drug

intraventricular—into a ventricle of the brain or heart

intravesicular—into the urinary bladder

intravitreal—into the vitreous chamber of the eyeball behind the lens

Investigational Device Exemption (IDE)—exemption to current law that allows an investigational device to be used in a clinical study in order to collect safety and effectiveness data

investigational new drug application (INDA)—the means by which a pharmaceutical company obtains permission to ship an experimental drug across state lines (usually to clinical investigators) before a marketing application for the drug has been approved
ionizing radiation—radiation that, when interacting with other atoms, ejects an electron, proton, or neutron, changing the ionization state of the atom
iso-osmotic—having the same osmotic pressure
isotonic—having the same tone
isotope—any of two or more species of an element with the same atomic number but a different mass number or atomic mass
just-in-time (JIT)—an inventory strategy that minimizes inventory levels, thus minimizing the tying up of large sums of money
Kefauver-Harris Amendments—amendments to the federal Food, Drug, and Cosmetic Act that required all new drugs marketed in the United States to be proven safe and effective
kiloelectron-volt (keV)—the unit of measurement for energy in an isotope
lacrimal fluid—tears
laminar flow hood—a sterile work area with a positive-pressure airflow system that filters the air
levigation—the mixing of particles with a base vehicle, in which they are insoluble, to produce a smooth dispersion of the drug by rubbing with a spatula on a tile
lipophilic—lipid-loving
liter—a basic unit of volume in the metric system
long-term care (LTC)—health care provided in an organized medical facility for patients requiring chronic or extended treatment
lotion—liquid preparation intended for external application
mail-order pharmacy—a pharmacy that fills prescriptions and refills by mail, online, by phone, or via smartphone apps anywhere in the United States; orders are delivered directly to the patient's home
Maimonides—Rabbi Moses ben Maimon, a Spanish-born Hebrew physician, pharmacist, and rabbi (1135–1204); physician to Sultan Saladin; author of a health book, *Book of Counsels*, and a handbook on poisons
malaria—an infectious fever-producing disease, transmitted by infected mosquitoes
materials management—the division of a hospital pharmacy responsible for the process of procurement, control, storage, and distribution of drugs and pharmaceutical products
matrix management—an organizational concept that emphasizes the interrelationship among departments and the common areas of decision making
Medical Device Amendment—legislation enacted in 1976 that amended the Food, Drug, and Cosmetic Act; it requires classification of medical devices according to their function and risk
medical information—information pertaining to health
medication administration record (MAR)—a record maintained by the nursing staff containing information about the patient's medication and its frequency of administration
medication management system—an organized, complex and controlled system of manufacturing, purchasing, distributing, storing, prescribing, preparing, dispensing, administering, using, controlling, and monitoring a drug's effects and outcomes to ensure that drugs are used safely and effectively
medication order—orders for all medications and intravenous solutions; they are written on an order sheet or recorded via computerized physician order entry on a hospital-wide computer system
medication regimen review (MRR)—the process established by the CMS to provide appropriate drug therapy for patients; it requires a licensed pharmacist to review medication use every month for all residents in a skilled nursing facility
medication therapy management (MTM)—(1) a distinct service or group of services that optimize therapeutic outcomes for individual patients; these services are independent of, but can occur in conjunction with, the provision of a medication product (2) program in which pharmacists offer nondrug services such as drug therapy management for diabetes, anticoagulation, anemia, hypertension, and renal failure
medication administration record (MAR)—a record maintained by the nursing staff containing information about the patient's medication and its frequency of administration
medication administrator—a person who administers or gives medications to patients
medication-related problem (MRP)—undesirable events a patient experiences as a result of drug therapy that interfere with a desired patient outcome
medium—the substance through with another substance is dispersed
MedWatch—a program that allows health professionals, manufacturers, and the public to report serious reactions and problems related to FDA-regulated medical products
meniscus—the shape of the outer surface of a liquid; it can be a concave or crescent shape, which is caused by surface tension
metabolism—the process by which an organism converts food to energy needed for anabolism
metabolite—a chemical synthesized within cells as part of a metabolic pathway
meter—a basic unit of length in the metric system
metric system—a system of weights based on the meter (length), the gram (weight), and the liter (volume)
mode of transmission—the way in which the disease-causing agent is moved between the portal of exit and the portal of entry to a susceptible host
molecular form—the drug form that elicits biological responses regardless of dosage form
monastery—a dwelling place for individuals under religious vows who live in ascetic simplicity
monograph—a compilation of information about a specific drug product; contains a list of and amounts of ingredients, instructions on usage, the circumstances under which it may be used, and any contraindications for use of the product
multidrug-resistant organisms (MDROs)—microorganisms, predominantly bacteria, that are resistant to one or more classes of antimicrobial agents (antibiotics)
multiple compressed tablets—tablets that are layered in multiple compression cycles
National Drug Code (NDC)—a unique 11-digit identifier for a drug's product, strength, and package size
National Formulary—a database of drugs of established usefulness not found in the U.S. Pharmacopeia
National Home Infusion Association (NHIA)—the trade organization for home infusion providers
National Pharmacy Technicians Association (NPTA)—professional organization dedicated to advancing the role of

pharmacy technicians in pharmaceutical care by providing education, advocacy, technological support, and leadership training; has practice sites in the community, hospital, home care, long-term care, nuclear sites, military sites, and prison facilities

National Association of Boards of Pharmacy (NABP)—an organization formed in 1904 to assist member boards in developing pharmacy standards to protect the public health

National Association of Chain Drug Stores (NACDS)—an association of corporations represented by chief executive officers, many of whom are not pharmacists; includes chain pharmacies, grocery store pharmacies, department store pharmacies, and discount outlets

National Community Pharmacists Association (NCPA)—formed in 1898 to represent the interests of independent pharmacy owners; formerly the National Association of Retail Druggists

Native American—a person who was an original resident of the Americas

new drug application (NDA)—vehicle through which drug sponsors formally propose that the Food and Drug Administration approve a new pharmaceutical for sale and marketing in the United States

no carbon required (NCR) form—carbonless copy paper, non-carbon copy paper, or NCR paper is an alternative to carbon paper, used to make a copy of an original, handwritten (or mechanically typed) document without the use of any electronics

nomogram—a chart that determines body surface area from height and weight

nonadherence—forgetting or purposefully not taking medications as prescribed

nonprescription medications—drugs available to patients who have conditions that are considered self-treatable; also known as over-the-counter medications (OTCs)

not-for-profit facility—a type of long-term care facility that does not pay a profit with its extra income, but rather reinvests the excess revenue back into programs or building improvements for the benefit of the serviced population; these facilities are not obligated to pay taxes and have the ability to raise funds for charitable purposes

nuclear pharmacy technician (NPT)—a pharmacy technician who has undergone special training to work in a nuclear pharmacy

nuclear pharmacy—a specialized pharmacy where radiopharmaceuticals are compounded and dispensed for patient use, usually on the same day they were compounded

Nuclear Regulatory Commission (NRC)—U.S. government agency that regulates the use of by-product nuclear material

nursing home or skilled nursing facility (SNF)—an institution that provides long-term care to individuals needing extensive medical care as well as personal care around the clock

Oath of a Pharmacist—pledge taken by graduating pharmacists to uphold a particular standard of practice

Occupational Safety and Health Act of 1970—federal law that ensures every working man and woman in the nation safe and healthy working conditions; established the Occupational Safety and Health Administration (OSHA)

Occupational Safety and Health Administration (OSHA)—organization created to decrease hazards in the workplace, to maintain a reporting system for monitoring job-related injuries and illnesses, and to develop mandatory job safety and health standards

off-label marketing—providing information regarding the use of a drug for other than its approved and intended use

ointment—an oil-based, semisolid, external dosage form, usually containing a medicinal substance

Omnibus Budget Reconciliation Act (OBRA)—mandated three provisions that affect the profession of pharmacy: drug manufacturers are required to provide their lowest prices to Medicaid patients, and pharmacists are to provide drug use reviews and patient counseling

orally dissolving tablet (ODT)—a tablet that disintegrates rapidly when contact with saliva is made without the need for water; also known as fast dissolving

Orphan drugs—drugs used for diseases and conditions considered rare in the United States, for which adequate drugs have not yet been developed and do not generate incentives for drug manufacturers to research and develop treatments

outcome competency—the measurable desired ability, knowledge, and skill achieved upon completion of a program

over-the-counter medications (OTCs)—drugs that can be sold without a prescription

pandemic—a global epidemic disease

parenteral product—a dosage form administered by injection

parenteral—a sterile, injectable medication; introduction of a drug or nutrient into a vein, muscle, subcutaneous tissue, artery, or spinal column; often refers to intravenous infusions of nutritional solutions

patent—an exclusive license, provided for in the U.S. Constitution, that provides an inventor with a statutory time period during which the inventor can exclusively market the patented product

pathogen—disease-causing organism

patient accounting system—a component of a hospital information system that allows the hospital to bill and collect for its services

patient package insert (PPI)—an informational leaflet written for the lay public describing the benefits and risks of a prescribed medication

patient confidentiality—the need for all personal information related to patient care to remain between the patient and the health care provider

patient's bill of rights—a declaration ensuring that all patients—inpatients, outpatients, and emergency service patients—are afforded their rights in a health care institution

payer—The pharmacy benefit manager

peptic ulcer disease (PUD)—ulceration of the stomach or duodenal lining

percentage—a number representing an amount per hundred (e.g., 5% represents 5 parts per 100)

percutaneous—through the skin

performance improvement (PI)—is the process of self evaluation whereby the organization can use results of assessments and audits to improve upon areas of practice

personal care and support services—the provision of nonprofessional services to patients in their place of residence

personal protective equipment (PPE)—protective gear worn by health care workers, made up of barriers used to prevent skin and mucous membrane exposure when contact with blood or other potentially infectious materials is anticipated

pharmaceutical care—the direct, responsible provision of medication-related care for the purpose of achieving definite outcomes that improve a patient's quality of life

pharmacogenetic polymorphism—a genetic variation accounting for changes in severely decreased drug metabolism, or when a normal dose is given, toxic concentrations can result

pharmacognosy—the study of therapeutic agents derived from natural sources (e.g., plants)

pharmacotherapy—the treatment of disease with medications

Pharmacy and Therapeutics Committee (P&T)—the liaison between the department of pharmacy and the medical staff, consisting of physicians who represent the various clinical aspects; this committee selects the drugs to be used in the hospital. The pharmacy director is the secretary and a voting member of this committee

pharmacy benefit manager (PBM)—a provider of prescription drug programs; can be a third-party administrator or part of an integrated healthcare system. Responsibilities include processing and paying prescription drug claims, developing and maintaining the formulary, contracting with pharmacies, and negotiating discounts and rebates with drug manufacturers

Pharmacy Technician Certification Board (PTCB)—established in 1995 to provide a voluntary mechanism for a national certification program for pharmacy technicians

Pharmacy Technician Educators Council (PTEC)—an organization with the mission of assisting the profession of pharmacy to prepare high-quality, well-trained technical personnel through education and practical training programs

phlegm—a viscous mucus secreted orally

phonetic alphabet—an alphabet that is used to prevent miscommunication by spelling a word out by the way it sounds; for example, "A is for alpha, B is for bravo," etc.

photon (gammaray)—a particle originating in the nucleus of an atom that is massless and chargeless, similar to light

physicochemical properties—the physical and chemical properties of a pharmaceutical

piggyback—refers to a small-volume IV solution (25 to 250 mL) that is run into an existing IV line over a brief period of time (e.g., 50 mL over 15 minutes)

pneumatic tube system—a method for sending a medication order from various locations in a hospital to its pharmacy by placing the order in a "tube" and sending it to a dispatcher, who then forwards it to a specific location

Poison Prevention Packaging Act—a federal law mandating special packaging requirements that make it difficult for children under the age of 5 to open the package or container

policy—a defined course to guide and determine present and future decisions; established by an organization or employer who guides the employee to act in a manner consistent with management philosophy

polymorphism—the property of a compound to exist in more than one crystalline form

portal of entry—the route by which a disease-causing agent enters a host; may be through breaks in the skin, inhalation of contaminants, or insect bites

portal of exit—the route by which an agent moves from a reservoir to a susceptible host; may be through body secretions such as saliva, blood, and urine

postmarketing surveillance—the reporting of adverse events to the FDA by manufacturers of drugs and devices whenever an adverse event may have led to or did lead to serious injury or death

preferred drug provider (PDP)—a gatekeeper between individual and government payers under Medicare Part D

prefix—a word element attached to the beginning of a word to modify its meaning

premarket approval (PMA)—the process of scientific and regulatory review to evaluate the safety and effectiveness of Class III medical devices; Class III devices are those that support or sustain human life, are of substantial importance in preventing impairment of human health, or present a potential, unreasonable risk of illness or injury

prescriber—a licensed person in health care who is permitted by law to order drugs that legally require a prescription; includes physicians, physician assistants, podiatrists, dentists, and nurse practitioners

prescription order form—a course of medication therapy ordered by a physician or other health care practitioner in an organized health care setting

prescription—permission, granted orally or in writing, from a physician for a patient to receive a certain medication on an outpatient basis that will help relieve or eliminate the patient's problem

preservatives—substance used to prevent the growth of microorganisms

primary resources—specific research resources and most current sources of information, including original research articles published in professional journals; also include descriptive patient case reports, observational studies, and experimental studies

prime vendor—a drug wholesaler who contracts directly with hospital pharmacies for the purpose of providing their high-volume pharmaceuticals

prior authorization—a request to a pharmacy benefit manager to cover the cost of a drug that is outside the formulary

PRN (*pro re nata*) order—order for drugs to be given as needed when a clinical situation arises

procedure—guideline on the preferred way to perform a certain function; particular actions to be taken to carry out a policy

prodrug—a class of drugs, the pharmacological action of which results from a chemical modification (or modifications) made by an organism on a chemical compound

product line management—an organizational concept that emphasizes the end product or category of services being delivered

propellant—a substance used to help expel the contents of a pressurized container

proportion—formed using two ratios that are equal (e.g., ½ = 5/10)

proprietary facility—a type of long-term care facility that is owned by one person, a family, a partnership, or a corporation; is run like a corporate business; and makes a profit for its investors

prospective drug review—a review of a patient's medication profile by a pharmacist to screen for any drug problems prior to a drug being dispensed

protected health information (PHI)—any individually identifiable health information, with the exclusion of employment records

protozoa—single-celled parasitic organisms with the ability to move

psychiatric—relating to the medical treatment of mental disorders

Pure Food and Drug Act of 1906—federal law passed by Congress because of concern about the risks to public health and safety associated with unsanitary and poorly labeled foods and drugs

pyrogen—an agent that causes a rise in temperature; produced by bacteria, molds, viruses, and yeasts

quality drug therapy—safe, effective, timely, and cost-effective drug therapy delivered with care
quasi-legal standard—recognized standards that are similar to laws
radiation safety officer (RSO)—the individual in charge of the safe use and handling of RAM; abides by the conditions of the facility's RAM license and has full authority over the nuclear pharmacy and its employees where RAM is concerned
radiation—the use of x-rays, ultraviolet rays, or short radio waves to sterilize, for example, hospital supplies, vitamins, antibiotics, steroids, plastic syringes, and needles
radio-frequency identification device (RFID)—is the wireless noncontact use of radio-frequency electromagnetic fields to transfer data, for the purpose of automatically identifying and tracking tags attached to objects. The tags contain electronically stored information
radioactive decay—process that occurs when unstable isotopes release energy in the form of waves or particles to achieve a more stable state
radioactive material (RAM)—a substance that emits radiant energy in the form of alpha, beta, or gamma particles
radiochemical purity—measure of the percentage of the total radioactivity is in the desired radiopharmaceutical form
radionuclidic purity—measure of the percentage of the total radioactivity is in the desired form
radiopaque—having the property of absorbing x-rays
radiopharmaceutical—substance used as a diagnostic or therapeutic agent to diagnose or treat disease and evaluate organ function and physiological processes
RAM license—license granted to a nuclear pharmacy that regulates the procuring, storing, handling, and disposing of RAM
ratio—the relationship of two quantities (e.g., 1:10 is read as one part in ten parts)
read-back verification—a process in which the recipient of a message speaks the message back to the sender of the message to confirm the message was received correctly
receptor—a cell component that combines with a drug or hormone to alter the function of the cell
recertification—a renewal of an individual's certification
reciprocity—a mutual exchange or interchange between two parties
refractory—resistance to treatment or a stimulus
regulated medical waste (RMW)—used syringes and vials returned from customers
regulation—process or procedure issued by a governing body
rehabilitation facility—an institution that provides services to patients recovering from acute or traumatic events on a short-term basis
reservoir—a place where a disease-causing agent can survive
restricted area—An area for the preparation and dispensing of compounded sterile products
retailer—a company responsible for delivering products to patients
rickettsia—intercellular parasites that need to be in living cells to reproduce
robotics—technology based on a mechanical device, programmed by remote control to accomplish manual activities, such as picking medications according to a patient's computerized profile
root—the primary building block of a word; in medical terminology, the core word used to identify fundamental anatomical and physiological nomenclature
rule—guideline that dictates particular actions and procedures as issued by a governing body
Safe Medical Devices Act of 1990—a federal law that requires all facilities that use medical devices (referred to as device-user facilities) to report serious injuries, serious illnesses, and deaths to the U.S. Food and Drug Administration and the manufacturer. The purpose of the act is to protect the public by ensuring that medical devices are not unsafe for their intended use
safety data sheets (SDS)—documents that provide workers and emergency personnel with procedures for handling or working with a substance in a safe manner; includes information such as physical data (melting point, boiling point, flash point, etc.), toxicity, health effects, first aid, reactivity, storage, disposal, protective equipment, and spill-handling procedures
sanatorium—an institution for the treatment of chronic diseases, such as tuberculosis or nervous disorders
Schedule III—a controlled substance whose abuse may lead to moderate or low physical dependence or highly psychological dependence
Schedule II—a controlled substance with a high potential for abuse, with severe psychological and/or physical dependence liability
Schedule IV—a controlled substance with less abuse potential and limited risk of physical and psychological dependence
Schedule I—a controlled substance with a high potential for abuse that currently has no approved medical use
Schedule V—contains preparations with limited quantities of certain narcotic drugs
script—an abbreviated form of the term *prescription*
secondary plant metabolite—derived from primary plant metabolites
secondary resources—research resources such as indexing and abstracting services; usually available electronically and quickly link the reader to the primary literature
side effects—known effects of a drug experienced by most people taking the drug; these are usually minor
site survey—a visit by representatives of the ASHP to review training programs and ascertain compliance with standards
sodium pertechnetate ($NaTcO_4$–)—eluted from a Mo-99/Tc-99*m* generator, it is a radiopharmaceutical used in nuclear medicine alone or bound to a pharmaceutical to diagnose a disease state or to evaluate organ function or a physiological process
solution—a homogeneous mixture of one or more substances dispersed in a dissolving solvent; clear liquid with all components completely dissolved
specialty pharmacy—a pharmacy that specializes in dispensing expensive injectable medications that require more than just distribution to the patient. In addition to the medication, they generally provide all of the necessary ancillary supplies the patient may need to administer the medication. Patient education is also included and, if necessary, injection training is provided by a nurse either by phone or in person
standard precautions—infection control safety measures developed by OSHA; designed to protect health care workers and patients from infections; also called universal precautions
STAT order—*statim*; order for drugs to be given immediately
state board of pharmacy—body established to ensure that the public is well served professionally by pharmacists
statute—enacted law
step therapy—a system designed to allow physicians to first try the least expensive drug alternative before progressing to more expensive alternatives to treat diagnosed conditions
sterile—free from living microorganisms
subcutaneous (SC)—under the skin

sublingual—under the tongue
suffix—a word element attached to the end of a word to create a new word with a specific meaning
suppository—a solid dosage form for insertion into a body cavity (e.g., rectum, vagina, urethral), where it melts at body temperature
survey meter—radiation detection instrument measuring exposure in millirems per hour; can be gas filled or a scintillation detector
susceptible host—must be present for the agent to be transferred; the host is usually vulnerable to disease due to lack of resistance
suspending agent—a chemical additive used in suspensions to "thicken" the liquid and retard settling particles
suspension—a liquid containing finely divided drug particles that are uniformly distributed
systemic action—affects the body as a whole
tablet—a solid dosage form of varying weight, size, and shape that contains a medicinal substance
tare—a weight used to counterbalance the container holding the substance being weighed
target tissue/organ—the tissue or organ of interest in a nuclear medicine study and the one that is the target for a dose of a given radiopharmaceutical
taring—the process of resetting an electronic balance to a zero reading
tertiary resources—general research resources, including package inserts, textbooks, compendia, computer databases, and review articles; commonly consulted when initiating a search strategy; usually used to educate oneself about a medical condition or medication
The Joint Commission—a not-for-profit organization that sets standards designed to ensure effective quality services (e.g., optimal standards for the operation of hospitals)
Theophrastus—a Greek philosopher and botanist who classified plants by pharmaceutical actions
therapeutic interchange—a policy that allows one drug product to be substituted for another that differs in composition but is considered to have the same or very similar pharmacologic and therapeutic activity
thermal sterilization—sterilization using heat; moist heat and dry heat are methods of thermal sterilization
thin-layer chromatography (TLC)—a method of quality control performed on compounded radiopharmaceuticals
tiered copayment schedule—a prescription drug payment schedule that aligns the amount of a copayment to the formulary tier of the drug dispensed
transdermal—entering through the dermis of the skin, as in administration of a drug applied to the skin in ointment or patch form
triple beam balance—a single-pan unequal arm balance used for weighing large amounts
triturate—to reduce particle size and mix one powder with another
tuberculin skin test (TST)—a test performed to identify exposure to the tuberculosis bacillus
turnaround time—the time required from order entry to delivery of medication to the patient care area
turnover rate—the rate of drug inventory; calculated by dividing the total dollars spent to purchase drugs in 1 year by the actual pharmacy inventory dollars
T_{max}—time required to reach maximum plasma drug concentration
U.S. Pharmacopeia- National Formulary (USP-NF)—the official pharmacopeia of the United States, published dually with the National Formulary as the USP-NF; prescription and over-the-counter medicines and other health care products sold in the United States are required to follow USP-NF standards
unit dose—a single-use package of a drug. In a unit-dose distribution system, a single dose of each medication is dispensed prior to the time of administration
unit-dose distribution system—a system in which medication is distributed in a single-dose or unit dose form from the pharmacy for use by the individual administering the drug
unit-of-use—prescription medication that contains a quantity designed and intended to be dispensed directly to a patient for a specific use without modification
utilization review—the work of a committee that determines if the use of resources has met certain established criteria and standards
vasodilator—an agent or drug that causes dilation of the blood vessels; increases the caliber of the blood vessels
vector-borne transmission—infection through contact with infection-carrying insects or animals
vehicle transmission—infection through contact with contaminated food or water
verbal order—an order for a drug or other treatment that is given verbally to an authorized receiver by an authorized prescriber
virus—a submicroscopic agent of infectious disease that is capable of reproduction
volatile—evaporates at low temperature
wetting agent—a substance that moistens the particles in a powder**well counter**—a scintillation detector, used for measuring test tubes housing package and area wipes
word elements—in medical terminology, the parts of a word such as roots, prefixes, and suffixes

INDEX

NOTE: Page references in *italics* refer to figures, illustrations, and tables.